ANNUAL PROGRESS IN
CHILD PSYCHIATRY AND
CHILD DEVELOPMENT
1987

ANNUAL PROGRESS IN CHILD PSYCHIATRY AND CHILD DEVELOPMENT 1987

Edited by

STELLA CHESS, M.D.

Professor of Child Psychiatry
New York University Medical Center

ALEXANDER THOMAS, M.D.

Professor of Psychiatry
New York University Medical Center

and

MARGARET HERTZIG, M.D.

Associate Professor of Psychiatry
Cornell University Medical College

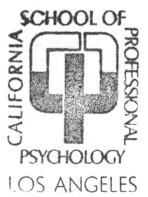

CALIFORNIA SCHOOL OF PROFESSIONAL PSYCHOLOGY LOS ANGELES

BRUNNER/MAZEL, *Publishers* • **New York**

Published by

BRUNNER/MAZEL, INC.

19 Union Square

New York, New York 10003

Library of Congress Card No. 68-23452

ISBN 0-87630-476-5

ISSN 0066-4030

MANUFACTURED IN THE UNITED STATES OF AMERICA

10 9 8 7 6 5 4 3 2 1

CONTENTS

PREFACE

This volume contains both an author and a subject index. The Author Index reflects the major contributions of the leading theorists, researchers, and clinicians to the fields of child psychiatry and child development. Beyond these, the list of authors also highlights the emergence of an impressive number of younger workers who have begun to make their mark in recent years, which augurs well for our progress in the next 20 years.

The Subject Index dramatizes the increasing breadth and scope of the concerns and activities of mental health professionals over the past 20 years. Unidimensional theories of development have given way to a recognition of the need for a multifactional approach which takes into account the interaction of biological, psychological, and sociocultural influences at all age-stage levels of functioning. Workers in our field, guided by theoretical interest, clinical relevance, and social concern have come increasingly to formulate specific investigative hypotheses capable of critical testing through the identification of appropriate samples and populations for study, with methods that are replicable, reliable, and statistically analyzable. Increasing emphasis has been laid by developmental psychologists and psychiatrists on the study of children in naturalistic life situations, rather than relying primarily on laboratory experiments and observations which could be carefully controlled but might bear little relevance to the real child in his real life.

For the clinician, the increasing emphasis on empirical precision in diagnostic criteria and judgments is reflected in the successive *Annual Progress* volumes and in the publication of DSM-III and DSM-III-R. These diagnostic manuals have provided clinical child psychiatrists as well as investigators with a developmentally oriented and phenomenologically based multiaxial system of diagnosis, which summarizes much of our available knowledge with respect to the clinical characteristics, natural history, associated factors, complications, predisposing factors, prevalence, familial patterns, and differential diagnosis of conditions that usually arise and are first evident in infancy, childhood, or adolescence. Indeed our knowledge base has been expanding so rapidly that there have been only seven years between the publication of DSM-III and DSM-III-R.

The progress of the past 20 years has given us a new perspective on the nature of the infant and her normal development and revised and expanded our concepts of prevention and treatment. At the same time, we also have a sharper understanding of what we do not know and a healthy skepticism regarding many of the "sacred cows" of theory and practice of even the recent past. Child psychiatry and child development have now come of age with innovative strategies, testable hypotheses, and an increasing pool of sophisticated researchers and clinicians with high standards of performance. We may not be able to predict the specific scientific breakthroughs in our field in the next 20 years, but we can be confident that they will be even more exciting and dramatic than the progress of the past 20 years.

A NOTE FROM THE EDITORS

This is the 20th year of our *Annual Progress in Child Psychiatry and Child Development* series. Editing these volumes has been a labor of love for us. Arduous it has been, especially in recent years, as the number of journals has proliferated and the number of papers in existing journals has expanded. Not only has the quantity of articles increased, but their quality has improved significantly over the years—a reflection of the steady progress in the fields of child psychiatry and child development.

This expansion in research and clinical expertise, which we can truly call explosive, has indeed made our editorial task more and more demanding and challenging. We now monitor some 100 journals yearly, which include many more articles of merit compared to the past. Harder decisions have to be made as to which papers to include, in order to keep each volume to a manageable size.

On the other hand, the increasing effort and time required to edit each volume underlies the value of such an annual survey of the literature on normal and pathological development. This judgment has been confirmed by the consistently favorable reviews the volumes have received, as well as the many appreciative personal comments by professional colleagues.

It is clear that this series should continue. However, each year we ourselves grow a year older. For *Annual Progress* to maintain the standards we have set for it, it becomes necessary to begin to share the editorial burden with a younger colleague. We have therefore asked Dr. Margaret Hertzig to join us and to take increasing editorial responsibility in succeeding years.

Dr. Hertzig is eminently qualified for this demanding task of editing the *Annual Progress* series. She is Associate Professor of Psychiatry at Cornell University Medical College. She is also Director of the Child and Adolescent Outpatient Department and Medical Director of the Nursery School Treatment Center of the Payne Whitney Clinic at New York Hospital. In addition, she is a member of the editorial board of the *American Journal of Orthopsychiatry*.

Dr. Hertzig has contributed a substantial number of research and clinical papers to various professional journals and books. She is astute and sophisticated in her judgment of research and clinical reports in both normal and pathological child development. We are pleased that she has accepted our invitation to work with us as a co-editor of the *Annual Progress* series.

Stella Chess, M.D.
Alexander Thomas, M.D.

ANNUAL PROGRESS IN
CHILD PSYCHIATRY AND
CHILD DEVELOPMENT
1987

Part I

INFANCY STUDIES

It is now clear from a number of studies that learning and memory are active from birth onward. The newborn's level of neurophysiological organization is already sufficiently advanced to permit the infant to perceive, integrate, and respond to a wide variety of environmental stimuli. Some workers have speculated further that perhaps this process of learning may actually begin in the fetus, even before birth. DeCasper and Spence review the research evidence that suggests that the fetus can learn in utero, and report their own study which confirms the possibility that prenatal auditory experience can influence postnatal auditory preferences.

Evidence has accumulated from a number of sources (see Rutter, M. 1972. *Maternal Deprivation Reassessed.* Middlesex: Penguin Books) which has effectively challenged the view that there is some special unique quality to the mother-infant attachment. Further data in this regard are provided in the study of social referencing by Klinnert and her associates. Previous studies have demonstrated that one-year-old infants look toward their mothers' facial expressions and use the emotional information these expressions convey. In this study, however, the authors report the infant's similar use of emotional signals from a friendly adult. The mother was also present but refrained from emotional expressiveness. In other words, the infant's responses can be influenced by other adults even in the presence of the mother. The mother is not necessarily always the most important guide for the infant's behavior.

Washington and her associates report a study of the development of preterm infants in the first year of life using a number of measures: perinatal and neonatal assessment, a semistructural parental psychiatric interview, home observations, maternal-infant interaction ratings, developmental assessment, and temperament ratings. These researchers provide rich data on the group interactions of mothers and infants, with particular emphasis on babies who switched temperamental categories in the first months of life. To obtain a more accurate comprehension of these statistical findings, they examined the "switchers," babies who moved from difficult to easy temperament and also the reverse, and the ratings of the specific mother's behavior. Thus, they were able to identify a particular set of mother-child dyads whose interactions were influential enough to be responsible for the statistical trend. This combination of quantitative and qualitative examination of data clarifies sequences of development that are obscured when only the standard correlations of a group as a whole are evaluated.

In the examination of EEG patterns of preterm infants and their relationship to later I.Q., Beckwith and Parmelee have concurrently examined the nature of the rearing environments. The EEG has, in this study, been found to be a predictive marker in prematures, vis-à-vis later intelligence, as long as the concurrent influence of the caregiving environment is given adequate consideration.

1

Prenatal Maternal Speech Influences Newborns' Perception of Speech Sounds

Anthony J. DeCasper and Melanie J. Spence
University of North Carolina, Greensboro

Pregnant women recited a particular speech passage aloud each day during their last 6 weeks of pregnancy. Their newborns were tested with an operant-choice procedure to determine whether the sounds of the recited passage were more reinforcing than the sounds of a novel passage. The previously recited passage was more reinforcing. The reinforcing value of the two passages did not differ for a matched group of control subjects. Thus, third-trimester fetuses experience their mothers' speech sounds and that prenatal auditory experience can influence postnatal auditory preferences.

Human newborns do not act like passive and neutral listeners. They prefer their own mothers' voices to those of other females, female voices to male voices, and intrauterine heatbeat sounds to male voices, but they do not prefer their fathers' voices to those of other males (Brazelton, 1978; DeCasper & Fifer, 1980; DeCasper & Prescott, 1984; Fifer, 1980;

Reprinted with permission from *Infant Behavior and Development,* 1986, Vol. 9, 133–150. Copyright 1986 by Ablex Publishing Corporation.

This research was supported by a research Council Grant from the University of North Carolina at Greensboro and a generous equipment loan by Professor Michael D. Zeiler. We wish to thank the medical and administrative staff of Moses H. Cone Hospital, Greensboro, NC and, especially, the mothers and their infants for making this research possible. Thanks also to G. Gottlieb, R. Harter, R. Hunt, R. Panneton, K. Smith, and, especially, W. Salinger for their helpful comments on drafts of the manuscript. Portions of this paper were presented at the Third Biennial International Conference on Infant Studies, March 1982, Austin, TX.

Panneton & DeCasper, 1984; Wolff, 1963). Why should newborns prefer some sounds over others? One hypothesis is that their auditory preferences are influenced by prenatal experience with their mothers' speech and heartbeats (DeCasper & Prescott, 1984). Several considerations suggest this hypothesis is plausible.

Third-trimester fetuses hear, or are behaviorally responsive to, sound (e.g., Bernard & Sontag, 1947; Birnholz & Benacerraf, 1983; Grimwade, Walker, Bartlett, Gordon, & Wood, 1971; Johansson, Wedenberg, & Westin, 1964; Sontag & Wallace, 1935). Intrauterine recordings taken near term indicate that maternal speech and heartbeats are audible in utero (Querleu & Renard, 1981; Querleu, Renard, & Crepin, 1981; Walker, Grimwade, & Wood, 1971). Nonmaternal speech, for example male speech, is less audible because of attenuation by maternal tissue and/or masking by intrauterine sounds (Querleu & Renard, 1981; Querleu et al., 1981).

The newborns' preference for their own mothers' voices requires that they had some prior experience with her voice, but there is no evidence that the necessary experience occurred after birth. Fifer (1980) failed to find any relation between maternal-voice preference and postnatal age, whether the newborns roomed with their mother or in a nursery, or whether they were breast fed or bottle fed. Since the maternal voice is audible in utero, and since third-trimester fetuses can hear, perhaps the necessary experience occurred before birth. In contrast, newborns show no preference for their own fathers' voices, even if they had explicit postnatal experience with his voice. Since male voices are not very audible in utero, perhaps the absence of a paternal-voice preference indicates the absence of prenatal experience with his voice (DeCasper & Prescott, 1984). The correlations between the presence or absence of specific-voice sounds before birth, and the presence or absence of specific-voice preferences after birth suggest that prenatal auditory experiences influence the earliest voice preferences.

Consider that complex auditory stimuli can function as positive reinforcers, neutral stimuli, or negative reinforcers of newborn behavior. Known reinforcers include vocal-group singing, solo female singing, prose spoken by a female, synthetic speech sounds, and intrauterine heartbeat sounds (Butterfield & Cairns, 1974; Butterfield & Siperstein, 1972; DeCasper, Butterfield, & Cairns, 1976; DeCasper & Carstens, 1981; DeCasper & Sigafoos, 1983). On the other hand, male speech and instrumental music lack reinforcing value, while white noise and faster-than-normal heartbeat sounds are aversive (Butterfield & Siperstein, 1972; DeCasper & Prescott, 1984; Salk, 1962). The differential reinforcing effectiveness of these sounds seems to covary more with their similarity to sounds that were present in utero than with any general acoustic characteristic(s), which further suggests that prenatal auditory experience influences postnatal auditory perception.

Finally, prenatal auditory experience has been shown to cause postnatal auditory preferences in a variety of infrahuman species (e.g., Gottlieb, 1981; Vince, 1979; Vince, Armitage, Walser, & Reader, 1982).

The hypothesis implies that prenatal experience with maternal speech sounds causes some property of the sounds to be differentially reinforcing after birth. Speech sounds enable at least two kinds of discriminations; some speech cues allow discrimination of language-relevant sounds, per se, or what is said, and some allow discrimination of the speaker or source of the speech sounds (Bricker & Pruzansky, 1976; Studdert-Kennedy, 1982). Thus, the prenatal experience hypothesis implies that newborns prefer their own mothers' voices, regardless of what she says, because of prenatal experience with her voice-specific cues. This implication, however, cannot be directly tested for obvious ethical and practical reasons. The hypothesis also implies that newborns will prefer the acoustic properties of a particular speech passage if their mothers repeatedly recite that passage while they are pregnant.

We directly tested the latter implication in the following way. First, pregnant women tape-recorded three separate prose passages. Then, they recited one of the passages, their target passage, aloud each day during the last 6 weeks of pregnancy. After birth their infants were observed in an operant learning task where recordings of the target passage and a novel passage, one their mothers had recorded but had not recited, were both available as reinforcers. Then their relative reinforcing effectiveness was evaluated. If the prenatal experience with the target passage increases its reinforcing value then: (a) the acoustic properties of the target passage will be more reinforcing than those of a novel passage; (b) the differential reinforcing value of the target passage should be carried by its language-relevant cues and, thus, should not require the presence of the infant's own mother's voice cues; and (c) the reinforcing values of the target and novel passages should not differ for control newborns who had never been exposed to either passage.

METHOD

Prenatal Phase

Pregnant subjects. Thirty-three healthy women approximately 7½ months pregnant were recruited from childbirth preparation classes after being informed about the project. All were experiencing uncompli-cated pregnancies.

Prenatal procedures. After becoming familiar with three short children's stories they tape-recorded all three. Recordings were made in a quiet room on an Akai 4000 stereophonic tape recorder. The tapes would be used as reinforcers in a postnatal learning task. Each woman was then assigned one of the stories as her target story. Assignment was made after all three had been recorded to prevent them from biasing the recording of their target, for example, by exaggerated intonation.

The women were instructed to read their target story aloud "two times through each day when you feel that your baby (fetus) is awake" and to "read the story in a quiet place so that your voice is the only sound that your baby can hear." They maintained a log of their daily recitations and were occasionally checked by the researchers.

Story materials. The stories were *The King, the Mice, and the Cheese* (Gurney & Gurney, 1965), the first 28 paragraphs of *The Cat in the Hat* (Seuss, 1957), and a story we called *The Dog in the Fog,* which was the last 28 paragraphs of the *The Cat in the Hat* with salient nouns changed. The three stories were about equally long, they contained 579, 611, and 642 words, respectively. Each could be comfortably recited in about 3 min. Each was also com-posed from equal size vocabularies of 152, 142, and 154 words, respec-tively. Salient, high-frequency nouns common to at least two stories were changed. For example, cat and hat in *The Cat* became dog and fog in *The Dog,* and cat and dog from those stories became turtle and zebra in *The King. The Cat* contained 46 unique words (i.e., words that appeared only in *The Cat*), which accounted for 22% of the total word count; *The Dog* con-tained 57 unique words, which accounted for 22% of the total word count; and *The King* contained 85 unique words, which accounted for 44% of the total word count. All three stories contained common high-frequency words. For example, *a, all, and, did, do, he, I, in, like, not, now, of, said, that, the, to, with,* and *you* occurred at least three times in each. The common high-frequency words accounted for 43% of *The Cat,* 38% of the *The Dog,* and 36% of the *The King.* The remaining words occurred at least once in at least two of the stories. The stories also differed in prosodic qualities, such as patterns of syllabic beats. Thus, they differed in the acoustic properties of individual words as well as in prosody. *The Cat* and *The Dog* sounded more similar to each other than either did to *The King,* but we could readily identify the origin of short (several seconds) segments from all three.

Postnatal Phase

Experienced newborns. Sixteen of the 33 fetal subjects completed testing as newborns. The 16 had been prenatally exposed to their target story an average of 67 times or for about 3.5 hours in all. They were tested at an average age of 55.8 hours (SD = 10). Each had to have had an uncomplicated full-term gestation and delivery, a birth weight between 3500–3900 grams, and APGAR scores of 8, 9, or 10 at 1 and 5 min after birth. If a subject was circumcised, he was not tested until at least 12 hours afterward. Parents gave informed consent for the testing and were invited to observe.

Seventeen infants were not tested or did not complete a test session: 5 because their mothers failed to return their logs, 4 because they encountered intrapartum or postpartum difficulties, 5 failed to meet state criteria at the time of testing or cried, and 3 subjects' sessions were unavoidably interrupted.

Apparatus. Sessions occurred in a quiet, dimly lit room adjacent to the nursery. The infants lay supine in their bassinets and wore TDH-39 earphones, which were suspended from a flexible rod. They sucked on a regular feeding nipple with the hole enlarged to 1 mm. Rubber tubing connected the nipple to a Statham P23AA pressure transducer that was connected to a Grass polygraph and solid state programming and recording components. Each infant heard a tape recording of his/her target story and a tape recording of a novel story, one of the others their mother had recorded but not recited. Both stories were recorded by the same woman, and each was played on separate channels of the stereo recorder. The tape ran continuously, and sound was electronically gated to the earphones by the automated programming equipment. Intensities averaged 70 dB SPL at the earphones.

Testing procedures. Sessions began about 2.5 hours after a scheduled feeding in order to maximize the chance of obtaining an awake, alert, and cooperative infant (Cairns & Butterfield, 1974). Each infant was brought to a quiet-alert state before testing could begin (Wolff, 1966) and had to visually fixate and follow an experimenter's face when he/she spoke to the infant. (If the infant was not alert and did not fixate or follow, he/she was returned to the nursery, and another attempt was made after a later feeding.)

The infant was then placed supine in the bassinet and the earphones were locked in place. One researcher, who could not be seen by the infant and who was blind to the exact experimental condition in effect, held the nonnutritive nipple loosely in the infant's mouth. Another monitored the equipment. The infant was then allowed 2 min to adjust to the situation and had to emit sucks having negative pressures of at least 20-mm Hg, a pressure normally exceeded by healthy infants. (If the infant failed to suck adequately, he/she was returned to the nursery, and another attempt was made after a later feeding.)

Testing began with 5 min of baseline sucking during which no voices were presented over the earphones. Unconstrained nonnutritive sucking occurs as groups or bursts of individual sucks separated by interburst intervals of several seconds. A sucking burst was defined as a series of individual sucks separated from one another by less than 2 s; when 2 s elapsed without a suck the equipment registered the end of the burst. Thus, interburst intervals (IBIs) began 2 s after the last suck of one burst and ended with the onset of the first suck of the next burst. This criterion accurately captures the burst-pause pattern of newborns' nonnutritive sucking (see Figure 1). IBIs tend to be unimodally distributed for individual infants, and modal values vary between infants. The baseline was used to estimate the distribution and median value of each infant's IBIs just before reinforcement began. Differential reinforcement of IBIs began after baseline had been established. (Hereafter, if the infant stopped sucking for two 1-min periods for any reason, he/she was returned to the nursery and not tested again.)

Reinforcement contingencies. For eight randomly selected infants, sucking bursts that terminated IBIs equal to or greater than the infants' baseline medians (t) produced the recording of a woman's voice reciting the target story. Bursts terminating IBIs less than the baseline median were reinforced with the same woman's recording of a novel story. Thus, only one of the two stories was presented binaurally with the first suck of a burst and remained on until the burst ended. Reinforcement contingencies were completely controlled by the solid-state equipment. Reinforcement contingencies were reversed for the other eight newborns, to control for the effects of any response bias that might arise from either of the contingencies or from changes in the behavioral dispositions of the infants, for example, arousal or fatigue. Differential reinforcement lasted about 20 min.

The same differential reinforcement procedures were used in earlier voice-preference studies (DeCasper & Fifer, 1980; DeCasper & Prescott, 1984). The rationale is based on well-established reinforcement procedures that differentiate the temporal properties of behavior: Differentially reinforcing a range of IBIs causes the shorter differentially rein-

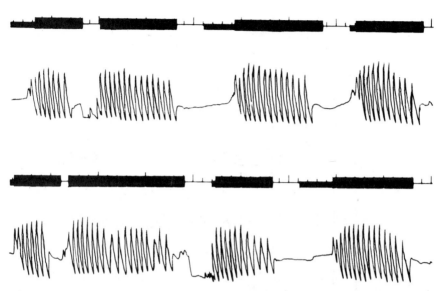

Figure 1. Polygraph record of a newborn's nonnutritive sucking. Wide horizontal marks indicate the onset and offset of a sucking burst. The time between the end of one burst and the beginning of the next denotes an interburst interval. Onset of the narrow event mark denotes that the time criterion, *t* seconds, has elapsed since the end of the last burst. Vertical lines indicate time in seconds.

forced IBIs to increase in frequency (see newborn studies by DeCasper & Fifer, 1980; DeCasper & Sigafoos, 1983; as well as animal studies by Anger, 1956; Catania, 1970; DeCasper & Zeiler, 1977; Malott & Cumming, 1964).

Subject controls. Twelve control newborns matched to a prenatally experienced counterpart on sex, race, and median interburst interval of baseline were also tested. They met the same selection criteria and were tested under exactly the same conditions as their counterparts, but their mothers had never recited any of the three stories.

Other experimental controls. The influence of mother-specific voice cues on the reinforcing effects of the target stories was controlled by having nine newborns reinforced with recordings made by their own mother and seven with recordings made by some other infant's mother. Both stories heard by an infant were recorded by the same woman to insure that their reinforcing value could not be unequally influenced by the speaker's voice characteristics. The acoustic properties of any one story could not systematically influence the reinforcing value of the target because each of the three stories had served as the target at least four

Table 1. Conditional Probability of Responding with (0.0t≤IBI<0.4t) and (1.0t≤IBI<1.4t) During Baseline and During Reinforcement for Experienced and Control Subjects

| | Story | Criteria | | Experienced Subjects | | | | Control Subjects | | | |
| | | | | Target | | Novel | | Target | | Novel | |
Sex	Target/Novel	for Target	Voice	C.P. Base	C.P. Reinf.	C.P. Base	C.P. Reinf.	C.P. Base	C.P. Reinf.	C.P. Base	C.P. Reinf.
F	Cat/Dog	<5	M	.11	.06	.18	.21				
F	Dog/Cat	<6	M	.06	.26	.26	.32				
F	Dog/King	<3	M	.12	.10	.18	.13				
M	King/Dog	<6	M	.10	.16	.33	.28				
F	Cat/King	<3	O	.14	.16	.33	.06	.16	.10	.06	.16
F	Dog/King	<4	O	.02	.15	.10	.07	.06	.05	.32	.11
M	Dog/King	<4	O	.09	.12	.19	.21	.04	.07	.19	.13
M	King/Dog	<6	O	.03	.09	.19	.11	.08	.10	.20	.23
M	Cat/Dog	≥3	M	.29	.37	.12	.13	.10	.17	.21	.16
M	Dog/Cat	≥5	M	.23	.21	.06	.05	.06	.04	.24	.11
F	Dog/King	≥3	M	.16	.17	.13	.11	.08	.22	.12	.13
M	King/Dog	≥3	M	.26	.32	.17	.18	.63	.35	.09	.16
M	Cat/King	≥5	M	.17	.31	.09	.10	.49	.16	.12	.07
F	King/Dog	≥3	O	.06	.08	.17	.08	.26	.05	.10	.05
M	Dog/King	≥3	O	.03	.20	.24	.29	.13	.12	.14	.19
F	Cat/King	≥6	O	.23	.28	.06	.18	.31	.16	.14	.03

times. No particular combination of target/novel pairings could systematically influence the reinforcing value of the target because five of the six possible target/novel pairings occurred at least twice. Unpredictable subject loss prevented precise counterbalancing of voices and target/novel pairings (see Table 1).

Data analysis. Interburst intervals were read off the polygraph records. Times between the event marks signalling the end of one burst and the beginning of the next burst were measured and rounded down to the nearest whole second (see Figure 1). Thus, the scorers (AJD and MJS), who were highly practiced, did not have to make detailed judgments about IBI values that might bias the data. Interscorer reliability approached 100%.

Next, each subject's IBIs from the baseline and reinforcement phases were converted to a proportion of their time criterion (t). For example, if $t = 4$ s then all 2-s IBIs had the value $0.5t$, and if $t = 6$ s then 2-s IBIs had the value of $0.33t$. Converted IBIs were grouped into bins that were $0.2t$ s wide; Bin 1 contained IBIs between $0.0t$ and $0.2t$ s, Bin 2 contained IBIs between $0.2t$ and $0.4t$ s, . . . , and Bin 10 contained IBIs between $1.8t$ and $2.0t$ s. Bin 11 contained all IBIs greater than $2.0t$ s. IBIs were assumed to be equally distributed within a bin. The conversion equates the relative size of IBIs across subjects and allows averaging over subjects.

RESULTS

Experienced Newborns

The hypothesis asserts that in utero exposure to the acoustic properties of the target story will make it more reinforcing than the novel story. If so, the relative frequency of short IBIs should increase over baseline when reinforced by the target stories in the IBI $< t$ condition and the relative frequency of IBIs slightly longer than the baseline median should increase when reinforced by target stories in the IBI $> t$ condition.

Baseline IBI distributions were examined first in order to determine whether they differed between reinforcement contingencies. They did not differ: A mixed ANOVA of the relative frequencies of baseline IBIs, with Contingencies ($< t$ vs. $> t$) and Bin (1–10) as factors, indicated a significant effect of Bin, $F(9, 126) = 13.3$, $p < .001$. The effect merely confirms that the IBIs were unimodally distributed. Most important, there was no Contingency effect, $F(1, 14)$ $p < 1.0$, and no Contingency $\times$ Bin interaction, $F(9, 126) = 1.67$, $p > .10$.

The predictions of the hypothesis were first assessed by examining the differences between the relative frequencies of IBIs that occurred during baseline and those that occurred during reinforcement. Difference scores were entered into a mixed ANOVA with Contingencies ($< t$ vs. $> t$) and Bin (1–10) as factors. There was no effect of Contingency, $F(1, 14) < 1.0$, and a significant effect of Bin, $F(9, 126) = 5.48, p < .025$. Most important, there was a significant Contingency $\times$ Bin interaction, $F(1, 126) = 2.07$, $p < .05$. Planned tests of simple effects confirmed that the interaction occurred because with the IBI $< t$ contingency the relative frequency of short IBIs increased over baseline levels, while those of all other IBIs either decreased or did not change. With the IBI $> t$ contingency the relative frequency of IBIs slightly greater than t seconds increased, while those of the others decreased or did not change. Any IBI between 0 and t seconds would have produced the target story under the IBI $< t$ contingency, and any IBI $\geq t$ seconds would have produced it under the IBI $> t$ contingency. But only the relative frequencies of the shorter IBIs reinforced by the targets systematically increased.

The differential reinforcement effects are more clearly revealed in the analysis of IBIs between $0.0t$ and $0.4t$ (the shorter IBIs) and those between $1.0t$ and $1.4t$ (IBIs slightly longer than t seconds). Conditional probabilities of baseline and reinforced IBIs in these classes were obtained by dividing the relative frequency of IBIs in each class by the relative frequency of that class and all longer IBIs (see Table 1). This is a sensitive measure of temporally differentiated responding because: (a) it adjusts the inherently unequal opportunity for infants to emit equal numbers of short and long IBIs in a limited period of time; (b) it measures the probability that an infant will emit a particular class of IBIs given the opportunity to do so (cf. Anger, 1956; DeCasper & Fifer, 1980); and (c) it renders the conditional probabilities of IBIs between $0.0t$ and $0.4t$, and those between $1.0t$ and $1.4t$, arithmetically independent of one another. The dependent variables for the target story and for the novel story were their reinforcement ratios: (conditional probability of IBIs during reinforcement) divided by (conditional probability of IBIs during reinforcement) plus (conditional probability of IBIs during baseline).

The average values of baseline conditional probabilities of target-story IBIs and novel-story IBIs did not differ, $t(15) = 1.37, p > .10$. However, their reinforcement ratios differed as expected. A mixed ANOVA with Contingency ($< t$ vs. $> t$) and Interval ($0.0t$–$0.4t$ vs. $1.0t$–$1.4t$) as factors, revealed no effect of Contingency, $F(1, 14) < 1.0$, and no effect of Interval, $F(1, 14) = 1.59, p > .20$, but a significant Contingency $\times$ Interval interaction, $F(1, 14) = 6.65, p < .025$ (Figure 2). Target-story reinforcement ratios were larger than novel-story reinforcement ratios, independent of the contingency and of the interval. The fact that 13 of the 16 infants

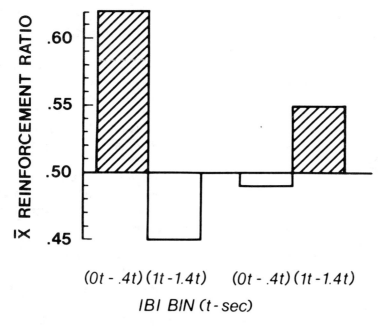

Figure 2. Mean reinforcement ratios of the target (hatched bars) and novel (open bars) stories for Experienced infants in the IBI $< t$ condition (left side) and in the IBI $> t$ condition (right side). The means are based on a total of 400 baseline and 1040 reinforced interburst intervals.

had larger target ratios than novel ratios ($p = .011$ by the binomial test) and 13 of the 16 had target-story ratios greater than .50 indicates this result was typical. The individual-subject consistency implies that maternal voice cues were not necessary for producing the differential reinforcement effect. Neither the target-story reinforcement ratios nor the difference between the target ratios and novel ratios differed between the 9 infants who heard their own mothers' voices and the 7 who heard unfamiliar voices, p-values of both t-tests $> .10$.

Control Subjects

The following analysis of control-subject performances parallels that of the experienced subjects. The relative frequency distributions of baseline IBIs did not differ between reinforcement contingency conditions. A mixed ANOVA with Contingency ($< t$ vs. $> t$) and Bin (1–10) as factors revealed a marginal effect of Bin, $F(9, 90) = 1.90$, $.10 < p > .05$, but no effect of Contingency, $F(1, 10) < 1.0$, or of the Contingency $\times$ Bin interaction, $F(9, 90) = 1.38$, $p > .10$. The subsequent mixed ANOVA on the difference scores of IBIs that occurred during the baseline and reinforcement phases revealed no effect of Contingency, $F(1, 10) < 1.0$, a significant effect of Bin, $F(9, 90) = 5.19$, $p < .001$, and a significant Contingency $\times$ Bin interaction, $F(9, 90) = 3.48$, $p < .005$. However, none of the follow-up tests of simple effects were statistically reliable; the interaction seemed to result from unsystematic variation in the difference scores of the two contingency conditions in Bins 1–5.

Subsequent analysis of conditional probabilities confirmed that the preceding interaction did not result from systematic effects of target-story reinforcement. The baseline conditional probabilities of target and novel stories did not differ, $t(11) < 1.0$; neither did their reinforcement ratios computed for the intervals $0.0t$–$0.4t$ and $1.0t$–$1.4t$. The mixed ANOVA with Contingency and Interval as factors revealed no reliable effects whatever, p values of all F statistics $> .10$ (Figure 3).

A comparison of the reinforcement ratios of matched-subject pairs revealed that experienced newborns had larger target-story ratios than their matched naive counterparts, $t(11) = 2.68$, $p < .05$, but that their novel-story ratios did not differ, $t(11) < 1.0$.

DISCUSSION

Three implications of the prenatal-experience hypothesis were confirmed: (1) For experienced subjects the target story was more reinforcing than the novel story when both were concurrently available; (2) the greater reinforcing value of the target story was independent of who recited the story; and (3) for matched-control infants the target story was no more reinforcing than the novel story. The only experimental variable that can systematically account for these findings is whether the infants' mothers had recited the target story while pregnant. Subject characteristics also seem unable to account for the results; the differential-reinforcement effect did not occur within the matched-control group, and the differential-reinforcing value of the target story differed between matched subjects, but the reinforcing effect of the novel story did not. The results also cannot be attributed to individual-subject and subgroup differences in baseline patterns of responding. The most reasonable conclusion is that the target stories were the more effective reinforcers, that is, were preferred, because the infants had heard them before birth. The conclusion is consistent with earlier, independent evidence that hearing becomes

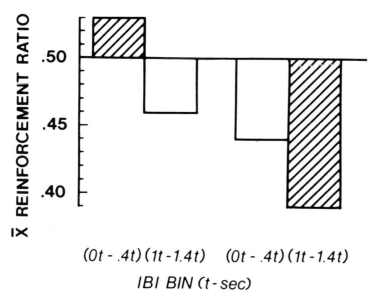

Figure 3. Mean reinforcement ratios of the target (hatched bars) and novel (open bars) stories for Control infants in the IBI < *t* condition (left side) and in the IBI > *t* condition (right side). The means are based on 300 baseline and 800 reinforced interburst intervals.

functional during the third trimester and that maternal speech attains audible in utero levels during this time. Thus, the study provides the first direct evidence that prenatal auditory experience with a particular maternally generated speech stimulus influences the reinforcing value of that stimulus after birth.

The conclusion implies that the fetuses had learned and remembered something about the acoustic cues which specified their particular target passage (e.g., prosodic cues such as syllabic beat, the voice-onset-time of consonants, the harmonic structure of sustained vowel sounds, and/or the temporal order of these sounds). Recall also that newborns prefer their mothers' voices over that of another female, when both speak the same novel material (DeCasper & Fifer, 1980; Fifer, 1980). The present results add to the evidence indicating that the maternal-voice preference also originated in utero. If so, then fetuses also register some specific information about their mothers' voices (e.g., spectra of nasals and vowels, glottal frequency and spectrum, and/or the temporal characteristics of pitch, intensity, and formants) (Bricker & Pruzansky, 1976). The specific acoustic cues that register in utero and which influence subsequent perception of speech and voice sounds are not known at present. However, whether language-relevant cues or voice-specific cues play an active role in newborns' perception has now been shown to depend upon: (a) which class of cues are differentially available, (b) the infants' prenatal experience with the cues, and (c) the circumstances attending postnatal perception (e.g., behavioral contingencies, infant state, or the presence or absence of other sounds).

The present study suggests noninvasive, ethically acceptable methods to further study the effects of prenatal auditory stimulation on postnatal auditory function and development, especially the development of speech perception. Such research might also benefit clinical treatment of the perinate, for example, by aiding in the diagnosis of fetal condition and by providing information for designing environments of preterm infants.

Some Post Hoc Considerations

Learning is generally and most satisfactorily inferred from a *change* in performance rather than from absolute measures of performance. However, change scores—the difference scores and reinforcement ratios used in this study—are almost always inversely related to prelearning performance, the baseline probabilities of responding (cf. Glass & Stanley, 1970, p. 182). The present discussion focuses on the extent to which the preceding inferences about differential-reinforcement effects were influenced by the relation between baseline levels of performance and the difference scores and reinforcement ratios. The issue is salient here because the hypothesis asserts that reinforcement would differentially affect specific IBIs whose baseline probabilities varied considerably.

The abscissa of Figure 4 shows the mean conditional probabilities of baseline IBIs for each of the eight subconditions represented in Table 1. The mean baseline conditional probabilities of IBIs between $0.0t$ and $0.4t$ (subconditions 1–4 in Figure 4) are lower than the mean baseline conditional probabilities of IBIs between $1.0t$ and $1.4t$ (subconditions 5–8). They differ simply because baseline IBIs between $0.0t$ and $0.4t$ come from the left of a unimodal distribution and IBIs between $1.0t$ and $1.4t$ come from near the median of the distribution. The primary means of experimentally controlling for the influence of these baseline differences was to counterbalance the reinforcers associated with the IBI $< t$ and IBI $> t$ contingencies: As Figure 4 suggests, and as reported earlier, when the values of baseline probabilities are pooled over IBI $< t$ and the

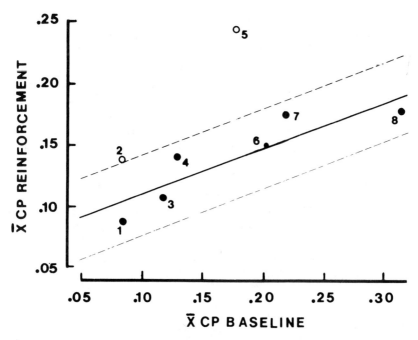

Figure 4. Mean conditional probability that subjects in the eight subconditions would emit IBIs between 0.0*t*–0.4*t* and between 1.0*t*–1.4*t* during reinforcement as a function of the mean conditional probability that they would do so during baseline. Open circles refer to Experienced subjects reinforced by the target story with IBI < *t* (2) and with IBI > *t* (5). Filled circles refer to Experienced subjects reinforced by the novel story with IBI < *t* (4) and with IBI > *t* (7); to Control subjects reinforced by the target story with IBI < *t* (3) and with IBI > *t* (8); and to Control subjects reinforced by the novel story with IBI < *t* (1) and with IBI > *t* (6). The solid line represents the regression equation (.07 + .38 [baseline probability]) for the six control subconditions (filled circles) and the dashed lines represent the 95% confidence interval around the regression line.

IBI > *t* contingencies (1 with 6; 2 with 5; 3 with 8; 4 with 7) the average baseline probabilities do not differ.

Figure 4 also shows the empirical relation between the mean baseline probabilities and the mean probabilities occurring with reinforcement for each subcondition. The solid line represents the regression equation relating the baseline and reinforcement probabilities for the six subconditions in which no differential-reinforcer effect was expected (filled

symbols), $r = .89, p < .02$. For these six subconditions the probability of
responding during reinforcement is almost completely determined by
the prior baseline probability. Their reinforcement probabilities do not
increase over baseline probabilities, but instead become increasingly
smaller than baseline as the baseline probability increases. Figure 5
shows that when reinforcement ratio (a change score) is substituted for
reinforcement probability (the absolute score), the strong linear relation
between baseline performance and reinforced performance is preserved,
but for statistical and mathematical reasons, the correlation is negative,
$r = -.93, p < .01$.

Since the means of the subcondition baselines were not equal, these
correlations raise an important question. Might the reinforcement probabilities and reinforcement ratios that resulted when Experienced newborns were reinforced with their target story be determined simply by

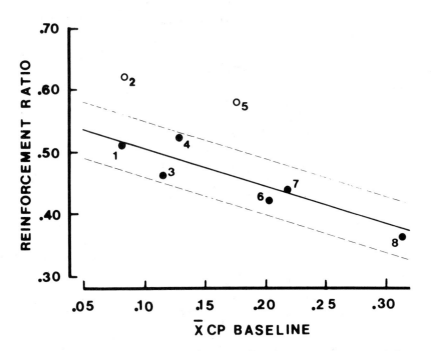

Figure 5. Reinforcement ratio as a function of baseline conditional probability
for the eight subconditions described in Figure 4. The regression equation is
(.57–.63 [baseline probability]) for the control subconditions and the dashed
lines represent the 95% confidence interval.

their baseline probabilities? That is, do the differences in the subgroups' terminal performances, as measured by reinforcement probabilities or difference scores and reinforcement ratios, reflect differential reinforcement effects or just the fact that the subgroups began with different baseline probabilities?

Figure 4 shows that the mean baseline probabilities of the two conditions where Experienced subjects were reinforced with their target story (open symbols) fall within the range of baseline probabilities entailed in the correlation. Significantly, however, the mean probabilities that occur with reinforcement by the target story are both above their baseline levels and above the 95% confidence interval of the regression line ($p < .0006$). Similarly, both reinforcement ratios are well above .50 and also above the 95% confidence interval of the regression line of Figure 5. Thus, the possibility that the reinforcement probabilities and reinforcement ratios occurring when Experienced subjects were reinforced with their target story were determined by or could be predicted by their baseline probabilities can be rejected. The favored alternative hypothesis, of course, is that prenatal experience increased the reinforcing effectiveness of their target stories: The effect of prenatal experience with the reinforcer was to increase the conditional probability of reinforced responding by 40% over the level predicted by baseline in the IBI $< t$ condition and by 76% in the IBI $> t$ condition. Reinforcement ratios were increased by 20% and 26% over the levels predicted by baseline performance.

It may still be argued, however, that the preceding analysis was based on subgroup means and that the pattern of individual-subject baseline probabilities within the subgroups was biased toward producing difference scores and reinforcement ratios that supported the prenatal hypothesis. That is, if the baseline probability of each Experienced subject reinforced with the target story had been the same as the baseline of a control subject, then their reinforcement probabilities and reinforcement ratios might not differ.

The following analyses addressed this possibility by comparing selected groups of subjects after matching individual infants on baseline probabilities. Subject matching was accomplished by applying the following three rules: (1) baseline probabilities had to be within $\pm .02$ of each other; (2) if possible, the subjects were to have the same reinforcement contingency; and (3) if more than one match was possible, pairs were matched so as to minimize the difference between conditional probabilities that occurred with reinforcement. No other factors were considered.

In the first comparison, 10 of the 16 baseline probabilities produced by Experienced infants in the conditions where they were reinforced with the target story were matched to the baseline probabilities of 10 of the 16 Experienced subjects in the conditions where they were reinforced with the novel story. The 10 baseline pairs were: (.06/.06), (.06/.06), (.09/.09), (.10/.10), (.12/.12), (.14/.13), (.16/.17), (.17/.17), (.23/.24), and (.26/.26). The mean baseline probability for each group was .14. The mean probability occurring with reinforcement by the target story (.20) was greater than that occurring with reinforcement by the novel story (.15), $t(9) = 2.61$, $p < .01$ (1-tail t test) $T = 4.5$, $p < .025$ (Wilcoxen test). The mean probability of responding with target-story reinforcement was greater than the baseline mean, $t(9) = 2.99$, $p < .005$; $T = 3$, $p < .01$, but the mean probability of responding with novel-story reinforcement did not differ from baseline, $t(9) = .58$; $T = 22.5$. In addition, the mean occurring with target-story reinforcement was well above the 95% confidence interval of Figure 4, but the mean occurring with novel-story reinforcement was well within the interval. The reinforcement ratio of the target story was well above the 95% confidence interval of Figure 5, but the reinforcement ratio for the novel story was within the interval.

Six infants from each reinforcement condition could not be matched. The mean of the unmatched baselines for the target-story condition was .12; the mean occurring with reinforcement was .18. For the novel-story infants these means were .22 and .17, respectively. The reinforcement mean and reinforcement ratio occurring with target-story reinforcement were above the 95% confidence intervals of Figures 4 and 5, but the analogous measures resulting from reinforcement with the novel story were well within the confidence intervals.

Next, baselines of Experienced subjects who were reinforced with the target story were matched to baselines of Control subjects reinforced with the target story. Nine pairs could be formed: (.03/.04), (.06/.06), (.06/.06), (.09/.08), (.10/.10), (.14/.13), (.16/.16), (.26/.26), and (.29/.31). The baseline mean of each group was .13. The mean reinforcement probability for the Experienced subjects (.19) was greater than that of Control infants (.10), $t(8) = 2.58$, $p < .01$; $T = 1$, $p < .005$. The Experienced subjects' reinforcement probabilities were larger than baseline probabilities, $t(8) = 2.94$, $p < .005$; $T = 0$, $p < .005$, but the Control subjects' were not, $t(8) = 1.19$, $p > .10$; $T = 15$. Here, too, the Experienced subjects' mean reinforcement probability and reinforcement ratio were both well above the 95% confidence intervals of Figures 4 and 5. The reinforcement probability of the Control group was within the interval of Figure 4. Their reinforcement ratio, however, fell below the 95% confidence interval of

Figure 5, even though the members of the group had exactly the same baseline probabilities as their Experienced counterparts.

Seven Experienced subjects' and three Control subjects' baselines could not be matched. The baseline means of these subjects are .13 and .40, respectively. Their respective means occurring with reinforcement by the target story were .19 and .20. The reinforcement mean and reinforcement ratio of the Experienced subjects both lay well above the 95% confidence intervals of Figures 4 and 5. Analogous scores for Control subjects were within the intervals.

Finally, Experienced subjects reinforced with the novel story were matched to Control subjects who were also reinforced with the novel story. The nine pairs of baseline probabilities were: (.06/06), (.09/.09), (.10/.10), (.12/.12), (.13/.13), (.19/.20), (.19/.19), (.24/.24), and (.33/.32). The mean for each group was .16. Neither the between-group difference nor the changes from baseline were statistically reliable (all *t* values < 1.0; all *T* values > 16). All reinforcement means and reinforcement ratios fell within the confidence intervals of Figures 4 and 5. Seven Experienced infants and three Control infants could not be matched. Their respective baseline means were .19 and .16, and their respective reinforcement means were .18 and .13. All reinforcement means and reinforcement ratios were within the confidence intervals of Figures 4 and 5.

After equating the baseline probability of IBIs of individual infants in specific conditions, the only consistent finding was that the target story was the more effective reinforcer for Experienced infants. In sum, the results of this study cannot be accounted for by differences in the baseline values of subconditions or individual subjects. The previous conclusion can be retained: The postnatal reinforcing value of a speech passage is increased by prenatal experience with the passage.

REFERENCES

Anger, D. (1956). The dependence of interresponse times upon the relative reinforcement of different interresponse times. *Journal of Experimental Psychology, 52,* 145–161.

Bernard, J., & Sontag, L.W. (1947). Fetal reactivity to tonal stimulation: A preliminary report. *Journal of Genetic Psychology, 70,* 205–210.

Birnholz, J.C., & Benacerraf, B.R. (1983). The development of human fetal hearing. *Science, 222,* 517–519.

Brazelton, T.B. (1978). The remarkable talents of the newborn. *Birth & Family Journal, 5,* 4–10.

Bricker, P.D., & Pruzansky, S. (1976). Speaker recognition. In N.J. Lass (Ed.), *Contemporary issues in experimental phonetics.* New York: Academic.

Butterfield, E.C., & Cairns, G.F. (1974). Whether infants perceive linguistically is uncertain, and if they did its practical importance would be equivocal. In R.L.

Scheifelbush & L.L. Lloyd (Eds.), *Language perspectives: Acquisition, retardation, and intervention.* Baltimore, MD: University Park Press.

Butterfield E.C., & Siperstein, G.N. (1972). Influences of contingent auditory stimulation upon nonnutritional sucking. In J. Bosma (Ed.), *Oral sensation and perception: The mouth of the infant.* Springfield, IL: Charles C Thomas.

Cairns, G., & Butterfield, E.C. (1974). Assessing infants auditory functioning. In B.Z. Friedlander, G.M. Sterritt, & G.C. Kirk (Eds.), *Exceptional infant: Vol. 3.* New York: Brunner/Mazel.

Catania, C.C. (1970). Reinforcement schedules and psychophysical judgments: A study of some temporal properties of behavior. In W.N. Schoenfeld (Ed.), *The theory of reinforcement schedules.* New York: Appleton-Century-Crofts.

DeCasper, A.J. Butterfield, E.C., & Cairns, G.F. (1976). *The role of contingency relations in speech discrimination by newborns.* Paper presented at the Fourth Biennial Conference on Human Development, Nashville, TN.

DeCasper, A.J., & Carstens, AA. (1981). Contingencies of stimulation: Effects on learning and emotion in neonates. *Infant Behavior and Development,* 4, 19–35.

DeCasper, A.J., & Fifer, W.P. (1980). Of human bonding: Newborns prefer their mother's voices. *Science,* 208, 1174–1176.

DeCasper, A.J., & Prescott, P.A. (1984). Human newborns' perception of male voices: Preference, discrimination and reinforcing value. *Developmental Psychobiology,* 17, 481–491.

DeCasper, A.J., & Sigafoos, A.D. (1983). The intrauterine heartbeat: A potent reinforcer for newborns. *Infant Behavior and Development,* 6, 19–25.

DeCasper, A.J., & Zeiler, M.D. (1977). Time limits for completing fixed ratios: IV. Components of the ratio. *Journal of the Experimental Analysis of Behavior,* 27, 235–244.

Fifer, W.P. (1980). Early attachment: Maternal voice preferences in one- and three-day old infants. Unpublished doctoral dissertation, University of North Carolina at Greensboro.

Glass, G.V., & Stanley, J.C. (1970). *Statistical methods in education and psychology.* Englewood Cliffs, NJ: Prentice-Hall.

Gottlieb, G.G. (1981). Roles of early experience in species-specific perceptual development. In R.N. Aslin, J.R. Alberts, & M.R. Petersen (Eds.), *Development of perception.* New York: Academic.

Grimwade, J.C., Walker, D.W., Bartlett, M., Gordon, S., & Wood, C. (1971). Human fetal heart rate change and movement in response to sound and vibration. *American Journal of Obstetrics and Gynecology,* 109, 86–90.

Gurney, N., & Gurney, E. (1965). *The King, the mice, and the cheese.* New York: Beginner Books/Random House.

Johansson, B., Wedenberg, E., & Westin, B. (1964). Measurement of tone response by the human fetus: A preliminary report. *Acta Oto-laryngologica,* 57, 188–192.

Malott, R.W., & Cumming, W.W. (1964). Schedules of interresponse time reinforcement. *Psychological Record,* 14, 211–252.

Panneton, R.K., & DeCasper, A.J. (1984). *Newborns prefer intrauterine heartbeat sounds to male voices.* Paper presented at the International Conference on Infant Studies, New York.

Querleu, D., & Renard, K. (1981). Les perceptions auditives du foetus humain, *Medicine & Hygiene,* 39, 2102–2110.

Querleu, D., Renard, K., & Crepin, G. (1981). Perception auditive et reactivite foetale aux stimulations sonores. *Journal de Gynecologie Obstetrique et Biologie de la Reproduction, 10,* 307–314.

Salk, L. (1962). Mothers' heartbeat as an imprinting stimulus. *Transactions of the New York Academy of Science,* 24, 753–763.

Seuss, D. (1957). *The cat in the hat.* New York: Beginner Books/Random House.

Sontag, L.W., & Wallace, R. (1935). The movement response of the human fetus to sound stimuli. *Child Development, 6,* 253–258.

Studdert-Kennedy, M. (1982). The beginnings of speech. In K. Immelmann, G.W. Barlow, L. Petrinovich, & M. Main (Eds.), *Behavioral development.* Cambridge: Cambridge University Press.

Vince, M.A., (1979). Postnatal effects of prenatal sound stimulation in the guinea pig. *Animal Behaviour,* 27, 908–919.

Vince, M.A., Armitage, S.E., Walser, E.S., & Reader, M. (1982). Postnatal consequence of prenatal sound stimulation in the sheep. *Behavior,* 81, 128–139.

Walker, D., Grimwade, J., & Wood, C. (1971). Intrauterine noise: A component of the fetal environment. *American Journal of Obstetrics and Gynecology,* 109, 91–95.

Wolff, P.H. (1963). Observations on the early development of smiling. In B.M. Foss (Ed.), *Determinants of infant behavior (Vol. 2).* New York: Wiley.

Wolff, P.H. (1966). The causes, controls and organization of behavior in the neonate. *Psychological Issues, 5* (1, Monograph No. 1).

2

Social Referencing: The Infant's Use of Emotional Signals from a Friendly Adult with Mother Present

Mary D. Klinnert

National Jewish Center for Immunology and Respiratory Medicine, Denver, Colorado

Robert N. Emde and Perry Butterfield

University of Colorado Health Sciences Center Denver, Colorado

Joseph J. Campos

University of Denver, Colorado

Previous studies have demonstrated that 1-year-old infants look toward their mothers' facial expressions and use the emotional information conveyed. In this study, 46 1-year-olds were confronted with an unusual toy in a context where an experimenter familiar to the infants posed either happy or fearful expressions and where their mothers were present but did not provide facial signals. Most of the infants (83%) referenced the familiarized stranger. Once the adult's facial signals were noted, the infant's instrumental behaviors and expressive responses to the toy were influenced in the direction of the affective valence of the adult's expression.

Reprinted with permission from *Developmental Psychology,* 1986, Vol. 22, No. 4, 427–432. Copyright 1986 by the American Psychological Association, Inc.

This work was supported by National Institute of Mental Health Project Grant #MH22803, Dr. Emde's Research Scientist Award #5 K02MH36808, and the Developmental Psychobiology Research Group at the University of Colorado Health Sciences Center.

26

The results indicate that infants may be influenced by the emotional ex-pressions of a much broader group of adults than has previously been recognized.

In this study we investigated whether infants would reference an adult other than their mothers and would make use of the affective information obtained. Emotional expressions of others provide important informa-tion about environmental events. Recent studies have shown that prever-bal infants engage in "social referencing"—they look to others when con-fronted with a variety of events and use the emotional reactions of others to regulate their own behavior. The infants' mothers provided the emo-tional signals in these studies, by giving either prototypical facial ex-pressions (Klinnert, 1984; Sorce, Emde, Campos, & Klinnert, 1985) or vocal signals (Svejda & Campos, in press) or by controlling the positive af-fect in multichanneled responses (Feinman & Lewis, 1983).

Although the purpose of these initial studies was to demonstrate that infant behavior is responsive to a social signaling process, the studies also reflect a basic assumption about infants' social referencing: If an infant is responsive to anyone's affective signals, the person most likely to in-fluence the infant is his or her mother. The central role of mothers in in-fants' social referencing was initially suggested by Campos and Stenberg (1981), who postulated that "mother becomes the target of social referencing" (p. 295). In fact, the term *maternal referencing* was sometimes used interchangeably with the term *social referencing.* In the same vein, Feinman (1982) discussed the "selectivity of the source of information" (p. 459) as a key aspect of social referencing. Although Feinman did not restrict the process to infants and their mothers, he suggested that the target of social references would be selected using the same parameters as those that influence the choice of a model in the imitation process (e.g., nurturance, similarity, and power). In any case, available data regard-ing infant visual behavior support the notion that infants select their mothers to reference. Lamb (1976) found that when a stranger entered the room, 1-year-olds looked toward their mothers more than toward their fathers, suggesting that the mother was the preferred source of in-formation. Field (1979) found that infants 10–14 months of age looked toward their own mothers more than they did toward infant peers or other infants' mothers. Furthermore, the literature on infant attachment is replete with examples of infants looking frequently toward their attach-ment figures in a variety of contexts, and it could be inferred that at least some of these looks functioned as social references.

In an attempt to define the role of emotional signaling within the attachment relationship, Bradshaw, Goldsmith, and Campos (1984) placed 12-month-old infants in a social referencing situation, the visual cliff. They hypothesized that the infants would look more toward their mothers than they would toward an equally available but unfamiliar adult. A preference to look toward their mothers would be regarded as an index of the attachment relationship. Surprisingly, the infants looked toward the stranger almost as much as they looked toward their mothers. The results did not indicate whether the infants behaved in accordance with the stranger's emotional signals, because the mother's signals and the stranger's signals were the same. Zarbatany and Lamb (1985) also found that infants looked about equally toward their mothers and toward strangers. In their study, regulation of 12-month-old infants' behavior by mothers' and strangers' signals was assessed, and the results showed that the infants' behavior was affected by the mother's signals, but not by the stranger's. However, the paradigm involved leaving the infants alone with the stranger, and the stress they experienced may have caused them to be unable to use the stranger's signals.

The evidence, then, is mixed as to whether infants are selective in their choice of a referencing target. To what extent might they use the affective signals of other adults? Increasing attention is now being given to the infant's developing capacity to socialize with adults other than attachment figures and members of their immediate family. For example, Bretherton, Stolberg, and Kreye (1981) found that most infants in a group 12–24 months of age initiated proximal interactions with unfamiliar adults. Clarke-Stewart (1978) described how in dealing with strange adults, 30-month-olds were straightforward in their use of the affective cues that the adults directed toward them. Regardless of their mothers' reactions to the strangers, the toddlers approached those adults who gave them positive affective signals and stayed away from those who responded negatively to them. Given this emerging picture in which infants are regarded as active participants in a broader social world, it seemed likely to us that social referencing would occur with a wider range of adults than had been studied to date.

In some circumstances it may be ecologically relevant for infants to look for information from a relatively unknown adult and to incorporate that information into a behavior plan. The specific circumstances would depend on the context. Sroufe, Waters, and Matas (1974) have demonstrated that contextual factors have an important effect on infants' social functioning, and we believe that such factors are probably quite important in social referencing situations. When a child is engaged in a positive, ongoing interaction with an adult and an ambiguous event occurs, that adult may well become the referencing target, regardless of the broader relationship he or she has with the child. Another contextual factor that necessarily determines emotional availability is physical proximity, and the geometry of a room may be a significant determinant of who becomes a referencing target.

We therefore decided to conduct a systematic study of social referencing involving a situation that included the factors just discussed. The setting was an unfamiliar playroom, and the situation was the entrance of an unusual remote-controlled toy. The toy approached the infant, who was playing with the friendly adult at some distance from the infant's mother. Following a pilot study with this context, we hypothesized that (a) infants would visually reference the friendly adult as well as the mother, (b) infants who received a smile signal would be more likely to approach the toy than those who received a fear signal, (c) infants who received a fear signal would be more likely to go to their mothers, and (d) infants' affect would be influenced by the friendly adult's emotional signal of smiling or fear.

METHOD

Subjects

The subjects were 46 infants between 12 and 13 months of age, drawn from a subject pool of middle-class volunteers from metropolitan Denver. The sample consisted of 25 female infants and 21 male infants.(Sixty-five infants and mothers actually took part in the study, but 19 (29%) were eliminated because of procedural problems.) Infants were randomly assigned to one of two experimental groups: (a) the smile group or (b) the fear group. References to the mother and to the familiarized adult (the experimenter) were assessed for all 46 infants, and these data showed that 8 infants failed to reference the experimenter. Because infant references to the experimenter were necessary to address a central question of the study, subjects were solicited and randomly assigned to the two conditions until there were two groups of 19 infants who had referenced the experimenter.

Setting

The setting was a comfortable playroom, 10 ft (3 m) by 20 ft (6 m), which was observable from two sides by one-way mirrors. A small table was placed on one side of the room and was covered with a cloth that hid a remote-controlled R2-D2 robot toy placed under the table. Opposite the table was a toy telephone that was secured to a chair so that its location was fixed. The toy telephone served to interest the infant until the robot appeared. A chair for the infant's mother was placed at the far end of the room, 9 ft (2.7 m) from both the table and the infant.

Procedure

Upon arrival for the experiment, the mother and the infant entered the playroom with a female experimenter. The experimenter invited the infant to play with interesting toys on the floor near the mother while she explained the study to the mother, trained her in the neutral facial expression she was to display, and had her sign a consent form. Following this introductory phase, which lasted about 10 min, the experimenter sat on the floor and engaged the infant in play for about another 10 min. The infant was then placed near the toy telephone, across from the small table, with his or her back to the mother. In this position the infant and the experimenter played together approximately 2 ft (.6 m) apart during a 15-s baseline period, after which the robot toy was activated by a second experimenter behind the one-way mirror. With this activation, the robot toy emerged, beeping, from under the table, pushing aside the cloth as it moved. The robot approached the infant in a graded manner, stopping just beyond the infant's reach. The robot approach typically lasted 1 minute. The infant's behavior was videotaped for 3 min, starting from the point when the robot began beeping and moving out from under the table.

Independent Variable

The independent variable was the facial expression displayed by the experimenter when the infant looked at her following the emergence of the robot. Each infant was randomly assigned to one of two facial expression conditions, smile or fear. The experimenter was trained to display patterns of facial expression components described by Izard (1971) and Ekman and Friesen (1975). For the smile condition, the experimenter's forehead was smooth, the corners of her mouth were lifted, her cheeks were raised, and her eyes were bright with crow's-feet visible. For the fear expression, her forehead was wrinkled transversely, her eyebrows were raised and contracted, her eyes were wide open and staring (upper lids raised), and the corners of her mouth were pulled back. The experimenter looked alternately at the infant and the robot, making no sounds or gestures. The mothers were instructed to appear neutral or slightly puzzled when the infants looked toward them during the trial.

Dependent Variables

The infants and mothers were videotaped using the two cameras behind separate one-way mirrors. Videotapes were scored by two observers who were naive to the independent variable. The observers produced a second-by-second record of each infant's behavior, focused on the direction of the infant's gaze and all instrumental behaviors. The visual behaviors of interest were looks toward the experimenter or the mother. Other behaviors recorded were presence or absence of movement in the direction of the robot toy or the mother, duration of touching or playing actively with the robot toy, and duration of physical contact with the mother.

We assessed the reliability for these variables by having both of the observers rate 14 of the videotaped infants. For the visual behavior, the observers agreed on the occurrence of a change in gaze and subsequent direction of a gaze for 94% of the gaze changes in the reliability sample. They achieved 100% agreement on the occurrence and type of instrumental behaviors displayed by the infants; agreement involved the two raters reporting the onset of the same type of behavior within 3 s of each other.

The infants' affective responses were rated by two separate observers, who were also blind to the independent variable condition. The observers rated infant affect every 5 s using a 9-point bipolar scale that ranged from *high positive involvement with the robot toy* (+4) through sober, interested expression (0) to *obvious fear of the robot toy* (−4). The scale took into account affective displays, such as smiling or crying, as well as the quality of behavior, such as kissing or kicking the robot toy. Both observers rated 14 of the videotaped infants. Reliability, assessed by calculating the percentage of 5-s periods for which the two raters were in perfect agreement on the rating scale, was 86%.

Mother's Facial Signals

To control for the influence of the infants' mothers, the mothers' facial expressions were rated during each reference to her. Global ratings of positive, neutral, or negative were obtained for each such reference. Positive ratings included smiles; eyebrow lifts; bright, expectant, or pleasant expressions; and forward movements. Negative ratings included intense concentration, tight lips, and frowns. Observers were in perfect agreement on 77% of these global ratings.

Facial expression ratings revealed that the mothers were generally well able to maintain neutral expressions when their infants referenced them during the trials. In the fear group, mothers' expressions were scorable for 59 of the 69 infant references. Of the 59 expressions, 79.7% were scored as neutral, 3.4% as negative, and 17.9% as positive. In the smile group, mothers' expressions were scorable for 78 of the 80 infant references. Of the 78 expressions, 70.5% were scored as neutral, 1.3% as negative, and 28.2% as positive. The higher percentage of positive expressions in the smile group proved to be largely accounted for by two mothers, who smiled broadly when their infants referenced them. Eliminating the infants of these two mothers from the smile group resulted in maternal emotional signals for this group that were comparable to those of the fear group, that is, 85.5% were scored as neutral, 1.6% as negative, and 12.9% as positive. Although eliminating the two infants made the groups more comparable, both of the infants had referenced the experimenter and made definitive movements prior to looking at their mothers. Therefore, the two infants were retained as subjects with the provision that only data reflecting their behavior prior to their first look at their mothers be included; the data for all other variables for the two infants were excluded.

RESULTS

Visual References

Our first hypothesis was that the infants would look at the experimenter in this context. Of the 46 infants in the study, 38 (or 83%) referenced the experimenter. The remaining 17% referenced only the mother. Further descriptions of looking behavior as well as analyses addressing differential reactions of the smile and fear groups will be reported only for the 38 infants who referenced the experimenter. During the 3-min trial, those infants who referenced the experimenter directed twice as many looks toward her as they did toward the mother; for the 38 infants in the final sample, the average number of looks toward the experimenter was 8.7, and the average number of looks toward the mother was 3.9. In addition, the infants' first references after seeing the robot toy were predominantly toward the experimenter; 30 of the 38 infants looked first toward her. However, most of the infants (22 of 38) also looked toward the mother at least once before they took action.

Initial Reaction

To determine whether the two groups of infants were similar at the start, we compared initial reactions for the time period following the entrance of the robot toy and prior to the infant's first reference to the experimenter. Because this time period varied across infants, a mean score of affective state was calculated for each infant, based on the number of 5-s affective ratings for the time period. We compared the two groups (38 infants) by conducting a t test on the scores. The mean affective rating for the fear group was 2.26, and the mean for the smile group was 2.79, $t(36) = 0.41, p = .69$. These data suggest that the initial reactions of the two groups of infants were similar prior to the introduction of the differential affective signals.

Behavioral Responses to the Robot Toy

Our second hypothesis was that infants who received the smile signal would approach the robot toy more than would infants who received the fear signal. As shown in Table 1, 13 of 19 infants in the smile group approached and touched the robot toy, whereas 8 of 19 infants in the fear group did—a marginally significant trend, $\chi^2 (1, N = 38) = 2.66, p < .10$. Moreover, the quality of behavior for the two groups of infants as they approached and touched the robot toy was very different. Of the infants who touched the robot toy, those in the smile group approached it significantly more quickly than those in the fear group did. For the smile group, the mean latency to touch the robot toy was 60 s, whereas for the fear group it was 98 s, $t(19) = 2.24, p = .025$. Furthermore, the smile-group infants (excluding the two who received positive maternal signals during the trial) touched the robot toy for a longer period of time: They touched it for 42 s, whereas the fear-group infants touched it for 11 s, $t(17) = 2.61, p < .01$.

Our third hypothesis predicted that more infants who received the fear signal would approach and touch their mothers within the 3 min of the trial. This hypothesis was supported: 13 infants in the fear group went to their mothers and touched them, whereas 6 of 17 infants in the smile group did, $\chi^2(1, N = 36) = 3.95, p < .95$.

Finally, we looked at the infants' affective reactions to the facial signals. We wanted to determine whether the infants' own affective states were influenced by these signals and if so, whether the affective changes preceded, accompanied, or followed the infants' instrumental behaviors. As stated earlier, the two groups showed similar (mostly positive) affect prior

Table 1. Behavioral Responses and Mean Affective Ratings of Infants Who Received Smile Signals and Those Who Received Fear Signals From Familiar Adult

	Group[a]		
Item	Smile	Fear	p
Behavioral response			
Number of infants who approached and touched robot toy[a]	13	8	$< .10$
Mean latency to approach robot toy in seconds, for subjects who approached ($n = 21$)	60	98	$< .025$
Mean length of time touching robot toy, in seconds, for subjects who touched ($n = 19$)	42	11	$< .01$
Number of infants who approached and touched mother[b]	6	13	$< .05$
Affective rating[b]			
Prior to first reference to experimenter	2.88	2.26	.197
First 15 s following reference to experimenter, unless first action occurred within 15 s	2.94	2.34	.126
5-s period when infants first took action	1.88	−1.16	$< .01$
15 s postaction	1.87	0.27	$< .05$

Note. Data for two infants in the smile group were excluded from some of the results because the infants received positive maternal signals.
[a] $n = 19$ for the smile group; $n = 19$ for the fear group. [b] $n = 17$ for the smile group; $n = 19$ for the fear group.

to the first reference to the experimenter. During the 15 s following that first reference, the affect of both groups remained positive but the smile-group infants tended to look more positive than the fear-group infants. However, later in the trial, during the 5-s period when the infants first moved toward either the robot toy or the mother, the affect of the fear-group infants became negative, whereas the affect of the smile-group infants became sober. The mean rating for the fear group was 3 points lower than the mean for the smile group. The difference in affect maintained during the 15 s following the action. The affective data for the four time periods were subjected to a repeated measures analysis of variance, with group and time period as the two factors. The overall interaction was significant, $F(3. 102) = 4.15, p < .01$, and a main effect for group was also significant, $F(1, 34) = 11.64, p < .002$. The changes in infant affect across the trial are illustrated in Figure 1. The simple effects for group for each time period are presented in Table 1, which shows a trend at the first post-reference point ($p = .126$) and significant effects at the second and third points ($p < .01$ and $p < .05$, respectively). On the whole, then, the infants in the fear group showed more negative affect throughout the trial.

DISCUSSION

Over the past decade there has been a great deal of emphasis on infants' reliance on attachment figures for a sense of security (e.g., Bowlby, 1969; Sroufe & Waters, 1977). Investigations of social referencing have focused on infants' propensity to visually check with their mothers when confronted with ambiguous circumstances and to respond behaviorally to their mothers' emotional signals. We questioned whether emotional signals influence the behavior of 1-year-old infants even when the source is a relatively unfamiliar adult.

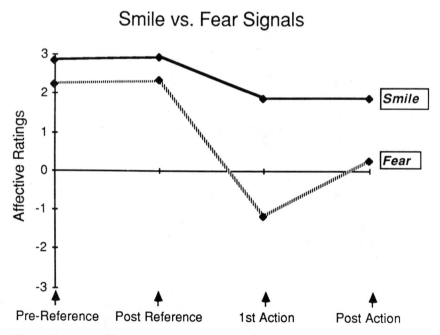

Figure 1. Mean affective ratings for time periods prior to and following infant references, for the time of the first infant action, and following the first action.

Our findings indicate that social referencing is not exclusively directed toward attachment figures. Social referencing consists of two components, social attention and behavior regulation, both of which were affected by the behavior of the familiarized adult in this study. More specifically, over 80% of the infants we tested looked toward the familiarized adult after the entry of the robot toy, and once the infant noted the adult's facial signals, his or her instrumental behaviors and expressive responses to the robot toy were influenced in the direction of the affective valence of the adult's expression.

In terms of instrumental behaviors, fear signals resulted in significantly more infants approaching the mother, whereas smiles resulted in a marginal trend toward more infants approaching the robot toy. Furthermore, within the subset of infants who approached the robot toy, those who received positive signals approached it more quickly and touched it longer than did those who received fearful signals. Anecdotal observations on the quality of touching behavior indicated that the infants who received positive signals were more likely to pat or kiss the robot toy, whereas those who received fear signals were more likely to swat it or knock it over.

The expressive states of the two groups of infants were also influenced by the emotional messages from the familiar adult. The infants who received smiles were more positive than those who received fear signals. Thus, not only did the infants adapt their behavior according to the information received from the familiar adult, but also their emotional state was influenced by the adult whom they had just met.

There were three other noteworthy findings in this study. First, facial expressions of the experimenter influenced behavior even when the infant's reaction to the toy was not initially uncertain. All too often, social referencing is assumed to operate only when primary appraisal fails. In the present study, the infant's initial reaction to the robot toy was predominantly positive, yet the adult's facial signals resulted in the infant's regulating his or her behavior in a manner appropriate to the posed affect. Although they may be clearest when events are maximally uncertain (e.g., Gunnar & Stone, 1984), social referencing effects are not restricted to conditions of uncertainty.

Second, emotional expressions of others do not necessarily produce all-or-none responses in infants. Although a substantial number of infants did approach the robot toy despite the adult's expression of fear, the effects of the fear signal were clearly evident in parametric analyses, such as latency to approach the robot toy, length of time touching the robot toy, and the quality of handling the robot toy.

Third, in this study we found that expressive changes corresponded in time with changes in the infant's instrumental behaviors. This finding thus leaves open the question of whether affective changes mediate (i.e., precede) the instrumental behavior changes or instrumental behavior results in expressive changes. We suspect that both processes are operating. Microanalytic techniques may be required to show that affective resonance or state correspondence occurs in response to the detection of emotional expressions in others prior to the occurrence of any instrumental behavior (Klinnert, Campos, Sorce, Emde, & Svejda, 1983; Stern, 1985) or that the subject's appraisal of the probable success or failure of an instrumental reaction will also determine the nature of the subject's expressive state (Lazarus, 1968).

We have suggested that the willingness of the infants to turn to slightly familiar adults was related to certain contextual components. The presence in the room of the infant's mother was a significant aspect of the social context and may have facilitated the infants' use of the stranger's signals. The availability of the mother constituted a major difference between this study and that of Zarbatany and Lamb (1985), in which the infants did not use the stranger's signals. Future investigations should pursue the systematic assessment of the relation between availability of the mother, infant stress level, and infants' use of emotional signals. A related contextual component is the practical issue of proximity; the experimenter was sitting only 2 ft (.6 m) from the infant, whereas the child's mother was sitting across the room. Pilot studies had showed that a play time during which the adult experimenter actively attempted to engage the infant went a long way toward establishing sufficiently friendly relations such that the baby would reference the experimenter. This finding is consistent with evidence that, like other people, infants are more likely to engage in social interactions with people who show a desire to engage in interaction with them. Still another factor is the positive exchange that took place between the mother and the experimenter before the test. An earlier study suggested that these positive exchanges influence the subsequent response of the infant to a stranger (Boccia & Campos, 1983). It is unclear how much of a role each of these contextual factors played in facilitating the infants' reliance on the familiar adult in the present study. Whatever the influence of each of the factors, it was possible to manipulate them within a single situation such that the majority of 1-year-old infants would reference and be influenced by a person they hardly knew. Perhaps what the infants responded to was the adult's *emotional availability;* that is, perhaps the contextual factors that enhanced the probability that the infants would reference the familiarized adult are some of the conditions that represent the emotional availability of one human being for another.

On the other hand, there are undoubtedly great individual differences in the extent to which 1-year-olds will rely on unknown adults after a short time of exposure. Within the present study there were infants who never referenced the mother, those who referenced both the mother and the experimenter, and those who referenced the experimenter only. This range of responses can probably be explained by many factors, including the infant's temperamental traits, such as sociability or fearfulness; the infant's experiences of being exposed to a variety of people and situations; and the infant's history of qualitative interactions, both with care givers and others which facilitate infants' development of trust in the broader social world (Feinman & Lewis, 1983).

In summary, the present study not only has demonstrated that infants are influenced by the emotional signals of relatively unknown adults, but also has illustrated that when theorizing about the social world of infants, it is no longer accurate to think solely in terms of the infants' attachment figures. The conditions under which extrafamilial emotional signaling takes place and the identification of sources of individual differences in response to emotional signals are exciting new areas of investigation.

REFERENCES

Boccia, M., & Campos, J.J. (1983, April). *Maternal emotional signals and infants' reactions to strangers.* Paper presented at the meeting of the Society for Research in Child Development, Detroit.

Bowlby, J. (1969). *Attachment and loss (Vol. 1).* New York: Basic Books.

Bradshaw, D.L., Goldsmith, H.H., & Campos, J.J. (1984). *Attachment, temperament, and social referencing: Interrelationships among three domains of infant affective behavior.* Unpublished manuscript, University of Denver.

Bretherton, I., Stolberg, U., & Kreye, M. (1981). Engaging strangers in proximal interaction: Infants' social initiative. *Developmental Psychology,* 17, 746–755.

Campos, J.J., & Stenberg, C. (1981). Perception, appraisal, and emotion: The onset of social referencing. In M.E. Lamb & L.R. Sherrod (Eds.), *Infant social cognition: Empirical and theoretical considerations* (pp. 273–314). Hillsdale, NJ: Erlbaum.

Clarke-Stewart, K.A. (1978). Recasting the lone stranger. In J. Glick & K.A. Clarke-Stewart (Eds.), *The development of social understanding* (pp. 109–176). New York: Gardner Press.

Ekman, P., & Friesen, W. (1975). *Unmasking the face.* Englewood Cliffs, NJ: Prentice-Hall.

Feinman, S. (1982). Social referencing in infancy. *Merrill-Palmer Quarterly,* 28, 445–470.

Feinman. S., & Lewis, M. (1983). Social referencing at ten months: A second order effect on infants' responses to strangers. *Child Development,* 54, 878–887.

Field, T.M. (1979). Infant behaviors directed toward peers and adults in the presence and absence of mother. *Infant Behavior and Development,* 2, 47–54.

Gunnar, M.R., & Stone, C. (1984). The effects of positive maternal affect on infant responses to pleasant, ambiguous and fear-provoking toys. *Journal of Child Development,* 55, 1231–1236.

Izard, C.E. (1971). *The face of emotion.* New York: Plenum Press.

Klinnert, M.D. (1984). The regulation of infant behavior by maternal facial expression. *Infant Behavior and Development,* 7, 447–465.

Klinnert, M.D., Campos, J.J., Sorce, J.F., Emde, R.N., & Svejda, M. (1983). Emotions as behavior regulators: Social referencing in infancy. In R. Plutchick & H. Kellerman (Eds.), *Emotions in early development: Vol 2. The emotions* (pp. 57–86). New York: Academic Press.

Lamb, M.E. (1976). Twelve-month-olds and their parents: Interaction in a laboratory playroom. *Developmental Psychology,* 12, 237–244.

Lazarus, R. (1968). Emotions and adaptations: Conceptual and empirical relations. In W.J. Arnold (Ed.), *Nebraska Symposium on Motivation* (pp. 175–266). Lincoln, NE: University of Nebraska Press.

Sorce, J.F., Emde, R.N., Campos, J.J., & Klinnert, M.D. (1985). Maternal emotional signaling: Its effect on the visual cliff behavior of one-year-olds. *Developmental Psychology,* 21, 195–200.

Sroufe, L.A., & Waters, E. (1977). Attachment as an organizational construct. *Child Development.* 48, 1184–1199.

Sroufe, L.A., Waters, E., & Matas, L. (1974). Contextual determinants of infant affective response. In M. Lewis & L. Rosenblum (Eds.), *The origins of fear* (pp. 49–72). New York: Wiley.

Stern, D.N. (1985). *Interpersonal world of the infant.* New York: Basic Books.

Svejda, M., & Campos, J.J., (in press). The mother's voice as the regulator of the infant's behavior. *Developmental Psychology.*

Zarbatany, L., & Lamb, M. (1985). Social referencing as a function of information source: Mothers versus strangers. *Infant Behavior and Development,* 8, 25–33.

PART I: INFANCY STUDIES

3

Temperament in Preterm Infants: Style and Stability

Jane Washington and Klaus Minde
Queen's University, Kingston, Ontario
Susan Goldberg
University of Toronto, Ontario

A sample of low birthweight preterm infants was assessed for temperamental characteristics at 3, 6, and 12 months of age by parent report. Results indicate that this sample contains a significantly higher percentage of "difficult" infants ($p < 0.02$) than reported in full-term samples. Infant characteristics such as severity of perinatal and postnatal complications and maternal characteristics, such as socioeconomic status and available support structures, were found to be unrelated to parent temperament reports. However, mother-infant interaction in the first year was shown to be related to both the style and stability of temperament reports. These findings suggest that temperament, at least during the first year of life, is a reflection of the transactions between the infant and his or her caregivers.

In recent years there has been a renewed interest in the identification and measurement of behavioral differences in young children, commonly referred to as temperament. This construct had quickly become popular among mental health professionals after it was identified and

Reprinted with permission from the *Journal of the American Academy of Child Psychiatry,* 1986, Vol. 25, No. 4, 493–502. Copyright 1986 by the American Academy of Child and Adolescent Psychiatry.

This research was supported by Grant 972–80/83 of the Ontario Mental Health Foundation and the Laidlaw Foundation.

validated by Thomas et al. (1963) and at present may well be one of the most frequently used psychiatric concepts of the practicing clinician. One reason for this popularity may be that the concept of different temperamental dispositions allowed the clinician to conceptualize the varying difficulties children of the same family have with their caretakers by using a more dynamic, yet apparently validated model. Early findings linking specific temperamental dispositions and later childhood behavior and adjustment problems (Graham et al., 1973; Rutter et al., 1964) also seemed to support the notion that certain temperamental characteristics make it more likely for the child to form a mismatch or "poor fit" (Thomas, 1981) with those who interact with him or her.

While there remains agreement that infants and children differ in their behavior, researchers during the past 5 years have increasingly questioned the best way to detect those differences. As parental ratings have been most commonly used to measure children's temperament, reviewers have particularly focused on the reliability of parent perceptions of their children (Bates, 1980; Goldsmith and Campos, 1982). Findings here have shown both a rather poor test-retest reliability of instruments currently used to measure temperament (Hubert et al., 1982) and poor correlations of parent reports against external criteria, especially of the category "difficult" temperament (Bates, 1980; Hubert et al., 1982). Carey, who developed the widely used Infant Temperament Questionnaire (Carey, 1970) pointed out that the rapid development of young children may well be responsible for the poor test-retest reliability (Carey, 1983). Indeed, recent confirmation of significant shifts in infants' biobehavioral organization (Emde and Harmon, 1984; McCall, 1981; Rutter, 1984) might well preclude behavioral consistencies, at least during the early years.

Some writers have also explained these poor correlations by asserting that parental perceptions of their children's temperament are primarily due to subjective factors such as parent personality, especially anxiety and social class (Sameroff et al., 1982; Vaughn et al., 1981).

While the measurement of temperament by parent reports obviously reflects a dynamic interaction between a parent and the instrument (Sameroff, 1983), one could still argue that parents who correctly or incorrectly perceive their infants as "difficult" or "easy" nevertheless would confirm this judgment in their behavior toward that infant. However, data here are also inconsistent. Difficult temperament has been associated with a more positive home environment and interactions (Peters-Martin and Wachs, 1981) as well as negative patterns of behavior such as lack of maternal responsiveness (Milliones, 1978). Still others have found no relationship between difficult temperament and the quality of mother-infant interaction (Bates et al., 1982; Vaughn et al., 1981) or a mother's treatment of her infant (Dunn and Kendrick, 1980).

In summary it appears that there is much controversy regarding the validity and reliability of temperament measures as well as the stability of temperament characteristics over time. However, there have been no previous studies in which a variety of parental background variables have been combined with repeated parental and observer ratings in establishing infant temperament. As our sample contains such data, we thought we might provide some more detailed information on possible objective and subjective components (Bates and Bayles, 1983) which go into a mother's perception of her young infant.

Finally, as our sample, in contrast to the majority of previous work, consisted of very low birthweight preterm infants from a variety of socio-economic backgrounds and included both twins and singletons, we felt we could also assess a number of disputed factors which potentially contribute to the measurement of temperament during the first year of life.

SUBJECTS AND PROCEDURES

The subjects for this research were preterm infants admitted to the Neonatal Intensive Care Unit of The Hospital for Sick Children within 12 hours of their birth between June 1980 and September 1982. Infants were recruited for the study if they weighed less than 1501 grams at birth and had no physical malformations. The total sample consisted of 76 infants; 22 sets of twins, 27 singleton controls and 5 surviving twins. Two families of singletons refused to participate, decreasing the final sample to 74 infants.

Table 1 presents a summary of the background data of the total sample and Table 2 a summary of the procedures employed which are relevant for the present study. There were no statistical differences between any of the groups on maternal or infant characteristics.

Perinatal and Neonatal Assessment

Information regarding the infants' birthweigtht, gestational age, type of delivery and early medical status was obtained from medical records. In addition, a research nurse kept detailed accounts of each infant's medical course throughout the period of hospitalization. These accounts

Table 1. Background Data

Mothers	Twins and Survivors (N = 49)			Singletons (N = 25)		
	Mean	N	s.d.	Mean	N	s.d.
Age of mother	27		4.8	27.1		5.3
No. of children:						
None		19			13	
1 or more		8			12	
Marital status:						
Married		23			20	
Other		4			5	
Socioeconomic class:						
1 and 2		7			9	
3		11			6	
4 and 5		9			10	
Previous abortions:						
None		18			17	
1 or more		9			8	

Infant	Twin A (N = 23)		Twin B (N = 26)		Singletons (N = 25)	
	Mean	s.d.	Mean	s.d.	Mean	s.d.
Birthweight (grams)	1125.5	262.5	1100.6	226.4	1078.2	183.5
Gestational age (weeks)	29.5	2.0	29.5	2.0	28.5	1.9
Total illness score	82.7	77.6	106.5	82.5	79.3	57.9
Days of hospital- ization	73.3	26.8	77.4	24.5	77.5	13.9
Sex (N)						
Male	15		15		16	
Female	8		11		9	

were quantified using a morbidity scale described elsewhere in detail (Minde et al., 1983). The scale measures the 19 most common diseases or pathophysiological states encountered in infants under1501 grams in our Neonatal Intensive Care Unit. Each medical conditon is given a daily score from 0 to 3 depending on how life-threatening the condition is to a premature infant. The daily scores are then summed to give a "total global score" which measures the overall severity of an infant's medical course in our hospital.

Table 2. Summary of Procedures

Procedure	Hospital	Time of Procedure (month)			
		3	6	9	12
Neonatal assessment	×				
Psychiatric interview	×				×
Discharge interview	×				
Observations	×	×	×	×	
Maternal-infant interaction ratings		×	×	×	
Developmental assessment			×		
Revised infant temperament questionnaire		×	×		
Toddler Temperament scale					×

Interviews

When the infants were 4 weeks old, the senior investigator (K.M.) gave all parents a semistructured psychiatric interview, assessing their social background, their experiences during the pregnancy, delivery and postnatal course of their infants, their attitudes, expectations toward the future and available support structures. Parent responses to 48 areas of information were quantified and recorded. Only 9 of these areas were used in the present analysis. The selection was made because other items of information (e.g., monthly income of mother or past criminal record of father) did not seem relevant to the issue at hand.

Before the infant's discharge from the hospital, a research assistant interviewed the parents to assess their knowledge about their infant's condition, the treatment they felt he or she had received at the hospital, their feelings of competence to care for their infant(s) at home and their knowledge about support structures available to them at home and in the community. Parental responses to 9 items on this discharge interview were quantified on a 5-point scale and summary scores were calculated. Four of these items were used in the present analysis.

Observations

A researcher visited the infants at home when they were 6 and 9 months corrected age (calculated from the expected date of delivery). The visits lasted from 1½ to 3 hours and were scheduled at a time when mother would be feeding her infant(s). The researcher observed the mother feeding her infant(s) and recorded the relative frequency of 17 maternal and 16 infant behaviors using a pencil and paper technique. The observation period was divided into 20-second intervals and the observer recorded the first instance of each of the target behavior performed by the mother or child during each interval. A transcript of the observation was then computer analyzed to give a relative frequency count of the target behaviors.

The same procedure was employed during the observation of a 10-minute play session between mother and child, using a set of standard toys supplied by us. The present analysis includes 10 infant and 9 maternal feeding behaviors and 10 infant and 14 maternal play behaviors. This selection was again made empirically by excluding behaviors; e.g., mother out of the room, which seemed unrelated to the task of this study.

Maternal-Infant Interaction Ratings

Following the home visits at 6 and 9 months, the observers completed two sets of interaction rating scales assessing 31 maternal care and play variables, such as facility in caretaking, appropriateness of interventions, accessibility, supportiveness in play and sensitivity, and 14 infant variables, such as responsivity to mother's interactions, social behavior, temperament, satisfaction with the play situation and amount of looking at mother's face during feeding. These scales were adapted from Ainsworth et al. (1978), Egeland and Brunquell (1979), and Egeland et al. (1977). Interrater reliabilities for these ratings were calculated for percent agreement from the two observers for the same observation. Agreements ranged from 0.72 to 1.00 with an average agreement of 0.90.

Developmental Assessment

One researcher visited the home and administered the Bayley Scale of Infant Development (Bayley, 1969) when the infant was approximately 6 months (corrected age). This test yields scores for mental development (MDI) and psychomotor development (PDI). The researcher also completed the 13-item Infant Behavior Record (IBR) which rates the infant's social orientation, activity, fearfulness, emotional tone, object orientation, cooperativeness, tension, goal directedness, attention span, endurance and reactivity.

Temperament Ratings

Mothers were asked to complete the Revised Infant Temperament Questionnaire (RITQ) (Carey and McDevitt, 1978) when their infants were 3 and 6 months old (corrected age). At 12 months, mothers and fathers completed the Toddler Temperament Scale (TTS) (Fullard et al., 1984). These temperament questionnaires are patterned after the Thomas and Chess interview style of assessment. The toddler form is seen by the authors as a logical addition "to fill the gap" (Fullard et al., 1984, p. 215) between the infant and preschool version of temperament scales presently available. Each type of questionnaire asks the mother to rate her infant's behavior in a number of relevant situations on a scale from 1 ("almost never") to 6 ("almost always"). These scores are then summed to give the child a score for each of the 9 characteristics identified by Thomas and Chess. Using 5 of these scores (for approach/withdrawal, rhythmicity, adaptability, intensity and mood) the child is assigned to a particular diagnostic cluster ranging from "easy" to "intermediate," "slow to warm up" or "difficult." We shortened the original questionnaire from 95 to 67 items by eliminating those items which yield scores for distractibility, persistence and threshold. There were two reasons for doing this. First, we were primarily interested in comparing the infants in our sample according to diagnostic clusters. Second, mothers in our sample were asked to complete these questionnaires three times and we felt that compliance, especially from mothers of twins, would be higher with the shortened questionnaire.

RESULTS

In analyzing our results we were initially interested in: (1) a comparison of parent reports of temperament in preterm infants with similar data derived from normal full-term samples, (2) an investigation of the stability of temperament in preterm infants during the first year of life, (3) examining inter-parent and interrater agreement in our sample, and (4) examining the relationship between mother-child interaction and the stability of temperament in preterm infants.

Comparison of Parent Report of Temperament in Preterm and Full-Term Infants

Description of the sample. Table 3 presents a distribution of the temperament ratings by diagnostic cluster obtained from mothers of our preterm sample at each of the three rating periods. For purposes of comparison

Table 3. Distribution of Temperament Ratings by Diagnostic Cluster at 3, 6 and 12 Months (in Percent)

	Easy	Intermediate Low	Intermediate High	STWU	Difficult
3 Months (N = 62)	16.1	29.0	32.3	6.5	16.1
6 Months (N = 54)	24.0	29.6	13.0	9.3	24.0
12 Months (N = 61)	23.0	36.1	21.3	8.2	11.5
4–8 Months (Carey and Mc-Devitt, 1978) (N = 203)	42.4	31.0	11.3	5.9	9.4

we have included the normative data reported by Carey and McDevitt (1978) on their sample of 203 infants between the ages of 4 and 8 months. The one difference between the two data sets is that our sample contains a significantly higher percentage of infants rated as difficult at 6 months ($\chi^2 = 11.97$, $df = 4$, $p < 0.02$) although this was less pronounced at 12 months.

Comparing the infants rated as easy and those rated as difficult with respect to birthweight, gestational age, degree of perinatal illness ("total global scores"), or length of stay in hospital revealed no significant differences between the groups. In addition Bayley scores for MDI and PDI showed no distinctions between easy and difficult infants at the time of the 6-month rating.

The only feature in the obstetric and newborn histories of our sample which distinguishes between those infants rated as easy and those rated as difficult was the type of delivery. As might be expected, our sample contained a high percentage of infants delivered by caesarian section (33%) compared to full-term samples. Table 4 shows that a significantly greater proportion of the infants rated as difficult at 3 months of age were surgically delivered ($\chi^2 = 5.38$, df 1, $p < 0.05$). Interestingly, these differences disappear at the time of the 6-month rating and became almost reversed by the time the infants reached 1 year.

Table 4. Type of Delivery

Infant Age and Type of Delivery[a]	Infant Behavior	
	Easy (%)	Difficult (%)
3 Months ($N = 62$)		
Vaginal	37	31
C/S	8	24
$\chi^2 = 5.38$, $p < 0.05$		
6 Months ($N = 54$)		
Vaginal	31.5	26
C/S	22.1	20.4
$\chi^2 = 0.34$, $p = NS$		
12 Months ($N = 61$)		
Vaginal	33	30
C/S	26	11
$\chi^2 = 3.62$, $p < 0.10$		

[a] C/S = caesarian section.

Stability of Temperament

Referring again to Table 3 we see that while a difficult temperament seems to be relatively common in preterm infants at 6 months, its incidence is reduced substantially by the time the infants are 1 year old. This raises questions about the stability of temperament in preterm infants, or at least the stability of maternal reports of temperament during the first year of life.

One method of measuring stability is to correlate the total temperament scores from maternal reports supplied at each of the rating periods. In our sample we have temperament ratings at 3, 6, and 12 months, on 42 infants. Pearson product moment correlations for scores between 3 and 6 months, 6 and 12 months, and 3 and 12 months showed a high correlation ($r = 0.52, p < 0.01$) between 6 and 12 month scores as well as between 3 and 6 months ($r = 0.50, p < 0.01$). There was a nonsignificant correlation ($r = 0.21$) between 3 and 12 months. Assessing temperament at 3 months, then, gives us some indication of how mothers will rate their infants at 6 months, but very little idea of their ratings at 1 year. Assessments at 6 months, however, seem to be more reliable indicators of maternal ratings at 1 year.

To compare the stability of temperament ratings in our sample with findings reported by other researchers using the same instruments on different samples we correlated characteristic scores for each of the infants over the three rating periods. Table 5 presents these findings along with data from Peters-Martin and Wachs (1981) who studied the correlations between the Revised Infant Temperament Questionnaire administered at 6 months and the Toddler Temperament Scale administered at 12 months. This comparison shows that our sample displays similar moderate to high longitudinal stability in all characteristics except adaptability between 6 and 12 months.

One may question to what extent the mixture of twins and singletons affected these findings. A more detailed analysis revealed that 44% of our singletons changed by 2 or more temperamental categories between 6 and 12 months while in 43% of our twin pairs did one twin change at least 2 categories while the other retained his initial rating. In 29% both twins remained in the same temperamental category between 6 and 12 months and in 28% both twins moved independently. This suggests that changes in Temperament ratings in our sample occurred with similar frequency in singletons and twins.

Table 5. Spearman Rank Order Correlations of Characteristic Scores at 3-6 Months, 6-12 Months and 3-12 Months ($N = 42$)

	Activity	Rhythmicity	Approach/Withdrawal	Adaptability	Intensity	Mood
3-6 Months	0.45[b]	0.28	0.39[a]	0.22	0.34[a]	0.45[b]
3-12 Months	0.20	0.14	0	0.18	0.14	0.39[a]
6-12 Months	0.35[a]	0.38[a]	0.48[b]	0.18	0.60[c]	0.62[c]
Peters-Martin and Wachs (1981) ($N = 29$)	0.49[b]	0.38[a]	0.32[a]	0.57[b]	0.04	0.46[b]

[a] $p < 0.05$.
[b] $p < 0.01$.
[c] $p < 0.001$.

Inter-Parent and Interrater Agreement

Validity of maternal reports of temperament has been assessed in several ways. In our study we had opportunities to compare reports of mothers with those of fathers on the same questionnaire measure. In addition, research assistants made judgments of infant temperament on the basis of home observations and in their scoring of the Bayley Infant Behavior Record (Bayley, 1969).

Mothers and fathers scored their infants independently on the Toddler Temperament Scale at 12 months. The correlation between their scores was moderately high (Pearson $r = 0.60$, $p < 0.01$) and comparable to that reported by others (Bates, 1980). Three items on the Infant Behavior Record at 6 months were compared with scores obtained from corresponding dimensions on the Infant Temperament Questionnaire at the same age. These correlations were moderate for activity ($r = 0.42$, $p < 0.05$) and approach ($r = 0.38$, $p < 0.05$) but negligible for mood ($r = 0.07$, NS).

Observers also rated "temperament" at home visits on a scale devised by Egeland and his colleagues (1977, 1979) from 1 (irritable) to 9 (cheerful). The correlations between these ratings and the RITQ scores were low ($r = 0.12$ at 3 months, $r = 0.02$ at 6 months). Since these ratings appear to assess "general disposition" or mood, we also examined correlations with the RITQ mood score and found little evidence of consistent relationships ($r = 0.19$ at 3 months and $r = 0.32$ at 6 months).

Maternal Reports of Temperament and Mother-Infant Interaction

The previous sections focused mainly on the impact infant characteristics such as medical complications may have on the style and variability of maternal temperament reports in the first year. However, maternal background variables and mother-infant interaction as observed and rated by researchers are equally important potential modifiers of parental perceptions.

The following analyses are based on temperament ratings obtained at 6 months of age as there appears to be greater stability in these reports as well as predictability to toddler temperament. Our first comparison involved those infants occupying the extreme categories of the temperament continuum. There were 12 infants in each of the easy and difficult groups at 6 months. Background information concerning pregnancy and delivery (from the psychiatric interview) and maternal competence, support from husband, socioeconomic status, and support structures available at home and in the community (from the psychiatric and discharge interview) showed no differences between easy and difficult groups.

Next we looked at some of the maternal and infant ratings (Ainsworth et al., 1969; Egeland and Brunquell, 1979; Egeland et al., 1977) made by observers following their home visit observations of a feeding and play situation at 6 and 9 months. Easy and difficult infants were compared on a variety of observer ratings such as responsivity to mother's interactions, social behavior, temperament and amount of looking at mother's face during feeding. Mothers of these infants were compared on ratings for facility in caretaking, response to crying and synchronization of interventions. In all, the infants were compared on eight of the fourteen ratings and the mothers on 19 of the 31 ratings. The ratings which were excluded from this analysis had to do with mother's availability and the amount of visual and auditory contact a child received as well as the stimulus potential of the environment. Infant ratings not used related to the child's state, position and muscle tone.

The mothers of difficult infants received more positive scores at 6 months on all of the 19 observer ratings ($p < 0.001$ by sign test). Table 6 shows that two of these ratings, facility in caretaking, and response to crying were significant at the 0.05 level. In contrast, observer ratings of the infants showed easy infants to be rated more positively on 6 of the 8 ratings compared, but none reached statistical significance.

A comparison of maternal and infant interaction ratings made by ob-

Table 6. Mother-Infant Interaction at 6 and 9 Months

Ratings and Behavior	Easy ($N = 12$) $\bar{X}$ (s.d.)	Difficult ($N = 12$) $\bar{X}$ (s.d.)
Ratings (6 months)		
Facility in caretaking	5.5 (1.76)	6.62[a] (1.08)
Response to crying	6.0 (1.47)	7.18[a] (0.94)
Ratings (9 months)		
Response to crying	5.82 (1.4)	6.92[a] (1.14)
Appropriateness of initiations	5.42 (1.44)	6.77[b] (0.97)
Synchronization of rate	5.82 (1.47)	7.00[b] (0.78)
Accessibility	6.08 (1.55)	7.15[a] (0.95)
Behaviors		
Smile (infant) 6 months	13.16 (11.4)	4.0[b] (5.0)
Smile (infant) 9 months	14.18 (11.3)	2.99[c] (4.28)

[a] $p < 0.05$.
[b] $p < 0.03$.
[c] $p < 0.01$.

servers following the 9-month home visit showed a similar trend. Mothers who had rated their infants as difficult 3 months earlier continued to receive more positive scores on 14 of the 19 observer ratings compared ($p < 0.04$ by sign test). Four of these ratings, mother's response to crying, appropriateness of mother's initiations or interaction, synchronization of her rate of feeding to baby's pace and mother's accessibility to her infant, differed significantly ($p < 0.05$) (Table 6). Easy infants received more positive scores on 4 of the 8 observer ratings compared, while difficult infants were scored more positively on the other 4. None of these reached statistical significance.

Table 6 also lists the frequencies of the 1 out of 16 infant behaviors (smiling) coded during the feed and play observations which showed a statistically significant difference between easy and difficult infants and their mothers.

As mothers who rated infants as temperamentally difficult at 6 months were rated to be more sensitive in their caretaking interactions, we wondered whether this pattern of behavior at 6 and 9 months would have any effect on the infants themselves or on maternal ratings of temperament at 12 months. In examining the Toddler Temperament Scale scores for these 24 infants we found that 8 of the 12 easy infants continued to be rated as easy at 1 year. However, 4 of them had switched to more difficult categories (intermediate high or slow to warm up). Of the 12 infants in the difficult category at 6 months, 8 continued to be rated as difficult or intermediate high, while 4 switched to the easy diagnostic cluster at 1 year.

This finding led us to reexamine the background and mother-infant interaction data to compare the "switchers" and "nonswitchers." Mothers of nonswitchers, whose infants were rated as easy or difficult at 6 months and continued to be rated that way at 12 months, showed no difference in background variables based on the psychiatric and discharge interviews.

However, when we looked at the observer ratings of the mothers of nonswitchers and their infants (Table 7) we found that consistently easy infants were rated as showing more positive reactions during free play with their mothers ($p < 0.05$) than were consistently difficult babies. In contrast to our previous findings, however, we also saw that the mothers of consistently easy infants received ratings which were equal to or higher than those for mothers of consistently difficult infants on 14 of the 19 observer ratings compared. This trend continued to be evident at the time of the 9-month home visit. Eleven of the 19 observer ratings were more positive with one, mother's supportiveness toward her infant's play, reaching statistical significance ($p < 0.02$).

Table 7. Mother-Infant Interaction at 6 and 9 Months

Ratings and Behavior	Easy → Easy ($N = 8$) $\bar{X}$ (s.d.)	Difficult → Difficult ($N = 8$) $\bar{X}$ (s.d.)
Ratings (6 months)		
Satisfaction (infant)	6.38 (.99)	4.88[a] (1.76)
Ratings (9 months)		
Supportiveness in play	6.5 (1.22)	4.57[c] (1.5)
Behaviors		
Hold (6 months)	7.54 (10)	67.78[b] (42.98)
Hold (9 months)	0 (0)	52.66[c] (50.8)
Vocalize (infant) (9 months)	22.9 (21.6)	43.3[b] (24.2)
Smile (infant) (9 months)	16.69 (13.1)	2.84[c] (4.87)

[a] $p < 0.05$.
[b] $p < 0.03$.
[c] $p < 0.02$.

Differences were also found in the directly observed frequency of behaviors during the feed and play session. At 6 and 9 months mothers of consistently difficult infants held their infants more ($p < 0.03$ and $p < 0.01$) and during the play session at 9 months consistently difficult infants vocalized more ($p < 0.03$) and consistently easy infants smiled more ($p < 0.02$).

It appeared then that it was the "switchers," those infants who changed diagnostic categories between 6 and 12 months, who were accounting for the differences noted in the first analysis (Table 6). Therefore, we compared the same background information, maternal and infant interaction ratings, and observed frequencies of discrete behaviors coded during the home visits for these two smaller groups of four infants each.

Table 8 summarizes the results of this analysis. Again we found no differences in maternal background variables between the groups. However, behavioral differences were evident. Mothers of infants described as difficult at 6 months but easy at 1 year were rated more positively on all of the 19 observer ratings ($p < 0.001$ by sign test) of behavior following the home visit at 6 months. In the case of four of these behaviors, facility in caretaking, negative regard, response to crying, and synchronization of rate of feeding, the differences were significant ($p < 0.03$).

Observer ratings of these infants and their mothers at the time of the 9-month home visit showed the same pattern with two ratings, facility in caretaking and the infants' responsivity to mothers' interactions reaching statistical significance ($p < 0.05$). There were no differences in observed frequency of behaviors during the home visits between the two groups.

From these findings it appeared that mothers who were rated by objective observers as putting a greater effort into their caretaking and play interactions ended up rating their infants more positively at 1 year.

Our final analysis involved comparing the switchers and nonswitchers within each of the easy and difficult categories. We wanted to know if there was any way of predicting which infants would become easier or more difficult based on observed interaction. Observer ratings of interactions based on the home visits were most positive for both infants and mothers (7 out of 8 for infants, $p < 0.04$ by sign test; 16 out of 19 for mothers, $p < 0.002$ by sign test) among the dyads where the infant shifted from difficult to easy temperament at 1 year although none reached statistical significance. Similarly there were no statistically significant differences in observed frequency of behaviors during the 6- or 9-month home visit.

Among the easy infants, however, there were a number of differences. Observers rated mothers of infants who remained easy at 1 year more

Table 8. Mother-Infant Interaction at 6 and 9 Months

Ratings	Easy → Difficult (N = 4) $\bar{X}$ (s.d.)	Difficult → Easy (N = 4) $\bar{X}$ (s.d.)
Ratings (6 months)		
Facility in caretaking	3.75 (1.09)	7.5[c] (1.11)
Negative regard	2.75 (1.3)	1.0[c] (0)
Response to crying	5.0 (1.41)	7.67[b] (0.94)
Synchronization of rate	5.0 (0.71)	6.75[b] (0.83)
Ratings (9 months)		
Responsivity (infant)	4.0 (1.73)	5.75[a] (0.43)
Facility in caretaking	4.5 (1.66)	7.5[a] (0.87)

[a] $p < 0.05$.
[b] $p < 0.03$.
[c] $p < 0.01$.

positively than mothers whose infants became difficult on all 19 of the behaviors compared ($p < 0.001$ by sign test).

Table 9 shows that three of these ratings, for facility in caretaking, positive regard and acceptance of their infants were significantly higher at the time of the 6-month home visit ($p < 0.05$). The infants in this group received higher ratings on 7 of the 8 behaviors ($p < 0.004$ by sign test) with one, responsivity to mothers' interactions during the feed, reaching statistical significance at both 6 and 9 months. Differences in observed frequency of behaviors included more fussing and object play during the 9-month feed among those infants who switched to more difficult categories at 1 year. This may explain why their mothers held them more.

DISCUSSION

The present study provides a number of unexpected findings which require an explanation. There is first of all the possibility that most of our findings result from the multiplicity of data sources which were employed in the study. For example, one could argue that 27 observational categories of mother-infant behaviors and 24 mother-infant ratings will provide a good number of significant chance associations. However, as both negative and positive findings in general are clustered in specific areas which hang together conceptually, we feel confident in the overall validity of our findings.

In discussing our results in more detail there is first of all the high percentage of infants rated as difficult compared to normal full-term samples, especially during the 3- and 6-month ratings. While it would seem reasonable that complications arising from our infants' prematurity may affect either the children's behavior or their mother's perception of them, we could not detect significant differences between the "easy" and "difficult" infants on infant characteristics such as birthweight, gestational age or degree of illness in hospital. However, one could argue that many of our mothers were highly anxious during part of their pregnancy, especially since the premature delivery in our sample on the average ocurred after the mother had spent 8 days in an obstetrical unit either for intermittent bleeding or in the hope of postponing the threatened delivery. This finding would give some credence to Vaughn et al.'s (1980) findings that 35% of the variables measured prenatally (and this included maternal anxiety) discriminated between mothers of "easy" and "difficult" infants. Some other preliminary work from our group (Walker et al., 1983) would lend some further support to this hypothesis. In Walker

Table 9. Mother-Infant Interaction at 6 and 9 Months

Ratings and Behavior	Easy → Easy (N = 8) $\bar{X}$ (s.d.)	Easy → Difficult (N = 4) $\bar{X}$ (s.d.)
Ratings (6 months)		
Facility in caretaking	6.38 (1.32)	3.75[b] (1.09)
Positive regard	6.75 (0.83)	5.25[a] (1.08)
Acceptance	7.5 (1.41)	5.75[a] (0.83)
Responsivity (infant)	5.88 (0.33)	4.25[a] (1.92)
Ratings (9 months)		
Responsivity (infant)	5.88 (0.60)	4.0[a] (1.73)
Behaviors (9 months)		
Fuss/cry (infant)	2.93 (4.04)	27.3[b] (12.5)
Object play (infant)	17.89 (16.99)	44.68[a] (11.83)
Hold (mother)	0 (0)	34.38[a] (39.24)

[a] $p < 0.05$.
[b] $p < 0.01$.

et al.'s study we found that mothers who rated their infants as difficult at 3 months were also given lower ratings on parental competence and available support structures during the psychiatric and discharge interviews. As these associations were not present for the 6- and 12-month temperament ratings, one could see them as reflections of maternal anxiety which influences the mothers' early but not later interactions with their babies. On the other hand, we also suggested that reliable estimates of temperament in preterm infants may not be possible at 3 months of age because of these infants' relative behavioral disorganization. Sameroff and his coworkers (1982) also speculate that even 4 months of age may be too early for mothers to have formed an accurate assessment of the child's temperament or for the child to have established stable patterns of behavior. The relative instability of certain temperament characteristics between 3 and 12 months in our sample (Table 5) supports this notion.

The finding that more infants delivered by caesarian section were reported to be difficult at the time of the 3-month temperament assessment is difficult to evaluate. The result may be a chance finding but could also relate to data reported by Grossman et al. (1980). In this study, surgically delivered infants scored significantly lower in psychomotor development (Bayley PDI) at 2, but not at 12 and 24 months than did infants delivered vaginally. Although we did not find any differences between 6-month Bayley scores for easy and difficult infants in our sample, it is possible that our mothers perceived delays at an earlier time and that these delays affected their early (3-month) ratings of temperament.

The most unexpected results of our study, however, were the mother-infant ratings obtained for infants rated as easy and as difficult at 6 months of age. While the clinical significance of all these findings has to be tempered with caution as we observed or rated 18 infant and 33 maternal characteristics or behaviors, the number of statistically significant associations was always above those expected by chance. As in addition many more observations or ratings were in the expected direction, we feel that our interactional findings represent valid data. Thus we were particularly surprised that while "easy" infants smiled more at their mothers during feeding, hence behaved in the expected way, it was the mothers of "difficult" babies who displayed more appropriate behavior toward their infants both at 6 and 9 months. It was only when we examined the toddler temperament ratings and found that one-third of the infants in each of the "easy" and "difficult" groups had shifted diagnostic categories between 6 and 12 months, that this finding became understandable. As Table 8 shows, mothers who rated their infants as difficult at 6 months but easy at 1 year were judged to be most adept and sensitive in their caretaking. Their high scores in fact raised the average score of all mothers with "difficult" children at 6 months above those of mothers with "easy" infants.

Similarly, mothers who rated their infants as easy at 6 months but difficult at 1 year were rated as far less competent and sensitive during our 6- and 9-month visits than were mothers who continued to perceive their infants as temperamentally easy at 1 year.

The conclusions which can be drawn from these findings are the following: Mothers' temperamental ratings in our sample were not biased by the effects of race or social class as is suggested by MacPhee (1983) although prenatal anxiety may have contributed to the high number of "difficult" infants, at least in the 3-month ratings. Furthermore, there is an important relationship between mother-child interaction and infants' future behavior patterns. Thus it seems suggestive from our data that some mothers, being confronted with an infant who shows signs of a difficult temperament, saw this as a challenge rather than a burden. As a consequence, they became especially attuned and sensitive to their babies and over 6 months managed to modulate some of their infants' temperament characteristics. While one could argue that the 12-month temperament ratings by these mothers are simply "rewards" which they gave themselves for their hard work, our data which suggest "easy" infants to smile more or cry and fuss less, would validate these mothers' judgments. It may also be that these mothers were generally more tolerant; i.e., could adjust to a wider range of infant characteristics and hence provide a "good fit" for their babies. On the other hand, our data also suggest that some mothers after 6 months became less adept at their caretaking, found their infants less pleasant and were less able or willing to respond appropriately to their crying or feeding needs. While it is not clear whether these changes occurred in response to some infant characteristics which we have not been able to measure, these data go along with results from another study from our group (Goldberg et al., 1986). Here Goldberg identified a group of infants who at 1 year, using Ainsworth's Strange Situation Paradigm (1978) were only marginally securely attached and had mothers who from 3 months onward had behaved in an increasingly insensitive and distant manner. In contrast, their securely attached peers all had mothers who remained sensitively attuned to their infants all during their first year of life.

In summary, our data suggest that temperament, at least early on in life, is not a fixed construct but a reflection both of the changing transactions between caretakers and infants accompanying growth and development, and the discontinuities of the infant's biobehavioral organization.

REFERENCES

Ainsworth, M., Blehar, M., Waters, E. & Wall, S. (1978), *Patterns of Attachment.* New York: Erlbaum.

Bates, J. E. (1980), The concept of difficult temperament. *Merrill-Palmer Quart.,* 26:299–319.

_____ & Bayles, K. (1983), Objective and subjective components in mothers' perceptions of their children from age 6 months to 3 years. Paper presented at SRCD, Detroit.

_____ Olson, S.L., Pettit, G.S. & Bayles, K. (1982), Dimensions of individuality in the mother-infant relationship at six months of age. *Child Develpm.,* 53:446–461.

Bayley, N. (1969), Bayley Scales of Infant Development, Institute of Human Development, University of California, Berkeley.

Carey, W.B. (1970), A simplified method of measuring infant temperament. *J. Pediat.,* 77:188–194.

_____ (1983), Some pitfalls in infant temperament research. *Infant Behav. Develpm.,* 6:247–254.

_____ & McDevitt, S.C. (1978), Revision of the infant temperament questionnaire. *Pediatrics,* 61:735–739.

Dunn, J. & Kendrick, C. (1980), Studying temperament and parent-child interaction: comparison of interview and direct observation. *Develpm. Med. Child Neurol.,* 22:484–496.

Egeland, B. & Brunquell, D. (1979), An at-risk approach to the study of child abuse: some preliminary findings. *This Journal,* 18:219–235.

_____ Taraldson, B. & Brunquell, D. (1977), Observations of waiting room and feeding situations (mimeographed report). Minneapolis, Minn: University of Minnesota.

Emde, R. N. & Harmon, R. (1984), Entering a new area in the search for developmental continuities. In: *Continuities and Discontinuities in Development,* ed. R. N. Emde & R. J. Harmon. New York: Plenum Press, pp. 1–11.

Fullard, W., McDevitt, S.C. & Carey, W.B., (1984), Assessing temperament in one-to-three year-old children. *J. Pediat. Psychol.,* 9:205–217.

Goldberg, S., Perrotta, M., Minde, K. & Corter, C. (1986), Maternal behavior and attachment in low birthweight twins and singletons. *Child Develpm.,* 57:34–46.

Goldsmith, H. H. & Campos, J. J. (1982), Toward a theory of infant temperament. In: *Development of Attachment and Affiliative Systems,* ed. R.N. Emde & R.J. Harmon. New York: Plenum Press.

Graham, P., Rutter, M. & George, S. (1973), Temperamental characteristics as predictors of behavior disorders in children. *Amer. J. Orthopsychiat.,* 43:328–339.

Grossman, F. K., Winickoff, S.A. & Eichler, L.S. (1980), Psychological sequelae of caesarian delivery. Paper presented at the International Conference on Infant Studies, New Haven, Conn.

Hubert, N.C., Wachs, T.D., Peters-Martin, P. & Gandour, M.J. (1982), The study of early temperament: measurement and conceptual issues. *Child Develpm.,* 53:571–600.

MacPhee, D. (1983), What do ratings of infant temperament really measure? Paper presented at SRCD, Detroit.

McCall, R.B., (1981), Nature-nurture and the two realms of developmental psychology: a proposed integration with respect to mental development. *Child Develpm.,* 52:1–12.

Milliones, J. (1978), Relationship between perceived child temperament and maternal behaviors. *Child Develpm.,* 49:1255–1257.

Minde, K., Whitelaw, A., Brown, J. & Fitzhardinge, P.M. (1983), The effect of neonatal complications in premature infants on early parent-infant interactions. *Develpm. Med. Child Neurol.,* 25:763–777.

Peters-Martin, P. & Wachs, T.D. (1981), A longitudinal study of temperament and its correlates in the first year of life. Paper presented at the SRCD, Boston.

Rutter, M. (1984), Continuities and discontinuities in socioemotional development: empirical and conceptual perspectives. In: *Continuities and Discontinuities in Development,* ed. R.N. Emde & R.J. Harmon. New York: Plenum Press, pp. 41–68.

_____ Birch, H.G., Thomas, A. & Chess S. (1964), Temperamental characteristics in infancy and later development of behavioral disorders. *Brit. J. Psychiat.,* 110:651–661.

Sameroff, A.J. (1983), Chair's comments for the symposium. Parent-report instruments for the assessment of infant temperament: what is being measured? Paper presented at SRCD, Detroit.

_____ Seifer, R. & Elias, P. K. (1982), Sociocultural variability in infant temperament ratings. *Child Develpm.,* 53:164–173.

Thomas, A. (1981), Current trends in developmental theory. *Amer. J. Orthopsychiat.,* 51:580–609.

_____ Chess, S., Birch, H.G., Herzog, M. & Korn, S. (1963), *Behavioral Individuality in Early Childhood.* New York: University Press.

Vaughn, B., Toraldson, B., Chrichton, L. & Egeland, B. (1981), The assessment of infant temperament: a critique of the Carey Infant Temperament Questionnaire. *Infant Behav. Develpm.,* 4:1–18.

Walker, L. Goldberg, S. & Minde, K. (1983), Maternal and infant characteristics related to temperament in low birthweight infants. Paper presented at the Hospital for Sick Children.

4

EEG Patterns of Preterm Infants, Home Environment, and Later IQ

Leila Beckwith and Arthur H. Parmelee, Jr.
University of California, Los Angeles

As part of a prospective longitudinal study of preterm infants, sleep state organization and EEG patterns were studied at term date in 53 preterm infants as an index of the maturity and integrity of neurophysiological organization that might have implications for their later development. The rearing environments of the infants were also assessed, using time sampling of caregiver-infant interaction during home observations when the infants were 1, 8, and 24 months. The infants were tested at 4, 9, and 24 months on the Gesell Developmental Scale. At age 5 the children were tested by the Stanford-Binet Intelligence Scale, and at age 8 by the Wechsler Intelligence Scale for Children. In general, children who at term date showed less 407-Tracé Alternant EEG pattern in the entire record and particularly in quiet sleep had lower IQs beginning at 4 months and continuing to age 8. There was an exception, however, for those children being reared in consistently attentive, responsive environments. They, by 24 months and continuing to age 8, had higher IQ scores, equal to those of

---

Reprinted with permission from *Child Development,* 1986, Vol. 57, 777–789. Copyright 1986 by the Society for Research in Child Development, Inc.

This work was supported by NIH-NICHD Contract no. 1-HD-3-2776, William T. Grant Foundation Grant no. B771121, National Foundation/March of Dimes Grant no. 6–25, and the Henry J. Kaiser Family Foundation and the John D. and Catherine T. MacArthur Foundation, which provided a fellowship for Arthur H. Parmelee, Jr., at the Center for Advanced Study in the Behavioral Sciences, 1984-85. Prior versions were presented at the International Study of Behavioral Development, University of Munich, West Germany, 1983, and the International Conference on Infant Studies, New York, New York, 1984.

infants with more 407-Tracé Alternant, even if they had shown decreased amounts of 407-Tracé Alternant earlier.

Preterm infants as a group are known to have more neurological and intellectual problems later in life than full-term infants (Caputo, Goldstein, & Taub, 1979; Drillien, Thomson, & Burgoyne, 1980; Hunt, 1981). Further, those preterm infants with the most neonatal complications have a greater incidence of developmental problems, and such neonatal complications are most frequent in infants with the lowest birth weights and gestational ages (Cohen & Parmelee, 1983). It has nevertheless been difficult to predict the outcome of individual preterm infants. A several-fold increase in incidence of developmental problems in preterm compared to fullterm infants is still a low enough incidence even among preterm infants to allow most of them to do well. In fact, many very low birth weight and early gestation preterm infants do well (Bennett, Robinson, & Sells, 1983; Hack, Caron, Rivers, & Fanaroff, 1983; Saigal, Rosenbaum, Stoskopf, & Sinclair, 1984). Even a number of preterm infants with identified intraventricular hemorrhages do well, except those with the severest hemorrhages, who generally have serious neurological problems if they survive (Dubowitz et al., 1984; Fitzhardinge, Flodmark, Fitz, & Ashby, 1982; Papile, Munsick-Bruno, & Schaefer, 1983).

Several studies have now demonstrated that social factors play an important role in the intellectual outcome not only of healthy fullterm and preterm infants but also of those who have suffered perinatal medical complications (Beckwith & Cohen, 1984; Beckwith, Cohen, Kopp, Parmelee, & Marcy, 1976; Broman, Nichols, & Kennedy, 1975; Drillien et al., 1980; Siegel, 1982; Smith, Flick, Ferriss, & Sellman, 1972; Werner & Smith, 1982). Those infants who may have neurophysiological changes may also be more vulnerable to adverse environments than neurophysiologically normal infants. We have found in our studies that the home environment is a strong predictor of the outcome of preterm infants (Beckwith & Cohen, 1984; Beckwith et al., 1976). The interactional effect of the home environment with neurophysiological variations in the infants has been more elusive. The course of development of a particular child is determined by the interaction between the neurophysiological functioning of the infant and his or her environment, and just as the infant's characteristics are likely to shape the response elicited from the environment, the environment may amplify or diminish the adverse effects of a neurophysiological difficulty (Sameroff & Chandler, 1975). Markers of neurophysiological variations in the neonatal period, except for those infants with serious neurological problems, have been difficult to establish. We are reporting on the use of EEG patterns and sleep states as neurophysiological markers.

EEG patterns of neonates and young infants have been studied frequently as a way to assess the maturation and integrity of neurophysiological organization. There is a rich literature that systematically documents the age-expected EEG patterns and state organization of prematures (Dreyfus-Brisac, 1964, 1968, 1970, 1979; Ellingson & Peters, 1980a; Parmelee et al., 1968; Parmelee, Wenner, Akiyama, Schultz, & Stern, 1967), fullterm neonates (Dreyfus-Brisac, 1979; Ellingson & Peters, 1980b; Parmelee et al., 1967; Prechtl, Akiyama, Zinkin, & Grant, 1968) and older infants (Ellingson & Peters, 1980a, 1980b; Parmelee et al., 1968). Investigators have shown that clinically deviant infants—those with seizures, untreated hypothyroidism, or Trisomy 21—show deviant or delayed EEG patterns (Ellingson & Peters, 1980c; Lombroso, 1979, 1982; Schultz, Schulte, Akiyama, & Parmelee, 1968; Tharp, Cukier, & Monod, 1981). Maturational delays or age-inadequate patterns have also been found in newborns exposed to biochemically abnormal intrauterine environments, for example, infants of diabetic mothers, small-for-dates infants of toxemic mothers, and "at risk" newborns (Dreyfus-Brisac, 1979; Haas & Prechtl, 1977; Schulte, Heinze, & Schrmepf, 1971). The implications for later development, however, particularly in neonates not displaying specific pathology, are unclear. Some studies find no relation between EEG or state organization and later development among infants without specific pathology at birth (Ellingson, Dutch, & McIntire, 1974; Tharp et al., 1981; Torres & Blaw, 1968). Other studies have shown that deviations in expected state and EEG patterns were linked to later medical and/or behavioral difficulties (Crowell, Kapuniai, Boychuk, Light, & Hodgman, 1982; Lombroso, 1982; Tharp et al., 1981; Thoman, Denenberg, Sievel, Zeidner, & Becker, 1980). In a retrospective study of a subsample of our subjects, we obtained similar findings using computer power spectral EEG analyses (Richards, Parmelee, & Beckwith, in press).

Within sleep, active sleep state (rapid eye movement, or REM sleep) and quiet (or non-REM sleep) alternate, with the proportion of quiet sleep increasing in the first months of life while the amount of active sleep decreases. Quiet sleep is a highly controlled state with significant cybernetic control systems necessary to maintain the defining parameters of regular respiration, absence of eye and body movements, regular heart rate, and the associated characteristic EEG patterns. The concordance of these parameters of quiet sleep increases, as does the amount of quiet sleep, in parallel with the growth of dendrites, axons, and synapses at all levels of the nervous system with their increasing potential for feedback loops and cybernetic controls. The development of quiet sleep, therefore, is potentially an important index of brain development and organization (Parmelee & Sigman, 1983; Parmelee & Stern, 1972). Active sleep also becomes more highly organized in the early months of life, but decreases in amount, and at all ages is characterized by marked variability within each parameter such as respiration, heart rate, and movements. Its developmental progression is therefore difficult to study.

Clinically one can identify quiet and active sleep quite well by observing respirations, eye movements, and body movements, and this has been a useful way of determining developmental organization (Thoman, Korner, & Kraemer, 1976). There is, however, considerable variability from hour to hour in the duration of each, so that long-term recordings are necessary to identify individual differences. In recording of sleep states determined only by respiration, eye and body movements, and heart rate, it is sometimes difficult to separate the semi-stupor of a very sick child from normal quiet sleep (Prechtl, Theorell, and Blair, 1973; Theorell, 1974). These children, however, also often have unexpected EEG patterns in this state. We decided that a recording of 1½ hours duration that included EEG, a measure of cortical activity, along with measures of the brain-stem-controlled activities of respiration and movement, was a practical approach for the study of a large number of infants. It was felt that concordance of brain stem and cortical activity would represent a significant level of cybernetic control even in a short record and avoid the spurious quiet sleep of sick infants who do not have the expected EEG patterns.

This article, therefore, addresses two questions: Can specific behavioral vulnerabilities be identified in early infancy within a preterm group by examining sleep state organization and EEG patterns? Are there significant protective factors within some caregiving environments that buffer vulnerable children against adverse outcomes?

METHOD

Subjects

The subjects in the study were all preterm infants born at the UCLA hospital or transferred to the nursery shortly after birth during the years 1972–1974 who met subject criteria and agreed to participate. They have been described previously (Cohen & Parmelee, 1983). Subjects were included in the prospective study who were born at 37 weeks gestation or less, and at birth weights of 2,500 grams or less, without obvious congenital anomalies. The physiological condition of the infants at birth was greatly variable. Obstetric and neonatal complications were recorded using the Prechtl optimality scoring system (Littman & Parmelee, 1978; Parmelee, Kopp, and Sigman, 1976). Additionally, the infants' families represented a broad range of social class and ethnic backgrounds, with approximately one-third of them being Hispanic. Because the outcome measures were depressed for the Spanish-language group, in order not to confound problems of bilingualism with neurophysiological organization, this report focuses on 53 infants born to English speaking parents with complete study data throughout their first 2 years of life who were then retested at age 5. The one child with cerebral palsy tested at all ages through 5 years was intentionally excluded to eliminate any child with manifest neurological problems. Of the 53 children tested through 5 years, 49 returned for retesting at age 8.

The subjects lost to follow-up at age 8 either could not be located or had moved out of the area and testing could not be arranged. A multivariate test, Hollingshead T^2, and univariate t tests were used to compare the subjects for whom 8-year scores were available with the 77 subjects of English-speaking parents initially enrolled in the study. The two groups did not differ on birth weight, gestational age, length of hospitalization, years of maternal education, social class, or birth order. Gestational ages of the 53 subjects ranged from 25 to 37 weeks, with a mean of 32.3 weeks, and birth weight from 800 to 2,495 grams, with a mean of 1,774 grams.

Although a number of infants suffered respiratory distress and required long hospitalizations, none developed chronic respiratory problems or were hospitalized past their expected date of birth. There were also some infants hospitalized only a short time and discharged to their homes quickly, one after only 2 days. The average hospitalization was 28.5 days. At the time the infants in this sample were enrolled, regular studies for intraventricular hemorrhages (IVH) were not done, so we do not know whether any had IVH or not. There was one child in this follow-up sample with hydrocephalus. This was corrected surgically by a ventricular-peritoneal shunt, and the child has developed normally. It is likely that during the period of the study, 1972–1974, most of the children with severe brain hemorrhage did not survive.

The subjects were 57% male, 51% firstborn. Approximately 60% of the subjects were from middle-class families and 40% from working-class families. Maternal education ranged from 8 to 17 years, with a mean of 12.9 years.

Procedures

EEG. A single sleep polygraph recording was made for each subject at 40 weeks conceptional age, based on maternal report, during day naptime in a sound-attenuated laboratory room. The electrodes were placed on the infants' heads using a fitted, soft rubber strap headgear. This allowed all of the electrodes to be put in place quickly with the least distress to the infants. The recordings were bipolar from the Frontal-Temporal, Frontal-Central, Temporal-Occipital, and Central-Occipital positions over both hemispheres following the "10–20" system. Respiration and heart rate were monitored electronically. Eye movements and body movements were noted by direct observation.

The recording time was 90 min, with the final 60 min used for analysis and the first 30 min considered to be adaptation to the strange situation. Records were visually analyzed by 20-sec epochs, with state and EEG codes determined independently, without knowledge of subjects' medical histories or subsequent development. State was coded for each 20-sec epoch on the basis of observable behavior and physiological functioning: awake (eyes open); quiet sleep (eyes closed, no eye movements, no body movements except for occasional body jerks, and regular respiration); active sleep (eyes closed, eye movements, body movements, irregular respiration); transitional sleep (eyes closed, but not fitting either of the other two sleep states). Each 20-sec period was coded in terms of the state that prevailed for most of the given period. Similar to some investigators (Prechtl, 1974) and unlike others (Thoman et al., 1976), we defined only one form of quiet sleep and one form of active sleep and coded all other sleep time as "transitional" or "indeterminate." The frequency of occurrence of each state was determined by the number of 20-sec epochs coded for each state without regard to sequential arrangement.

The EEG was coded without knowledge of the sleep states using a three-digit numbering system. The last digit in the code identified the general nature of the pattern, while the first two digits indicated the specific form of the pattern expected at 40 weeks conceptional age (Parmelee, Schulte, et al., 1968). In our previous studies, four patterns have been readily identified in the sleep of infants at term. Since others had similar findings, an international committee was formed to establish agreement on the characteristics of these four patterns in order to facilitate comparisons of findings in various laboratories (Anders, Emde, & Parmelee, 1971). The following are descriptions of these patterns (Fig. 1):

402-Low Voltage Irregular (LVI). This pattern consists of irregular activity

TERM EEG PATTERNS

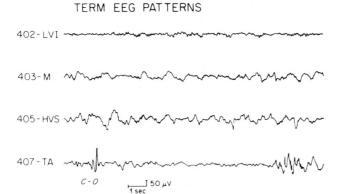

Figure 1. Examples of the EEG patterns at 40 weeks conceptional age. Each is from a bipolar Central-Occipital (C-O) lead recorded at a paper speed of 15 mm/sec.

of low voltage (14–35 uV), sometimes with periods of 3–8 sec duration of very rhythmical 4–8-Hz activity of 20–50 uV.

403-Mixed (M). This is characterized by both high-voltage slow and low-voltage polyrhythmic components. The frequencies of the wave range from 0.5 to 13 Hz and are of 30–100 uV.

405-High Voltage Slow (HVS). This pattern is one of continuous high-voltage slow waves of 0.5–4 Hz of 50–150 uV. The overall amplitude of the waves is greater than in the 403–Mixed pattern.

407-Tracé Alternant (TA). This pattern consists of bursts of high-voltage slow waves (0.5–3 Hz) of 3–8 sec duration separated by 4–8 sec of attenuated activity of mixed frequency. The high-amplitude slow waves occasionally have superimposed low-voltage rapid waves, and between the slow waves are interspersed sharp waves of 2–4 Hz.

EEG patterns that did not meet the criteria for the above codes were called unclassifiable and were either immature patterns expected at younger than 40 weeks conceptional age or deviant patterns not consistent with the four basic patterns even in immature form.

Each record was then tabulated as to the percentage of sleep in the last 60 min of observation and percentage of quiet, active, and transitional sleep states within sleep. Further, each record was coded as to the percentage of each EEG pattern in each sleep state and in all sleep states combined.

Caregiving environment. Assessments of the rearing environment were derived from naturalistic home observations made when the infants were 1, 8, and 24 months. The observers did not know the children's EEG records, medical histories, or developmental test scores. At the 1-month visit the infants were observed on an average for 73 min of awake time; at 8 months, 1½ hours of awake time, and at 24 months, 50 min of play time. The observer used a precoded check list, and every 15 sec recorded presence of a set of infant behaviors, caregiver behaviors, and events defined as contingent or reciprocal interactions between caregiver and child, as well as behaviors of other persons toward the infant (the specifics of this coding have been described elsewhere; see Beckwith et al., 1976, and Beckwith & Cohen, 1984).

Because we believe that caregiver responsiveness to the infant's signals is instrumental in providing meaning and predictability in the infant's experience, only some of the interactive events were selected a priori for study as indicators of responsive caregiving. At 1 month, these were maternal positive attentiveness to infant, face-to-face talk, mutual visual regard, and maternal contingency to distress; at 8 months, contingency to distress was omitted and contingency to nondistress vocalization was added. At 24 months, positive attentiveness and reciprocal interaction were used. Additionally, being held upright at 1 month, floor freedom at 8 months, and time spent in intellectual tasks (dramatic play, books, puzzles, and blocks) at 24 months were included because we believed them to be developmentally facilitating. Observer reliabilities were determined before the study started for 10 pilot subjects across the three ages by computing Pearson correlation coefficients for the total frequency of a specific behavior that each of three observers had recorded in an observation. Coefficients obtained for behaviors ranged from .80 to .98, with the majority being greater than .90. The codes of each of these indices were converted to standardized scores at each age and summed to make a single score per observation for each child that assessed the degree to which the environment was responsive and facilitating to the infant (Beckwith & Cohen, 1984).

Since we considered that the cumulative influence of the rearing environment over time would be most potent in shaping the child's development, we grouped the subjects according to the degree of responsiveness in their environment over the appropriate ages observed. For analyses of developmental level at 4 months, the more and less responsive caregiving group was determined by dividing the subjects at the median of the composite score of the 1-month observation. For analyses of developmental level at 9 months, the more responsive caregiving group contained those subjects who had been above the median at both the 1-

and 8-month observations compared to the less responsive group containing all other subjects. For analyses of later development, the more responsive caregiving group contained those subjects (above the median at 1-, 8-, and 24-month observations) who had experienced consistently responsive caregiving compared to the less responsive group containing all other subjects. Although shifts in patterns did occur, the environments tended, to a degree significantly greater than chance, to be either consistently responsive and facilitating (approximately 30% of the subjects) or consistently unresponsive (26%) during the three observations (Beckwith & Cohen, 1984).

Developmental and IQ tests. The Gesell Developmental Test, administered by testers trained in child development, was used to assess the developmental level of the infants at 4, 9, and 24 months. The Stanford-Binet Test, form L-M, was administered at age 5 by a clinical psychologist, and another clinical psychologist administered the Wechsler Intelligence Scale for Children—Revised at age 8. No tester was aware of the subjects' scores on other measures.

RESULTS

EEG Patterns

Several strategies have been used in the analysis of EEG patterns to determine deviance in the neonatal period. One is to specify unusual or deviant EEG patterns (Dreyfus-Brisac, 1979; Lombroso, 1979, 1982; Tharp et al., 1981). A second way is to code a persistent delay in the maturation of an expected EEG pattern (Ellingson & Peters, 1980c; Hass & Prechtl, 1977; Schultz et al., 1968). A third way, and the strategy we have used, is to describe the distribution of EEG patterns within and across states in order to identify differences in the occurrence of expected patterns across subjects and to further define sleep states by EEG patterns in addition to respiration and eye and body movements (Anders & Hoffman, 1973; Crowell et al., 1982).

On the average, the infants were asleep 93% of the observed time. About half of the sleep time ($M = 56\%$) was coded as transitional sleep, and half as more organized states of quiet and active sleep. Active sleep (26% of sleep time) exceeded quiet sleep (18%) as expected at this age (Parmelee et al., 1967). As shown in Table 1, 403-M activity was the most common EEG pattern during the recording as a whole and during active sleep, with 407-TA the most frequent pattern during quiet sleep. The 407-TA and 405-HVS waves rarely occurred during active sleep but did

Table 1. EEG Pattern Within Sleep States (%)

	SLEEP STATES							
	Total		Active		Quiet		Transitional	
EEG PATTERN	M	SD	M	SD	M	SD	M	SD
402–LVI	22.2	18.2	36.3	29.6	3.4	6.9	21.7	18.3
403–M	39.8	17.6	53.0	29.2	14.2	18.1	45.3	24.3
405–HVS	6.3	7.6	2.5	7.3	8.7	14.5	8.2	10.5
407–TA	22.4	13.3	2.1	8.0	54.0	29.8	21.9	16.2
Unclassifiable ...	9.3	17.6	4.1	16.1	15.9	25.5	2.8	2.4

appear during transitional sleep. The range of individual variability was wide, however. For example, infants had from 0% to 100% of quiet sleep with the 407–TA as the associate EEG pattern.

There were no significant correlations between any of the EEG patterns during quiet sleep or the amount of any EEG pattern in quiet sleep and its presence in active sleep. The percent 407–TA in quiet sleep did correlate with the percent 407–TA in the total record, $r(51) = .76, p < .01$, and with the percent in transitional sleep, $r(51) = .62, p < .01$. Since the amount of the 407–TA pattern in the total record is almost entirely in quiet sleep and transitional sleep, this suggests a relation of some portion of transitional sleep to quiet sleep.

EEG Patterns, State Organization, and Developmental Status

A correlation matrix was obtained between the developmental test scores at the successive ages and the percent of EEG code 402-LVI during active sleep, 403–M during active sleep, unclassifiable during active sleep, 405–HVS during quiet sleep, 407–TA during quiet sleep, unclassifiable during quiet sleep, and 402–LVI, 403–M, 405–HVS, 407–TA, and unclassifiable throughout the recording independent of state. As shown in Table 2, the percentage of 402–LVI and 403–M during active sleep or during the entire sleep record was unrelated to later developmental status, whereas the percentage of 405–HVS and 407–TA during quiet sleep and during the entire sleep record did show significant correlations with outcome. The percentage of EEG activity during quiet sleep that was unclassifiable and the percentage of active sleep during the entire recording also showed significant correlations. However, only 407–TA in quiet sleep showed significant correlations with all developmental measures across the age span from 4 months to 8 years.

As stated in the introduction, quiet sleep is a highly controlled state re-

Table 2. Correlations of Test Performance with % Sleep State and EEG Pattern

	4 Months	Gesell, 9 Months	24 Months	Stanford-Binet, 5 Years	Wechsler Intelligence Scale for Children, 8 Years
Total sleep:					
Active	.27	.05	.17	.24	.35*
Quiet	.07	−.07	.07	.07	−.06
402–LVI	−.08	.07	.01	.12	−.10
403–M	−.01	−.07	−.15	−.23	−.01
405–HVS	.30*	.08	−.06	−.18	−.23
407–TA	.23	.28*	.24	.34*	.37*
Unclassifiable	−.21	−.25	−.02	−.07	−.08
Active sleep:					
402–LVI	.17	.15	.11	.20	−.04
403–M	.14	−.02	.01	−.12	.10
Unclassifiable	−.14	−.08	.05	.12	.08
Quiet sleep:					
405–HVS	.30*	.03	−.17	−.24	−.26
407–TA	.32*	.33*	.28*	.38*	.36*
Unclassifiable	−.23	−.28*	−.08	−.09	−.11

*$p < .05$.

quiring significant cybernetic control systems to maintain even briefly the concordance of regular respiration and absence of eye and body movements along with a particular EEG pattern. Of the two EEG patterns seen in quiet sleep as determined by the non-EEG parameters, 407–TA is the most common at term. We had therefore anticipated that quiet sleep with the additional criterion of the 407–TA EEG pattern would be the most likely state organization to predict later outcome. We did not anticipate that the 407–TA EEG pattern independent of state would be equally predictive. Since 49% of all 407–TA was in quiet sleep, 50% in transitional sleep, and only 1% in active sleep, with the percentage in quiet and transitional correlated, we concluded that a significant amount of transitional sleep was a variant of quiet sleep with irregular respiration rather than the expected regular respiration. This is consistent with the quiet sleep defined by Thoman et al. (1976) as irregular quiet sleep. This type of quiet sleep occurs most frequently in the transition from quiet to active sleep after the irregular respirations have started and eye movements are not yet present (Shirataki & Prechtl, 1977).

The association with later competence of the children was not mediated by the amount of quiet sleep determined by observed absence of eye and body movements and presence of regular respiration. Even though a mean of 54% observationally determined quiet sleep co-occurred with the EEG pattern 407–TA, quiet sleep observationally determined by itself had no relation to outcome.

In order to further study the relation of 407–TA to later performance, the subjects were divided at the median, with those who generated less 407–TA during quiet sleep compared by Hotelling T^2 and univariate t tests to those who generated more. The test scores of subjects grouped by the median with respect to the percentage of 407–TA they generated during quiet sleep at 40 weeks conceptional age are shown in Table 3. Those infants who generated less than the median 407–TA in quiet sleep scored significantly lower on the developmental and IQ tests from 4 months to 8 years than did those infants who generated more than the median 407–TA. Within each group, however, the range of scores was large, with less competent and highly competent children in both groups.

EEG Patterns and Demographic and Perinatal Factors

There was no evidence that demographic factors or perinatal factors mediated the association between 407–TA and later developmental status. The two groups divided at the median on proportion of 407–TA during quiet sleep, were compared by Hotelling T^2 as to birth order, maternal age, maternal education, and social class status of the families and found not to differ. They also did not differ on birth weight, gestational age, Apgar scores at 1 and 5 months, and length of hospitalization (see Table 4).

Table 3. Test Performance of Children with Low or High % Tracé Alternant (407–TA) During Quiet Sleep

	GROUP							
	Low 407–TA (407–TA 0%–57%)				High 407–TA (407–TA 58%–100%)			
TEST	N	Score	SD	Range	N	Score	SD	Range
Gesell, 4 months	27	102.1	10.5	76–124	26	108.5	8.4	83–124
Gesell, 9 months	27	97.3	5.4	90–115	26	102.5	6.4	89–115**
Gesell, 24 months	27	97.7	13.8	71–138	26	104.7	9.5	88–125***
Stanford-Binet, 5 years	27	101.4	19.4	57–138	26	108.5	13.0	82–134
Wechsler Intelligence Scale for Children, 8 years	24	104.2	16.5	75–128	25	112.2	13.7	89–141*

*$p < .08$.
**$p < .05$.
***$p < .01$.

Table 4. Demographic and Perinatal Factors for Children with Low and High % Tracé Alternant (407–TA) During Quiet Sleep

	GROUP			
	Low 407–TA (407–TA 0%–57%) (N = 27)		High 407–TA (407–TA 58%–100%) (N = 26)	
FACTOR	M	SD	M	SD
Firstborn (%)	50	...	44	...
Maternal age	25.8	5.4	24.9	4.7
Maternal education	12.9	2.0	12.8	2.1
Social class status (Hollingshead 4-factor)	44.1	14.0	43.6	14.3
Birth weight	1732.3	511.7	1784.2	526.1
Gestational age	32.4	3.4	31.7	3.5
Apgar at 1 min	6.2	2.0	5.7	2.9
Apgar at 5 min	7.6	1.6	6.8	2.9
Length of hospitalization	32.1	26.5	26.3	20.7
Postnatal complications[a]	85.9	28.2	90.5	30.1

NOTE.—No significant differences were found.
[a] Higher score represents fewer complications.

EEG, Caregiving Environment, and Developmental Scores

In order to test for developmental differences that might be associated with the interaction between the EEG 407–TA pattern with caregiving environment, a series of 2 (responsiveness of caregiving environment) × 2 (amount of 407–TA in quiet sleep) ANOVAs were computed with the developmental test scores as dependent variables, using the 49 cases with complete data. The mean scores at each testing for each of the four groups are shown in Table 5.

For the Gesell scores at 4 months, there was a significant main effect for 407–TA, $F(1,45) = 7.55$, $p < .01$, but not for caregiving environment. Infants with more 407–TA had better developmental scores at 4 months. For Gesell scores at 9 months, there was again a significant main effect for 407–TA, $F(1,45) = 14.86$, $p < .001$. Additionally, a significant main effect for the caregiving environment appeared, $F(1,45) = 3.92, p < .06$. Thus, infants with more 407–TA had better developmental scores at 9 months, and infants in more responsive homes also had better scores at 9 months. Gesell scores at 24 months again showed a significant effect for 407–TA, $F(1,45), = 7.23$, $p < .01$, and a significant main effect for the caregiving environment, $F(1,45) = 10.43$, $p < .01$. The interaction of 407–TA with caregiving environment was not significant, $F(1,45) = .02$, $p > .10$. At age 5, since Levene's Test for Equal Variances indicated a significant deviation from equality, $F(3,45) = 3.02$, $p < .04$, a one-way

Table 5. Test Performance for Children with More or Less Responsive Caregiving and with Low or High % Tracé Alternant (407–TA) During Quiet Sleep

| | Group | | | | | | | | ANOVA $p < .05$ | | |
| | Low 407–TA | | | | High 407–TA | | | | | | |
Test	More Responsive Caregiving	N	Less Responsive Caregiving	N	More Responsive Caregiving	N	Less Responsive Caregiving	N	407–TA	Caregiving	Interaction
Gesell, 4 months	104.6	15	101.1	9	110.0	10	107.5	15	X	...	...
Gesell, 9 months	97.7	10	96.0	14	105.1	8	100.7	17	X	X	...
Gesell, 24 months	105.5	8	94.2	16	113.4	7	100.8	18	X	X	...
Stanford-Binet, 5 years	115.0[b]	8	93.9[a,b]	16	115.5[a]	7	105.8	18	...	...	X
Wechsler Intelligence Scale for Children, 8 years	116.6[c]	8	98.9[a,b,c]	16	118.5[a]	7	109.7[b]	18	...	...	X

Note.—Matching superscripts (a,b,c) denote pairwise mean differences with < .05 Bonferroni significance levels.

analysis of variance was computed for within-group variances not assumed to be equal, $F(3,41) = 8.46$, $p < .001$. Pairwise comparisons among the four groups, using the Bonferroni test to adjust for the multiple comparison of all pairs of means, showed the group with low 407–TA scores and less responsive caregivers to score significantly lower than the group with low 407–TA and consistently responsive caregivers, $t(21,31) = 3.71$, $p < .002$, and the group with high 407–TA and consistently responsive caregivers, $t(24,30) = 4.06$, $p < .001$.

By age 8, a significant interaction was recorded for EEG × caregiving, $F(1,45) = 5.89$, $p < .02$. The Bonferroni test was used to adjust for multiple comparison of all pairs of means, and indicated that the group with low 407–TA and less responsive caregiving was significantly less competent on the Wechsler Intelligence Scale for Children than all other groups, $F(1,45) = 3.88$, $p < 001$; $F(1,45) = 3.17$, $p < .003$; $F(1,45) = 3.42$, $p < .002$.

EEG, Caregiving Environment, and Perinatal Factors

A series of one-way ANOVAs was used to examine possible differences among the 407–TA by caregiving subgroups on other biological factors such as gestational age, birth weight, Apgar scores at 1 and 5 min, length of hospitalization, and degree of postnatal medical complications (Littman & Pamelee, 1978). None mediated the association between 407–TA, caregiving, and later developmental status. The groups divided at the median; those who generated more or less 407–TA during quiet sleep further divided into those reared in more or less responsive homes either at 1 month or at 1 and 8 months, or at 1, 8, and 24 months, did not differ significantly on the above measures, as tested by the one-way analyses of variance (Table 6).

DISCUSSION

The results indicate a positive relation between the amount of Tracé Alternant EEG pattern, 407–TA, that preterm infants had at term during sleep and IQ measurements made at intervals up to 8 years of age. Infants who had more of this EEG pattern during quiet and transitional sleep states performed more competently up to 8 years. The research extends the findings of other investigators that linked characteristics of state organization and EEG patterns during early infancy to developmental and medical status at 1 year (Crowell et al., 1982; Thoman et al., 1980). Our study also indicates that the relation can be modulated by environ-

Table 6. Perinatal Factors for Children with More or Less Responsive Caregiving and with Low or High % Tracé Alternant (407–TA) During Quiet Sleep

| | Low 407–TA | | High 407–TA | |
| | More Responsive Caregiving | Less Responsive Caregiving | More Responsive Caregiving | Less Responsive Caregiving |
FACTOR				
Gestational age (weeks)	32.2	32.2	30.2	32.8
Birth weight (grams)	1,766.7	1,715.1	1,625.7	1,845.9
Apgar score at 1 min	5.1	6.8	6.8	5.4
Apgar score at 5 min	7.0	8.0	7.2	6.7
Length of hospitalization (days) ..	26.6	34.9	31.0	24.5
Postnatal complications[a]	103.6	77.1	75.7	96.2

NOTE.—No significant differences were found.
[a] Higher score represents fewer complications.

mental factors. To our knowledge, the present study is the first to show the buffering effect of family environments in ameliorating early risk factors expressed in brain activity in young infants.

Less 407–TA EEG at term date may indicate either a transient or a more persistent deviation in brain development. As has been pointed out by others, the degree to which the deviation for either reason affects later behavior depends on the individual's transactions with the environment (Sameroff & Chandler, 1975; Werner & Smith, 1982). Less 407–TA EEG pattern was associated with lowered developmental scores during the first year, regardless of the home environment. By age 2, however, the beneficial effects of a consistently responsive social environment became apparent. Infants being reared in consistently responsive environments showed a marked increase in IQ scores, which was maintained through the early school years. By age 5 and continuing at age 8, children reared in consistently responsive homes, regardless of early EEG patterns, performed very competently on IQ tests. In those rearing environments, children with less 407–TA EEG patterns could not be distinguished from children with more of this pattern. Only in less responsive rearing environments could children with less 407–TA EEG activity be seen to have significantly lower IQ scores, although even within that group some children did well. It is likely that single risk factors are insufficient in determining outcome for most infants. As has been pointed out (Sameroff & Chandler, 1975; Werner & Smith, 1982), only an accumulation of risk factors, which include not only biological vulnerabilities but enduring adverse environments, interferes with development for most infants.

Although the concept that biological deviance in the neonatal period can adversely affect behavioral outcome even in an interactional model of behavioral development is obvious and well accepted, it has been difficult to identify neonatal markers of biological deviance. Preterm birth has been used as a prototype of a general marker for biological deviance that could affect behavioral outcome, and group data support this concept (Caputo et al., 1981; Drillien et al., 1980; Hunt, 1981). It is, however, a very general marker including a wide range of biological hazards for the infant from severe to none. Further refinement of the preterm model has included consideration of only very low birth weight preterm infants who are also likely to suffer more frequent and more severe perinatal problems than the larger preterms, increasing the probability of biological deviance that might cause brain dysfunction and poor outcomes. However, as stated in the introduction, many of these infants do well. In part this may be because we intervene medically with all of them, and, to the extent that we are successful, we may prevent the adverse effects, particularly on brain development, of a large number of the perinatal problems. This is supported by the improving survival and outcome of very low birth weight preterm infants in recent years (Bennett et al., 1983; Hack et al., 1983; Saigal et al., 1984). More recently, computer tomography and ultrasonography have made it possible to identify brain hemorrhages of various types, including severe intraventricular hemorrhages that extend into brain substance. This now specifies a biological deviance within the brain, but even with this specificity some of these infants recover and appear to be functioning normally on follow-up examination (Dubowitz et al., 1984; Fitzhardinge et al., 1982; Papile et al., 1983).

We have needed measures of deviant brain function to identify those infants significantly affected by hemorrhages, respiratory difficulties, or other perinatal difficulties. For example, the presence of seizures is generally associated with a poor outcome, particularly when persistent over several days and difficult to control medically (Lombroso, 1979; Tharp et al., 1981). Other approaches are needed for the children with less evident or severe brain dysfunction. These should also be applicable after the infant has recovered from the acute phase of the perinatal problem. Brain stem and cortical evoked potentials and EEG offer such possibilities. It has been difficult to identify the range of EEG variations that might be considered pathological in the neonatal period, but computer tomography and sonography may advance these studies. Evoked brainstem and cortical evoked potentials are also promising markers of brain functioning in the neonate, though these are limited to specific sensory pathways and stimuli (Lombroso, 1982; Parmelee & Sigman, 1983).

Another alternative has been the study of the development of state organization, particularly in sleep and with a combination of behavioral and EEG parameters. This takes into consideration the development of cybernetic control of respirations and body and eye movements coincident with specific EEG patterns generated in the cortex (Parmelee & Sigman, 1983). State organization is a general from of behavior but critical to the early interactions of infants with their environments.

The method we used to analyze the EEG recording was to note the distribution of normally expected EEG patterns independent of behavioral state and to code sleep states by the observational criteria of respiratory pattern and body and eye movements. Coding behavioral state and EEG patterns independently allowed their association to be investigated empirically. Our findings indicate that some degree of concurrence at term date is a marker of neurophysiological integrity. That is, whereas the presence of 407–TA during quiet sleep was positively correlated with later developmental status, the presence of 407–TA during active sleep proved to be unrelated. On the other hand, scoring quiet sleep independently of the 407–TA EEG pattern indicated that in these short recordings the degree of association at term date was not sufficient to support our previously held hypothesis that an increasing amount of observationally determined quiet sleep was a favorable maturational indicator in early life. Although the 407–TA pattern does tend to occur with quiet sleep, we found that quiet sleep, scored independently of EEG pattern, was unrelated to later developmental status. It was infants who generated the 407–TA EEG pattern during a larger portion of their quiet sleep irrespective of absolute amount of quiet sleep who showed the more optimum development, not infants who were in quiet sleep much of the recording but showed the 407–TA pattern in only a small portion. We believe, therefore, that the EEG pattern 407–TA, particularly in quiet sleep, is a useful marker of neonatal neurophysiological functioning in preterm infants.

REFERENCES

Anders, T., Emde, R., & Parmelee, A.H. (Eds.). (1971). A *manual of standardized terminology, techniques, and criteria for scoring of states of sleep and wakefulness in newborn infants.* Los Angeles: UCLA Brain Information Service/BRI Publications Office.

Beckwith, L., & Cohen, S.E. (1984). Home environment and cognitive competence in preterm children during the first 5 years. In A. Gottfried (Ed.), *Home environment and early cognitive development* (pp. 235–271). New York: Academic Press.

Beckwith, L., Cohen, S.E., Kopp, C.B., Parmelee, A.H., & Marcy, T.G. (1976). Caregiver-infant interaction and early cognitive development in preterm infants. *Child Development,* 47, 579–587.

Bennett, F.C., Robinson, N.M., & Sells, C.J. (1983). Growth and development of infants weighing less than 800 grams at birth. *Pediatrics,* 71, 319–323.

Broman, S.H., Nichols, P. L., & Kennedy, W.A. (1975). *Preschool IQ: Prenatal and early development correlates.* Hillsdale, NJ: Erlbaum.

Caputo, D.V., Goldstein, K.M., & Taub, H.B. (1981). Neonatal compromise and later psychological development: A 10-year longitudinal study. In S. Friedman & M. Sigman (Eds.), *Preterm birth and psychological development* (pp. 353–386). New York: Academic Press.

Cohen, S.E., & Parmelee, A.H. (1983). Prediction of five-year Stanford-Binet scores in preterm infants. *Child Development,* 54, 1242–1253.

Crowell, D.H., Kapuniai, L.E., Boychuk R.B., Light, M.J., & Hodgman, J.E. (1982). Daytime sleep state organization in three-month old infants. *Electroencephalography and Clinical Neurophysiology,* 53, 36–47.

Dreyfus-Brisac, C. (1964). The electroencephalogram of the premature infant and full-term newborn: Normal and abnormal waking and sleeping patterns. In P. Kellaway & I. Petersen (Eds.), *Neurological and electroencephalographic correlative studies in infancy* (pp. 186–207). New York: Grune & Stratton.

Dreyfus-Brisac, C. (1968). Sleep ontogenesis in early human prematurity from 24 to 27 weeks of conceptional age. *Developmental Psychobiology,* 1, 162–169.

Dreyfus-Brisac, C. (1970). Ontogenesis of sleep in human prematures after 32 weeks of conceptional age. *Developmental Psychobiology,* 3, 91–121.

Dreyfus-Brisac, C. (1979a). Neonatal electroencephalography. In E. M. Scarpelli & E. V. Cosmi (Eds.), *Reviews in perinatal medicine* (Vol. 3, pp. 397–472). New York: Raven.

Dreyfus-Brisac, C. (1979b). Ontogenesis of brain bioelectrical activity and sleep organization in neonates and infants. In F. Falkner & J.M. Tanner (Eds.), *Human Growth* (Vol. 3, pp. 157–182). New York: Plenum.

Drillien, C.M., Thoman, A.J. M., & Burgoyne, K. (1980). Low-birthweight children at early school-age: A longitudinal study. *Developmental Medicine and Child Neurology,* 22, 26–47.

Dubowitz, L.M.S., Dubowitz, V., Palmer, P.G., Miller, G., Fawer, C.L., & Levene, M.I. (1984). Correlation of neurologic assessment in the preterm newborn infant with outcome at 1 year. *Pediatrics,* 105, 452–457.

Ellingson, R.J., Dutch, S.J., & McIntire, M.S. (1974). EEGs of prematures: 3–8-year follow-up study. *Developmental Psychobiology,* 7, 529–538.

Ellingson, R.J., & Peters, J.F. (1980a). Development of EEG and daytime sleep patterns in low risk premature infants during the first year of life: Longitudinal observations. *Electroencephalography and Clinical Neurophysiology,* 50, 165–171.

Ellingson, R.J., & Peters, J.F. (1980b). Development of EEG and daytime sleep patterns in normal full-term infants during the first three months of life: Longitudinal observations. *Electroencephalography and Clinical Neurophysiology,* 49, 112–124.

Ellingson, R.J., & Peters, J.F. (1980c). Development of EEG and daytime sleep patterns in Trisomy-21 infants during the first year of life: Longitudinal observations. *Electroencephalography and Clinical Neurophysiology,* 50, 457–466.

Fitzhardinge, P.M., Flodmark, O., Fitz, C.R., & Ashby, S. (1982). The prognostic value of computed tomography of the brain in asphyxiated premature infants. *Journal of Pediatrics,* 100, 476–481.

Hack, M., Caron, B., Rivers, A., & Fanaroff, A.A. (1983). The very low birth weight infant:

The broader spectrum of morbidity during infancy and early childhood. *Developmental and Behavioral Pediatrics, 4,* 243-249.

Hass, G.H., & Prechtl, H.F.R. (1977). Normal and abnormal EEG maturation in newborn infants. *Early Human Development,* 1, 69-90.

Hunt, J.V. (1981). Predicting intellectual disorders in childhood for high-risk preterm infants. In S. Friedman & M. Sigman (Eds.), *Preterm birth and psychological development* (pp. 329-351). New York: Academic Press.

Littman, B., & Parmelee, A.H. (1978). Medical correlates of infant development. *Pediatrics,* 61, 470-474.

Lombroso, C.T. (1979). Quantified electrographic scales on 10 pre-term healthy newborns followed up to 40-43 weeks conceptional age by serial polygraphic recordings. *Electroencephalography and Clinical Neurophysiology,* 46, 460-474.

Lombroso, C.T. (1982). Some aspects of EEG polygraphy in newborns at risk for neurological disorders. In P. A. Buser, W. C. Cobb, & T. Okuma (Eds.), *Kyoto symposia* (EEG Suppl. No. 36) (pp. 652-663). Amsterdam: Elsevier Biomedical Press.

Papile, L. Munsick-Bruno, G., & Schaefer, A. (1983). Relationship of cerebral intraventricular hemorrhage and early childhood neurologic handicaps. *Journal of Pediatrics,* 103, 273-277.

Parmelee, A.H., Akiyama, Y., Schultz, M.A., Wenner, W.H., Schulte, F.J., & Stern, E. (1968). The electroencephalogram in active and quiet sleep in infants. In P. Kellaway & I. Petersen (Eds.), *Clinical Electroencephalography of children* (pp. 77-88). New York: Grune & Stratton.

Parmelee, A.H., Kopp, C.B., & Sigman, M. (1976). Selection of developmental assessment techniques for infants at risk. *Merrill-Palmer Quarterly,* 22, 177-199.

Parmelee, A.H., Schulte, F.J., Akiyama, Y., Wenner, W.H., Schultz, M.A., & Stern, E. (1978). Maturation of EEG activity during sleep in premature infants. *Electroencephalography and Clinical Neurophysiology,* 24, 319-329.

Parmelee, A.H., & Sigman, M. (1983). Perinatal brain development and behavior. In M.M. Haith & J.J. Campos (Eds.), P.H. Mussen (Series Ed.), *Handbook of child psychology: Vol. 2. Infancy and developmental psychobiology* (pp. 95-156). New York: Wiley.

Parmelee, A.H., & Stern, E. (1972). Development of states in infants. In C. Clemente, D. Purpura, & F. Meyer (Eds.), *Sleep and the maturing nervous system* (pp. 199-228). New York: Academic Press.

Parmelee, A.H., Wenner, W.H., Akiyama, Y., Schultz, M.A., & Stern, E. (1967). Sleep states in premature infants. *Developmental Medicine and Child Neurology,* 9, 70-77.

Prechtl, H.,F.R. (1974). The behavioral states of the newborn infant (a review). *Brain Research,* 76, 185-212.

Prechtl, H.F.R., Akiyama, Y., Zinkin, P., & Grant, D.K. (1968). Polygraphic studies of the full-term newborn: I. Technical aspects and qualitative analysis. In R. MacKeith & M. Bax (Eds.), *Studies in infancy* (Clinics in Developmental Medicine No. 27). Lavenham: Spastics International Medical Publications and Heinemann Medical Books.

Prechtl, H.F.R., Theorell, K., & Blair, A.W. (1973). Behavioral state cycles in abnormal infants. *Developmental Medicine and Child Neurology,* 15, 606-615.

Richards, J.E., Parmelee, A.H., Jr., & Beckwith, L. (in press). Spectral analysis of infant EEG and behavioral outcome at age five. Electroencephalography and Clinical Neurophysiology.

Saigal, S., Rosenbaum, P., Stoskopf, B., & Sinclair, J.C. (1984). Outcome in infants 501-1000 gm birth weight delivered to residents of the McMaster Health Region. *Journal of Pediatrics,* 105, 969-976.

Sameroff, A.J., & Chandler, M.J. (1975). Reproductive risk and the continuum of caretaking casualty. In F.D. Horowitz, E.M. Hetherington, M. Seigel, & S. Scarr-Salapatek (Eds.), *Review of child development research* (Vol. 4, pp. 187–244). Chicago: University of Chicago Press.

Schulte, F.J., Heinze, G., & Schrempf, G. (1971). Maternal toxemia, fetal malnutrition, and bioelectric brain activity of the newborn. *Neuropaediatrie, 2,* 439–460.

Schultz, M.A., Schulte, F.J., Akiyama, Y., & Parmelee, A.H. (1968). Development of electroencephalographic sleep phenomena in hypothyroid infants. *Electroencephalography and Clinical Neurophysiology, 25,* 351–358.

Shirataki, S., & Prechtl, H.F.R. (1977). Sleep state transitions in newborn infants: Preliminary study. *Developmental Medicine and Child Neurology, 19,* 316–325.

Siegel, L.S. (1982). Reproductive, perinatal and environmental factors as predictors of the cognitive and language development of preterm and full-term infants. *Child Development, 53,* 963–973.

Smith, A.C., Flick, G.L., Ferriss, G.S., & Sellman, A.H. (1972). Prediction of developmental outcome at seven years from prenatal, perinatal, and postnatal events. *Child Development, 43,* 495–507.

Tharp, B.R., Cukier, F.,, & Monod, N. (1981). The prognostic value of the electroencephalogram in premature infants. *Electroencephalography and Clinical Neurophysiology, 51,* 219–236.

Theorell, K. (1974). Clinical value of prolonged polygraphic recordings in high-risk newborn infants. *Neuropaediatrie, 5,* 383–401.

Thoman, E.G., Denenberg, V.H., Sievel, J., Zeidner, L., & Becker, P. (1980). Behavioral state profile in infancy are predictive of later medical or behavioral dysfunction. *Neuropaediatrie, 12,* 45–54.

Thoman, E.G., Korner, A.F., & Kraemer, H.C. (1976). Individual consistency in behavioral states in neonates. *Developmental Psychobiology, 9,* 271–283.

Torres, F., & Blaw, M.E. (1968). Longitudinal EEG—clinical correlations in children from birth to 4 years of age. *Pediatrics, 41,* 945–954.

Werner, E.E., & Smith, R.S. (1982). *Vulnerable but invincible: A study of resilient children.* New York: McGraw-Hill.

Part II
DEVELOPMENTAL ISSUES

In his paper "Child Psychology: The Future," H.R. Schaffer, a leading research worker in the field of child development, first points out the remarkable growth of developmental psychology in the past few decades. Not only has there been an impressive quantitative increase in the amount of research, but also studies have become increasingly sophisticated technically and conceptually. Schaffer then devotes his discussion to a number of fundamental issues that require serious attention if further research is to be fruitful. His review covers a wide range of methodological and conceptual issues, with a number of pertinent critiques of the methods and ideas in these areas. Only a few issues will be mentioned here for additional emphasis, but all the questions he raises deserve serious attention. He gives first consideration to our lack of knowledge regarding the mechanisms of development, since we cannot specify as yet the processes responsible for children's progression from one stage to another. He criticizes aptly the excessive reliance on laboratory studies, which may or may not correspond to the child's behavior in real life. He is therefore skeptical of the assumption that the child's reactions in the Ainsworth Strange Situations can be assumed to be "typical" of the child's attachment behavior—a skepticism that many of us share.

Schaffer also points out that the exploration of the ways in which parents influence their children cannot rely on the study of single relationships, such as the mother-child dyad, but must take into account the multiplicity of factors and influences that are operating simultaneously. He describes the many ways in which the contemporary family is changing and will continue to change, so that any single fixed notion of a presumably typical normal family structure becomes a stereotype. Of special interest to clinicians is his criticism of those studies that are content with reporting group trends but fail to explore many cases that go contrary to the overall group correlations. As Schaffer points out, the clinician must deal with individual children, whose behavior may or may not correspond to the average expectation. It is these individual differences that must be identified if the research data are to be really useful to the clinician. Schaffer takes up these and other issues concisely but definitively, and his paper represents a most salutory challenge to the field of developmental psychology.

The paper by Sameroff on the environmenal context of child development expands and spells out in detail one of the important issues raised by Schaffer. Sameroff reviews the literature on this question systematically and critically and points out the disproportionate lack of attention given to the study of the specific environmental factors that may enhance or hinder healthy child development. As he stresses, prevention can now be seen as a complex endeavor because no single environmental factor along determines outcome. Finally, Sameroff emphasizes that this complexity should not lead to pessimism regarding prevention and treatment. Rather, he takes an optimistic view based on the variety of possibilities that can be identified, and the ones that are pertinent to any one child or group of children can then be applied with the necessary focus and emphasis.

Ragan and McGlashan report a study comparing a substantial series of psychiatric inpatients, who had experienced the death of a parent in childhood, with a large matched control group who had not been subject to childhood parental death. No association with psychiatric diagnosis was found in comparing the two groups. The patients with a childhood parental death did, however, have significantly greater family pathology and impaired social and sexual functioning. But, as the authors point out, many stressful family factors may be involved in either precipitating the parent's death or emerge as a consequence of the death. The authors conclude that psychopathology is multidetermined and that any single event by itself, such as childhood parental death, while it may have various consequences for the child's further development, cannot play a decisive etiologic role in major psychiatric syndromes.

Sonis and his coworkers report a study of the effects of precocious puberty, which provides an experiment in nature that can give us information regarding the effects of early and continuous exposure to sex steroids on human behavior. They present systematic analyses of their data, which indicate a number of significant effects of this precocity. They emphasize that their findings have concentrated on the biological factors and indicate the need for additional studies of the reactions of parents and others to this disorder, as well as its effects on the youngster's self-image.

A great deal of controversy has raged over the significance of minor neurological indicators (a better term than the previously popular label, "soft neurological signs"). In a careful study, Landman and his associates report that although five-year old children with these mild neurological indicators had a high likelihood of experiencing difficulty with visual-perceptual, fine motor, and gross motor tasks, no relationship has been found with performance on linguistic, memory, sequencing, quantitative, or preacademic functions. As the authors emphasize, these findings suggest caution in evaluating the significance of these indicators in young children with academic difficulty. Caution is also imperative in evaluating the predictive value of such minor neurological indicators, especially in view of the current emphasis in many communities on programs of preschool screening.

Over the past 10 decades, a number of studies have reported that a specific behavior pattern, labeled "Coronary Type A," represents a high risk factor for heart disease in adults. This pattern is characterized by extremes of agressiveness, easily aroused hostility, a sense of time urgency, and competitive achievement striving. The opposite behavior pattern, "Coronary Type B," is at low risk for heart disease, and there are many who fall into an intermediate category. These studies have produced more convincing evidence of a specific relationship between a personality type and the occurrence of a physical illness than has been the case with previous efforts in the field of psychosomatic medicine.

A question of great interest in the studies of Type A behavior is whether this pattern can be identified in children, and, if this is the case, whether it correlates with Type A behavior in adults. If so, this could open the way for promising preventative measures to change the behavior of Type A children and thus reduce their risk of heart disease in adult life. A scale for rating Type A behavior in children, which appears satisfactory and is being extensively used, has been developed by Matthews. This scale, however, still leaves open the question of whether there is continuity between the childhood and adult ratings. Only a proper longitudinal study can answer this question. In the paper by Steinberg he reports that the teacher interviews in the first and second grades from our New York Longitudinal Study provided adequate data for rating the children according to the Matthews scale. He was also able to rate the subjects at adolescence and early adult life from the subject interviews. He found that Type A behaviors were stable between adolescence and early adulthood but not between childhood and adolescence or between childhood and adulthood. These findings are important, though not surprising, given the multidimensional factors that interact continuously through childhood to shape differences in behavioral patterns in adolescence and adulthood.

5

Child Psychology: The Future

H. R. Schaffer

University of Strathclyde, United Kingdom

Knowledge regarding the mechanisms of development is the aspect in most urgent need of attention, so that we can specify the processes responsible for children's progression from one stage to another. In particular, social influence processes need to be clarified, for past attemps to provide adequate socialisation theories have been hampered by various conceptual and methodological problems. Care must also be taken not to tie such theories to outdated sterotypes of the family; recent social changes and developments in the field of reproductive technology are raising new issues that need to be taken into account in attempts to explain the social context of child development.

INTRODUCTION

The growth of developmental psychology in the last few decades has been most impressive. This is expressed in a number of ways, of which the following may be singled out as particularly noteworthy.

(1) The sheer quantitative increase in the amount of research. One need only consider the successive editions of the *Carmichael Handbook of Child Psychology* to appreciate this point; thus in the 30 years between the 1954 edition and the recent 4th edition the amount of material for review increased from one volume of 1300 pages to four volumes totalling around 4000 pages. The growth in sheer factual knowledge, and in the in-

Reprinted with permission from the *Journal of Child Psychology and Psychiatry*, 1986, Vol. 27, No. 6, 761–779. Copyright 1986 by the Association for Child Psychology and Psychiatry, Pergamon Journals Ltd.

dustry generating that knowledge, is thus perhaps the most obvious aspect of recent trends.

(2) The increasing technical sophistication of research. Take the enormous surge of work on infancy which occurred during the 1960s and 1970s: to a considerable extent this was brought about by techniques becoming available which enabled investigators to find a way "into" the infant—techniques such as Fantz's visual preference procedure, the recording of sucking and headturning responses, the measurement of physiological indices such as heart rate, and so forth. As a result our conception of the infant changed drastically, from that of a passive, psychologically disorganised being to an active, in many respects highly competent organism biologically prepared to meet the most important challenges of its environment. We have here but one example of the way in which shifts in basic paradigms may be brought about by technical developments.

(3) The increasing conceptual sophistication of developmental psychology. The two most striking instances (involving cognitive and social development respectively) are Piagetian theory and Bowlby's attachment theory, both of which have massively transformed the research scene. Unlike some other approaches such as social learning theory these accounts were not imported into child psychology from the study of other types of organisms (rats, human adults, etc.), but derive their influence from their origins in the study of children *per se*. No wonder they have proved to be of so much greater heuristic value!

(4) The gradual blurring of the dividing line between "pure" and "applied" research. It has always been difficult to maintain this division, yet professional organisation and funding policies tended only too frequently to categorise work under one or the other heading and to erect barriers that prevented communication and cross-fertilisation. To some extent this situation is still with us, though no longer in as marked a form. The emphasis on "ecological validity", with its stress on situational determinants and consequent reservations about laboratory experiments, is one reason for this improvement; the demonstration by (above all) attachment theory that basic concepts are equally applicable to the "normal" and to the "pathological" arena is another.

I have no doubt that these trends will continue and will be found in even more marked form in the future, providing the backcloth to our further efforts to understand the nature of child development. There is no doubt, looking back, that a great deal has already been accomplished in gaining such understanding within a relatively short period; the task ahead nevertheless remains enormous. Under the circumstances there are many themes that one can pick out as candidates for further work in the next few decades. I make no pretence to being a prophet; present needs do not necessarily dictate the shape of the future, and entirely unexpected developments are by no means uncommon in scientific progress. What is presented here is therefore very much a personal choice, reflecting my own beliefs and hopes as to what needs to be done. And far from attempting to cover the whole field of child development I will confine myself to a number of themes that reflect my own competencies and interests.

PUTTING THE "DEVELOPMENTAL" INTO DEVELOPMENTAL PSYCHOLOGY

A great deal of information has been amassed now as to the nature of children's behaviour at different ages and stages. As a result we can compare and contrast different age groups with respect to many psychological functions and so gradually build up an overall descriptive account of development over the course of childhood. This task is far from complete; it is, for example, only recently that emotional development has begun to be plotted in precisely defined behavioural terms (Lewis & Rosenblum, 1978), and much of this effort is still confined to the earliest years and thus requires extension into later childhood. Nevertheless, our knowledge as to the "how" of children's development has leapt ahead at an enormous rate in the last few decades and can provide parents, professional workers and researchers with some most useful guidelines on which to base expectations and demands.

What is missing, however, is knowledge regarding the mechanisms of development. We may know how children behave at point A and how they behave at point B, but we have little idea as to how they get from A to B. The "why" of psychological development, i.e. the mechanisms responsible for developmental change, remains elusive. Not that there has been any lack of attempts to put forward explanations: Piaget in particular comes to mind, for he was not just content to provide insight into the characteristics of the various cognitive stages found during childhood but he has also set about, by means of the concept of equilibration, to account for the transition from one stage to the next. Yet this has remained one of the least satisfactory parts of Piagetian theory: it is an explanation based on intuition that remains impervious to empirical testing and thus condemned to the same fate as that of so many psychoanalytic concepts that similarly could not be either proved or disproved.

To provide satisfactory explanations for the facts of developmental change is surely the greatest challenge facing us at present. Up to now both conceptual and methodological problems have made it extraordinarily difficult for developmental scientists to focus on *change* as such. Where change over time has received attention it has generally been done in a rather crude manner, i.e. by means of correlations between "early" events and "late" events—correlations which do not, of course, have anything informative to say about the *processes* on which development is based. To know, for instance, that two-year-olds high in behavioural compliance with parental directives become children who, several years later, score high on tests of moral internalisation (Lytton, 1980), or that frequency of smiling in infancy is related to measures of reflection-impulsivity at age 10 (Kagan, Kearsley & Zelano, 1978), provides one with knowledge about associations (useful certainly for predictive purposes) but not with insight into why the latter event arises out of the former. Thus at present we do not even know about the mechanisms for proceeding from one stage to an immediately adjacent one (e.g. from being unable to retrieve a hidden object at sensori-motor stage 3 to possessing this capacity at sensori-motor stage 4, or from thinking along primarily egocentric lines during the preoperational period to being able to decentre once the period of concrete operations is reached). Far less are we able to explain in what way continuities can be postulated between events in infancy and "outcomes" in later childhood or adulthood. Truly developmental accounts remain conspicuous by their absence.

If we are to make progress in this respect we need clarification as to the concept of development as such, and in this respect there is now some encouraging progress that helps us at least to state the sorts of questions we should be asking. Thus it is becoming increasingly clear that development is best conceived in terms of sequential reorganisation rather than steady quantitative accretion. The child's mental life, that is, will periodically and relatively suddenly show transitions to new psychological levels that, in certain respects at least, are qualitatively different from preceding levels. As Piaget above all has shown, new sets of capacities emerge from time to time which drastically alter the child's mode of adaptation to the environment and which thus reveal major changes in psychological organisation. Whether these take the across-the-board form which Piaget believed in or whether they apply to much more specific functions as Fischer (1980) has argued is one of the issues that future research must settle. Another is the identification of the major transition points, though the various attempts that have already been made to list these, at least for the early years (e.g. by Emde, Gaensbauer & Harmon, 1976; McCall, Eichorn & Hogarty, 1977; Fischer, 1980; Schaffer, 1984), show a most welcome degree of agreement. In all these accounts development is conceived of as a step-like course, where transitions to qualitatively different modes of behaviour occur from time to time, bringing about new modes of adaptation on the part of the child. Each break represents a period of instability when (according to a suggestion by Emde *et al.,* 1976, which needs to be confirmed) the child is especially vulnerable to psychological and physiological stress. Each involves a large and rapid advance in many response patterns across various behavioural domains, giving rise to qualitatively new and more complex response patterns (though these rarely arise *de novo* but are generally tied to earlier processes which are the necessary prerequisites for their emergence; Hinde & Bateson, 1984).

To locate these transition points and describe the nature of the psychological changes which they usher in is one task: another is to identify the mechanisms responsible for the various transformations. One reason why we are still so ignorant in this respect is the continuing unease about the respective influence of endogenous and exogenous forces (the old heredity-environment argument). It may be widely agreed that psychological development is inevitably a function of both sets of forces and that it is their interaction that accounts for the particular course which development takes in any individual child. However, to pay lip-service to such an interactionist view is easy; to spell out in convincing detail the nature of that interaction and the specific process involved is still extraordinarily difficult. Under these circumstances it is perhaps not surprising that most writers continue to concentrate on one or the other set of determinants. Thus accounts of *cognitive* development have focused on endogenous forces, calling upon maturation to "explain" the onset of new competencies; even when a more epigenetic view has been taken (as by Piaget) statements have rarely gone beyond acknowledging in general terms the need for a supportive environment, without spelling out how such support interlinks with the child's current developmental status. Accounts of *social* development, on the other hand, have tended to go to the opposite extreme, concentrating on the shaping influence of exogenous forces (parental rearing patterns in particular) without taking into consideration any organismic factors that mediate the impact of the environment. A more even-handed approach is clearly required.

We can perhaps appreciate the nature of this problem better by examining in detail one particular transition point, i.e. that which takes place around the age of eight months—a specially important one from many points of view (Schaffer, 1986a). There is evidence (Diamond, 1983; Passingham, 1985) that many of the changes occurring at this time are directly linked to the maturation of precortical mechanisms; there is further evidence (Konner, 1982) that the age at onset for these new competencies shows considerable similarity across a wide range of cultures and of child-rearing practices. Thus separation protest, fear of strangers, object permanence, means-ends differentiation, goal-corrected behaviour, recall memory and a variety of relational abilities all seem at first sight to emerge according to some predetermined timetable dependent solely on the maturation of certain cortical structures; once these are ready it is thought the child is bound to make the psychological transition and manifest the respective set of abilities in overt behaviour. Attention is thus focused wholly on developments within the child; structural maturation is said to "cause" behavioural change, and the social context in which the psychobiological developments occur is brushed aside as without significance. Such a formulation is, however, questionable. There is also evidence—albeit of a suggestive nature only—that experiential factors in the period preceding the eight-months transition play a vital role in bringing about the respective changes. That there are social *consequences* to such changes can perhaps be readily accepted: the infant becomes in many respects a different being, makes different demands on his caretakers and the nature of social exchanges accordingly becomes transformed. That there are also social *antecedents,* on the other hand, which act as integral facilitating factors to mental reorganisation, is rarely acknowledged—*vide* Piaget's almost entirely asocial account of psychological growth. But children's developmental agendas do not run off in a vacuum; maturation always occurs in an environmental context of a specifically supportive nature. The problem is that this support is near-universal; it is usually an integral part of all caretaker–child interactions and its role therefore only becomes evident under grossly deviant conditions such as those produced by extremely depriving institutionalisation. As suggested elsewhere (Schaffer, 1986a), social facilitation may take both a general and a specific form: general in the sense of an energising function that plays a part in brain growth, specific in that parents may be found to indulge in "anticipatory" behaviour whereby they involve infants in interaction formats well before the child is in fact ready properly to participate—an involvement, however, which provides the child with plenty of experience of the part he is in due course expected to play.

   Whether these particular social antecedents indeed have the aetiological significance I have attributed to them remains to be established. I have used the eight-months transition point merely as one example of the type of analysis required to gain insight into the mechanisms of developmental change. That analysis is based on the assumption that human development is fundamentally a *joint* enterprise: joint, that is, between child and caretaker (Schaffer, 1984). Most accounts of psychological development have been individual-based: their concern has been with the child as such, everything outside his skin being considered extraneous. Even where the social context has been duly acknowledged as an essential ingredient there has been failure so far to describe the role it plays in specific terms. Take Vygotsky's (1978) proposal that the direction of development proceeds from the interpersonal to the intrapersonal, i.e. that new capacities initially appear in social context which is needed to support the manifestations of that behaviour before the capacities become internalised as part of the individual's mental repertoire. As yet we have very little indication as to how adults go about providing such support. Thus Bakeman & Adamson (1984) have shown that co-ordinated attention to both a person and an object is much more likely when infants aged 6 to 18 months play with the mother than when they play with a peer. The mother, that is, takes action to "scaffold" the infant's early attempts to embed objects in social interaction; without the presence of a mature partner the infant is much less capable of such sophisticated behaviour. What we do not know, however, is the form that such scaffolding actually takes; what is more, such studies are concerned with abilities that have already emerged in the child's repertoire: the action required by adults to help bring forth the ability in the first place needs to be investigated in its own right. Thus we have to keep an eye on child and caretaker simultaneously in any attempt to spell out the mechanisms of development; both endogenous and exogenous factors must be taken into account and their interaction becomes the major focus of enquiry.

SOCIALISATION PROCESSES

Development, it has been argued, can only be understood if it is seen as a joint enterprise involving parent as well as child; the role of *both* needs to be specified. The failure to take an interactionist view is probably the single most important reason why we do not as yet have an adequate socialisation theory, the provision of which is surely one of the more important requirements for the future. We need to understand, that is, how social influence processes work in a developmental context in order to learn how they produce particular long-term outcomes in children.

As to those outcomes, most attention has been given to the topics of moral development, sex role acquisition and (more recently) the development of prosocial behaviour. As is apparent from recent reviews of these three areas (Rest, 1983; Huston, 1983; Radke-Yarrow, Zahn-Waxler & Chapman, 1983), an enormous amount of research has been carried out in each; despite all this effort, however, we remain ignorant as to *how* socialisation influences produce socialised children. There are various reasons for this failure; to identify them is necessary for the sake of future work.

(1) Most of the relevant studies have been based on the assumption that either modelling or some form of direct instruction are the means whereby children are influenced by their caretakers and that observational learning and reinforcement are the primary mechanisms to account for the effects on their behaviour. There is no doubt that research adopting such paradigms has demonstrated that effects can indeed be produced in this way; one need only consider the vast number of studies which, influenced by Bandura (1977), showed all sorts of social learning to follow demonstrations by models. However, that such effects *can* be produced under the constrained and ephemeral conditions of the laboratory does not mean that they *are* produced in this way in real life; the phenomena have been forced into the straight-jacket of traditional learning theories as though the very use of the term "learning" will help us to understand how parental influences produce particular child outcomes. Learning, that is, has been used as an explanatory concept (Schaffer, 1986b), as though the demonstration of environmental influences means that we understand the processes at work, yet justifiably it can only be regarded as an umbrella term to cover a vast array of different kinds of external influences that bring about effects in ways about which we are still extraordinarily ignorant. The present usage of "learning" cloaks that ignorance; it is a descriptive term and future research concerned with socialisation effects should recognise it as such.

(2) Failures to take into account the influence of setting provides another source of difficulty. Thanks largely to Bronfenbrenner (1977) we have now become aware of the need for caution in generalising from one situation to another. For instance, a mother's patterns of visual attention to her child are likely to be totally different when observed in the playroom of a laboratory compared with the living room of her own home (Schaffer, 1984), the demand characteristics of each setting are such that generalisation from one to the other is unwarranted. Yet the present vogue for the Strange Situation as a means of assessing a child's attachment (Ainsworth, Blehar, Waters & Wall, 1978) neglects these constraints, and especially so as it goes on the assumption that "typical" behaviour is produced by the two reunion episodes built into this procedure, each of marked brevity. More cross-situational comparisons are badly needed; they may well show that assessments ought to be carried out in a variety of contexts if they are to have credibility. And if there is

anything in the proposal put forward by Whiting (1980), that the primary way in which parents influence children is by assigning them to specific settings (i.e. to particular places, particular tasks, the company of certain people, etc.) and that the children then develop the characteristics elicited by such settings, it becomes even more important to give due prominence to situational variables in our studies.

(3) One particular feature of past work has been the failure to study socialisation in the context of social interaction. Investigators have tended to pay attention to final products (impulse control, moral internalisation, self-regulation, etc.) without attempting *directly* to examine the processes that give rise to these products; in fact a research methodology was frequently used that involved a considerable time gap between the (assumed) antecedent and the consequent conditions, sometimes investigating the former only by retrospective, indirect and global means. No wonder that the socialisation literature and the social interaction literature have come up with quite different views as to the nature of parent–child influences: the former concentrating on conflict between an egocentric, uncooperative child and a basically antithetical social environment; the latter stressing the essential compatibility of parent and child and concentrating on mutuality rather than antagonism. The two bodies of literature need to be brought together by means of longitudinal studies, which would include a much more precise analysis of what transpires between parent and child at particular "early" points, together with specification of intervening processes, before long-term consequences are ascribed to those early events. Due recognition must thus be given to the complexity of developmental antecedent-consequent relationships.

(4) Most of the recent socialisation literature has been characterised by a cognitive bias, being concerned with the learning of contingencies, the acquisition of self-control, compliance to directives, awareness of reciprocities, and other such "intellectual" achievements. The socialisation of affect, on the other hand, has received comparatively little attention—a situation of which Maccoby & Masters (1983) have recently made us aware by means of a most timely and provocative statement. There is some evidence, as they point out, that cognition and affect may be regarded as two separate systems running along different developmental courses and shaped by different sets of determinants. What we have learned about the one may not therefore necessarily apply to the other. Thus it may well be that the most powerful and lasting forms of early learning are of an affective rather than a cognitive nature, possibly resulting from the emotional "tags" that parents attach to particular events by

means of their own responses to them [the so-called social referencing phenomenon (Feinman, 1982) is presumably one example thereof], and that the emphasis placed hitherto on the cognitive content of parental communications is therefore unduly one-sided. The work that has been carried out on emotional development (cf. Lewis & Rosenblum, 1978) has tended to focus on such individual-based topics as the emotional expressiveness of infants, the development of empathy, and the measurement of temperamental qualities. As an aspect of early interpersonal communication, however, affect has received little recognition, yet the way in which parents induce positive or negative moods, the ability of infants and young children to learn to share affect, the consequences of emotional "tagging", the relationship between such tagging and cognitive components in control–compliance sequences—these are but some of the problems to which research could most profitably address itself.

(5) Socialisation research has also unduly restricted itself to the study of single relationships, whose impacts are examined one at a time as though children deal with them purely as isolated entities. It is, of course, only quite recently that relationships other than that with the mother have received their due recognition and that the potential socialising influences of fathers, siblings, peers, teachers and even the media have come to be investigated. Yet either the various kinds of relationships have been studied in isolation from one another or, where they have been brought together, they have been compared and contrasted in order, for example, to determine whether fathers' speech to young children is similar to that of mothers, whether peer interaction serves a different function to that served by interaction with adults, or whether teachers' conversations with children are of a different order compared with mothers' conversation. These are all, of course, useful questions to ask, but by themselves they do not do sufficient justice to the complexity of the child's interpersonal world. The very fact that a child is exposed to a multiplicity of child-rearing strategies and expectations raises questions about the ability to cope with such diverse demands; it also suggests that long-term outcome for the child's personality may be not so much a function of the sum of specific relationships as of the extent and nature of the divergencies between them. Thus mothers and fathers do not impinge on the child separately, with additive effects, but have combined influence to which the child responds. That combination needs to become the focus of research. And the same applies to the child's incorporation in particular systems—that of the family, the peer group, the school, etc. Again it is only recently that the child's membership of systems other than that of

the family has been given its proper acknowledgement; again these systems are still treated in isolation. Yet the differene in values between family and nursery, for example, that many children encounter may in itself be a highly significant feature of their experience; whether such discrepancies are to be seen as conflicts leading to undesirable consequences or whether they are better thought of as challenges that children attempt to reconcile, thereby benefiting in terms of sociocognitive understanding, is but one of the questions that follow.

SOME METHODOLOGICAL CONSIDERATIONS

There are a number of methodological problems which have bedevilled socialisation research in the past and which will need to be dealt with if progress is to be made. The greatest of these concerns the difficult issue of cause–effect relationships: to what extent are particular parental practices responsible for particular child outcomes? The realisation that reciprocal effects can be found in parent-child relationships, that children affect parents as well as vice versa, has made the interpretation of correlations a much more difficult task. Unfortunately the bulk of findings on parents and children is in a correlational form and hence subject to ambiguity. Take the role of parental sensitivity, which has emerged as possibly one of the most crucial dimensions of parents' behaviour (Schaffer & Collis, 1986): variations in this respect are associated with a great many aspects of child behaviour, but whether adults "cause" these or whether individual differences in children bring about parental variations in the first place remains unsettled. Equally obscure is the relationship between parental speech input and children's language development, despite a lengthy and continuing debate about the role of "motherese" (Furrow, Nelson & Benedict, 1979; Gleitman, Newport & Gleitman, 1984). Cross-lag techniques have unfortunately failed to live up to their promise as a way out of this quandary (Rogosa, 1980); systems theory, the proponents of which frequently appear to eschew the need for all cause–effect statements, is in danger of merely turning its back on this important issue.

That parents do have an effect on children may seem obvious, yet in practice it has often proved extraordinarily difficult to demonstrate such an effect. It is ironic that despite the enormous amount of research in this area we still face the challenge of specifying as to what really goes on between parent and child that has such an impact on the child's development. It may be argued that much of the past research has been too simplistic in its expectation of one-to-one relationships between environmental input and child outcome. The usual strategy has been to examine variations in parental behaviour (in disciplinary techniques, attitudes, rearing practices, and so forth) and then to relate these to variations in child behaviour at either a concurrent or a future point of development, with at least the implicit assumption that the parental action is the initiator of change. As we have already seen, that assumption fails to take into account the fact that socialisation practices need to be geared to the unfolding of the child's developmental timetable; as Maccoby (1984) has also recently argued, socialisation so-conceived does not have a developmental dimension to it. The child too, that is, must be considered as the initiator of change. And once one focuses on the child as a contributor to his own development it becomes apparent that it is not sufficient to take into account parental practices *per se* as antecedent conditions, but that one must also pay attention to the *meaning* of these to the child, i.e. to the interpretation put on them by the individual and the kinds of internal representations of the social world to which they give rise. This is why some of the latest developments in attachment theory are so exciting, for in their much more sophisticated approach to antecedent-consequent relationships they are surely a sign of a new willingness to face the complexities of the child's interaction with the social world (Bretherton & Waters, 1985). As pointed out by Bowlby (1969), children come to construct internal working models of their attachment figures; these evolve out of experienced relationships but are no passive reflection of such events: the child actively construes his experience and consequently there is no reason to expect simple, universal one-to-one relationships between parental behaviour and child behaviour. Thus, the focus needs to swing away from an exclusive concern with overt action to a consideration also of internal representation, i.e. to the child's working model of self in relation to significant others. That model is, of course, by no means a static one; it is formed in the first place by the child's early interactions with caretakers but is subsequently transformed both by cognitive growth and further social experience. If that is so the end result is unlikely to be related to early events in some simple, straightforward manner; the working model of attachment figures formed in infancy may well, for instance, play a part in governing behaviour in new relationships but not as the sole determinant, and there is therefore no reason why, say, future peer relationships (Waters, Wippman & Sroufe, 1979) should be directly predictable from the quality of early attachments.

Methodologically, the implications of this approach once again call for a move away from the search for correlations between pairs of antecedent-consequent factors to a much more complex undertaking of a detailed longitudinal nature, in the course of which measures are repeatedly obtained of both experiential variables and aspects of child functioning. In this way the epigenetic pathways are traced from the original interactive experiences in infancy, through their resulting internal representations and the subsequent transformations thereof, to eventual psychological functioning in interpersonal and other situations. In order to undertake this we require more tools of assessment; the study of social interactions at a behavioural level has yielded a considerable range of suitable techniques in recent years (Schaffer, 1977; Sackett, 1978), but the new emphasis on the investigation of internal models badly requires a similar methodological push (though see the promising start made by the study of event schemes and scripts, Mandler, 1984; Nelson & Gruendel, 1981). One can then turn to answering such questions as the age when the child first becomes capable of forming internal models of the social world, how these are structured and in what way their structure changes in the course of development, what role affective components play in their formation and functioning, what determinants (cognitive and experiential) are responsible for their change and reorganisation, and in what way individuals differ in both content and form of representations. The area of "meta-sociability" (Schaffer, 1984), i.e. how the child conceives of other people, of the self and of the relationship between self and others, is likely to be a highly profitable one to pursue, providing an extra dimension to traditional studies of children's interpersonal relationships and also bringing about a further rapprochement between studies of cognitive and of social processes.

THE CHANGING FAMILY

The primary context for development is, of course, the family, and writers from Freud onwards have formulated their theories accordingly. But the kind of family to which these conceptions are tied has for long been a stereotype—one where the mother is inevitably the primary caretaker, where the father is a somewhat distant and definitely secondary figure, and where the whole unit is permanent and in continuous existence throughout the years of childhood. It is a well-documented fact that this sterotype no longer applies to a vast number of children, what with the divorce rate, single-parenthood, working mothers, non-working fathers, role reversibility, and so on. Yet many of our theories about phenomena such as the identification of children, their sex role development and their moral development continue to assume largely outmoded conceptions of the family; justice is not thereby done to either the diversity of family styles to which children may be exposed or to the impermanence of their interpersonal arrangements.

The importance of continuity of personal relationships throughout childhood is a theme on which particular emphasis has been placed in the past. Such continuity has been regarded as desirable, even essential to mental health; if a child did not experience it various pathological consequences were expected to appear as a matter of inevitability. It is important to note, however, that past research concerned with the effects of disrupting bonds has in fact dealt almost entirely with somewhat special populations, such as institutionalised children suffering from multiple deprivation or children coming from already disturbed social backgrounds—in short, with samples where a lot of other pathogenic influences prevail (Rutter, 1981). Conclusions derived from such groups about the role of continuity cannot be automatically generalised to children where only one of the two parental bonds is disrupted (and that perhaps not entirely so), where the child stays in the accustomed home environment, and where the break may actually alleviate a very tense home atmosphere (and in this latter respect it is worth bearing in mind the conclusions of both Rutter, 1981, and Hetherington, 1979, with regard to the effects of maternal deprivation and of divorce respectively, that is not so much the breaking of bonds as the earlier experience of family tension and turmoil that tends to be associated with any pathology that develops in the children concerned). It means that much still needs to be found out about children's multiple but *consecutive* attachments, about their identifications with different individuals at different periods, and about their experience of various patterns of shared care. Above all one should be prepared to consider life styles that deviate from the expected stereotypes not just from a negative but also from a positive point of view, searching for benefits as well as losses. Thus whatever undoubted traumata parental divorce may entail, it is surely at least conceivable that there are gains to be documented which, under the influence of society's present blinkered attitude, researchers tend not to notice—gains which, for example, subsequent parental remarriage brings, such as access to a larger kinship network, a more varied social experience as a result of becoming incorporated in a "blended" family, the opportunity to acquire a greater repertoire of social skills as part of the need to interact with a greater range of key figures including step-parents, and so forth.

From a cold-blooded theoretical point of view there is the opportunity for the developmental scientist to capitalise on this range of patterns— rather in the manner of the cross-cultural investigator who makes use of natural variations in order to put to the test theoretical propositions derived in the first instance from the study of one particular culture. And from a practical point of view, instead of assuming consistency of the social environment as the norm and using that as the baseline for action, it is clearly important to pay far more attention to adaptation to *change* in social circumstances, asking such questions as: 'How do children cope with various kinds of change at different ages?', 'Under what circumstances do they fail to cope?', 'What guidelines can one provide to parents and professional workers to help children cope?'. These are likely to be some of the issues of a practical nature that students of development will increasingly be asked to address.

Some of these considerations, as they apply to changes overtaking our notion of the family, have been given extra weight recently by what is happening in the much publicised area of reproductive technology. The Warnock Report (1984) was primarily concerned with medical, legal and ethical aspects and had little to say about psychological implications. This is hardly surprising, because at present these are still difficult to identify. And yet there is considerable apprehension among members of the mental health professions as to what is in store for them. Some of it may seem fanciful: what about the child whose parents died, 5, 10, or even 100 years ago? After all, sperm and ovum can now be preserved for such periods and the moment of conception be accordingly delayed. Or what about the fact that siblings no longer need a minimum age separation of 9 months? In theory at least, it will possible for a couple to bring into the world any number of children all at the same time, whether by means of surrogate mothers or by means of artificial wombs—a development that may well become technically feasible in the not too distant future. There are other aspects that do receive some mention in the Warnock Report, though very briefly: for instance, the effects of artificial insemination by donor on the relationship between the parents, where the Report wonders whether the husband might not feel inadequate and excluded and where not only the marital but also the parent-child relationship will therefore be adversely affected. Then again there are the effects on the child of finding out that it was conceived and/or born under unusual circumstances: might this not make such children feel different from their peers and so give rise to psychological difficulties? Obviously what is unusual depends, by definition, on the sheer frequency of that particular occurrence, and at the moment we have no idea how popular and morally acceptable some of the options of procreation are going to be that will be technically feasible. It is worth bearing in mind, however, that by the end of 1985 over a thousand test tube babies had already been born worldwide; what is unusual today need not be so tomorrow.

What is certain is that the concept of parenthood is becoming vastly more complex and fragmented. In theory at least the genetic mother, the woman who bears the child and the psychological mother may be three different people. Add to that the fact that the child's genetic father may be a different person from the psychological father, and it becomes clear that (to quote Warnock) " . . . there are thus many possible combinations of persons who are relevant to the child's conception, birth and early environment." The implications of all this for the child's sense of identity and belongingness is just one question that is certain to arise.

In addition, questions are bound to be asked as to what such fragmentation does to the sheer efficacy of parenting. Does it matter if the mother misses out on the experience of pregnancy and births? Or for that matter, will parents' faith in their child-rearing capabilities be adversely affected by having required an outside party to help in bringing the child into the world? Some of these questions are in fact no different from those that arise in cases of adoption; others, however, are unique to the area of reproductive technology and show how the range of possible patterns of family experience is likely to be greatly extended beyond the present stereotyped notions of parenthood, childhood and family life. In the past we have tended to regard these stereotypes as a *sine qua non* for normal development, with all deviations automatically viewed as pathogenic. In the future our norms in the area of family relationships may well have to undergo profound change.

INTEGRATING THE DIVERSE

One prediction about future work can safely be made: topics that are presently treated as though they refer to separate entities and are pursued without consideration of developments elsewhere will increasingly become integrated into more encompassing schemes. In this respect scientific progress is rather like the acquisition of a skill by an individual person (Bruner, 1973): attention is initially given to specific components of the skill, and it is only when these have been mastered one at a time and each in its own right that attempts are made to combine and integrate them into a unitary whole. Thus the psychological study of children has so far involved the setting up of boundaries that in many respects are arbitrary; it is highly likely that much of our future conceptual effort will go into dismantling these boundaries and integrating presently diverse areas of enquiry. Here are some of the more obvious candidates:

(1) Cognitive and Social-Affective Aspects

In the past the study of cognitive development and the study of social development have been pursued as though they refer to completely separate aspects of human functioning, each with its own tradition of research strategy and theoretical orientation (Maccoby, 1984). The recent surge of work on social cognition (Shantz, 1983) is one indication that such separation is artificial; thus how children construe their social experiences by means of the cognitive processes available to them at various developmental stages will certainly have implications for the nature of their interpersonal relationships and the successive transformations that these undergo. In fact every social activity implicates cognitive functions such as perception, memory and representation (Lamb & Sherrod, 1981), though the further suggestion that social development becomes only possible as a result of primary cognitive achievements (e.g. that separation protest is only possible after object permanence has been attained) has turned out to be more difficult to sustain than originally anticipated (Bates, Benigni, Bretherton, Camaioni & Volterra, 1977). For that matter, under the influence of Vygotsky's resurrected ideas, consideration has been given (e.g. by Doise & Mugny, 1984) to the possibility that cognitive functions require a social context for their initial emergence and subsequent facilitation before they eventually become internalised as "properties" of individuals. Relevant studies to examine how this comes about are now needed; reports such as those by Bakeman & Adamson (1984) and Wertsch, McNamee, McLane & Budwig (1980) are a beginning, but a great deal more has to be done in order to show that certain kinds of social input are necessary for particular cognitive developments to emerge (Schaffer, 1986a). Vygotsky's was an interesting idea that still has to be made into a convincing one.

(2) Overt Behaviour and Inner Representation

Again these two spheres have in the past been treated as separate enterprises; historically one or the other has even been totally denied as a legitimate field of enquiry. Yet, as the above comments on current trends in attachment research indicate, the bringing together of these two aspects is likely to be most fruitful. This will be especially necessary if one is to carry out longitudinal studies: as long as attachment work was confined to infancy it was at least feasible to confine investigations to overt behaviour; research on older ages, however, can hardly avoid the role which representational processes increasingly play in regulating interpersonal activities (though such processes may well be operative from a surprisingly early age—certainly by the second year of life). It is worth reminding ourselves, however, that it is not only children but also their parents in whom central processes play a part. As Park (1978) pointed out, there seems to be an assumption underlying many observational studies of parent–child interaction that the parent reacts to the child's behaviour in a mechanical, unthinking fashion—the parent, that is, tends to be treated as a black box reactor. But parents ought to be recognised as thinking organisms, with cognitions, perceptions, attitudes and knowledge relating to the child that guide their behaviour in the course of the interaction. Parental reports as objective measures of parental behaviour may be unsatisfactory but as indices of attitudes and feelings they are legitimate, telling us something about the filters through which the behaviour of the child is processed. The inclusion of both kinds of data, behavioural and central, for both partners, parent and child, should considerably enrich our understanding of the relationship.

(3) Genetic and Environmental Determinants

The nature-nurture debate has in recent years taken a more sophisticated form, yet here too such things as professional affiliation and personal loyalties are responsible for the maintenance of two camps, one considering development exclusively in terms of environmental and the other exclusively in terms of genetic factors. Lip-service is paid to the role of both sets of forces yet their interaction is rarely the focus of direct examination, despite the fact that the nature of human development can only be understood by the joint efforts of environmentalists and behaviour geneticists. To take one example: the many correlations that have been produced between measures of parental practices and children's development have almost invariably been interpreted in environmental terms, i.e. as input–output relationships that reflect the influence of experience on the child. Yet Plomin, Loehlin & DeFries (1985), in a most though-provoking study, have found evidence that such correlations can be genetically mediated to a substantial extent (approximately 50% on the average for their data derived from a comparison of parent–child correlations in adopted and non-adopted families). It is likely that the genetic effect is stronger for some relationships than for others: for example, Plomin *et al.* found that between infant soothability and certain parental practices is largely a genetic effect and not, as so many writers automatically assume, an environmental one. The implications for intervention efforts are obvious: knowledge about the basis for observed parent–child correlations has different consequences depending on the way in which they are produced. The blinkered attitude, whereby all such relationships are interpreted in environmental terms, needs to give way to a willingness to consider genetic mediating influences as well. As Wachs (1983) has put it: "What is lacking is not a knowledge base of the separate influences of genes and environment but rather a concentrated attempt to integrate the evidence from both areas and move forward to attack the question of *how* genetic and environmental influences transact to influence development."

(4) Different Levels of Analysis

There have always been debates as to the most suitable types of units to be adopted in developmental studies. There is, of course, no absolute answer to such a question; the level of analysis chosen must be appropriate to the questions being asked (Schaffer, 1986b). Thus investigations are justified at various levels; there must, however, also be concerted efforts to relate different levels to each other. Let us take recent trends in the study of early social development. For long, social behaviour was exclusively investigated in terms of what *individuals* did (when infants begin to smile; whether boys are more aggressive than girls; whether empathy can be detected in preschoolers, etc.). Rather more recently the focus shifted to the study of *dyads*: the structure, length, content and complexity of interactions (mostly between mothers and infants) were of interest and statements were accordingly made about the dyad as an interacting unit rather than about the interacting individuals (Schaffer, 1977). Still more recently, however, it has come to be appreciated that processes in dyads may not be generalisable to larger groups (Schaffer & Liddell, 1984), i.e. that interactions in *polyads* need to be investigated in their own right and cannot necessarily be understood in terms of lower levels (Schaffer, 1984). Each of these different levels still requires a great deal of study in order to determine what sort of statements one can make about each; it is also apparent, however, that future work needs to address itself to the inter-relationships of individual, dyadic and polyadic levels. For instance: 'What aspects of dyadic interactions are dependent on the characteristics of individual participants and what aspects are independent?', 'To what extent do children's social skills developed in dyadic contexts contribute to their ability to interact in larger groupings and to what extent are there uniquely polyadic skills?', 'What mixture of individual, dyadic and polyadic kinds of experiences should children of different ages be given (say, in the context of nurseries) if, as seems possible, each fosters somewhat different sets of competencies?'. Some of these issues are now being discussed by proponents of systems theory in relation to, for instance, the concept of the family as an integral unit (Minushin, 1985), though whether one can justify the uncompromising statement that the individual child cannot under any circumstances be meaningfully isolated for study from the system of which he is a part is just one of the issues in this area that needs to be debated.

(5) Group Trends and Individual Differences

Research publications frequently report their data purely in terms of group means, paying scant attention to individual variability. Let us quote one example among many: in a study concerning the nature of attachment to the mother in children who had been physically abused by that mother (Schneider-Rosen & Cicchetti, 1984) it was found that there were marked differences between the abused group and a normal, non-abused control group. A majority, namely about two-thirds, of the maltreated children were found to be markedly insecure in their attachments to the mother, whereas this was observed in only a minority, that is about a quarter, among the control children. This was statistically a highly significant difference, and the authors go on to discuss the results entirely in terms of this group difference. But what about the one third of the abused children who apparently had normal attachment? And for that matter, what about the 25% of the control group children who did *not* have normal attachments? No mention was made of these, and yet they represent quite substantial minorities. Analysis of such exceptions should be particularly useful because it requires the research worker to take into account individual difference variables and combine these with group effects. Treating groups as though they are homogeneous and neglecting variability within the group produces results of considerably reduced predictive power; concern for the individual, on the other hand, forces one to extend the nature of one's enquiry and take into account additional factors—concerning other relationships, the child's temperament, situational circumstances and so on—that so frequently tend to be neglected as determinants. If we are searching for a slogan for the future perhaps we should adopt "Let's mop up the variance!"

CONCLUSIONS

It is inevitable that our research into the nature of human development will become more and more complex as we attempt increasingly to do justice to the complexity of the processes involved. Cognitive aspects will need to be related to socio-emotional aspects; genetic as well as environmental influences will have to be considered in explaining particular sets of results; representational processes should be investigated concurrently with overt behaviour; individual differences can no longer be neglected when presenting group data; and attempts must be made to bring different levels of analysis into some sort of relationship with each other. The one-variable type of research is thus going to become less common as an organism-in-its-environment approach comes to prevail; it is therefore most fortunate that the advent of modern computing facilities makes possible the analysis of the large bodies of data that are likely to be generated by future research projects.

There are several implications of this trend. One is organisational: the lone researcher, equipped with only limited sets of skills, will no longer provide adequate resources for as large a proportion of the total research effort as is found at present. Many research workers are still firmly wedded to one particular methodology (observational techniques, or psychometric testing, or interviewing, etc.) which they spend their lives applying to various topics (indeed I would hazard a guess that many more change their field of interest than change their favourite methodology). The need for training courses (especially at the Ph.D. level) to be far more flexible in the range of skills taught to individual students is clear; the need for more post-experience courses, aimed at imparting new sets of skills, is also obvious. Above all, however, team research is likely to become a more prevalent feature of the psychological scene, providing an opportunity to tackle a widely varied set of problems in the context of any one study and with an armoury of skills and techniques.

The other implication takes us back to efforts aimed at "mopping up the variance", and in particular to doing justice to individual variability as well as to group trends. One of the reasons why practitioners so frequently find research findings unhelpful is that research workers are generally concerned with group comparisons and probabilities whereas practitioners are confronted with the need to make decisions about individuals. Thus clinicians, social workers and others require information that will provide them with grounds for predicting the course of *particular* children's development; statements about probabilities based on group means are insufficient when there are so many exceptions to general trends. The example mentioned above of abused children's attachments makes the point: decisions about removing the child from home, for instance, clearly cannot be based on the fact of abuse alone but must take into account other considerations prevailing in each family. Once research addresses itself to these other considerations and is prepared to do justice to the full complexity of circumstances defining each case, a much more adequate and helpful set of guidelines can be presented. If research is indeed going to become more wide-ranging and integrative with respect to the phenomena it tackles, then one welcome consequence will be a narrowing of the gap between research and practice. There are, of course, many reasons for this gap and efforts are badly needed to pin-point them. It does seem probable, however, that practitioners and research workers will be able more easily to communicate with each other once both parties deal with the same range of varied circumstances that define the conditions under which children's development takes place.

REFERENCES

Ainsworth, M.D.S., Blehar, M.C., Waters, E. & Wall, S. (1978). *Patterns of attachment.* Hillsdale, New Jersey: Erlbaum.

Bakeman, R. & Adamson, L.R. (1984). Coordinating attention to people and objects in mother–infant and peer–infant interaction. *Child Development,* 55, 1278–1289.

Bandura, A. (1977). *Social Learning Theory.* Englewood Cliffs, New Jersey, Prentice-Hall.

Bates, E., Benigni, L., Bretherton, I., Camaioni, L. & Volterra, V. (1977). From gesture to the first word: on cognitive and social prerequisites. In M. Lewis & L. Rosenblum (Eds.), *Interaction, conversation and the development of language.* New York: Wiley.

Bowlby, J. (1969). *Attachment and loss, Vol. 1: Attachment.* London: Hogarth Press.

Bretherton, I. & Waters, E. (Eds, 1985). Growing points of attachment theory and research. *Monographs of the Society for Research in Child Development,* 50, Nos. 1–2 (Serial No. 209).

Bronfenbrenner, U. (1977). Towards an experimental ecology of human development. *American Psychologist,* 32, 513–531.

Bruner, J.S. (1973). Organization of early skilled action. *Child Development,* 44, 1–11.

Diamond, A., (1983). Behavior changes between 6-12 months of age: what can they tell us about how the mind of the infant is changing? Unpublished doctoral dissertation, Harvard University.

Doise, W. & Mugny, G. (1984). *The social development of the intellect.* Oxford: Pergamon Press.

Emde, R.N.., Gaensbauer, T.J. & Harmon, R.J. (1976). Emotional expression in infancy: a behavioral study. *Psychological Issues,* 10, (1, Whole No. 37).

Feinman, S. (1982). Social referencing in infancy. *Merrill-Palmer Quarterly,* 28, 445–470.

Fischer, K.W. (1980). A theory of cognitive development: the control and combination of hierarchies of skills. *Psychological Review,* 87, 477–531.

Furrow, D., Nelson, K. & Benedict, H. (1979). Mothers' speech to children and syntactic development: some simple relationships. *Journal of Child Language,* 6, 423–442.

Gleitman, L.R., Newport, E.L. & Gleitman, H. (1984). The current status of the motherese hypothesis. *Journal of Child Language,* 11, 43–79.

Hetherington, E.M. (1979). Divorce: a child's perspective. *American Psychologist,* 10, 851–858.

Hinde, R.A. & Bateson, P. (1984). Discontinuities versus continuities in behavioural development and the neglect of process. *International Journal of Behavioural Development,* 7, 129–143.

Huston, A.C. (1983). Sex-typing. In E.M. Hetherington (Ed.), *Handbook of child psychology, Vol. IV: Socialization, personality and social development.* New York: Wiley.

Kagan, J., Kearsley, R. B. & Zelazo, P.R. (1978). *Infancy: its place in human development.* Cambridge, Massachusetts: Harvard University Press.

Konner, M. (1982). Biological aspects of the mother-infant bond. In R.E. Emde & R.J. Harmon (Eds.), *The development of attachment and affiliative systems.* New York: Plenum Press.

Lamb, M.E. & Sherrod, L.R. (Eds, 1981). *Infant social cognition.* Hillsdale, New Jersey: Erlbaum.

Lewis, M. & Rosenblum, L.A. (Eds, 1978). *The development of affect.* New York: Plenum Press.

Lytton, H. (1980). *Parent–child interaction: the socialization process observed in twin and singleton families.* New York: Plenum Press.

McCall, R.B., Eichorn, D.H. & Hogarty, P.S. (1977). Transitions in early development. *Monographs of the Society for Research in Child Development,* 42, No. 3 (Serial No. 171).

Maccoby, E.E. (1984). Socialization and developmental change. *Child Development,* 55, 317–328.

Maccoby, E.E. & Matin, J.A. (1983). Socialization in the context of the family: Parent–child interaction. In E.M. Hetherington (Ed.), *Handbook of child psychology, Vol IV: Socialization, personality and social interaction.* New York: Wiley.

Mandler, J. (1983). *Stories, scripts and scenes: aspects of Schema Theory.* Hillsdale, New Jersey: Erlbaum.

Minushin, P. (1985). Families and individual development: provocations from the field of family therapy. *Child Development,* 56, 289–302.

Nelson, K. & Gruendel, J. (1981). Generalised event representations: basic building blocks of cognitive development. In A. Brown & M. Lamb (Eds.), *Advances in developmental psychology* (Vol. 1). Hillsdale, New Jersey: Erlbaum.

Parke, R.D. (1978). Parent-infant interaction: progress, paradigms and problems. In G.P. Sackett (Ed.), *Observing behavior, Vol 1: Theory and applications in mental retadation.* Baltimore: University Park Press.

Passingham, R.E. (1985). Cortical mechanisms and cues for action. *Philosophical Transactions of the Royal Society of London,* B308, 101–111.

Plomin, R., Loehlin, J.C. & DeFries, J.C. (1985). Genetic and environmental components of "environmental" influences. *Developmental Psychology,* 21, 391–402.

Radke-Yarrow, M., Zahn-Waxler, C. & Chapman, M. (1983). Children's prosocial dispositions and behavior. In E.M. Hetherington (Ed.), *Handbook of child psychology, Vol. IV: Socialization, personality and social development.* New York: Wiley.

Rest, J.R. (1983). Morality. In J.H. Flavell & E.M. Markman (Eds.), *Handbook of child psychology, Vol. III: Cognitive psychology.* New York: Wiley.

Rogosa, D. (1980). A critique of cross-lagged correlation. *Psychological Bulletin,* 88, 245–258.

Rutter, M. (1981). *Maternal deprivation reassessed.* Harmondsworth: Penguin.

Sackett, G.P. (1978). Measurement in observation research. In G.P. Sackett (Ed.), *Observing behaviour, Vol II: Data Collection and analysis methods.* Baltimore University Park Press.

Schaffer, H.R. (Ed. 1977). *Studies in mother–infant interaction.* London: Academic Press.

Schaffer, H.R. (1984). *The child's entry into a social world.* London: Academic Press.

Schaffer, H.R. (1986a). Psychobiological development in a social context. In H. Ruch &

H.C. Steinhausen (Eds.), *Psychobiology and early development.* Amsterdam: North-Holland/Elsevier.

Schaffer, H.R. (1986b). Some thoughts of an ordinologist. *Developmental Review, 6,* 115–121.

Schaffer, H.R. & Collis, G.M. (1986). Parental responsiveness and child behaviour. In W. Sluckin & M. Herbert (Eds.), *Parental behaviour in animals and humans.* Oxford: Blackwell.

Schaffer, H.R. & Liddell, C. (1984). Adult-child interaction under dyadic and polyadic conditions. *British Journal of Developmental Psychology, 2,* 33–42.

Schneider-Rosen, K. & Cicchetti, D. (1984). The relationship between affect and cognition in maltreated infants: quality of attachment and the development of visual self-recognition. *Child Development, 55,* 648–658.

Shantz, C.U. (1983). Social cognition. In J.H. Flavell & E.M. Markman (Eds.), *Handbook of child psychology, Vol. III: Cognitive psychology.* New York: Wiley.

Vygotsky, L.S. (1978). *Mind in society.* Cambridge, Massachusetts: M.I.T. Press.

Wachs, T.D. (1983). The use and abuse of environment in behavior-genetic research. *Child Development, 54,* 396–407.

"Warnock Report" (1984). *Report of the Committee of Inquiry into Human Fertilisation and Embryology.* London: H.M.S.O.

Walters, E., Wippman, J. & Sroufe, L.A. (1979). Attachment, positive affect and competence in the peer group. *Child Development, 50,* 821–829.

Wertsch, J.V., McNamee, G.D., McLane, J.B. & Budwig, N.A. (1980). The adult–child dyad as a problem-solving system. *Child Development, 51,* 1215–1221.

Whiting, B. (1980). Culture and social behavior: a model for the development of social behavior. *Ethos, 8,* 95–116.

6

Environmental Context of Child Development

Arnold J. Sameroff
University of Illinois, Chicago

Pediatrics has been the discipline most concerned with the prevention of developmental disabilities. Among these disabilities are a variety of physical and behavioral disorders that require long-term intervention and treatment at great social cost. It has always been clear that disabilities affect the family and the community by the enormous drain on emotional and financial resources. It has been less obvious that the disabilities are in turn affected by parents and society. Prevention approaches that focus on the affected individual alone frequently have been found to be inadequate. The usual explanation for the ineffectiveness of such intervention programs is that the wrong treatment is being used. Another interpretation is that the treatment did not extend to a wide enough social context. In many cases, family and cultural factors may be more important than factors in the child for preventing developmental disabilities. This review is devoted to providing a balanced perspective on the factors that contribute to healthy psychologic outcomes in children. In this view, the biologic condition is only one ingredient in the developmental formula that will lead to intellectual and social-emotional competence.

Whereas linkages have been found between some "germs" and specific biologic disorders, this has not been true for behavioral disorders. Attempts to prevent developmental disabilities in the sense of deterring a biologic factor will have meaning in a very small percentage of

Reprinted with permission from *The Journal of Pediatrics,* 1986, Vol. 109, No. 1, 192–200. Copyright 1986 by the C.V. Mosby Company.

cases, although these cases may be the most severe and profound. On the other hand, the vast majority of identified handicaps are the result of factors more strongly associated with psychologic and social environment than of any intrinsic characteristics of the child. Between these two categories lie the high-risk graduates of neonatal intensive care units, whose risk for retardation is a complex function of the interplay between their biologic development and experience. New approaches to biologic and behavioral development emphasize causal analyses based on probabilistic interactions of multiple factors.[1] These approaches were required to explain paradoxes that occurred when explanations for a variety of disorders were restricted to linear causal models. Agent-disease models were most effective in understanding acute, primarily infectious diseases, in contrast to more chronic disorders.[2] For chronic disorders, whether heart disease, cancer, or mental retardation, unfavorable outcomes are produced by a combination of biologic, psychologic, social, and environmental risks, usually involving complex interactions among these factors.

The complexity of the relationships between germs, context, and disorder is illustrated by the study of cytomegalovirus.[3] Congenital cytomegalovirus infections are found in about 1% of babies born in the United States, with the highest rates in infants of teenage mothers of low socioeconomic status.[4] Of those infected, fewer than 5% have symptoms. As a group, infants with subclinical infections had lower IQ scores than did noninfected comparison infants, and about 10% to 20% had later central nervous system deficits. However, these differences were found only between infected lower socioeconomic status (SES) children and their peers. When similar comparisons were made between groups of infected and noninfected middle-class children, no IQ differences were found.[5] For such disorders, at least two factors and probably more are involved in producing clinical symptoms. Because the combination of these factors varies in each individual, the probability that a disorder will result will vary.

If we turn directly to the study of developmental disabilities, especially mental retardation, the necessity for the consideration of nonbiologic factors becomes even more apparent. Epidemiologic surveys in Sweden have found a prevalence of severe mental retardation in childhood of about 3:1000, compatible with rates of severe mental retardation in the United States. On the other hand, the prevalence of mild mental retardation in Sweden is about 4:1000, eight or ten times lower than rates recorded in the United States. Susser et al.[6] point out that these rates are related to the reduction in Sweden of cultural-familial retardation and evidence the powerful impact of the social environment on mental performance.

Another indication of the role of environment in mild mental retardation is the percentage of such children with detectable clinical abnormalities. In Sweden, 40% of mildly retarded children have identifiable conditions,[7] whereas the comparable proportion in the United States is only 10%. In the Collaborative Perinatal Project of the National Institute of Neurological Diseases and Stroke, the proportion of cases with mild mental retardation and detectable abnormalities was 14% for white children and 6% for blacks.[8] Similarly, in an English study that compared rates of mild mental retardation in schools with high or low social standing, the rate for children with organic conditions was twice as high in the schools with low social standing, but the rate for mildly retarded children without clinical abnormalities was 15 times as high.[9] It can be argued that there are subtle biologic factors yet to be discovered that will explain mental retardation in all children, but there is a great deal of evidence to support an alternative hypothesis. This evidence is reviewed below.

IDENTIFYING TARGETS FOR TREATMENT

To prevent developmental disabilites, a clear idea of the causes of the disorder is necessary. Because intellectual functioning requires cerebral activity, a biologic orientation would lead one to conclude that mental retardation must result from damage to the brain. Targets for treatment then become those factors that produce brain damage.

The basis for the connection between developmental disabilities and perinatal factors was laid more than a century ago in the work of Little,[10] who first focused attention on asphyxia as a cause of brain damage in the child. The mechanism of such a connection remained elusive, but this did not prevent many investigators from proposing various cause-effect models. Gesell and Amatruda[11] popularized the concept of "minimal cerebral damage" as the causal link. The inability to document the linkage was attributed to the adjective "minimal, " that is, undetectable.

The empirical basis for such a connection was provided in the work of Pasamanick and Knobloch[12] when they proposed the existence of a "continuum of reproductive casualty." In a series of retrospective studies in which they examined the delivery of birth histories of children with a variety of subsequent disorders, they were able to find a number of significant relationships. From these data they postulated a dimension running from gross neurologic disorders such as cerebral palsy and epilepsy at one extreme to a range of minor motor, perceptual, learning, and behavioral disabilities at the other. The more severe the disability (e.g., cerebral palsy in contrast to tics) the more severe the causal perinatal complication (e.g., maternal bleeding in contrast to cesarean section).

TESTING CAUSAL HYPOTHESES

Retrospective studies, such as those of Pasamanick and Knobloch, are important for generating hypotheses; however, other approaches are necessary to test them. In a typical retrospective study, persons are identified who already have the disorder, and then the investigator looks into their early history to find some cause. Retrospective approaches, however, entail serious problems in subject selection, because only those subjects who have the later disorder are studied. By contrast, prospective research permits the selection of subjects with early characteristics thought to be implicated in the cause of the later disorder. If indeed asphyxia leads to brain damage and mental retardation, and if a group of infants who had asphyxia at birth were followed up, a significantly greater amount of retardation would be found in this group than in a control group of infants who did not have anoxia.

Even if such a prospective connection were found, another explanation is possible. One of the ancillary findings of Pasaminick and Knobloch's epidemiologic work was that the absolute number of abnormalities of pregnancy was higher among poorer groups. Children from poorer families have poorer intellectual and social outcomes.[13] Later lower intelligence scores could be a consequence of earlier medical problems, or they could be a consequence of the fact that poorer families have both more medical problems and children with intellectual problems.

In one of the better of the longitudinal studies of the consequences of birth complications, Graham et al.[14] tried to overcome the inadequacies of previous studies that used either poor measures of anoxia at birth or poor measures of intelligence at follow-up. They argued that if a large variety of measures, including neurologic, personality adjustment, and perceptual-motor tasks, were utilized in a longitudinal study, the significant differences between the affected and control groups should be revealed. Several hundred infants from a St. Louis hospital were seen in the newborn period[15] and were followed up at 3 and 7 years of age.[16,17] As expected, when examined during the first days of life, anoxic infants were found to be impaired on a number of behavioral indices.[14] When the performance on these measures was compared with a prognostic score based on the degree of anoxia experienced by the children, those infants with the poorest prognostic scores performed most poorly on the newborn assessments.

At 3 years of age the children were tested with a battery of cognitive, perceptual-motor, personality, and neurologic tests.[16] The group of anoxic infants scored lower than did controls on all tests of cognitive function, had more positive neurologic findings, and showed some personality differences, but there were no differences on tests of perceptual-motor functioning. At 7 years of age the children were again tested.[17] Surprisingly, significant IQ differences had disappeared between the anoxic group and the control population; of the 21 cognitive and perceptual measures, only two showed differences. The investigators were forced to conclude that anoxic newborn infants showed minimal impairment of functioning at 7 years and that efforts to predict current functioning on the basis of the severity of newborn medical status were highly unreliable.

Many advances were made in diagnostic and assessment technology during the 1960s, but there was little change in the pattern of results among prospective studies of birth complications. Gottfried,[18] in a review of 20 investigations of the longitudinal effects of anoxia, came to conclusions similar to those of the St. Louis study, among which were that (1) intellectual consequences of perinatal anoxia are more prevalent in infants and preschoolers than in older children and adolescents; (2) anoxic subjects as a group are not mentally retarded; and (3) whether anoxic subjects are deficient in specific intellectual abilities is not known.

The most compelling of the prospective longitudinal studies in neonates, if only for its magnitude, is the Collaborative Perinatal Project of the National Institute of Neurological Diseases and Stroke in the United States.[19] Between 1959 and 1965, more than 50,000 women and their infants were recruited at birth, primarily from clinic population in 12 medical centers, to investigate the relationship between birth condition and later neurologic or behavioral deficits. The first major report of developmental outcome was the analysis of the IQ scores of the sample when the children were 4 years of age.[8] The effects on intelligence of 169 prenatal, delivery, infant, and family variables were examined. The implicit causal hypotheses of the collaborative study were reflected in this set of measures: Only eight of the 169 variables examined were related to family characteristics; the remaining 161 were assessments of the medical and developmental condition of the mother and child through the first year of life. The surprising result of the 4-year analysis was that the intellectual outcome for children was far better explained by the small set of family factors than any combination of the multitude of biomedical variables.

In the second major report on the intellectual development of the children from the collaborative study the focus moved from the general case of mental retardation to examine the cause of more specific learning disabilities.[20] It is not surprising that children with low IQs do poorly in school. But what about children with normal intelligence who do poorly? The analysis of the development of these children was expected to offer new hope for the identification of specific biomedical causes of these school-age disorders. Whereas the cause of general mental retardation did not seem to be illuminated by analysis of the early medical condition of the child, perhaps more specific entities, such as learning disabilities, dyslexia, minimal brain dysfunction, hyperkinetic syndrome, or attention deficit disorder, might be better targets for biologic causal models.

From a sample of 35,000 children tested at 7 years of age in the collaborative study, about a thousand were identified as having normal intelligence but poor school performance. This cohort was compared with a demographically matched sample of more than 6000 children with normal school performance to evaluate the contribution of perinatal conditions, behavior during the preschool period, and the child's social environment to problems of learning, reading, and hyperactivity.

The most compelling result of the 7-year follow-up analysis was that even when specific conditions are studied, the primary causal factors reside not in the child's biomedical history but in the environment, that is, the social context of development. The authors concluded that their major findings support and augment the conclusions of others that "lower socioeconomic status, less maternal education, higher birth order, and larger family size are related to higher rates of academic failure" (Broman et al.,[20] p 92).

The report of the school behavior of the large sample in the collaborative project supported the findings of many other studies that followed the development of smaller groups of children who had experienced perinatal complications. If social variables are ignored, there seems to be a correlation causal connection between birth complications and later lower IQ. When social status is included in the analysis, children from poorer SES groups are found to have the most perinatal difficulties and the lowest IQ scores. In fact, an adverse medical condition and an adverse social condition frequently act synergistically to worsen the fate of these children compared with children who experience only one of these detrimental conditions.[21]

A new generation of advances in neonatology has produced a new breed of intensive care nursery graduates. Not only are these infants of far lower birth weight than in previous samples, but diagnostic procedures have moved from inferred relations between birth complications and brain development to actual examinations of the brain through a variety of imaging techniques. New questions can be asked about the relation of birth condition to developmental disabilities. One such question is whether biologic factors play a greater role in the behavioral outcome of these very low birth weight (VLBW) infants than in heavier groups of infants. Another question is whether more sophisticated assessments of neurologic conditions can provide clearer causal links to later disabilities.

In regard to the question of whether VLBW infants have worse outcomes than LBW infants, the data are not completely clear. Because of the recency of many medical innovations, there is a necessary lag before extensive longitudinal data will be available. Furthermore, the introduction of some changes in high-risk infant care practices may have produced increases in morbidity while the appropriate applications were being tested. In a survey of the world literature on follow-up of VLBW babies, Stewart et al.[22] concluded that the chances of a healthy survival have increased steadily, whereas the prevalence of handicap has remained stable. It would not be unreasonable to assume from these data that the role of social factors in the development of VLBW infants will be similar to their role in previous studies of high-risk infants.

The studies reviewed give clear evidence that there is no deterministic relationship between perinatal medical status and later outcome. Further data from the Collaborative Perinatal Project indicate that the biologic condition of the child even a year after birth is not strongly related to later disability. Of 229 children in whom cerebral palsy was diagnosed at one year of age, more than half were free of motor handicap at age 7 years.[23] In most of the children who were judged to be nonhandicapped at follow-up, mild cerebral palsy had been diagnosed, but the group included more than one fourth of those with moderate or severe cerebral palsy.

The second question was whether more sophisticated diagnostic techniques can more accurately identify those children who will have later disabilities. Neonatal neurologic examinations continue to produce many false positive results in the light of follow-up studies, indicating a high degree of transient neonatal morbidity.[24] Brain lesions have been hypothesized to have a strong connection with developmental disabilities. A common method of determining cerebral intraventricular hemorrhage has been use of computed tomographic brain scans. In a 24-month follow-up of VLBW infants with varying degrees of hemorrhage, Papile et al.[25] found more major handicaps to be associated with higher grades of hemorrhage. However, the majority of infants with hemorrhage grades 1 through 3 had no major handicap, and not a few infants with the most extensive grade 4 hemorrhage were found to have no evidence of handicap. In a similar study,[26] a large proportion of infants with moderate ventriculomegaly showed spontaneous regression or stabilization, with normal development in a high percentage of cases.

Despite the lack of linear connections between birth status and measures of later general cognitive functioning, such as IQ scores, there is evidence from a number of studies that differentiated cognitive assessments may reveal subtle specific deficits in behavior at later ages. For example, deficits have been found in visual recognition memory.[27,28] In these cases, however, it is not clear that such deficits are maintained in development independent of environmental conditions. Sigman[28] reported that for full-term infants there were relationships between caretaking patterns and visual attentiveness. For preterm infants the relationship was only evident in a female subsample; visual attention performance was correlated to the amount of verbal and social interaction with caretakers. Rose[29] found that preterm infants performed more poorly at differentiating novel from familiar stimuli in an attention task at 6 months of age. However, if the preterm infants received extrasensory stimulation during the first weeks of life, their later performance was indistinguishable from that of full-term infants. Rose suggested that visual recognition memory is negatively affected by prematurity and that performance can be improved by altering early environmental conditions. In a study that compared preterm infants' performance on a complex perceptual processing task at 1 year with that of lower and middle-class full-term infants, Rose et al.[30] found that the preterm and lower SES full-term infants performed similarly, with neither doing as well as the middle SES full-term babies. These studies indicate that environment is able to facilitate or inhibit even specific aspects of cognitive functioning throughout the first year of life.

The need to study the developmental course of specific functions is evidenced by the differential impact of perinatal events on separate aspects of behavior. Siegel[31] examined the relation between child language and intellectual competence at 3 years and reproductive, perinatal, and demographic risk factors. A measure of the home environment in terms of cognitive and social-emotional stimulation, the Home Observation for Measurement of the Environment (HOME) scale,[32] also was made at 3 years. Children who were classified as being at risk at 12 months but who had scores in the normal range at 3 years came from families with significantly higher scores on the HOME scale. Children not detected as being at risk in infancy, but whose development was delayed at 3 years, came from families with lower scores on the HOME scale. In a further follow-up of this sample at 5 years, Siegel[33] added specific tests of perceptual-motor functioning to the earlier measures of language and general intelligence. She found that environmental and demographic variables continued to contribute more to the prediction of language functioning and delay, but that perinatal and reproductive variables contributed more to the prediction of perceptual-motor functioning.

In the absence of frank disorder, major questions remain as to the nature of the developmental risk to which LBW and VLBW infants are subject. In those who show no later deficits, a case can be made for biologic resiliency or recovery. In those that do have later difficulties, it is not altogether clear that there was a direct connection with the biologic risk. An explanation is needed for the discrepancy between the retrospective and prospective studies of perinatal risk factors reported above.

CASUALTY AND CONTEXT

How do we explain the later disappearance of the effects of severe trauma to the early physiologic functioning of the brain? Moreover, how do we explain the retrospective data that tends to show that children with a variety of deficits do have more perinatal complications in their histories than children without these disorders? The answers to these questions require the study of children in their environmental context. This context is invisible in most follow-up studies of perinatal complications because it is rarely assessed. Luckily, some studies have examined both sets of factors: the developmental progress of high-risk infants, and the family and social context.

An excellent example of such research is the Kauai study of child development. Werner et al.[34] reported on the growth of all 670 children born in 1955 on Kauai in the Hawaiian Islands. The multiracial nature of Hawaii and the total sampling of social class involved in the Kauai sample permitted the investigators to provide ample controls for both racial and social class variables. During the newborn period, each infant was scored on a 4-point scale for severity of perinatal complications. At 20 months and again at 10 years of age these scores were related to assessments of physical health, psychologic status, and such environmental variables as socioeconomic status, family stability, and mother's education.

As in the St. Louis study, during early childhood, Kauai infants who had had severe perinatal stress were found to have lower scores. In addition, however, a clear interaction was found between the impairing effect of perinatal complications and environmental variables, especially socioeconomic status. For infants living in a high SES environment with a stable family structure or with a mother who was well educated, the IQ score differences between children with and without complication was only 5 to 7 points. For infants living in a low SES environment, with low family stability or with a mother of poor educational background, the difference in mean IQ scores between infants with and without perinatal complications ranged from 19 to 37 points. The results of the Kauai study seem to indicate that perinatal complications taken alone are not consistently related to later physical and psychologic development, but only when combined with and supported by persistently poor environmental circumstances.

In the infants of the Kauai sample there was no correlation between the perinatal stress score and the measures at 10 years.[35] Some correlation was found, however, between the 20-month and 10-year data, especially when SES and parents' educational level were taken into consideration. The stability of intellectual functioning was much higher for those children who had IQ scores < 80 at the 10-year testing period. All of these children had 20-month scores of ≤ 100, with almost half < 80, and the majority had parents with little education and low SES. The Kauai study seems to suggest that risk factors operative during the perinatal period disappear during childhood as more potent familial and social factors exert their influence. Werner et al.[34] extrapolated their findings to predict that of every 1000 live births in Kauai, by age 10 years only 66% of children would be functioning adequately without a recognized physical, intellectual, or behavioral problem in school. In the 34% who had problems at the age of 10 years, only a minor proportion could be attributed to the effects of serious perinatal stress. The authors concluded that "ten times more children had problems related to the effects of poor early environment than to the effects of perinatal stress."

How are we to understand a situation where perinatal complications have a greater impact on later development in children raised in poor environmental conditions? These data imply that the biologic outcome of pregnancy is worse for those in poorer environments. The level of later disability is clearly not the result of the delivery complications alone; children with identical complications raised in good environmental situations show fewer consequences of such problems. The few studies of infant development that have examined environmental factors typically have used global variables, for example, family SES or mother's education. When a more differentiated view of the developmental context is examined, we can appreciate the multiplicity of factors that have an impact on the child's progress. Social status is only a summary variable that incorporates a variety of risk factors that exert both independent and interactive influences on outcome. These variables include enduring characteristics of the family (e.g., number of children; marital and minority status), psychologic characteristics of the parents (e.g., mental health, education, child-rearing attitudes, beliefs and coping skills), and stressful life events that interfere with the family's ability to provide a nurturant context for the child. Sameroff and Seifer [36] have shown that the developmental outcome for young children is determined by these multiple variables. The greater the number of these factors that are in the risk category, the poorer the outcome for the child. No single factor is always present or always absent when high levels of social-emotional and intellectual incompetency are found. If the child also is at risk by virtue of biologic condition, this must be added to the existing list of risk factors in the family. To understand how these risk factors operate, we can turn to specific studies of the interaction between biologic risk and caregiver behavior.

Several investigations have been directed at identifying specific factors that may differentiate caregiver interactions with normal infants from those with infants who had medically complicated newborn periods.[37] In a review of this work, Goldberg et al.[38] found consistent group differences in the developing parent-infant relationship. At discharge preterm infants were less alert and responsive and their motor coordination and state control were less organized. Their parents appeared to be less actively involved, made less body contact, and smiled, talked to, and touched them less. Goldberg concluded that the parent-preterm infant relationship may follow a different course of development than do full-term dyads.

The continuation of these differences in interaction patterns through 2 years of age was confirmed in a study by Barnard et al.[39] They found that by 8 months of age preterm infants had caught up to full-term babies in their ability to participate in the mother-infant interaction, but the mothers continued to treat them differently. The mothers of preterm infants were less positive in teaching interactions and described themselves as less involved with the child.

One cause of these differences is the separation of high-risk infants from their parents.[40] The separation effects are somewhat confounded by the effects of the illness that cause the separation. In an innovative study, Field et al.[41] compared interactions of mothers with preterm, full-term, and post-term infants. If the preterm infants behaved differently from both full-term and post-term infants, the explanation would be based on their relative biologic immaturity or in the fact that they were the only group separated from the mother during the lying-in period. The results were that both post-term and preterm infants differed from the full-term control group in attentive behavior and mother caregiving behavior. The hypothesized common factor was that both groups of infants had physical problems, albeit different ones. To explore directly the effects of illness, Minde et al.[42] compared relatively sick with relatively well VLBW infants. Not suprising, the sick infants were less interactive than the well ones. Somewhat more surprising was the finding that mothers visited the sicker infants less than the well ones, and were still interacting less with them several months after discharge. In a study of twins with birth weights < 1500 gm, Minde et al.[43] found that mothers developed preferences within the first month for the healthier twin that were expressed in more positive behavior for at least 6 months afterward.

Illness affects the behavior of newborn infants and their parents. Would these behavioral differences be consistently related to later developmental problems? Cohen et al.[44] compared the development of sick and well preterm infants in their UCLA longitudinal study. They found that a postnatal illness rating alone did not relate to outcome at 5 years of age, but that children who were doing poorly all had had a number of such hazardous events. They explained this paradox by hypothesizing two paths from illness to outcome. One path reflected the negative consequences of illness for development; the other reflected the ameliorating and fostering effects of good caregiving. Better parental caregiving interactions were related to better outcome. None of the sick infants who received good caregiving had below average intelligence scores at 5 years.

INTERVENTION EFFECTS

The relations that have been described between child development and environmental effects are primarily based on correlational analyses of risk factors and longitudinal outcomes. To test these interactive causal models, experiments that manipulated environmental factors would be necessary. Such studies can be found in attempts at early intervention with infants at high biologic risk, primarily preterm infants. This rich literature[37] cannot be extensively reviewed in this context, but several examples give an indication of the results of intervention efforts. To the extent that environmental risks are found in demographic variables such as SES or minority status, effective intervention strategies lie primarily in the political rather than the health domain. However, developmental risks associated with parental lack of knowledge or cognitively and emotionally impoverished parent-child interaction patterns can be suitable targets for behavioral interventions.

One group of mothers generally defined as high-risk are lower SES, single teenagers. Field[45] reviewed several approaches for working with this population. In one study the mothers were given demonstrations of the Brazelton Neonatal Behavioral Assessment Scale[46] during their pre-term baby's first month of life and were asked to administer a version of the examination independently.[47] The treated mothers had better interactions with their infants, and by the end of a year their infants were attaining higher developmental scores than a control group of infants. Another group of low SES teenage mothers were visited at home every 2 weeks and were trained to do a variety of age-appropriate baby exercises and simple developmental assessments. At the end of a year, infants in the intervention group were heavier and longer than control infants, did better on developmental assessment mental scales, and were rated by their mothers as having a less difficult temperament; their mother-child interactions were more playful and verbally stimulating. In a third study, an attempt was made at more substantial impact on the teen-age mother's life. A new group of such mothers brought their infants to a center-based infant nursery, where they carried out the exercise program from the previous home intervention and were employed as part-time teacher aide trainees for 20 hours a week. Thus the teenage mothers received free day care for their infants, a paid job, training, and an incentive to continue schooling. At the end of a year the infants of those mothers were heavier and taller than the home intervention group of infants, and they performed significantly better on both mental and motor scales of developmental assessments. Of possibly more important long-term value to their infants, the mothers in the center-based program had a much higher rate of return to school and a lower rate of repeat pregnancy. Such extensive interventions would not be necessary or appropriate for many groups of mothers with better personal or social resources. On the other hand, the extent of the intervention needs to be determined more by the deficits in the caregiving context than by the biologic condition of the child. Field[45] concludes her review by noting that the reported effects are suggestive of a transactional phenomenon whereby teaching parents other ways of caregiving, or altering their perceptions, attitudes, and behaviors, appears to mediate developmental strides in their infants, which in turn reinforce and elicit more of the parenting skills necessary for fostering development.

SUMMARY

In the summary of a recent report to the National Institute of Neurologic and Communicative Disorders and Stroke, and the National

Institute of Child Health and Human Development on current knowledge about prenatal and perinatal cause of neurologic dysfunction, Freeman[48] states, "It once seemed simple to say that a specific insult, such as birth trauma, asphyxia or obstetric maneuvers, were each the cause of brain disorders, and that prevention of these insults would substantially decrease the number of afflicted children. Our indepth review of available information shows that while each of these insults, either alone or together, can cause brain damage, they are not alone frequent causes of mental retardation . . . In the area of mental retardation, we despair of disentangling the individual environmental factors that interact with the individual child's biologic potential to produce a given level of function. Yet we continue to believe that optimizing environment and minimizing risk factors will result in better function and adaptability for the individual" (pp 13–15).

The despair felt by the authors of the report is in part a consequence of the disproportionate lack of attention that has been paid to the study of the environment's role in enhancing or hindering child development. Much of the research reviewed above has pointed to fruitful directions for further research efforts in the analysis of environmental influences. Many factors, including family social context, parental child-rearing attitudes and practices, the school system, and the availability of medical and educational services to the disabled, have been identified as playing a role in the child's outcome.

For many years the theory of a continuum of reproductive casualty played a major role in filling the gap between early medical risk and later developmental disabilities by hypothesizing as yet unmeasurable biologic insults. As our understanding of the developmental process has advanced, a new continuum has been hypothesized to fill the gap. Sameroff and Chandler[49] proposed a "continuum of caretaking casualty" to describe the range of developmental disorders that could be attributed to poor parenting, that is, to the socioeconomic and familial factors that tend to overshadow the effects of early perinatal difficulties in producing emotional and intellectual problems in children. Prevention has become a much more complex enterprise because, as in the analysis of biomedical factors thought to lead to mental retardation, no single environmental factor alone determines outcome. On the other hand, this conclusion has been interpreted optimistically because it permits a variety of possibilities for either prevention or treatment.

REFERENCES

1.   Gollin ES. Development and plasticity. In: Gollin ES, ed. Developmental plasticity. New York: Academic Press, 1981.

2. Scott KG, Carran DT. Prevention of mental retardation. Am Psychol (in press).
3. Eisenberg L. Overview. In: Parron DL, Eisenberg L eds. Infants at risk for developmental dysfunction health and behavior: a research agenda. Interim Report No. 4, Institute of Medicine. Washington D C · National Academy Press, 1982.
4. Hanshaw J. Cytomegalovirus infections. Pediatr Rev 1981; 2(8):245–251.
5. Hanshaw J, Scheiner A, Moxley A, et al. School failure and deafness after "silent" congenital cytomegalovirus infection. N Engl J Med 1976; 295:468–470.
6. Susser M, Hauser WA, Kiely JL, et al. Quantitative estimates of prenatal and perinatal risk factors for perinatal mortality, cerebral palsy, mental retardation and epilepsy. In: Freeman JM, ed. Prenatal and perinatal factors associated with brain disorders. Washington D.C.: National Institutes of Health, 1985, Publ. No. 85–1149.
7. Hagberg B, Hagberg G, Lewerth A, et al: Mild mental retardation in Swedish school children. I. Prevalence. Acta Paediatr Scand 1981; 70:445–452.
8. Broman SH. Perinatal anoxia and cognitive development in early childhood. In Field TM, ed. Infants born at risk. New York: Spectrum Publications, 1979.
9. Stein ZA, Susser M. The social distribution of mental retardation. Am J Mental Defic 1963;67:811–821.
10. Little WJ. On the influence of abnormal partuition, difficult labor, premature birth, and asphyxia neonatorum on the mental and physical condition of the child especially in relation to deformities. Lancet 1861;2:378–380.
11. Gesell A, Amatruda C. Developmental diagnosis. New York, Hoeber, 1941.
12. Pasamanick B, Knobloch H. Epidemiologic studies on the complications of pregnancy and the birth process. In: Caplan G, ed. Prevention of mental disorders in children. New York: Basic Books, 1961.
13. Broman SH, Nichols PL, Kennedy WA. Preschool IQ: prenatal and early developmental correlates. Hillsdale, N.J., Lawrence Erlbaum Associates, 1975.
14. Graham FK, Pennoyer MM, Caldwell BM, et al. Anoxia as a significant perinatal experience: a critique. J Pediatr 1957; 50:556–569.
15. Graham FK, Matarazzo RG, Caldwell BM. Behavioral differences between normal and traumatized newborns. II. Standardization, reliability, and validity. Psychol Monogr 1956;70:21(428).
16. Graham FK, Ernhart CB, Thurston DL, et al. Development three years after perinatal anoxia and other potentially damaging newborn experiences. Psychol Monogr 1962; 73:3(522).
17. Corah NL, Anthony EJ, Painter P, et al. Effects of perinatal anoxia after seven years. Psychol Monogr 1965;79:3(596).
18. Gottfried AW. Intellectual consequences of perinatal anoxia. Psychol Bull 1973; 80:231–242.
19. Broman S. The Collaborative Perinatal Project: an overview. In: Mednick SA, Harway M, Finello KM, eds. Handbook of longitudinal research, vol 1. New York: Praeger, 1984.
20. Broman S, Bien E, Shaughnessy P. Low achieving children: the first seven years. Hillsdale, N.J.: Lawrence Erlbaum Associates, 1985.
21. Escalona SK. Babies at double hazard: early development of infants at biologic and social risk. Pediatrics 1982;70:670–768.
22. Stewart AL, Reynolds EOR, Lipscomb AP. Outcome for infants of very low birthweight: survey of world literature. Lancet 1981;1:1038–1041.
23. Nelson KB, Ellenberg JH. Children who "outgrew" cerebral palsy. Pediatrics 1982;69:529–536.

24. Bierman-van Eendenburg MEC, Jurgens-van der Zee AD, Olinga AA, et al. Predictive value of neonatal neurological examination: a follow-up study at 18 months. Dev Med Child Neurol 1981;23:296–305.

25. Papile L-A, Munsick-Bruno G, Schaefer A. Relationship of cerebral intraventricular hemorrhage and early childhood neurologic handicaps. Pediatric 1983;103:273–277.

26. Liechty EA, Gilmo RL, Bryson CQ, Bull MJ. Outcome of high-risk neonates with ventriculomegaly. Dev Med Child Neurol 1983;25:162–168.

27. Rose SA, Gottfried AW, Bridger WH. Effects of haptic cues on visual recognition memory in full-term and preterm infants. Infant Behav Dev 1979;2:55–67.

28. Sigman M. Individual differences in infant attention: relations to birth status and intelligence at five years. In Field T, Sostek A, eds. Infants born at risk: physiological, perceptual, and cognitive processes. New York: Grune & Stratton, 1983.

29. Rose S. Enhancing visual recognition memory in preterm infants. Dev Psychol 1980;16:85–92.

30. Rose SA, Gottfried AW, Bridger W. Cross-modal transfer in infants: relationship to prematurity and socioeconomic background. Dev Psychol 1979;14:643–652.

31. Sigel LS. Reproductive, perinatal, and environmental factors as predictors of the cognitive and language development of preterm and full-term infants. Child Dev 1982;53:963–973.

32. Bradley RH, Caldwell BM. The relation of home environment, cognitive competence, and IQ among males and females. Child Dev 1980;51:1140–1148.

33. Siegel LS. The prediction of possible learning disabilities in preterm and full-term children. In: Field T, Sostek A, eds. Infants born at risk: physiological, perceptual, and cognitive processes. New York: Grune & Stratton, 1983.

34. Werner EE, Bierman JM, French FE. The Children of Kauai. Honolulu: University of Hawaii, 1971.

35. Werner EE, Honzik M, Smith R. Prediction of intelligence and achievement at ten years from twenty months pediatric and psychologic examinations. Child Dev 1968;39:1036–1075.

36. Sameroff AJ, Seifer R. Familial risk and child competence. Child Dev 1983; 54:1254–1268.

37. Sameroff AJ. The psychological needs of the parent in infant development. In: Avery G, ed. Neonatology, 3rd ed. New York: Lippincott, 1986.

38. Goldberg S, Brachfield S, DiVitto B. Feeding, fussing and play: parent-infant interaction in the first year as a function of prematurity and perinatal medical problems. In: Field TM, Goldberg S, Stern D, eds. High-risk infants and children: adult and peer interactions. New York: Academic Press, 1980:133–153.

39. Barnard KE, Bee HL, Hammond MA. Developmental changes in maternal interactions with term and preterm infants. Infant Behav Dev 1984;7:101–113.

40. Klaus MH, Kennell JH. Parent-infant bonding. St. Louis: Mosby, 1982.

41. Field T, Dempsey J, Schuman HH. Developmental follow-up of pre- and post-term infants. In: Friedman S, Sigman M, eds. Preterm birth and psychological development. New York: Academic Press, 1981.

42. Minde K, Whitelaw A, Brown J, Fitzhardinge P. Effect of neonatal complications in premature infants on early parent-infant interactions. Dev Med Child Neurol 1983;25:763.

43. Minde K, Perrotta M, Corter C. The effect of neonatal complications in same-sexed premature twins on their mothers' preferences. J Am Acad Child Psychiatry 1982;21:446.

44. Cohen SE, Sigman M. Parmelee AH, Beckwith L. Perinatal risk and developmental outcome in preterm infants. Semin Perinatol 1982;6:334–339.

45. Field TM. Infants born at risk: early compensatory experiences. In: Bond LA, Joffe JM, eds. Facilitating infant and early childhood development. N.H.. University Press of New England, 1982;251–283.

46. Brazelton TB. Neonatal Behavioral Assessment Scale. London: Spastics International Medical Publications, 1973.

47. Widmayer S, Field T. Effects of Brazelton demonstrations on early interactions of preterm infants and their mothers. Infant Behav Dev 1980;3:79–89.

48. Freeman JM. Summary. In Freeman JM, ed. Prenatal and perinatal factors associated with brain disorders. Washington D.C.: National Insitutes of Health, 1985, Publ. No. 85–1149.

49. Sameroff A, Chandler M. Reproductive risk and the continuum of caretaking casualty. In: Horowitz FD, Hetherington M, Scarr-Salapatek S, Siegel G. Review of Child Development Research, vol 4. Chicago: University of Chicago Press, 1975.

7

Childhood Parental Death and Adult Psychopathology

Paul V. Ragan
Naval Hospital, Bethesda, Maryland
Thomas H. McGlashan
Chestnut Lodge, Rockville, Maryland

Childhood parental death has frequently been linked with adult mental disorders—mostly depression. The authors found no association with psychiatric diagnosis among 72 inpatients who had experienced the death of a parent when they were children, compared with 460 other patients in the Chestnut Lodge Follow-Up Study. The patients with a childhood parental death did, however, have significantly greater family pathology and impaired social and heterosexual functioning. These results refute the view that childhood parental death is singularly causal of adult psychopathology but support its role in multidetermining matrix of contributing factors.

Since Freud (1) and Abraham (2) emphasized the role of loss and early experiences, respectively, in the development of adult depression, it has been widely held that the death of a parent during childhood represents a

Reprinted with permission from the *American Journal of Psychiatry,* 1986, Vol. 143, No. 2, 153–157. Copyright 1986 by the American Psychiatric Association.

Presented at the 138th annual meeting of the American Psychiatric Association, Dallas, May 18–24, 1985.

Supported in part by NIMH grant MH-35174 and by the fund for psychoanalytic research of the American Psychoanalytic Association.

The opinions expressed in this paper are those of the authors and are not to be construed as reflecting the views of the Navy Department, the Naval Service at large, or the Department of Defense.

trauma predisposing the individual to later psychopathology. For more than 40 years, researchers have investigated the incidence of childhood parental death in a wide variety of psychiatric disorders, especially depression (3-17). Two reviews, however, came to opposite conclusions about the role of childhood parental death and subsequent adult depression: Lloyd (18) noted that "parental bereavement during childhood increases the risk of depression in adulthood by a factor of about two or three" (p. 534). Crook and Elliot (19), however, concluded, "There is no sound base of empirical data to support the theorized relationship between parental death during childhood and adult depression or any subtype of adult depression" (p. 258).

Other studies have investigated the link between childhood bereavement and schizophrenia (20-22), antisocial behavior (23-27), and a variety of other psychiatric difficulties (28-33). Overall, no clear relationships emerge, in part because of methodologic pitfalls such as diagnostic vagueness, inadequate characterization of study populations, and shifting definitions of childhood "trauma."

We considered again the issue of parental death and adult psychopathology using a sample of patients participating in a recently completed follow-up study (34, 35). Our sample is unique in this field of investigation in that all patients were systematically rediagnosed according to current nosology, information was available concerning long-term functional outcome, and most of the patients studied were relatively young, chronically ill patients from higher socioeconomic classes. Three principal research questions were addressed: 1) Is childhood parental death a general risk factor for the subsequent development of severe mental illness? 2) Is parental death associated with particular diagnostic syndromes and/or psychopathological behaviors? 3) Is parental death associated with any particular nondiagnostic factors, either before or after the development of illness (i.e., either premorbid or outcome)?

METHOD

The subjects in this study were severely ill psychiatric inpatients at a long-term residential treatment facility who underwent follow-up examination an average of 15 years after discharge. As outlined previously (34), outcome data and diagnostic-demographic data were collected independently.

Outcome data were collected following provision of informed consent by interviews with the patients and/or significant others. The majority of the interviews were conducted by telephone and averaged 2 hours in length. These interviews were conducted and rated by one of us (T.H.M.) or by research-trained social workers. Interviews contained structured and unstructured segments and assessed multiple dimensions of outcome over the entire period of time since discharge. The information gathered was sufficient to rate approximately 40 outcome dimensions, with an average reliability of .71 (kappa and intraclass correlations).

Diagnostic-demographic assessment involved abstracting the patient's medical record into a 25-page document called the chart abstract. From this each patient was rated on approximately 60 demographic-predictor variables and 50 sign and symptom variables, all with a missing data rate of only 12% and with interrater reliabilities averaging .67 (kappa and intraclass correlations). By use of these data, all study patients were rated according to eight current operational diagnostic systems as detailed elsewhere (34).

Eight nonoverlapping study diagnostic categories were assigned by use of these diagnostic systems. Five were psychotic categories: Schizophrenia, schizoaffective psychosis, schizophreniform psychosis, bipolar affective disorder, and unipolar affective disorder. Two were personality disorder categories: schizotypal personality disorder and borderline personality disorder. The final category was nonspecified and labeled "other."

Major comparisons involved two groups, patients who had experienced the death of one or both parents before age 18 and the rest of the follow-up sample. These groups were tested across three families of variables or hypotheses: diagnostic, demographic-predictor, and outcome. Statistical analysis used chi-square tests for categorical variables and t tests for continuous variables. Sample sizes fluctuated depending on the variable tested. Outcome variables, of course, involved patients about whom we obtained follow-up data. Diagnostic and demographic-predictor variables, on the other hand, often involved larger samples because chart abstracts were available for additional patients missing to follow-up. The chart abstract histories did not reliably include the causes of the parents' death. Therefore, no further breakdown and analysis by reason for the parents' death was possible.

RESULTS

In the overall study sample (N = 532), 72 patients (13.5%) were identified as having lost a parent in childhood. Table 1 presents the cumulative frequency and percent of patients who had lost a parent in the total sample across four age periods from birth to 18 years of age. For com-

Table 1. Cumulative Frequency of Parental Death in Four Childhood Age Periods for 532 Adult Patients in the Chestnut Lodge Follow-Up Study and a Population Control Sample[a]

Age of Child by Which One or Both Parents Were Dead (years)	Chestnut Lodge Patients		Control Sample (%)
	N	%	
0–4	15	2.8	2.7
5–9	31	5.8	7.3
10–14	42	7.9	12.7
15–17[b]	72	13.5	17.6

[a]These figures are from a large sample of the U.S. population surveyed in 1940 and reported by the Metropolitan Life Insurance Company in 1944; cited by Gregory (23).
[b]15–18 years for Chestnut Lodge patients.

parison, table 1 also presents a similar breakdown for a normative U.S. sample surveyed from a roughly comparable period of history (23). Although statistical analysis was not possible here, the relative rates fail to suggest that the frequency of childhood parental death was any greater in our severely ill psychiatric patients than in the general population.

The diagnoses of the 72 patients who had experienced parental death are shown in table 2. Rates of patients who experienced parental death in each diagnostic group ranged from 6% to 18%. Chi-square analysis failed to demonstrate any significant differences in these rates. Although antisocial personality disorder was not a study diagnosis, antisocial behaviors and traits (e.g., drug abuse, sexual deviation, trouble with the law, and assaultiveness) were assessed for each patient. Comparisons between patients who had and patients who had not experienced childhood parental death in childhood did not yield any significant differences.

Differences between the two groups of patients emerged most frequently in the realm of family characteristics. As shown in table 3, patients who had experienced childhood parental death scored significantly worse than those who had not on paternal psychopathology, pathology of mothering, family nurturing capacity, family leadership, family global functioning, and family history of substance abuse.

No demographic variable (age, sex, marital status, etc.) discriminated between the patients who had or had not experienced childhood parental death. No differences were found or expected in socioeconomic status because the entire sample was so homogeneous on this variable. Most measures of premorbid functioning also failed to discriminate between

Table 2. Diagnoses of Adult Patients in the Chestnut Lodge
Follow-Up Study

Diagnosis	All Patients (N=532)		Patients With Parental Death (N=72)	
	N	%	N	% of Patients Given Diagnosis
Schizophrenia	188	35	24	13
Schizoaffective psychosis	87	16	16	18
Schizophreniform psychosis	15	3	1	7
Schizotypal personality disorder	33	6	2	6
Borderline personality disorder	94	18	14	15
Bipolar affective disorder	23	4	4	17
Unipolar affective disorder	58	11	6	10
Other	34	6	5	15

the patients, with one exception: patients who had experienced child-hood parental death scored significanly worse on a measure of hetero-sexual functioning before their first episode of illness (table 3). They also formed intense, unstable interpersonal relationships and complained of chronic feelings of emptiness and boredom more frequently than the patients who had not experienced loss of a parent. Finally, at index ad-mission they displayed significantly more severe levels of psycho-pathology—whatever their diagnosis.

Only one outcome measure among the many tested significantly dis-criminated the two groups of patients: frequency of social contacts in the follow-up period (table 3). Another measure, intimate relationships, reached trend level. On both dimensions, the patients who had experi-enced childhood parental death were inferior to those who had not. Im-portant negative outcome results were no different from those reported in the literature for alcohol abuse, legal trouble, or suicidal thoughts and behaviors.

The possible influence on outcome of the child's age at the time of parental death was examined. Preliminary analysis revealed, unex-pectedly, that it was the 32 patients who were adolescents (12–18 years old) rather than the 17 who were children (0–6 years old) or the 23 who were in latency (6–12 years old) who had the worst outcome as measured by the amount of hospitalization, time employed, number of meetings with friends, and the overall level of their functioning.

Table 3. Characteristics of Adult Patients in Chestnut Lodge Follow-Up Study Who Had (N = 72) or Had Not (N = 460) Experienced Childhood Parental Death

Characteristic	Experienced Death	Had Not Experienced Death	Analysis
Baseline			
Paternal psychopathology (mean score[a])	3.8	3.3	t=−2.40, df=496, p=.019
Pathology of mothering (mean score[b])	1.5	1.9	t=3.06, df=482, p=.002
Family nurturing capacity (mean score[c])	1.7	2.0	t=2.04, df=459, p=.042
Family leadership (mean score[c])	1.0	1.3	t=1.99, df=413, p=.047
Family global functioning (mean score[a])	4.2	3.7	t=−3.05, df=492, p=.002
Family history of substance abuse (%)	70	46	χ²=5.43, df=1, p=.020
Premorbid and morbid			
Heterosexual functioning before first episode of illness (mean score[d])	2.1	2.4	t=2.22, df=499, p=.027
Intense, unstable interpersonal relationships (%)	89	74	χ²=6.93, df=1, p=.01
Chronic feelings of emptiness or boredom (%)	48	35	χ²=3.84, df=1, p=.05
Severity of psychopathology at index admission (mean score[a])	5.5	5.3	t=−2.18, df=530, p=.032
Social outcome			
Frequency of social contacts (mean score[e][f])	1.6	2.2	t=2.50, df=438, p=.013
Intimate relationships (mean score[d][f])	1.2	1.6	t=1.84, df=438, p=.066

[a]7-point scale: 1=normal; 7=extremely ill or most pathologic.
[b]5-point scale: 0=extensive; 4=normal.
[c]5-point scale: 0=absent; 4=intact.
[d]5-point scale: 0=none; 4=married or dating regularly.
[e]5-point scale: 0=no contact; 4=weekly contact.
[f]Only 61 patients who had and 385 who had not experienced childhood parental death were included in this analysis.

DISCUSSION

A substantial proportion (13.5%) of our inpatient population sample had lost one or both parents by the time they reached 18 years of age. This rate, however, was not unusual or excessive in comparison with normative rates of parental death during childhood and adolescence in the general population from roughly the same period of history. If anything, the patients in our sample had a lower rate of early parental death (a difference that may be explained by their much higher mean socioeconomic status). These results certainly fail to support any hypotheses about early parental death as a nonspecific risk factor in the development of severe mental illness. They do not, of course, rule out the importance of parental death to specific patients. Since our population consisted of severely and largely chronically mentally ill patients, this study cannot address the effects of early parental death on milder forms of psychopathology such as the neuroses, dysthymias, and less severe personality disorders.

Our results fail to demonstrate any significant association between childhood parental death and diagnosis ("choice" of psychopathology). Patients experiencing childhood parental loss did not cluster preferencially within any study diagnostic group, including schizophrenia and the affective disorders. They also were not significantly associated with antisocial symptoms or behaviors, either around the time of index admission or through the follow-up period.

Although our findings refute any linkage between childhood parental death and the types of psychiatric disorder seen in our population, our results concerning severity of illness at index admission do suggest an association between early parental loss and a quantitative factor in expressed psychopathology. Although childhood loss through parental death may not bear etiologically on the form of mental illness that develops, it may bear pathogenically on its severity and extent in ways as yet not understood.

The nature of any psychological "trauma" associated with premature parental death is unclear and likely to be heterogeneous. Our ratings of parental and family functioning demonstrated the existence of multiple problems in affected families. These were not detailed but generally involved a variety of physical and/or emotional difficulties often leading to or resulting from the mother's or father's demise.

We cannot judge the effects of childhood parental death using a single determination theory. Psychopathology is multidetermined. We must also look beyond negative conditions to positive, compensatory influences when assessing the role of early "traumatic" events. Parental object loss falling on the fertile soil of an impaired family unit, for example, may be what is pathogenic rather than early parental death per se. This view is consistent with the findings of Soloff and Millward (36) that both separation trauma and pathological family structure occurred more frequently in the developmental histories of borderline patients.

How can we account for the strong tradition of associating adult psychopathology and childhood parental death? Three possibilities present themselves. First is state-dependent association and recall. Depressed patients, for example, are likely to ruminate selectively about sad and depressing personal historical events like parental loss. Second is retrospective justification, or the need to construct etiologic hypotheses that externalize to past events responsibility for mental illness in order to defend against personal feelings of blame, guilt, and shame. Third is retrospective rationalization and closure, or the need to render certain (i.e., have an answer for) that which is unknown and therefore frightening.

Although early parental death is not associated with diagnostic diathesis in our study cohort, it is associated with important dimensions of personality functioning in the social and sexual sphere. Patients growing up in families where one or both of the parents died appear more compromised in their interpersonal relationships, both premorbidly and at follow-up, which may reflect premorbid differences. That is, these patients are more likely to have impairment in achieving stable, mature adult attachments regardless of diagnosis. This, in turn, may be linked to their more chaotic familial backgrounds. These findings at least suggest such an association, although its nature (i.e., genetic or environmental or both) remains undetermined.

In summary, our findings suggest that early parental death can have an impact on one's subsequent life, but not in ways heretofore suggested. It appears to be associated with negative familial, social, and interpersonal functioning, both premorbidly and at long-term follow-up. It does not, however, appear to be a risk factor for the development of severe mental illness generally, nor does our evidence support its role in determining the specific diagnostic class of psychopathology. Although these findings by no means rule out the importance of early loss to later emotional problems in individual cases, they do not support the general notion that early environmental trauma, at least of this type, regularly plays an etiologic role in major psychiatric syndromes.

ACKNOWLEDGMENTS

The authors wish to acknowledge the help of many people who have contributed to the project: Polly Curry and Linda Berman for project coordination; Ellen Boren and Patricia Kelly for manuscript preparation; Allison Benesch for chart abstraction and diagnostic evaluation; Renee Marshel and Victoria Solsberry for outcome evaluation; Michael Koontz and John Bartko for statistical consultation; Lawrence Abrams, John Cook, William Flexsenhar, Kathleen Free, Lee Goldman, Anita Gonzalez, Wendy Greenspun, Brian Healy, Tom Martin, Jim Miller, Jack O'Brien, Terry Polonus, Steven Richfield, Rochelle Spiker, Holly Taylor, Barry Townsend, Denise Unterman, Susan Voisinet, Robert Welp, and Donald Wright for chart abstraction; and Dexter Bullard, Jr., William T. Carpenter, Jr., Robert A. Cohen, David Feinsilver, and Wells Goodrich for general consultation and manuscript review.

REFERENCES

1. Freud S: Mourning and melancholia (1917 [1915]), in Complete Psychological Works, standard ed, vol 14, London, Hogarth Press, 1957
2. Abraham K: Notes on the psycho-analytical investigation and treatment of manic-depressive insanity and allied conditions (1911), in Selected Papers on Psycho-Analysis. London, Hogarth Press, 1927
3. Krugeger DW: Childhood parent loss: development impact and adult psychopathology. Am J Psychother 37:582–592, 1983
4. Brown F: Depression and childhood bereavement. J Ment Sci 107:754–777, 1961
5. Sethi BB: Relationship of separation to depression. Arch Gen Psychiatry 10:486–496, 1964
6. Dorpat TL, Jackson JK, Ripley HS: Broken homes and attempted and completed suicide. Arch Gen Psychiatry 12:213–216, 1965
7. Levi LD, Fales CH, Stein M, et al: Separation and attempted suicide. Arch Gen Psychiatry 15:158–164, 1966
8. Hill OW, Price JS: Childhood bereavement and adult depression. Br J Psychiatry 113:743–751, 1967
9. Dizmang LH: Loss, bereavement and depression in childhood. Int Psychiatry Clin 6:175–195, 1969
10. Birtchnell J: Depression in relation to early and recent parent death. Br J Psychiatry 116:299–306, 1970
11. Birtchnell J: The relationship between attempted suicide, depression and parent death. Br J Psychiatry 116:307–313, 1970
12. Brown GW, Harris T, Copeland JR: Depression and loss. Br J Psychiatry 130: 1–18, 1977
13. Roy A: Vulnerability factors and depression in women. Br J Psychiatry 133:106–110, 1978
14. Parker G: Parental deprivation and depression in a non-clinical group. Aust NZ J Psychiatry 13:51–57, 1979

15. Roy A: Role of past loss in depression. Arch Gen Psychiatry 38:301–302, 1981

16. Tennant C, Hurry J, Bebbington P: The relation of childhood separation experiences to adult depressive and anxiety states. Br J Psychiatry 141:475–482, 1982

17. Pfohl B, Stangl D, Tsuang MT: The association between early parental loss and diagnosis in the Iowa 500. Arch Gen Psychiatry 40:965–967, 1983

18. Lloyd C: Life events and depressive disorder reviewed, I: events as predisposing factors. Arch Gen Psychiatry 37:529–535, 1980

19. Crook T, Elliot J: Parental death during childhood and adult depression: a critical review of the literature. Psychol Bull 87:252–259, 1980

20. Watt NF, Nicholi A: Early death of a parent as an etiological factor in schizophrenia. Am J Orthopsychiatry 49:465–473, 1979

21. Hildgard JR, Newman MF: Parental loss by death in childhood as an etiological factor among schizophrenic and alcoholic patients compared with a non-patient community sample. J Nerv Ment Dis 137:14–28, 1963

22. Granville-Grossman KL: Early bereavement and schizophrenia. Br J Psychiatry 112:1027–1034, 1966

23. Gregory I: Studies of parental deprivation in psychiatric patients. Am J Psychiatry 115:432–442, 1958

24. Gregory I: Anterospective data following childhood loss of a parent, I: delinquency and high school dropout. Arch Gen Psychiatry 13:99–109, 1965

25. Gregory I: Anterospective data following childhood loss of a parent, II: pathology, performance, and potential among college students. Arch Gen Psychiatry 13:110–120, 1965

26. Brown F: Childhood bereavement and subsequent psychiatric disorder. Br J Psychiatry 112:1035–1041, 1966

27. Brown F, Epps P: Childhood bereavement and subsequent crime. Br J Psychiatry 112:1043–1048, 1966

28. Dennehy CM: Childhood bereavement and psychiatric illness. Br J Psychiatry 112:1049–1069, 1966

29. Gay MJ, Tonge WL: The late effects of loss of parents in childhood. Br J Psychiatry 113:753–759, 1967

30. Jacobson G, Ryder RG: Parental loss and some characteristics of the early marriage relationship. Am J Orthopsychiatry 39:779–787, 1969

31. Birtchnell J: Early parent death and mental illness. Br J Psychiatry 116:281–288, 1970

32. Birtchnell J: Early parent death and psychiatric diagnosis. Soc Psychiatry 7:202–210,1972

33. Bowlby J: The making and breaking of affectional bonds, I: aetiology and psychopathology in the light of the attachment theory. Br J Psychiatry 130:201–210, 1977

34. McGlashan TH: The Chestnut Lodge Follow-up Study, I: follow-up methodology and study sample. Arch Gen Psychiatry 41:573–585, 1984

35. McGlashan TH: The Chestnut Lodge Follow-up Study, II: long-term outcome of schizophrenia and affective disorders. Arch Gen Psychiatry 41:586–601, 1984

36. Soloff PH, Millward JW: Developmental histories of borderline patients. Compr Psychiatry 24:574–588, 1983

8

Biobehavioral Aspects of Precocious Puberty

William A. Sonis
University of Minnesota, Minneapolis
Florence Comite and Ora H. Pescovitz
National Institute of Child Health and Development,
National Institutes of Health
Karen Hench
Clinical Center, National Institutes of Health
**Charles W. Rahn, Gordon B. Cutler, Jr.,
D.L. Loriaux, and Robert P. Klein**
National Institute of Child Health and Development,
National Institutes of Health

Precocious puberty is an experiment in nature from which we can learn about the effects of early and continuous exposure to sex steroids on human behavior. We studied the relationships between behavior problems, brain lesions, height, and two measures of sex steroid exposure in 77 children with precocious puberty. Behavior problems were assessed using the Child Behavior Checklist. We found that the diagnosis of precocious puberty regardless of the etiology was a risk factor for increased behavior problems. Although there may be important effects related to en-

Reprinted with permission from the *Journal of the American Academy of Child Psychiatry,* 1986, Vol. 25, No. 5, 674–679. Copyright 1986 by the American Academy of Child and Adolescent Psychiatry.

This research took place while Dr. Sonis was a Medical Staff Fellow in the Child and Family Research Section, LCE, NICHD, NIH.

vironmental and psychological variables, we found that older girls with idiopathic precocious puberty who looked closer to expected peer height and who had less pubic hair had more behavior problems.

Precocious puberty is defined as the development of secondary sexual characteristics before age 9 in girls, and before age 10 in boys (Rosenfield, 1982). In response to increased levels of sex steroids, these children develop breasts, pubic hair, and maturation of the external genitalia. This disorder is a natural experiment from which we can learn about the effects of early and continuous exposure to sex steroids on human behavior (Rubin et al., 1981).

Two behavior problems seem to occur consistently while these children experience precocious puberty: social difficulties related to an age/appearance discrepancy, and moodiness (Conner and McGeorge, 1965; Hampson and Money, 1955; Money and Alexander, 1969; Money and Hampson, 1955; Money and Walker, 1971; Solyom et al., 1980). The descriptions of these developmental problems, however, are based upon individual case reports or analysis of semistructured interviews of primarily retrospective experience from small, clinically heterogenous populations without controls. We have reported elsewhere a study comparing 33 girls with true precocious puberty (TPP) with matched controls using the Child Behavior Checklist (Sonis et al., 1985). Girls with TPP had at least 10 times the expected prevalence of behavior problems. They differed significantly in the total number of behavior problems reported and scored higher in several areas of behavior, including social withdrawal, depression, and aggression, than matched controls. They also exhibited less social competence than peers. Despite the large group differences between girls with TPP and the control girls, there was also considerable within group variation. Indeed, a majority of the girls with TPP scored within the normal range. Although environmental and psychological variables may account for the observed within group variation, biological mechanisms may also be important. Biological aspects of this disorder that may influence behavior include: (1) effects related to the specific diagnostic etiologies that cause sexual precocity, (2) effects secondary to an age/appearance discrepancy, and (3) effects secondary to chronic CNS exposure of pubertal levels of sex steroids.

Precocious puberty is a descriptive diagnosis, with several etiologies, each of which may have specific behavioral effects. Precocious puberty can occur as a result of various CNS lesions, such as hypothalamic hamartomas, optic gliomas, and hydrocephalus; as part of a syndromal constellation, as in the McCune-Albright syndrome (sexual precocity,

pigmented skin lesions and polyostotic fibrous dysplasia) or neurofi-
bromatosis (Von Recklinghausen's syndrome); as a genetic disorder with
several male generations affected (familial); or as an idiopathic disorder
without a definitive etiology despite extensive medical evaluation (Rosenfield, 1982). Because of the diagnostic heterogeneity of the syndrome,
there may be behavioral effects related to the etiologic diagnosis, in
general, and relative integrity of the individual's central nervous system,
in particular.

Shaffer (1976) demonstrated that CNS lesions above the brainstem
predisposes to an increased prevalence of nonspecific behavior problems. Rutter et al. (1970) showed an increased prevalence of behavior disorder in children with lesions above the brainstem even when compared
to other chronically ill children, for example, those with asthma. This
may also hold true for children with precocious puberty. Thus, one might
expect that children with both brain lesions and precocious puberty to
have more behavior problems than children with idiopathic precocious
puberty alone. Comparison of children with precocious puberty but
without brain lesions (idiopathic group—IPP) to children with precocious puberty and brain lesions (CNS group) is necessary to determine
the relative contribution of the CNS lesion to observed within group
differences.

Regardless of etiology of precocious puberty, these children look different from their peers. Several authors have published studies showing a
relationship between height, behavior problems and personality characteristics in children with precocious puberty (Money and Alexander,
1969; Money and Walker, 1971) or short stature (Money and Politt, 1966;
Rotnem et al., 1977, Steinhausen and Stahnke, 1976). These authors
believe the behavior problems in children with statural anomalies arise as
a reaction to their age/appearance discrepancy. Although virtually all
children with precocious puberty are taller than peers, there is variability
in the relationship between the child's height age equivalent (HA) and
their chronologic age (CA). This can be expressed as a height age to
chronological age ratio (HA/CA). One might then expect that children
with a higher HA/CA ratio, i.e., look much taller than expected for age, to
have more behavior problems, since these children have the most pronounced age/appearance discrepancy.

Although height is a measureable aspect of chronic exposure to pubertal levels of sex steroids, sex steroids cross the blood brain barrier and
may directly influence behavior by their effects on brain receptors (Rubin
et al., 1981). Cross-sectional information about sex steroids such as single
measures of estradiol and testosterone provide only limited information

about the temporal relationship between brain development, behavior, and sex steroids. Tanner staging, however, provides an overall index of pubertal development and represents the final common pathway between exposure to sex steroids and end organ sensitivity (Rosenfield, 1982). Thus, Tanner stage is the variable that most accurately measures the degree of secondary sexual development and is a measure of the chronicity and concentration of sex steroid exposure. Children with more advanced sexual development have been exposed to more sex steroids over a longer time and may be expected to have more problems.

This paper will examine the relationship between brain lesions, height and two measures of sex steroid exposure and the behavior of 77 children with precocious puberty using the Child Behavior Checklist. In this manner, we will explore the hypothesis advanced by Money and Walker (1971) that early exposure to sex steroids affects behavior.

SUBJECTS

All children participating in this study were evaluated as part of an approved National Institute of Child Health and Human Development (NICHD) protocol to halt or reverse pubertal maturation in childen with precocious puberty using a synthetic luteinizing hormone releasing hormone analogue ($LHRH_a$). The etiologic diagnosis of precocious puberty was established by the procedure described by Comite et al. (1981).

The sample consisted of 77 children, 22 boys and 55 girls, aged 4–11 years. The children's mean age at enrollment in the study was 83.5 months (6.8 years). Mean parental socioeconomic status (SES) was 5.7 (Hollingshead, 1975). The etiologic categories in our subjects with precocious puberty are listed in Table 1. At the time of presentation 85% of the sample had heights and weights greater than the 95h percentile in the NCHS growth curves (NCHS, 1978). Pubertal maturation and develop-

Table 1. Etiology of Precocious Puberty

Etiology	Boys	Girls	Total
Idiopathic	2	37	39
Central nervous system	6	10	16
Other (includes Mac-Cune Albright, precocious adrenarche, contenital adrenal hyperplasia, and familial precocious puberty)	14	8	22

ment ranged from Tanner stage II–V. Bone age was advanced by 2–5 years over chronological age. At the time their parent was asked to fill out the CBCL, none of the children had begun LHRH$_a$ treatment. Children with multiple medical problems or with an uncertain etiology for their precocious puberty were excluded from the data analysis. Each family was seen by a clinical social worker who consulted a psychiatrist when needed.

Children were recruited from across the country from physicians who knew about the NIH study. As such, any generalizations based on our findings should be restricted to the appropriate population.

METHOD

The child's parents were asked to fill out the CBCL as a routine part of the protocol. The CBCL is a 120-item parental report of children's behavior problems and social competence. The CBCL and the scoring norms were developed at the National Institute of Mental Health (NIMH) using 1200 children from the Washington, D.C., area. The Social Competence section consists of 7 domains while the Behavior Problem section consists of 113 items. The Social Competence items are scored according to both the number and relative competence of th individual activities in each domain. The items in the Behavior Problem section are scored 0, 1, or 2 where 0 is considered "not to be true" of a particular child and 2 is considered to be "almost always true."

Where possible, the parent accompanying the child was approached in the first few days of the child's initial hospitalization, prior to beginning treatment. They were told that we were interested in learning about the psychological consequences, if any, of having a chronic disorder such as precocious puberty. The CBCL was then hand checked and scored for omissions or errors. Interrater reliability for coding the CBCL was greater than 0.95 for each child.

The Child Behavior Profile (CBP) is generated from the CBCL. The CBP consists of 3 social competence scales (Activities, Social Activities, School) and 8 or 9 behavior problem scales (depending on the child's age and sex), and two second order factors (Internalizing or Externalizing scales) (Achenbach, 1978; Achenbach and Edelbrock, 1979). In their broadest nosologic interpretation the Internalizing scale is felt to represent "overcontrolled or neurotic symptoms," e.g., worry, withdrawal, nail biting, and similar behaviors, while the Externalizing scale is felt to represent "undercontrolled or conduct disturbance symptoms," e.g., lying, stealing, fighting, and similar behavior. All the social competence items are summed to get a Total Social Competence score, and all the behavior problems items are summed to get a Total Behavior Problem score. The social competence and the behavior problem scales are expressed as both percentile and T-scale scores (Achenbach, 1978; Achenbach and Edelbrock, 1979). Only the Total Behavior Problem score and scores on the Internalizing and Externalizing Scales were used as outcome measures.

Diagnostic age (DXAGE) was the age at which the child was initially seen at NIH. In most, but not all cases, the DXAGE was identical to enrollment in the behavioral section of the study, and thus the two variables were highly correlated ($r = 0.967$). We chose to use DXAGE in all the analyses.

Height, in bare feet, was measured on a stadiometer at 8:00 A.M. on the second hospital day. Ten sequential measurements of height were obtained and the average was taken as the final height. The child's height age (HA) was considered to be the age at which the child's height was at the 50th percentile on the NCHS growth charts. The height age/chronological age ratio (HTRAT) was found by dividing the child's height age (HA) in months by the child's chronological age (CA) in months at the date of the height determination. Tanner staging for pubic hair and breast development was performed by independent observers (K.H., O.P.). Differences between observers were averaged and recorded as a single score. Interrater reliability for Tanner staging was $r = 0.753$ for breast staging and $r = 0.967$ for pubic hair staging.

Analysis of variance was used to test for associations between the different diagnostic groups and the Total Behavior Problem score, the internalizing scales and the externalizing scales. Multiple regression analysis was used to test the relationship between height and Tanner stage and the outcome measures. Significance level was set at $p < 0.05$.

RESULTS

We divided the sample into three main etiologic groups. Comparisons were made among girls with idiopathic precocious puberty (IPP) ($N = 35$), children with precocious puberty and CNS lesions (CNS) ($N = 16$), and children with other forms of precocious puberty, such as McCune-Albright syndrome, familial precocious puberty, and secondary precocious puberty (Other) ($N = 22$). Analysis of variance by etiologic group showed no significant group differences in any of the main CBP scales (Total Behavior Problem Score, Internalizing Scale Score, or Externalizing scale score) among the three etiologic groups (Table 2).

Table 2. Mean Dependent Variables by Etiology

Variable	Total Group (N = 75)	Idiopathic (N = 37)	CNS (N = 16)	Other (N = 22)	F
DXAGE (year)	6.69	6.48	6.76	7.00	
(S.D.)	(1.81)	(1.54)	(1.55)	(2.35)	<1
Total	59.43	59.19	58.19	60.75	
(S.D.)	(12.43)	(11.45)	15.23	12.28	<1
Internal	59.23	59.97	56.75	59.77	
(S.D.)	(12.21)	(10.94)	(14.88)	(12.48)	<1
External	37.70	57.50	36.69	58.82	
(S.D.)	(11.60)	(11.60)	(11.93)	(11.84)	<1

We examined the correlations between DXAGE, diagnosis and the outcome variables. There was a significant positive correlation for the entire sample ($N = 77$) between DXAGE, Total Behavior Problem Score, and both the Internalizing and Externalizing scales. Both the IPP and the Other group showed a significant correlation between DXAGE and the outcome variables, while the CNS group did not.

There were significant differences in the correlations between and the outcome variables and age at diagnosis among the different etiologic groups (Table 3). Girls with IPP had the strongest correlation between etiologic group and the dependent measures, and had the most uniform etiologic diagnosis. Subsequent analyses of height and Tanner stage were based on the group of girls with IPP since the CNS and OTHER groups were etiologically heterogenous.

Preliminary analysis of the height measure data showed a possible curvilinear effect. To test for this relationship both a linear (HTRLIN) and a quadric (HTRQUAD) form were included in the analysis. DXAGE was used as a covariate in the analysis. After controlling for DXAGE, the quadratic term (HRTQUAD) but not the linear term (HTRLIN) showed a

Table 3. Correlation Matrix of CBP Scales vs. Age at Diagnosis by Etiology of Precocious Puberty

	Total Group (N = 75)	Idiopathic (N = 37)	CNS (N = 16)	Other (N = 22)
Total	0.310**	0.542***	−0.153	0.356*
Internal	0.362**	0.546***	−0.056	0.461*
External	0.303**	0.561**	−0.092	0.214

$* p < 0.05.$ $** p < 0.01.$ $*** p < 0.001.$

significant relationship with the outcome measure. HTRQUAD had a slightly greater negative correlation with the Internalizing scale than with the Total Behavior Problem scale or the Externalizing scale. Controlling for DXAGE in the regression analysis showed that HTRAT accounted for about 40% of the total variance in the major CBP scales.

Analysis of the Tanner Stage measures showed that Pubic Hair staging (PH) and Breast Staging (BREAST) were significantly positively correlated to each other ($r = 0.445$), and PH mildly correlated with DXAGE ($r = 0.461$).

We carried out a stepwise regression analysis using as candidate variables DXAGE, BREAST, and PH to analyze the relationship between the Tanner stage measures and CBP scales (Table 4). DXAGE entered first, followed by PH which contributed significantly. Breast stage showed essentially no relationship. Table 5 shows the results of the stepwise regression for DXAGE and PH. Like the HTRAT, less pubic hair was significantly associated with more behavior problems.

Table 4. Correlations between DXAGE, CBP Scales, and HTRAT (N = 35)

Correlate	DXAGE	Total	Internal	External
Total	0.523***			
Internal	0.519**			
External	0.563**			
HTRLIN	−0.384*	−0.289	−0.258	−0.307
HTRQUAD	−0.339*	−0.498**	−0.510**	−0.420**

*$p < 0.05$.   **$p < 0.01$.   ***$p < 0.001$.

Table 5. Partial Correlation Coefficients: CBP by DXAGE and PH

Step	Total		Internal		External	
	DXAGE	PH	DXAGE	PH	DXAGE	PH
0	0.51***	−0.191	0.49**	−0.17	0.57***	−0.13
1	*0.51***	−0.43**	*0.49**	−0.40*	*0.57***	−0.39*
2	*0.61***	−0.43**	*0.58***	−0.40*	*0.65***	−0.39*

*$p < 0.05$.   **$p < 0.01$.   *** < 0.001.   *Italics* = variable in equation.

DISCUSSION

In this study, we attempted to identify those biological variables that might account for some of the variation in behavior reported by parents of children with precocious puberty. We initially hypothesized that: (1) children with brain lesions and precocious puberty, (2) children who looked much taller than expected for age, and (3) who also had been exposed to more gonadal steroids would have more behavior problems than other children with precocious puberty. On the basis of our analysis, we rejected all our hypotheses. We found that older girls with idiopathic precocious puberty (IPP) who looked closer to expected peer height, and who had less pubic hair, scored highest on the behavior problem scales.

Children with precocious puberty were at risk for behavior problems regardless of etiologic diagnosis. Children with precocious puberty and brain lesions fared no worse than girls with IPP alone, nor than children with various other etiologic causes for precocious puberty. The lack of main effects for DX may be related to differences between our CNS group and brain-injured groups reported by Rutter and Shaffer. In their studies, the brain-injured group consisted of children with clinical central nervous system disorders, for example, epilepsy and hydrocephalus. In our group, a majority (approximately 75%) of the children had small hypothalamic hamartomas, without clinical neurologic symptoms. Prior to the advent of high resolution CAT scans, these children would have been classified as having idiopathic precocious puberty, and would not have been considered "neurologically impaired." Thus our CNS groups may be considered more neurologically intact than brain-injured children reported by Rutter et al. (1970) and Shaffer (1976).

Relative clarity of the medical explanation for the precocious puberty may also be important in understanding the relationship between age, etiologic diagnosis and the dependent variables. Girls with IPP had the strongest positive correlation between age and the three dependent measures than any other etiology. Children with "Other" diagnoses had an intermediate correlation between age and behavior problems and children with brain lesions and precocious puberty had the lowest correlations. One explanation for these findings may be the relative clarity of the medical explanation for the cause of precocious puberty. Children with brain lesions and precocious puberty have a relatively understandable medical explanation for their symptoms. That is, a structural brain abnormality caused the symptoms. Children with "Other" diagnoses and children with IPP have more ambiguous explanations for the onset of symptoms. Solyom et al. (1977) found that girls with precocious adrenarche and precocious thelarche had more behavior problems than girls with idiopathic precocious puberty. She accounted for the the between group differences on the basis of lack of specific medical explanation in the adrenarche and thelarche group with a concomitant increase in the child and family's anxiety. Similar reasoning has been used to account for the low prevalence of behavior problems in growth hormone deficient (GHD) boys compared to boys with constitutional short stature (Gordon et al., 1982).

Older children with IPP can better comprehend their condition and its lack of medical explanation, with a possible increase in behavior problems. This explanation may account for the positive correlation between age and behavior problems of these girls. In both Solyom et al.'s (1977) and Gordon et al.'s (1982) studies the authors believed that there was a positive but unmeasured, effect of medical treatment, for both idiopathic precocious puberty and GH deficiency, which both "legitimized" the disorders and provided nonspecific support for the children and their parents. Unlike the children in these studies, all children in our study were equally likely to receive treatment, thus any systematic bias arising from additional medical attention was minimized.

We also rejected the hypothesis that children with a greater age/appearance discrepancy would have more behavior problems. Age was positively related to behavior problems but the HA/CA ratio was inversely related to both age and behavior problems. That is, older girls had a lower HA/CA ratio than younger girls and also had more behavior problems. The inverse relationship was held even when we corrected for age. Although the relative height discrepancy between older girls with idiopathic precocious puberty and peers is not as great as the discrepancy in younger girls, the perception of the difference rather than the actual difference may account for the older girls' high scores.

We also rejected the hyothesis that children with greater exposure to sex steroids, as evidenced by their breast and pubic hair staging, will have more behavior problems. We found no relationship between Tanner breast staging and behavior problems; however, there was a positive relationship between age and pubic hair development and an inverse relationship between pubic hair development and behavior problems. Older girls had more pubic hair compared to younger girls while girls with less pubic hair had more behavior problems, even when we controlled for age. If we then look at the group of girls with the highest scores on the behavior problem section of the CBP, they were older girls whose height age was closer to their chronologic age and who also have less pubic hair. Hormonally, less pubic hair implies lower androgen levels or a shorter duration of androgen exposure.

Several factors may explain the lack of association between breast development and behavior. First, estrogen effect as measured by breast development may not be related to behavior problems. Secondly, there was both a greater error of measurement and less variability in breast measurement than there was with pubic hair staging. Thus measurement problems and a restricted range may weaken whatever relationship may be present.

Despite the influence of biologic factors, self-perception may be a major mediating variable between behavior and pubertal development. Older girls may be more aware of the differences between themselves and peers than younger children, and thus have more problems. This may hold true both for the problems related to the diagnosis of precocious puberty as well as the positive association between behavior problems, age and a lower HA/CA ratio. Older children experience a wider range of social situations involving peers and thus may be more sensitive to their age/appearance discrepancy than younger children. Other investigators have found similar patterns in short children, particularly during adolescence (Money and Pollitt, 1966; Steinhausen and Stahnke, 1976).

We are aware that there are several potential explanations for the behavior problems observed in children who have precocious puberty. In this paper we explored biological factors which explained only part of the variance observed in the behaviors of children with precocious puberty. We are in the process of exploring other factors, including familial and parental reactions to the disorder as well as the child's self-perception which may explain additional variance. Behavior problems in children with statural and sexual developmental anomalies may be mediated by self-perception as well as be influenced by sex steroids.

REFERENCES

Achenbach, T.M. (1978), The Child Behavior Profile; I. In boys aged 6-11. *J. Consult. Clin. Psychol.,* 46:478–488.

———— & Edelbrock, C.S. (1979), The Child Behavior Profile; II. Boys aged 12-16 and girls aged 6-11 and 12-16. *J. Consult. Clin. Psychol.,* 47:223–233.

Comite, F., Cutler, Jr., G., Rivier, J., Vale, W.W., Loriaux, D.L. & Crowley, W.F. (1981), Short-term treatment of idiopathic precocious puberty with a long-acting analogue of leutinizing hormone releasing hormone. *New Eng. J. Med.,* 305:1546–1550.

Conner, D.V. & McGeorge, M. (1965), Psychological aspects of acelerated pubertal development. *J. Child Psychol. Psychiat.,* 6:161–177.

Gordon, M., Crouthamel, C., Post, E.M. & Richman, R.A. (1982), Psychosocial aspects of constitutional short stature: social competence, behavior problems, self-esteem and family functioning. *J. Pediat.,* 101:477–480.

Hampson, J.G. & Money, J. (1955), Idiopathic sexual precocity in the female. *Psychosom. Med.,* 18:16–35.

Hollingshead, A. (1975), *Four Factor Index of Social Status.* New Haven, Conn.: Department of Sociology, Yale University, Yale Station.

Money, J. & Alexander, D. (1969), Psychosexual development and absence of homosexuality in males with precocious puberty. *J. Nerv. Ment. Dis.,* 148:111–123.

_____ & Hampson, J. G. (1955), Idiopathic sexual precocity in the male. *Psychosom. Med.,* 18:1–15.

_____ & Pollitt, E. (1966), Studies in the psychology of dwarfism. *J. Pediat.,* 68:381–390.

_____ & Walker, P. (1971), Psychosexual development, maternalism, nonpromiscuity and body image in 15 females with precocious puberty. *Arch. Sexual Behav.,* 1:45–60.

National Center for Health Statistics, NCHS *Growth Curves for Children,* (DHEW Publication No. (PHS) 78-1650, 37.

Rosenfield, R.L. (1982), The ovary and female sexual maturation. In: *Clinical Pediatric and Adolescent Endocrinology,* ed. S.A. Kaplan. Philadelphia: W.B. Saunders, pp. 242–259.

Rotnem, D., Genel, M., Hintz, R.L. & Cohen, D.J. (1977), Personality development in children with growth hormone deficiency. *This Journal,* 16:412–426.

Rubin, R.T. Reinisch, J.M. & Haskett, R.F. (1981), Postnatal gonadal steroid effects on human behavior. *Science,* 211:1318–1324.

Rutter, M, Tizard, J. & Whitmore, K. (ed) (1970), *Education, Health and Behavior.* London: Longmans.

Shaffer, D. (1976), Brain injuries. In: *Child Psychiatry,* ed. M. Rutter & M. Hersov. Oxford: Blackwell Scientific Publication, pp. 185–228.

Solyom, A., Austad, C.C., Sherick, I. & Bacon, G.E. (1980), Precocious sexual developmental in girls: the emotional impact on the child and her parents. *J. Pediat., Psychol.,* 5:385–393.

Sonis, W.A., Comite, F., Blue, F.J., Pescovitz, O., Rahn, C., Hench, K., Cutler, Jr., B. Loriaux, D. & Klein, R. (1985), Behavior problems and social competence in girls with true precocious puberty. *J. Pediat.,* 106:156–160.

Steinhausen, H.C. & Stahnke, N. (1976), Psychoendocrinological studies in dwarfed children and adolescents. *Arch. Dis. Child,* 51:778–783.

PART II: DEVELOPMENTAL ISSUES

9

Minor Neurological Indicators and Developmental Function in Preschool Children

Gary B. Landman

Johns Hopkins Hospital, Baltimore, Maryland

Melvine D. Levine, Terrence Fenton, and Bethany Solomon

Boston Children's Hospital, Massachusetts

An attempt was made to determine whether neuromaturational indicators (soft neurological signs) were associated consistently with specific areas of developmental function in 5-year-old children. Fifty-eight children were assessed over two diagnostic sessions. One involved administration of the Pediatric Exam of Educational Readiness (PEER) by pediatric fellows; the other consisted of administration of the McCarthy Scales of Children's Abilities (MSCA) by trained psychoeducational specialists. Data indicate that children who exhibited a greater number of minor neurological indicators had a high likelihood of experiencing difficulty with visual-perceptual, fine motor, and gross motor tasks of the PEER and the MSCA. What is more important, no relationship was found between aggregates of minor neurological indicators and performance on linguistic, memory, sequencing, quantitative, verbal, or preacademic sections of these diagnostic instruments. This information suggests that physicians should limit their interpretation of such signs when

Reprinted with permission from *Developmental and Behavioral Pediatrics,* 1986, Vol. 7, No. 2, 97–101. Copyright 1986 by Williams & Wilkins Co.

Paper presented in part at the Annual Meeting of the Society for Behavioral Pediatrics, Washington, D.C., May 10-11, 1985.

evaluating young children with academic difficulties. Additional data must be accumulated before the role of neuromaturational signs can be fully understood.

The neurological examination of children with learning disorders has been a matter of some controversy. Relatively few findings have emanated from the traditional scrutiny of cranial nerves, deep tendon reflexes, and sensory intactness.[1] On the other hand, there is a considerable literature suggesting that there exists a series of neurological "indicators" (sometimes called "soft neurological signs") that may be more revealing, and probably associated with impaired school performance and/or behavioral abnormalities in school children[2-4] (i.e., choreiform movements, dysdiadochokinesis, and synkinesias or associated movements) and markers of deficient somatosensory interpretation (i.e., astereognosis and finger agnosia). There currently exist conflicting data regarding the significance of these indicators, and their precise developmental and academic correlates.[5-7] Much of the research performed so far has focused on elementary school-aged children in whom neurological dysfunction may have had an opportunity to interact with educational experience and cultural factors that influence the acquisition of skills.[8] The present study was designed to investigate the developmental correlates of these indicators in children between 4 and 5 years old, i.e., prior to the teaching of academic skills. In particular, there was an attempt to determine whether neuromaturational indicators were associated consistently with specific areas of developmental delay.

BACKGROUND

Various studies have demonstrated that school children with low severity developmental delays (so-called "learning-disabled youngsters") display a greater number of "soft signs" than their appropriately achieving peers.[2] Ordinarily, most of these signs disappear over the normal course of maturation. Their persistence beyond age seven or eight has sometimes been characterized as "neuromaturational delay," the delay being linked to a likelihood of developmental dysfunction and impaired learning.[3,9]

The present study afforded several unique opportunities. First, it allowed for an evaluation of individual neuromaturational signs and their associated findings in a community population not thought to be socially or academically vulnerable. Second, it focused exclusively on prekindergarten children. Third, the methodology allowed for the compilation of observations on the minor neurological indicators, as well as specific areas of development, overall cognition, and preacademic skill. This permitted the investigators to address the following questions. Are these indicators confined largely to youngsters who have specific kinds of developmental delays, such as language disabilities, gross motor weaknesses, fine motor, or visual-perceptual deficits? Are the indicators in any way related to general cognitive level or intelligence? Finally, is there a relationship between gender and the prevalence of specific minor neurological indicators in preschool children?

METHOD

A volunteer sample of 58 children was recruited by mail from Brookline, Massachusetts, as part of a study standardizing a newly developed neurodevelopmental examination. Children were white, middle-class, and English-speaking. Volunteers were not paid, but were provided a "snapshot" of processing strengths and weaknesses. Children with a past history of observed developmental abnormalities were excluded. All children were tested during the summer before their entry into kindergarten. Assessmnents were performed over two diagnostic sessions. One involved the administration of the Pediatric Exam of Educational Readiness (PEER),[10] and the other consisted of administration of the McCarthy Scales of Children's Abilities (MSCA).[11] Two trained educational specialists were employed to administer the MSCA, and the PEER was administered by fellows in the Department of Ambulatory Pediatrics at The Children's Hospital Medical Center, Boston, Massachusetts. Measures of interrater reliability for the PEER were conducted prior to this testing (85 to 95% agreement). All 58 children (34 males and 24 females) from the sample received both the PEER and MSCA. Their mean age was 59 months with a standard deviation (SD) of 5 months. The sample had a mean I.Q. of 111 with a SD of 15 (as measured by the MSCA).

Tools

The PEER is a recently developed, multidimensional assessment procedure for preschool and kindergarten-aged children. It was designed to assess six areas of development: orientation, gross motor, fine motor, visual motor, language, and preacademic knowledge. Processing efficiency, selective attention, and neuromaturational indicators are also evaluated as part of the large examination (see Levine for a more extensive description).[12] For the purposes of this study, only the developmental skill areas and neuromaturational scores were analyzed.

Developmental attainment scores were computed by adding the total score for each subtest (see Fig.1). Orientation was not scored, since many of the items directly overlapped with the neuromaturational subtest. A score of 0 represented performance below the 4½-year-old level: 1 was indicative of a 4½-year-old; 2 was noted when the child performed at the 5-year-old level; and 3 was assigned when the performance was at the 5½-year-old level of competency. The scores from each item were totaled to yield a subtest score.

Neuromaturation scores were derived from the PEER scoring sheet (Fig 1). The indices of neuromaturational status are well established and normed. They include: associated movements (AM), visual tracking (VISTR), agraphesthesia (AGRAPH), astereognosis (ASTEREO), dystonic posturing (DISTONIC), choreiform movements (CHOREIF), mixed preference (MIX PREF), and dysdiadochokinesis (DYSDIA). A score ranging between 1 and 3 was given on each of the 23 separate minor neurological indicator items. A score of 1 was given when a child demonstrated unquestionable evidence of an indicator (e.g., associated movements). A 2 was assigned when the child's performance was strongly suggestive of an indicator (e.g., partial but not complete "mirror movement"). A score of 3 was noted when there was no evidence at all for an indicator. A mean composite rating was then computed for each child by dividing the total score by the number of potentially eliciting minor neurological indicators. This was done because recent data suggest that combining neuromaturational indicators, rather than analyzing them separately, provides a more satisfactory method of assessing neuromaturation.[13]

The MSCA is a standardized and widely used psychoeducational instrument. Profiles of processing strengths and weaknesses, as well as a measure of general cognitive functioning, are derived from this examination. The MSCA is comprised of 18 subtests, scores from which combine to form composites for five skill areas: verbal, perceptual-performance, quantitative, memory, and motor. All five skill area weighted scores and the general cognitive score were analyzed for the purposes of this study. The MSCA test data were scored according to the manual.[11]

RESULTS

The extent to which the presence of multiple minor neurological indicators varied as a function of sex was investigated by means of an *F*-test

pediatric examination of educational readiness (peer)

TASK	DEVELOPMENTAL ATTAINMENT					NEUROMATURATION	
	BELOW LEVELS	LEVEL ONE	LEVEL TWO	LEVEL THREE	REFUSED TASK	ASSOCIATED MOVEMENTS 3 2 1	OTHER MINOR NEUROLOGICAL SIGNS 3 2 1
ORIENTATION							
Identify Body Parts	□ 1-3	□ 4-5	□ 6-7	□	□		
Imitative Finger Movement	□ 1-2	□ 3-4	□ 5	□	□	AM* □□□	DYSKINESIA □□□
Graphesthesia	□ 1-2	□ 3	□ 4	□	□		AGRAPH* □□□
Stereognosis	□ 1-2	□ 3	□ 4	□	□		ASTEREO* □□□
Visual Tracking	□ Err. x2-4	Erratic x1 □	Smooth □		□	AM* □□□	VISTR* □□□
GROSS MOTOR							
Walk on Heels (6 feet)	□ 3 lapses	□ 2 lapses	0-1 lapse □		□	AM* □□□	DYSTONIC* □□□
Walk on Toes (6 feet)	□ 3 lapses	□ 2 lapses	0-1 lapse □		□	AM* □□□	DYSTONIC* □□□
Stand on One Foot (10 secs.)	□ 3 losses	□ 2 losses	0-1 loss □		□	AM* □□□	
Pronation-Supination	□ >45°	□ 10-45°	<10°dev'n □		□	AM* □□□	DYSDIA* □□□
Motor Stance	□ 2-5 sec.	□ 6-9 sec.	10 sec. □		□		CHOREIF* □□□
Catch Ball	□ 1-2	□ 3-4	□ 5		□	AM* □□□	
VISUAL-FINE MOTOR							
Visual Matching	□ 1-3	□ 4-7	□ 8-10		□		
Manipulate Sticks	□ Inacc.	□ Awkward	□ Proficient		□	AM* □□□	MIX PREF* □□□
ASSOCIATED OBSERVATIONS			CHECKPOINT A				
Copy Figures	□ A	□ B	□ C		□	AM* □□□	MIX PREF* □□□
Draw from Memory	□ A	□ B	□ C		□	AM* □□□	
Block Construction	□ Inacc.	□ Awkward	□ Proficient		□	AM* □□□	
SEQUENTIAL							
Finger Opposition	□ A	□ B	□ C		□	AM* □□□	DYSKINESIA □□□
Object Span	□ 3	□ 4	□ 5		□		
Word Span	□ 1-2	□ 3	□ 4-5		□		
LINGUISTIC							
Spatial Directions	□ 1-2	□ 3-4	□ 5		□		
Name Pictures (# uncued & correct)	□ 5-9	□ 10-12	□ 13-15		□		
Complex Sentences	□ 1-2	□ 3-4	□ 5-6		□		
Categorize	□ 1<3	□ 3-4	□ >4		□		
Temporal Directions	□ 1-2	□ 3-4	□ 5		□		
PREACADEMIC LEARNING							
Name Symbols	□ 1-2	□ 3-4	□ 5-7		□		
Name Days of the Week	□ 1-2	□ 3 or more	In order □		□		
Count Fingers	□ 1-2	□ 3-4	□ 5		□		
Count Aloud	□ 1-9	□ 10-19	□ 20		□		
Write Letters	□ 1st name	ABCD	□ Full name		□		
ASSOCIATED OBSERVATIONS			CHECKPOINT B				
Totals:							
Maximum Obtainable:	29	29	29	29	29	36	33

comments:

AM* —Associated Movements
VISTR* —Visual Tracking
AGRAPH* —Agraphesthesia
ASTEREO* —Astereognosis
DYSTONIC* —Dystonic Posturing
CHOREIF* —Choreiform Movements
MIX PREF* —Mixed Preference
DYSDIA* —Dysdiadochokinesis

Figure 1. PEER scoring form.

(see Table 1). Results indicated that there were no significant differences between cohorts; therefore, data from boys and girls were grouped for all other analyses.

The relationship between minor neurological indicators and PEER and MSCA measures was examined by a series of stepwise multiple

Table 1. The Relationship between Sex and the Presence of Neuromaturational Indicators

Sex	N	Mean	SD	F	p
Male	34	2.35	0.23	2.22	NS
Female	24	2.44	0.22		

regression analyses. Each analysis studied the regression of a separate section from the PEER or MSCA on two predictors: age and minor neurological indicator rating. In each analysis, age was placed into the regression equation as the first step, while the rating was entered on the second. The increment in R^2 between steps one and two was recorded, and the statistical significance of the increment was examined by means of an F-test. The size of this R^2 increment provided an indication of the proportion of covariance between minor neurological indicator ratings and any given PEER or MSCA section, controlling for the potentially mediating effects of age.

Table 2 presents the results of the analyses in which the PEER subtests were regressed on age and minor neurological indicator ratings. The ratings made substantial contributions toward accounting for the variance on the gross motor subtest (R^2 increment = 0.11) and on the visual fine motor subtest (R^2 increment = 0.06). The R^2 increment in the gross

Table 2. PEER Subtests Regressed on Age and Minor Neurological Indicator Ratings

Peer Subtests	df		R^2	R^2D	F	p
Gross motor	1/55	age	0.18	0.18		
		NI[a]	0.29	0.11	8.93	< 0.01
Visual fine motor	1/55	age	0.09	0.09		
		NI	0.16	0.06	3.61	0.06
Sequencing	1/55	age	0.05	0.05		
		NI	0.06	0.00	0.22	NS
Linguistic	1/55	age	0.09	0.09		
		NI	0.09	0.00	0.15	NS
Academic	1/55	age	0.17	0.17		
		NI	0.19	0.02	1.50	NS

[a]NI = neurological indicator.

motor area proved to be statistically significant ($F = 8.93$, $df = 1/55$, $p < 0.01$), whereas the results in the visual fine motor area just missed significance at the 0.05 level ($F = 3.61$, $df = 1/55$, $p = 0.06$). The minor neurological indicator rating made virtually no contribution toward accounting for the variance on the sequencing (R^2 increment = 0.01), the linguistic (R^2 increment = 0.00), or the preacademic section (R^2 increment = 0.02). In each of these areas, the small increment in R^2 fell far short of statistical significance.

Table 3 presents the results of the analyses in which the MSCA subtests were regressed on age and neuromaturational status scores. The minor neuological indicator ratings made significant contributions toward accounting for the variance on the motor subtest (R^2 increment = 0.24, $F = 17.17$, $df = 1/55$, $p < 0.01$), and on the perceptual subtest (R^2 increment = 0.09, $F = 5.13$, $df = 1/55$, $p < 0.05$). However, the ratings did not contribute toward accounting for the variance on the quantitative, verbal, and memory subtest where R^2 increments of 0.01 were observed in each analysis and F-tests results fell short of statistical significance. Finally, minor neurological indicator ratings failed to make a significant contribution toward accounting for the variance in the general cognitive score (R^2 increment = 0.03).

Table 3. McCarthy Subtests Regressed on Age and Minor Neurological Indicator Ratings

McCarthy Subtests	df		R^2	R^2D	F	p
		age	0.00	0.00		
Motor	1/55	NI[a]	0.24	0.24	17.17	< 0.01
		age	0.00	0.00		
Perceptual	1/55	NI	0.09	0.09	5.13	< 0.05
		age	0.01	0.01		
Quantitative	1/55	NI	0.01	0.00	0.06	NS
		age	0.00	0.00		
Verbal	1/55	NI	0.01	0.01	0.53	NS
		age	0.01	0.01		
General	1/55	NI	0.03	0.03	1.44	NS
		age	0.00	0.00		
Memory	1/55	NI	0.01	0.00	0.24	NS

[a]NI = neurological indicator.

DISCUSSION

One finding of this study was that children who exhibited a greater number of minor neurological indicators had a high likelihood of experiencing difficulty with visual-perceptual, fine motor, and gross motor tasks of the PEER and the MSCA. On the other hand, no relationship was found between aggregates of minor neurological indicators and performance on linguistic, memory, sequencing, quantitative, verbal, or pre-academic sections of these diagnostic instruments. Confidence in these results was reinforced by the fact that similar sections of the two examinations revealed an identical pattern of correlation with minor neurological indicators. Not only were the test items different, but the two assessments were administered by different professionals at different times. Moreover, the results followed a very clear-cut pattern. Those subtests which were not significant in their correlations with minor neurological indicators had extremely low *F*-values, wheras fine motor, gross motor, and visual-perceptual function related strongly to the ratings used.

The relationship between specific developmental dysfunctions and academic performance delays is unclear. In the past, many investigators concluded that reading disabilities often were associated with visual-perceptual deficiencies.[14] However, recent research has suggested that many children with such handicaps read well and, in fact, there may be no significant differences when seriously delayed readers are compared with their normal peers on tasks that measure visual-perceptual function.[15] In recent years, there has been a greater emphasis on language facility and the capacity to form rich visual-to-verbal associations as being more relevant to reading ability than visual perception as such.[15] Thus, although a high loading of minor neurological indicators correlated strongly with visual-perceptual sections of the PEER and the MSCA, such findings may not be predictive of reading problems in early elementary school. The lack of a correlation between minor neurological indicators and performance in sequential organization and various linguistic and memory functions is significant, since these areas of development are more likely to have an impact upon reading. The lack of correlation with overall cognitive functioning ("general" category of the MSCA) is important because minor neurological indicators have been seen as indicators of cognitive abilities.[16]

IMPLICATIONS

The finding that neuromaturational signs are related to performance in visual perceptive and motor areas may have remedial or curriculum implications if supported by further investigations. The most important finding from this study is *negative*; that is, the lack of relationship between neuromaturational signs in 5-year-old children, and measures of language functioning, memory, quantitative thinking, sequencing, and overall intelligence as measured by the PEER and MSCA. Thus, physicians should limit their interpretation of such signs. Neuromaturational indicators should constitute only one component of a broad evaluation of function.

It may be time to begin to do another kind of research, namely, the assessment of neuromaturation findings as part of a cluster. A recent study has shown that adding processing skills, such as short-term memory and language items, can improve their diagnostic usefulness.[17] This approach appears to be fruitful, and should be continued.

Throughout North America there is a growing emphasis on preschool screening.[18] Communities are implementing such programs at a rapid rate. The neurodevelopmental content of assessments demands careful scrutiny. Further research is needed to demonstrate the concurrent and predictive validity, as well as the therapeutic implications of all such observations, whether they entail minor neurological indicators or other components of neurodevelopmental description.

REFERENCES

1. Werry J, Klaus M, Guzman A, Weiss G, Degan K, Hoy E: Studies on the hyperactive child. VII. Neurological status compared with neurotic and normal children. Am J Orthopsychiatry 42:441–450, 1972.
2. Peters JE, Romaine JS, Dykman RA: A special neurological examination of children with learning disabilities. Dev Med Child Neurol 17:63–78, 1975.
3. Meltzer LJ, Levine MD, Palfrey JS, Aufseeser CL, Oberklaid F: Evaluation of a multidimensional assessment procedure for preschool children. J Dev Behav Pediatr 2:67–73, 1981.
4. Wolff PH, Hurwitz I: The chorieform syndrome. Dev Med Child Neurol 8:160–165, 1966.
5. Rutter M, Graham P, Bireh H: Interrelations between the chorieform syndrome, reading disability and psychiatric disorder in children of 8–11 years. Dev Med Child Neurol 8:149–159, 1966.
6. Adams RM, Kocsis JJ, Estes RE: Soft neurological signs in learning disabled children and controls. Am J Dis Child 128:614–618, 1974.
7. Hart P, Rennick P, Klinge V, Schwartz ML: A pediatric neurologist's contribution to evaluations of school underachievers. Am J Dis Child 128:319–323, 1974.
8. Hertzig M: Neurological "soft" signs in low-birthweight children. Dev Med Child Neurol 23:778–791, 1981.
9. Bortner M, Hertzig ME, Birch HG: Neurologic signs and intelligence in brain damaged children. J Special Ed 6:325–333, 1972.

10. Levine MD: Pediatric Exam of Educational Readiness. Cambridge, MA, Ed. Publishers Services, Inc., 1982.
11. McCarthy D: Manual for the McCarthy Scales of Children's Abilities. New York, The Psychological Corp., 1982.
12. Levine MD, Oberklaid F, Ferb T, Hanson MD, Palfrex JS, Aufseeser CL: The pediatric examination of educational readiness: Valid data of an extended observation procedure. Pediatrics 6:341–349, 1980.
13. Rasmussen P, Gillberg P, Waldeenstrom E, Suenson B: Perceptual, motor and attentional deficits in seven year old children: Neurological and neurodevelopmental aspects. Dev Med Child Neurol 25:315–333, 1983.
14. Birch HG: Dyslexia and maturation of visual function, in Money J (ed.): Reading Disability: Progress and Research Needs in Dyslexia. Baltimore, MD, Johns Hopkins Press, 1962.
15. Vellutino FR: Toward an understanding of dyslexia, in Benton A, Pearl D (eds.): Dyslexia: An Appraisal of Current Knowledge. New York, Oxford University Press, 1978.
16. Bennett IC, Sherman R: Management of childhood "hyperactivity" by primary care physicians. J Dev Behav Pediatr 4:88–93, 1983.
17. Shaywitz SE, Shaywitz BA, McGraw K, Grall S: Current status of the neuromaturational examination as an index of learning disability. J Pediatr 104:819–825, 1984.
18. Dworkin PH, Levine MD: The preschool child: Prescribing and predicting, in Scheiner A, Adams K (eds.): The Practical Management of the Developmentally Disabled Child. St. Louis, MO, C.V. Mosby Co., 1980.

PART II: DEVELOPMENTAL ISSUES

10

Stability (and Instability) of Type A Behavior from Childhood to Young Adulthood

Laurence Steinberg
University of Wisconsin, Madison

This article examines the stability, from childhood to young adulthood, of overt Type A behaviors. The Type A behavior pattern has been established as a risk factor for coronary heart disease. Measures were taken from interviews conducted with individuals' teachers during the first or second grades, with the participants during adolescence, and with the participants during young adulthood. Analyses indicate that (a) the Type A behavior pattern is composed of a prosocial dimension, best characterized as achievement striving, and an antisocial dimension, best characterized as impatience aggression; (b) the correlation between the prosocial and antisocial components shifts as individuals age, from significantly positive (during elementary school), to unrelated (during adolescence), to significantly negative (during young adulthood); and (c) Type A behaviors are stable between adolescence and adulthood but not between

Reprinted with permission from *Developmental Psychology,* 1986, Vol. 22, No. 3, 393–402. Copyright 1986 by the American Psychological Association, Inc.

This research was carried out during the author's tenure as a William T. Grant Foundation Faculty Scholar under the foundation's program in the Mental Health of Children. Data from the New York Longitudinal Study were made available through a grant from the James A. and Catherine T. MacAuthur Foundation to Jacqueline V. Lerner and Richard M. Lerner.

I am exceedingly grateful to Athena Droogas for her painstaking coding of the interview transcripts, to Jacqueline Lerner and Richard Lerner for their assistance in obtaining access to the New York Longitudinal Study archive, and to two anonymous reviewers whose thoughtful comments on an earlier draft of this article were extremely helpful.

childhood and adolescence or between childhood and adulthood. Although
there may exist Type A children, these children do not necessarily grow up
to be Type A adults.

Over the past two decades, the Type A behavior pattern has been con-
vincingly established as a major risk factor for coronary heart disease. The
Type A pattern, now richly described in the psychological, medical, and
epidemiological literatures, is characterized by extremes of aggressiveness, easily aroused hostility, a sense of time urgency, and competitive
achievement striving a sense of time urgency, and competitive achievement striving (Matthews, 1982). Now that the association between adult
Type A behavior and coronary heart disease has been confirmed,
researchers have begun more recently to turn their attention to the study
of the development and etiology of the behavior pattern, with an eye
toward understanding the core underpinnings of the Type A construct
and the treatment and prevention of coronary proneness.

One line of research in this spirit has been the examination of Type A
behaviors in children. Matthews and her colleagues, for example, have
demonstrated in a series of studies that it is possible to measure during
childhood behavior that is analagous to adult Type A behavior—that is,
competitive achievement striving, impatience, and easily aroused anger—and that scores on a questionnaire measure of Type A behavior
developed for use with children are meaningfully related to children's
behavior in situations designed to elicit the Type A pattern. For example,
children categorized as Type A are more likely than are their Type B peers
to behave impatiently and aggressively, work harder in the absence of a
deadline, exert greater efforts to excel in achievement situations, choose
to evaluate their performance in achievement situations against the performances of superior competitors, and exert stronger efforts to maintain
control when threatened with the possibility of failure (Matthews, 1979;
Matthews & Angulo, 1980; Matthews & Siegel, 1983; Matthews &
Volkin, 1981).

Demonstrating that there exist Type A children is one thing; demonstrating that these children grow up to be Type A adults is quite another.
For, despite the burgeoning literature on the identification of children
who exhibit overt Type A behaviors, these studies do not explicitly link
Type A behavior prior to adolescence (when its consequences for coronary disease have not been established) with Type A behavior during
adulthood (which has been shown to be predictive of coronary disease).
Thus, we do not know whether the constellation of behaviors that has

come to be labeled Type A when observed among adults necessarily has, as its early developmental precursor, an analogous behavior pattern.

Although it is reasonable to propose that the behavioral manifestations of an underlying disposition (for instance, having a Type A personality) are similar during different developmental periods, such is not always the case. To draw upon a distinction made by Kagan (1980), although some characteristics (e.g., aggression) are *homotypically* stable over time (that is, the observable manifestations of the characteristic are similar across different periods), other characteristics (e.g., dependency)—with underlying psychological cores that may be just as stable—are *heterotypically* stable (that is, the observable manifestations are dissimilar across different periods). Although most recent research on the development of the Type A behavior pattern has proceeded from the assumption that the pattern is homotypically stable, this assumption may not prove to be correct. For example, one recent report (Bergman & Magnusson, 1985) linked young adult Type A behavior with aggression and overambition among adolescent boys (consistent with the notion that the pattern is homotypically stable), but not with these traits and instead, with hyperactivity among adolescent girls (consistent with the view that the pattern may be heterotypically stable).

Previous studies of Type A behaviors have suggested that the Type A pattern is actually composed of several more or less distinct components, although the specific components have varied somewhat from one study to another. Matthews and Angulo (1980) reported, for example, that among elementary school children, Type A behavior ratings derived from the Matthews Youth Test of Health (MYTH) cluster into two othogonal factors: competitive achievement striving and impatience aggression. The Jenkins Activity Scale (JAS), perhaps the most widely used paper-and-pencil measure of Type A behavior among adults, yields three factor-analytically derived subscales: speed and impatience, hard-driving competitiveness, and job involvement (Jenkins, Zyzanski, & Rosenman, 1971). Steinberg (1985, 1986), using data collected as a part of the New York Longitudinal Study (NYLS), also found that Type A behaviors clustered into two distinct components similar to those observed by Matthews. Indeed, the accumulating evidence that Type A behavior is multidimensional prompted Matthews (1982) to propose that "future research should take care to assess *individual Type A behaviors*" [italics added] (p. 316).

Viewing Type A behavior as a multidimensional construct has several important implications for developmental research examining the developmental course of the behavior pattern. First, it is possible that the components of the Type A behavior pattern cluster differently at one point in the life span than at another; thus, in order to examine the continuity of the behavior pattern across developmental periods, it is necessary to examine the structure of the Type A behavior pattern at different ages and to construct Type A profiles accordingly. Second, different dimensions of the behavior pattern themselves may show different degrees (and different patterns) of stability during various developmental periods. Thus, it is important to ask whether some dimensions of the Type A pattern are more stable than others. Third, it is possible that the different components of the adult Type A behavior pattern may be differentially predictable from early measures.

Existing longitudinal studies of relevant personality dimensions (e.g., achievement striving, competitiveness, anger arousal) provide indirect evidence that at least some aspects of the Type A behavior pattern should be expected to enjoy differential degrees of continuity between adolescence and adulthood, and that most aspects of the behavior pattern may be more stable among males than among females (Block, 1971; Kagan & Moss, 1962). For example, the greater stability of Type A behaviors among males may be attributable to the more consistent and continuous socialization of both achievement and aggression that males are likely to receive across different developmental periods (cf. Kagan & Moss, 1962). Among girls, the aspect of Type A behavior shown to be most stable is reactivity (Bronson, 1967). Taken together, these studies suggest that it may be important to examine the developmental course of the Type A pattern separately for males and females.

Few studies have examined the stability of Type A behavior directly. Matthews and Avis (1983) reported that Type A behavior assessed via the MYTH is relatively stable over one-year intervals during the elementary school years. Although suggestive of continuity in the behavior pattern, their findings unfortunately, do not establish the stability of Type A behaviors over a period of time during which changes in the form or expression of such behaviors might more reasonably be expected to occur. More important, it remains to be demonstrated that the behavior pattern is stable between two developmental periods in which individuals change environments (and presumably, their exposure to stimuli likely to elicit the behavior pattern).

The present research provides evidence relevant to the question of the *homotypic* stability of the Type A pattern from childhood to young adulthood. Specifically, this article examines the stability, over time, of the Type A behavior pattern measured and conceptualized similarly across different developmental periods.

METHOD

Subjects

The subjects of this study were drawn from a sample of 133 individuals, now young adults, who compose the core sample of the ongoing NYLS. The NYLS was initiated in 1956 by Alexander Thomas and Stella Chess. Originally, the sample consisted of 138 individuals, but in the early years of the study, 5 subjects were dropped, or withdrew, from the study. Remarkably, there has been no further sample attrition since that time, some 25 years ago.

Detailed information on the sample and its recruitment has been reported elsewhere by the NYLS principal investigators (Thomas & Chess, 1977; Thomas, Chess, & Birch, 1968; Thomas, Chess, Birch, Hertzig, & Korn, 1963). The core NYLS sample is composed of 66 male and 67 female subjects from 84 middle- or upper-middle-class families. Although the sample is in no way representative of the general population, it represents an ideal group within which to examine the development of Type A behaviors, because of the likely emphasis these highly educated, highly successful, urban families placed on achievement striving during the course of their children's socialization.

The data presented in this report were derived from three sources of information: (a) measures of Type A behaviors derived from interviews conducted with the youngsters' elementary school teachers during the first or second grades (mean age: 7 years, 2 months), (b) measures of Type A behaviors derived from interviews conducted with the participants during adolescence (mean age: 16 years, 9 months), and (c) measures of Type A behaviors derived from interviews with the participants during young adulthood (mean age: 21 years, 0 months). Virtually all of the subjects were enrolled in school (high school or college) at the time of the adolescent and young adult interviews.

Complete interview transcripts were available for 101 individuals (76%) during childhood (52 males, 49 females), for 96 individuals (72%) at adolescence (46 males, 50 females), and for 108 individuals (81%) at young adulthood (53 males, 55 females). Complete, codable transcripts for *both* childhood and adolescence were available for 84 individuals (44 males, 40 females); for both childhood and young adulthood, 77 individuals (40 males, 37 females); and for both the adolescence and young adult interview dates, 73 individuals (35 males, 38 females). Reductions in sample size from the original NYLS sample of 133 to the present samples of between 84 and 73 are due chiefly to the loss of individuals who had completed only one of the two measures of interest, rather than to large-scale attrition over the course of the NYLS investigation.

Measures

The original directors of the NYLS were not specifically interested in the development of Type A behaviors per se. But their interest in temperament and adjustment over the life cycle led them to include in their impressive battery of measures a series of interview schedules designed to elicit information on a range of topics relevant to the study at hand (e.g., achievement striving, aggression, susceptibility to frustration). It was therefore possible to return to the original interview transcripts, review a sample of them with an eye toward determining which, if any, relevant information might be extracted, and then develop a coding scheme to fit the aims of the present study. Thus the reader should note that the Type A data discussed in this article were coded specifically for this study from interviews designed by other investigators and conducted for other research purposes. Childhood, adolescent, and young adult interview transcripts were all approximately 20 pages in length.

Existing measures of Type A behavior available for use with children, adolescents, and young adults (e.g., the JAS, Jenkins, Rosenman, & Friedman, 1967; the MYTH, Matthews & Angulo, 1980; the Hunter-Wolf A-B Rating Scale, Hunter, Wolf, Sklov, Webber, Watson, & Berenson, 1982) were reviewed in order to guide the selection of variables. Although there continues to be debate over the relative importance of various traits as components of the Type A pattern (and, in particular, over whether achievement striving is, or is not, a key component), I decided to cast a wide, rather than narrow, net over the array of potentially relevant attributes.

All of the interviews were coded by a single rater, a member of a team of researchers who had been working with the NYLS archive for some time. Thus, the rater was a highly experienced judge who was quite familiar with the style and nature of the interviews and with the design and intent of the NYLS. Childhood, adolescent, and young adult interviews were coded independently; codings of each wave of transcripts were separated by at least a 3-month interval, and all identifying information was removed from interview transcripts in order to minimize contamination.

Childhood measures. Because the childhood interviews were conducted with the participants' elementary school teachers, the data set presented an opportunity to operationalize childhood Type A behavior in a way as similar as possible to that used by Matthews and her colleagues

(Matthews & Angulo, 1980) in the development of the MYTH, the most widely used measure of Type A behavior during childhood. The MYTH includes 17 items for which teachers are asked to characterize their students' behavior on a 5-point scale (from *extremely uncharacteristic to extremely characteristic*). After a preliminary review of the elementary school teacher interview transcripts, it was decided that it was indeed possible to code the transcripts for the 17 items contained in the MYTH, rating the teacher's description of each child's behavior on a 5-point scale, from *extremely characteristic to extremely uncharacteristic.*

Note that although the information coded from the teacher interviews is quite similar to that obtained via the MYTH, the data were gathered and presented in a different manner from that used by Matthews and her colleagues. In both instances, teachers, rather than parents or the individuals under investigation, provided the assessment of Type A behavior, on the assumption that many of the behaviors assumed to compose the Type A pattern are displayed relatively frequently in school settings. But in the standard use of the MYTH, teachers provide their assessments by completing a structured questionnaire used to rate students on the 17 predetermined items. In the present study, in contrast, interviews covering a variety of topics and originally conducted for multiple purposes (of which the assessment of Type A behavior was *not* one of them) were recoded using Matthews and Angulo's (1980) 17-item scheme. In a subsequent section of this article, the comparability of information derived from the MYTH and from the present approach is discussed; at this juncture, suffice it to say that the clustering of items obtained through a factor analysis of the interview-derived data in the present study was virtually identical to that reported by Matthews in her studies using the MYTH.

Adolescent and young adult measures. Identical interview protocols and coding schemes were employed for the adolescent and young adult data. On the basis of existing measures of Type A behavior, as well as previous studies of Type A behavior, and after reviewing the adolescent and young adult interview transcripts, 14 variables were selected for inclusion in the coding scheme used to assess Type A behavior during these developmental periods: (a) perseveres, (b) concentrates intently, (c) self-motivated, (d) strives to achieve, (e) assumes leadership positions, (f) competitive, (g) serious about schoolwork, (h) impatient, (i) hurries/rushes, (j) high activity level, (k) impulsive, (l) easily annoyed, (m) easily angered, and (n) easily frustrated (see Appendix).

For each variable, a global score was assigned on the basis of the information contained in the entire interview, using a 5-point scale ranging from *very characteristic* (5), "This trait is mentioned frequently and prominently . . . a characterization of this individual would not be complete without reference to this trait," to *very uncharacteristic* (1), "This trait is not at all a part of this person's character; if anything, its opposite is true." Coders were instructed to use the scale midpoint, (3), in cases in which a trait, or behaviors relevant to a trait were discussed but where the trait seemed "neither characteristic nor uncharacteristic of this person." The characteristic/uncharacteristic continuum was chosen in order to maximize comparability between the coding scheme employed in the present study and the format of several existing measures of Type A behavior (cf., the MYTH, the JAS). In each of these measures, individuals are rated (either by themselves or by others) as to their usual or characteristic behavior. Recall that the MYTH asks teachers to judge how "characteristic" each of 17 items is of the student being evaluated; similarly, the JAS asks respondents to report how they "usually," "ordinarily," or "frequently" behave.

Reliability

A second rater was employed in order to establish reliability. Reliability was calculated on the basis of ratings of the two coders for 20 childhood interviews, randomly selected from among the interviews of 10 male and 10 female subjects, and on the basis of 10 (5 men and 5 women) randomly selected young adult interviews. The young adult and adolescent interview protocols and coding schemes were identical.

With regard to the childhood interviews, interrater agreement on whether codable information for a specific variable was present in the transcript averaged 87% across the 14 variables. Exact interrater agreement on codings for codable variables (i.e., variables for which information was determined to be present) averaged 44%. Reliabilities determined by essential percentage of agreement (instances in which the two raters agreed within one point of each other, cf. Kagan & Moss, 1962) averaged 92%. On only two of the 17 items was essential agreement below 75%: "This child likes to argue or debate" (essential agreement = 70%), and "It is important for this child to win, rather than to have fun in games or schoolwork" (essential agreement = 71%). Average interrater reliability as determined by product-moment correlation was .74 with only two of the correlations falling below .62: "This child gets irritated easily" ($r = .43$), and "This child tends to get into fights" ($r = .56$).

With regard to the adolescent and young adult interviews, interrater agreement on whether codable information for a specific variable was present in the transcript averaged 75% across the 14 variables. Exact interrater agreement on codings for codable variables (i.e., variables for which information was determined to be present) averaged 66%. Reliabilities determined by essential percentage of agreement averaged 94%; raters agreed within one point of each other in 100% of the cases for 12 of the 14 variables, the two exceptions being *easily angered* (essential agreement 71%) and *impulsive* (essential agreement = 50%). Average interrater reliability as determined by product-moment correlation was .87. Only the reliability coefficient for the variable *impulsive* fell below .70. Because this variable was used infrequently in subsequent analyses (see ahead), however, its low level of interrater agreement does not present a major problem.

RESULTS

Structure of the Type A Behavior Pattern

Childhood, adolescent, and young adult Type A data were examined via factor analyses, separately for each developmental period. Somewhat different procedures were followed for the treatment of the childhood data, on the one hand, and the adolescent and young adult data, on the other. In both cases, intercorrelation matrices of the relevant set of variables were subjected to factor analytic procedures using principal components analyses with orthogonal rotation of factors. (Orthogonal, rather than oblique, rotation was used because previous factor analytic studies of Type A behaviors, e.g., Matthews & Angulo 1980, have suggested that this method is appropriate.) In the case of the childhood data, the number of factors was limited to two and the data for male and female subjects were treated together (in order to examine comparability between the present data and those reported by Matthews & Angulo, 1980). In the case of the adolescent and young adult data, no limit was imposed on the number of rotated factors to be extracted (all factors with eigenvalues above 1.0 were rotated), and the analyses were conducted separately for male and female subjects within each period.

Childhood data. Table 1 presents the loadings for the two factors obtained in the present analysis and for those reported by Matthews and Angulo (1980). The factor analyses of the data for elementary school children resulted in two factors that closely resemble those reported by Matthews and her colleagues (Matthews and Angulo, 1980). One factor is best characterized as competitive achievement striving and the other as impatience aggression. Indeed, the similarity of factor loadings between

Table 1. Factor Loadings of MYTH-Form O Items and Interview-Derived Elementary School Type A Items

Item	MYTH		Interview	
	Factor 1	Factor 2	Factor 1	Factor 2
1. Competitive in games	.725	.304	.786	.308
2. Works quickly and energetically	.449	.095	.338	.043
3. Impatient when waiting	.250	.617	.147	.648
4. Does things in a hurry	.239	.354	.360	.052
5. Takes a lot to anger	-.073	-.546	-.174	-.760
6. Interrupts others	.116	.688	.312	.454
7. Leads in activities	.764	-.045	.412	.122
8. Easily irritated	.155	.790	.184	.331
9. Performs better when competing with others	.686	.094	.632	.206
10. Likes to argue/debate	.270	.763	.292	.524
11. Patient with slower children	-.005	-.594	-.023	-.632
12. Tries to better others	.794	.162	.819	.158
13. Can sit still long	.178	-.500	-.069	-.402
14. Important to win, rather than have fun	.544	.448	.672	.257
15. Others look to as leader	.813	-.187	.320	-.112
16. Competitive	.775	.336	.814	.310
17. Gets into fights	.169	.735	.037	.822

Note. MYTH = Matthews Youth Test of Health. Factor loadings for MYTH-Form O are reported in Matthews and Angulo (1980).

those obtained in the present analysis and those reported in studies using the MYTH in its standard format are remarkable, given the differences in sample and procedures used to generate the two sets of data. The similarity lends credibility both to the coding scheme employed in the present analysis and to the two-factor (achievement striving and impatience aggression) conceptualization of Type A behavior in the literature on children. Although it is conceivable that this structure was in part unconsciously imposed on the data by the rater, it is unlikely that such unconscious processes could have yielded factor loadings so similar to those reported by Matthews and Angulo (1980).

For each child, scores on two subscales were calculated using unweighted item scores. Following Matthews, scores on Items 1, 2, 7, 9, 12, 14, 15, and 16 were summed to yield a competitive achievement-striving subscale; scores on the remaining items were summed to yield an impatience-aggression subscale. Both subscales were combined to yield an overall Type A score. In the few cases in which data were missing for a specific item, the item mean for that gender was substituted in the calculation of the individual's subscale scores.

For purposes of comparison with findings reported by Matthews and Angulo (1980), the reliability coefficients (alpha) of the competitive achievement-striving, impatience-anger, and Type A scales used in the present study are .66, .74, and .76, respectively. Not unexpectedly, the alphas reported by Matthews are somewhat higher (.82, .79, and .82, respectively). Finally, in the present study, the correlation between the competitive achievement-striving and impatience-anger subscales is $r(101) = .45$ $p < .001$). Matthews and Angulo reported a comparable between-scale correlation of .41.

Adolescent data. The factor analysis of the data for adolescent boys resulted in two factors with eigenvalues greater than 1.0 after rotation; the two factors accounted for 80% of the common variance after rotation. Table 2 presents the factor loadings for the two factors. The two factors closely resemble those derived from the elementary school data: The first factor is best characterized as competitive achievement–striving; the second, as impatience–aggression. For each adolescent boy, scores on two subscales were calculated using unweighted item scores: competitive achievement-striving (perseveres, concentrates, self-motivated, achievement striving, leadership, competitive, serious about schoolwork, hurries, and high activity) and impatience-anger (impatient, easily annoyed, easily angered). Overall Type A scores were computed by summing the subscale scores. In cases in which data were missing for a specific item, the item mean for the adolescent male sample was substituted in the

Table 2. Factor Loadings of Overt Type-A Behaviors During Adolescence

	Males			Females		
Behavior	Factor 1	Factor 2	Behavior	Factor 1	Factor 2	Factor 3
Perseverance	.83	.07	Perseverance	.71	-.45	.01
Concentration	.48	.03	Self-motivation	.66	-.17	-.13
Self-motivation	.57	.04	Achievement striving	.79	-.30	.02
Achievement striving	.90	.13	Leadership	.47	.02	-.15
Leadership	.28	.01	Competitiveness	.46	.09	.21
Competitiveness	.53	-.17	Serious about schoolwork	.68	-.45	.00
Serious about schoolwork	.78	.12	Hurries	.73	.14	.13
Hurries	.72	.09	High activity	.73	.27	-.17
High activity	.67	-.02	Impatience	-.19	.58	.02
Impatience	.17	.66	Easily frustrated	-.02	.95	.04
Easily annoyed	.04	.79	Impulsivity	-.48	.03	.46
Easily angered	-.06	.74	Easily annoyed	.01	.04	.86
Easily frustrated	-.70	.03	Easily angered	-.01	.00	.84
Impulsivity	-.28	.06	Concentration	.10	-.00	-.03

calculation of subscale scores. (Missing data were treated comparably in the calculation of subscale scores for adolescent girls and for the young adult men and women.)

The factor analysis of the data for adolescent girls resulted in three factors with eigenvalues greater than 1.0 after rotation. The three factors accounted for 89% of the common variance after rotation. The factor loadings are also presented in Table 2. Inspection of the loadings reveals a competitive achievement-striving cluster similar to that extracted from the boys' data. However, the make-up of the second and third factors suggests that impatience and anger may be less interrelated among adolescent girls than among adolescent boys. For adolescent boys, the display of anger and irritability may be part of the same overall arousal/reactivity dimension, but for adolescent girls—among whom sanctions against the display of anger and annoyance are likely to be far stronger—reactivity may manifest itself more as impatience or frustration, separate from anger. For girls, therefore, three subscale scores were computed: competitive achievement striving (perseveres, self-motivated, achievement striving, leadership, competitive, serious about schoolwork, hurries, high activity); impatience (impatient, easily frustrated); and anger (impulsive, easily angered, easily annoyed). (In some subsequent analyses, the impatience and anger subscales were combined to yield an impatience-anger score for adolescent girls in order to examine sex differences on comparable dimensions.) Overall Type A scores were computed by summing the subscale scores.

Among adolescent boys, the competitive achievement striving and impatience–anger dimensions are unrelated, $r(46) = .08$, $p > .05$; among adolescent girls, competitive achievement striving and anger are, similarly, not significantly correlated, $r(50) = -.18$, $p > .05$, but competitive achievement striving and impatience are negatively correlated, $r(50) = -.24$, $p > .05$.

Young adult data. The results of the factor analyses of the data for young adults in this sample have been reported previously (Steinberg, 1985). Among young adult men, achievement striving and competitive drivenness cluster on two different factors, whereas the third factor, impatience aggression, is similar to that extracted from the adolescent boys' data. These three clusters parallel those derived from studies of Type A behavior among adults employing the JAS (job involvement, hard-driving competitiveness, and speed and impatience; Jenkins et al., 1971). Among young adult women, two factors are found: achievement striving and impatience–aggression. As is the case for young men, competitiveness is not a part of the achievement-striving factor for young women. It may be the case that as individuals move into adulthood (and leave high school environments that often explicitly link achievement with competition), achievement per se begins to be more tied to internally produced performance standards and less to direct competition with others. Among young adult men and women both, the achievement-striving and impatience-anger dimensions are significantly negatively correlated (for young men, $r(53) = -.25, p < .05$; for young women, $r(55) = -.31, p < .01$).

Taken together, the three sets of factor analyses lend strong support to the notion that the Type A behavior pattern is actually composed of two distinct, but related, dimensions of personality: a prosocial dimension, best characterized as achievement-striving, and an antisocial dimension, best characterized as impatience-aggression. The preceding analyses also indicate that, across all three developmental periods, individuals who are achievement strivers are also likely to be competitive, self-motivated, persevering leaders, and individuals who are easily annoyed are also likely to be impatient, easily frustrated, and quick to anger. The prosocial and antisocial dimensions are differentially related during childhood, adolescence, and young adulthood, however.

Stability (and Instability) of Type A Behavior Clusters

The stability across childhood, adolescence, and young adulthood, of the factor analytically derived prosocial and antisocial Type A behavior clusters was examined separately for male and female subjects by correlating subscale scores derived from the elementary school data with comparable scores derived from the adolescent and young adult data, and by correlating scores derived from the adolescent data with comparable subscale scores derived from the young adult data. These correlations are presented in Table 3.

Overall, Type A behaviors show an impressive degree of stability over the period between adolescence and adulthood. Indeed, virtually all of the correlations between conceptually similar clusters (e.g., achievement striving with achievement striving) measured during adolescence and young adulthood reach statistical significance (the only exception is the correlation between adolescent impatience and young adult impatience–anger among female subjects), whereas virtually none of the correlations between conceptually different clusters (e.g., achievement striving with impatience–anger) attains significance.

When we examine the correlations between the adolescent and young adult assessments, we find that, generally speaking, the achievement-striving clusters appear to be more stable than do the impatience-anger clusters, especially among male subjects. Stability coefficients for the impatience-anger clusters are of about the same magnitude for male and female subjects, although it is worth pointing out that among female sub-

Table 3. Pearson Correlations Among Child, Adolescent, and Young Adult Type A Behavior Clusters

Behavior cluster	Competitive achievement–striving	Impatience–anger	Type A total
	Childhood: Males		
Adolescence			
Achievement striving	.08	−.07	.00
Impatience–anger	−.01	−.17	−.12
Type A total	.06	−.15	−.07
Young adulthood			
Achievement striving	−.26*	−.18	−.26*
Competitive drivenness	−.10	−.01	−.06
Impatience–anger	.31*	.14	.26*
Type A total	−.06	−.04	−.06
	Adolescence: Males		
Young adulthood			
Achievement striving	.75****	−.09	.60****
Competitive drivenness	.31*	−.20	.16
Impatience–anger	−.17	.34*	.04
Type A total	.55****	.01	.48***
	Childhood: Females		
Adolescence			
Achievement striving	.08	−.01	.03
Impatience	.11	.15	.14
Anger–irritation	.02	.04	.04
Type A total	.12	.08	.10
Young adulthood			
Competitive achievement–striving	.17	.22	.22
Impatience–anger	−.05	−.09	−.08
Type A total	.08	.09	.10

Behavior cluster	Competitive achievement striving	Impatience	Anger–irritation	Type A total
	Adolescence: Females			
Young adulthood				
Competitive achievement striving	.41**	.16	.25	.26
Impatience–anger	.08	−.07	.35*	.25
Type A total	.32*	.04	.12	.37*

**** $p < .001$, one-tailed. *** $p < .005$, one-tailed.
** $p < .01$, one-tailed. * $p < .05$, one-tailed.

jects the adolescent anger cluster is a significant predictor of young adult impatience-anger, whereas the adolescent impatience cluster is not. Overall Type A scores also show moderate stability, although they are somewhat higher among male, $r(35) = .48, p < .005$, than among female subjects, $r(38) = .37, p < .05$. For the purposes of comparison, the reader should bear in mind that Matthews and Avis (1983) reported *one-year* stability coefficients of approximately .57 and .53 for the MYTH scores of elementary school boys and girls, respectively.

On the other hand, Type A behaviors are not stable between childhood and adolescence, or between childhood and adulthood, for either male or female subjects. None of the correlations between childhood and adolescent Type A behaviors reached statistical significance, and, among male subjects, some of the correlations between childhood and young adult Type A behaviors are actually negative. For example, the correlation between achievement striving assessed in childhood and again in young adulthood is $r(40) = -.26$, $p < .05$, and the correlation between overall Type A scores in childhood and young adult achievement striving is $r(40) = -.26, p < .05$. It is interesting that both overall Type A scores as well as competitive achievement-striving assessed during childhood are significantly positively correlated with young adult impatience-anger among male subjects, $r(40) = .26$, $p < .05$, and $r(40) = .31, p < .05$, respectively. Among female subjects, in contrast, childhood indicators of Type A behavior and impatience-anger are predictive (albeit marginally so) of young adult achievement striving, $r(37) = .22, p < .10$, and $r(37) = .22$, $p < .10$, respectively.

Stability (and Instability) of Type A Classifications

Many previous studies of Type A behavior have categorized individuals as Type A or Type B according to their relative standing on the measure of Type A behavior employed. In the present analysis, individuals were classified into Type A and Type B groups at adolescence and at young adulthood on the basis of median splits within the male and female subsamples for each age. Contingency analyses indicated that among male subjects, Type A classifications remained highly stable over the period from adolescence to young adulthood ($\chi^2(1, N = 35) = 8.06$, $p < .005$); nearly three-fourths of the male subjects scoring above the median at adolescence scored above the median as young adults. This is true not only for overall Type A scores, but for achievement-striving as well (the median-split analysis yields $\chi^2(1, N = 35) = 7.90, p < .005$). This was not the case for impatience-anger, however (i.e., male subjects scoring above the median on this dimension as adolescents did not necessarily score above the median as young adults).

Among female subjects, Type A classifications were not stable between adolescence and adulthood, $\chi^2(1, N = 38) = .422, ns)$, although it is interesting that median split classifications with regard to achievement striving and impatience-anger were $\chi^2(1, N = 38) = 6.73, p < .01$, and $\chi^2(1, N = 38) = 5.09, p < .05$, respectively). This finding further supports the view that the antisocial and prosocial dimensions of the Type A pattern function quite independently of each other. Combining the two dimensions and examining only overall Type A scores would not reveal what happens to be an interesting developmental pattern: Even though female subjects who are highly achievement striving or highly impatient and angry as adolescents are likely to be so as young adults, remaining high on one dimension is not associated with remaining high on the other.

In view of the correlational findings reported earlier, it is not surprising to find that Type A classifications made on the basis of the elementary school data are not at all predictive of classifications made during adolescence or young adulthood. Neither of the median split analyses of overall Type A scores (i.e., childhood to adolescence or childhood to young adulthood) suggested stability of classifications. This is also the case for analyses examining individuals who scored above or below the median on achievement striving and impatience-anger. These analyses were repeated after trichotomizing the samples and including only the highest and lowest tertiles. Again, however, no significant trends emerged.

DISCUSSION

Several words of caution regarding the generalizations one might draw from this investigation are in order. First, because the sample of individuals studied in this research compose a very homogeneous and special group, it would be unwise to generalize the findings presented here to populations of individuals whose socioeconomic and regional backgrounds differ from those of the sample studied in this research.

Second, it is not clear whether the results obtained in the present analysis would be replicated if comparable analyses were conducted using standardized measures of Type A behavior. Although this is an important concern that will need to be addressed in future studies of the behavior pattern, it is worth pointing out that even among researchers using so-called *standard* measures of Type A behavior, there exist considerable differences of opinion as to which of the different measures should be considered standard. Indeed, one recent report (Jackson & Levine, 1983) indicated that intercorrelations among existing measures are not at all high. More research directly examining sources of method variance in the assessment of Type A behavior is sorely needed.

These caveats notwithstanding, the findings of the present study suggest four important conclusions. First, the Type A behavior pattern appears to be composed of two distinct, but related, dimensions of personality: a prosocial dimension, best characterized as achievement striving, and an antisocial dimension, best characterized as impatience aggression. This bidimensional nature of the Type A pattern is evident among males as well as females, and is apparent during a wide range of developmental periods.

Second, the correlation between the prosocial and antisocial components of the Type A pattern shifts, as individuals age, from significantly positive (during elementary school), to unrelated (during adolescence), to significantly negative (during young adulthood). What this pattern suggests is that the behaviors that have come to be viewed as composing the Type A pattern become increasingly more differentiated over the lifespan. Whereas for children, achievement striving is often accompanied by an irritable sort of impatience, the two dimensions are separated over the course of late childhood and adolescence. Perhaps as individuals become more socialized into "appropriate" achievement roles, they learn, for example, that one can work energetically and strive to succeed without being impatient with others or frustrated by occasional impediments to one's progress. Indeed, it may well be the case that individuals learn, with age and experience, that the antisocial aspects of the Type A pattern (e.g., being easily annoyed) actually interfere with the prosocial aspects of the pattern (e.g., striving to succeed).

The differentiation of the prosocial and antisocial components of the Type A pattern is especially pronounced during young adulthood and represents a finding that has important etiological and developmental implications. With regard to the former, it indicates that some individuals are able to maintain high levels of achievement striving (which may benefit themselves and society) without having to suffer the consequences of impatience, anger, and irritability (which probably benefit neither). Moreover, in light of some speculation that it is specifically the antisocial component of Type A behavior, and not the prosocial component, that is most strongly related to coronary disease, the finding that the two dimensions function somewhat independently suggests that individuals may be able to maintain hard-working, achievement-striving profiles without endangering their health.

Third, this study provides evidence that Type A behaviors show an impressive degree of stability over the period between adolescence and adulthood, among both male and female subjects. Indeed, virtually all of the correlations between conceptually similar clusters (e.g., achievement striving with achievement striving) measured during adolescence and young adulthood reach statistical significance, whereas virtually none of the correlations between conceptually different clusters (e.g., achievement striving with impatience-anger) attains significance. The finding that different dimensions of the Type A pattern may evidence different degrees of continuity between adolescence and adulthood—with the achievement striving (or prosocial) component of the pattern more stable than the impatience-anger (or antisocial) component—lends further support to the suggestion that researchers proceed with a multidimensional framework in mind. Whether this differential stability is peculiar to the specific developmental eras studied, or whether it is also characteristic of other lifespan periods, awaits further investigation.

It would be erroneous, of course, to draw the conclusion that the Type A pattern is best conceived as a more or less immutable trait or predisposition after adolescence. Stability over time in any characteristic may be reflective of both intraindividual stability on the dimension in question as well as environmental stability—and, in all likelihood, of the combined effects of both (cf. Scarr, 1981). But whatever the mechanism through which Type A behavior may be maintained over time—through the persistence of a behavioral style, through continuity in socialization, or through a tendency for individuals to maintain patterns of niche-picking that reinforce already existing styles of behavior—the findings suggest that it may be possible to identify individuals during adolescence who may end up driving themselves toward serious coronary disease as adults.

Finally, and perhaps most important, the results suggest that Type A behaviors do not show stability between childhood and adolescence or between childhood and young adulthood. None of the correlations between childhood and adolescent Type A behaviors reaches statistical significance, and, among male subjects, some of the correlations between childhood and young adult Type A behaviors are actually negative. This apparent lack of stability may have important implications for researchers who believe that assessing youngsters' Type A behavior during elementary school has predictive significance. It suggests that although the apparent structure of Type A behavior observed among elementary school children resembles the structure of Type A behavior observed among adults—a conclusion derived from previous research and clearly supported by the present study—this does not guarantee that individual differences in the behavior pattern remain stable over the same developmental period. Yes, there are Type A children—that is, children who, like Type A adults, are competitive, achievement striving, impatient, and angry—and yes, these children can be reliably identified. But, no, these children do not necessarily grow up to be Type A adults.

Previous studies have indicated that the adult Type A behavior pattern may have underpinnings in the domain of temperament that are apparent early in childhood (Steinberg, 1985), but that these underpinnings become increasingly predictive of Type A behavior as one moves up the lifespan (Steinberg, 1986). One interpretation of this pattern of findings, in light of the results reported in the present investigation, is that the Type A behavior pattern may begin to stabilize sometime between middle childhood and early adolescence and may become increasingly stable over time. The pattern may become more stable because individuals who perceive themselves and are perceived by others as Type A may select, and be directed toward, experiences that reinforce and strengthen the behavior pattern.

It is important to ask whether the lack of stability between childhood and adulthood found in the present investigation is a methodological artifact owing, perhaps, to the use of a nonstandard procedure for the assessment of Type A behavior. Ultimately, the question can be answered only through a prospective study of children who have been assessed via the MYTH and whose Type A behavior is assessed at some later point in time. But several lines of evidence in the present article suggest that the instability found in this sample should not be summarily dismissed as a methodological artifact. First, the comparability of factor loadings obtained in this study and those reported for the MYTH provides support for the construct validity of the coding scheme used in the present investigation. Along similar lines, the correlation between factors reported in this study is also very similar to that obtained with the MYTH. Finally, the alpha coefficients and measures of interrater reliability reported in the present study, although not overwhelming, are at least comparable to those reported by investigators using the MYTH (Jackson & Levine, 1983; Matthews & Volkin, 1981).

It could be the case, of course, that the higher stability coefficients between the adolescent and adult assessments of Type A behavior than between the childhood and adolescent, or childhood and adult, assessments are due to the fact that the adolescent and adult assessments both derive from interviews with subjects, whereas the childhood data derive from interviews with the subjects' teachers. Measures derived from similar sources would be expected to be more highly correlated than are measures derived from different sources. In order to examine this possibility, an additional set of analyses was performed using *temperament* ratings derived by the original NYLS investigators from the elementary school interviews in an effort to predict young adult and adolescent Type A scores.* As noted earlier, previous analyses had shown that early childhood temperament is predictive of later Type A behavior. If the low correlation between childhood and later Type A scores is indeed due to source variance, we would expect to find the same problem of source variance operating here and hypothesize that temperament scores derived from the teacher interviews are *not* predictive of later Type A behavior.

This is not the case, however. Regression analyses indicate that measures of temperament taken during the early elementary school years generally are significantly predictive of young adult Type A behaviors. Among male subjects, for example, elementary school temperament accounts for approximately 30% of the variance in young adult Type A scores, 11% of the variance in young adult achievement striving, and close to 20% of the variance in young adult impatience-anger (the first and third regression equations are significant at $p < .05$). Among female subjects, elementary school temperament accounts for about 20% of the variance in young adult Type A scores, 23% of the variance in young adult achievement striving, and 15% of the variance in young adult impatience-anger (all three equations are significant at or beyond $p < .10$). The magnitudes of the multiple correlations are similar to those reported in analyses examining early childhood temperament (Steinberg, 1985), and as was the case in those analyses, the present analyses once again point to low sensory threshold, low adaptability, negative mood, and high approach as important temperamental underpinnings of the Type A behavior pattern. More to the point, however, despite the fact that the temperament assessments were derived from interviews with persons other than the subjects themselves, they nevertheless are significantly related to assessments of Type A behavior derived from self-report measures several years later.

---

*Temperament ratings were derived by the original investigators from interviews with elementary school teachers and from interviews with parents. Nine dimensions of temperament were assessed (rhythmicity, adaptability, approach/withdrawal, sensory threshold, intensity, quality of mood, distractibility, persistence, and activity level) and global ratings were made for each dimension for each child on the basis of information contained in both interviews. Unfortunately, it was not possible to obtain temperament ratings derived *solely* from the teacher interviews. Nevertheless, these temperament assessments can be used to examine whether the absence of self-report data during the elementary school assessment has attenuated the correlation between childhood and adult measures.

The findings presented in this article should not be taken to mean that Type A classifications made during childhood are without etiologic value. It may be the case that the *health* outcomes of childhood Type A behavior are important independent of whether the behavior pattern itself persists over time. For instance, it has been shown that early adolescents classified as Type A individuals show greater systolic blood pressure variability and greater heart rate variability than do their Type B peers. Such variability may damage the inner layer of coronary arteries and increase the likelihood of the development of atherosclerosis and coronary heart disease (Krantz & Manuck, 1984). It is not known however, whether such hemodynamic variability is maintained over time in the absence of a maintained Type A style, or, more to the point whether hemodynamic variability during childhood is, in and of itself, a cause of coronary heart disease during adulthood. Both issues await prospective longitudinal investigation. Until such questions are resolved, researchers should not abandon the assessment of Type A behavior during childhood but should proceed with the proper amount of caution.

Nor does the absence of stability found in the present study mean that investigators should abandon the goal of identifying , before adulthood, individuals likely to develop the adult Type A pattern. The present findings suggest only that this goal may not be best realized through research that assumes homotypic stability in the Type A pattern—that is, through research that attempts to identify potential Type A adults by searching for children who exhibit behaviors analagous to their older counterparts.

REFERENCES

Bergman, L., & Magnusson, D. (1983). Type A-related behavior in childhood and adult Type A behavior: A longitudinal study. Unpublished report (No. 612). Department of Psychology, University of Stockholm, Stockholm, Sweden.

Block, J. (1971), *Lives through time*. Berkeley, CA: Bancroft.

Bronson, W. (1967). Adult derivatives of emotional expressiveness and reactivity-control: Developmental continuities from childhood to adulthood. *Child Development,* 38, 801–817.

Hunter, S. Wolf, T. Sklov, M., Webber, L., Watson, R., & Berenson, G. (1982). Type A behavior pattern and cardiovascular risk factor variables in children and adolescents: The Bogalusa heart study. *Journal of Chronic Disease,* 35, 613–621.

Jackson, C., & Levine, D. (1983 August). *Comparison of two measures of Type A behavior in children.* Paper presented at the annual meeting of the American Psychological Association, Anaheim, California.

Jenkins, C., Rosenman, R., & Friedman, M. (1967). Development of an objective psychological test for determination of the coronary-prone behavior pattern in employed men. *Journal of Chronic Disease,* 20, 371–379.

Jenkins, C., Zyzanski, S., & Rosenman, R. (1971). Progress toward validation of a computer-scored test for the Type A coronary-prone behavior pattern. *Psychosomatic Medicine, 33,* 193–202.

Kagan, J. (1980). Perspectives on continuity. In O. Brim, Jr. & J. Kagan (Eds.), *Constancy and change in human development.* Cambridge, MA: Harvard University Press.

Kagan, J., & Moss, H. (1962). *Birth to maturity.* New York: Wiley.

Krantz, D., & Manuck, S. (1984). Acute psychophysiologic reactivity and risk of cardiovascular disease; A review and methodologic critique. *Psychological Bulletin, 96,* 435–464.

Matthews, K. (1979). Efforts to control by children and adults with the Type A coronary-prone behavior patten. *Child Development, 50,* 842–847.

Matthews, K. (1982). Psychological perspectives on the Type A behavior pattern. *Psychological Bulletin, 91,* 293–323.

Matthews, K., & Angulo, J. (1980). Measurement of the Type A behavior pattern in children: Assessment of children's competitiveness, impatience-anger, and aggression. *Child Development, 51,* 466–475.

Matthews, K, & Avis, N. (1983). Stability of overt Type A behaviors in children: Results from a one-year longitudinal study. *Child Development 54,* 1507–1512.

Matthews, K., & Siegel, J. (1983). Type A behaviors by children, social comparison, and standards for self-evaluation. *Developmental Psychology, 19,* 135–140.

Matthews, K., & Volkin, J. (1981). Efforts to excel and the Type A behavior pattern in children. *Child Development, 52,* 1283–1289.

Scarr, S. (1981). Testing for Children: Assessment and the many determinants of intellectual competence. *American Psychologist, 36,* 1159–1166.

Steinberg, L. (1985). Early temperamental antecedents of adult Type A behaviors. *Developmental Psychology, 2,* 1171–1180.

Steinberg L. (1986). Stability of Type A behaviors from early childhood to young adulthood. In P. Baltes, D. Featherman, & R. Lerner (Eds.) *Lifespan development and behavior* (Vol. 8). Hillsdale, NJ: Erlbaum, in press.

Thomas A., & Chess, S. (1977). *Temperament and development.* New York: Brunner/Mazel.

Thomas, A., Chess, S., & Birch, H. (1968). *Temperament and behavior disorders in children.* New York: New York University Press.

Thomas, A., Chess, S., Birch, H., Hertzig, M., & Korn, S. (1963). *Behavioral individuality in early childhood.* New York: New York University Press.

APPENDIX

Because the 14 variables chosen to assess Type A behavior resemble in spirit, but not necessarily language, those components of Type A behavior generally measured via standard assessment instruments, a few words about their operational function is in order. The variables were defined as follows.

1. Perseveres: reports persistence with regard to work, schoolwork, or interpersonal problems; evidence of ability to complete projects once started; persistence and perseverance in the face of obstacles or interrup-

tions; persistence in response to failure; and persistence in response to elusive success.

2. Concentrates: reports ability to concentrate or resist being distracted while engaged in a work or school task, especially with regard to concentration in the face of noise and other external distractors, and concentration in the face of internal distractors, such as physical restlessness or a lack of interest in the subject at hand.

3. Self-motivation: describes patterns of academic, career, and social goal-setting without excessive regard for the rewards and promptings of others; evidence of self-initiated major projects or involvement in time-consuming nonrequired activities; evidence of self-initiated acceleration in school (i.e., carrying extra classes in order to graduate early).

4. Achievement striving: devotes large amount of time and energy to attainment of short- and long-term academic and career goals; strives for success in social and leisure activities; demonstrates achievement behavior in response to societally or institutionally imposed performance standards.

5. Leadership: reports taking (rather than avoiding) formal leadership positions and responsibilities; and the assumption of informal leadership roles with friends, peers, or siblings.

6. Competitive: exhibits competitive behavior in athletic situations; places importance on winning; prefers and seeks out competitive as opposed to noncompetitive sports and activities; exhibits competitiveness in academic situations, including showing interest in comparisons between own and others' performance.

7. Serious about schoolwork: believes in intrinsic importance of school; reports patterns of disciplined study; evidence of much time and energy devoted to schoolwork; high salience of school in interviewee's life.

8. Impatience: reports inability or difficulty in waiting or remaining placid in the face of temporary or minor obstacles to behavior or immediate goals.

9. Hurries and rushes: reports unwillingness or difficulty in relaxing and behaving in an unhurried, unpressured fashion; reports little interest in leisure activities; does things quickly including activities for which hurrying is not required.

10. High activity: maintains high level of activity in work and leisure activities; avoids sedentary activities; reports of restlessness; fills days with high-pressured schedule.

11. Impulsivity: shows patterns of spontaneity, rather than deliberateness, across a variety of behaviors, including potentially dangerous

behaviors; makes decision quickly; rarely establishes and implements long-term plans and goals.

12. Easily annoyed: is quick to feel irritated; reports frequently feeling annoyed at minor irritations; describes self as difficult to get along with.

13. Easily angered: loses temper easily; experiences intense anger; frequently fights or argues with others, feels angry when uncontrollable circumstances interfere with goals or plans.

14. Easily frustrated: is quick to feel frustrated or blocked by minor obstacles; expresses exasperation or frustration easily and frequently.

Part III

COGNITION AND LEARNING

The first article, "Inside Intelligence," by Robert J. Sternberg provides a lucid explanation of metacognition as distinct from cognition, and a pointed review of recent studies in this area.

To gain a historical perspective, most psychometricians have forgotten that Alfred Binet devised the first psychologically based estimate of intelligence in order to provide practical aid for poor learners. In the city of Paris, in 1904, Binet insisted that his test was a practical device and should not be reified, that it was not intended for ranking normal children, that the children identified by his scores as being in need of special training should be given it, since they were capable of improvement, and that low scores should not be used as markers of innate incapacity. (Stephen Jay Gould, 1981. *The Mismeasure of Man.* W.W. Norton & Co.: New York, p. 155.)

While Binet's original intentions and warnings against misuse of his test were promptly forgotten with their translation into English as the Stanford-Binet test of intelligence, periodically workers in this area either recall or rediscover that these heterogeneous tasks are a useful base for general identification of learning disability, but require more specific indicators in order to design a useful program of instruction for a specific pupil in learning difficulty.

Attempts to capture the basic nature of intelligence range from Spearman's "g" put forth in 1904 as a unitary quality underlying all intelligence, to a host of studies since then in which many separate areas are defined, such as verbal intelligence as differentiated from mathematical intelligence, and the like.

In recent years, still another set of elements has gained interest in a psychologically significant division of intelligence into (1) cognitive processes and (2) metacognitive strategies. The distinction between these two processes is a relatively new focus of research by cognitive scientists.

How a child or adolescent habitually solves a problem is cognition. The extent to which he or she first maps out a strategy, makes a plan, and steps back to evaluate step by step the success of accomplishment of the cognitive task is metacognition.

These distinctions are more than theoretical, they are functionally useful. For one, Sternberg, as had Binet, found that children who did not habitually utilize metacognitive skills, in contrast to gifted children who did, achieved lower scores on cognitive problem solving. With training, however, these less gifted youngsters learned to utilize metacognition and consequently began to show significant improvement on their scores on intellectual problem solving. The gifted children, with similar training, also improved their scores.

These data have clear applications to learning in all areas. Not only do they bear upon education, but they also are relevant to psychiatric and psychological intervention. Helping a child or adolescent disentangle him or herself from self-defeating behaviors can be done in many ways. Determining whether metacognitive strategies can be acquired by the youngster may indeed speed the progress of therapy.

Some 40 years ago, motivational factors were given dominant and even exclusive attention in explaining a host of psychological problems and psychiatric ills. As applied to the field of learning, a child whose reading skills fell well behind the ability to comprehend concepts presented in the oral mode was assumed by psychiatrists and psychologists, and also by sophisticated educators, to need psychotherapy. Things have changed, but by 15 years ago the concept that learning disability was not necessarily motivational in origin was well accepted. The concept was not a unified one. Workers in this field included amongst the causative factors such problems as perceptual difficulties, perceptual-motor inadequacy, difficulties in sequencing of letters and numbers, and faulty short-term and long-term memory. All these have to be differentiated from mild mental retardation.

In the paper, "Future of the LD Field: Research and Practice," by Barbara K. Keogh, this confusion in the definitions of Learning Disability, (LD) is summarized. But, alas, the confusions that require clarification today sound extraordinarily like those of 15 years ago. The contradictory proportions of the school population identified in different states, in the data which Keogh supplies, attest to differences either in definition or in methods of sample identification, or both. Different assumptions as to whether elements of learning difficulty appear separately or are usually clustered in an LD child are still in the forefront of unanswered questions—in fact, at times this issue is not even raised. It is certain that curricula devised under these circumstances will not be helpful for many individual children. And, mainly, the results of treatment are unclear because they have not been sufficiently researched in an orderly fashion. The fallacy of conceiving LD to be a single entity is reviewed lucidly and forthrightly by Keogh. For the field of LD, she has outlined the steps by which order can be brought both to symptom identification and to interventions intended to assist the LD pupil.

While this article is addressed primarily to educators, it has great relevance to those working with the psychological aspects of those children. These professionals must know when to suspect the presence of Learning Disability and must be familiar with the resources for its detailed diagnosis and programmatic assistance. And it is also necessary to be alert to (1) the feelings of shame and embarrassment such a difficulty brings to the school child, and (2) the defensive behaviors children bring to the fore in the attempt to conceal their "dumbness," not realizing that they are in fact concealing their need for help. It is important that parents, teachers, school nurses, pediatricians, educators, as well as child development psychologists and child psychiatrists, all recognize such defensive behavior for what it is and identify and treat the educational and the psychological needs that underlie such behavior.

On January 18, 1987, *The New York Times* published an item indicating that educators have become deeply concerned over the shortcomings of the learning achievements of American school children in comparison with children in a number of other countries. Limited mathematical mastery leads the list. In last year's issue of *Annual Progress in Child Psychiatry and Child Development,* we republished a 1985 report by Stevenson and his associates comparing both cognitive performance and academic achievement of Japanese, Chinese, and American children. In this section, we have included a further report from the same investigative group using the same schools in the same three cities: Sendai, Taipei, and Minneapolis. While each article is understandable in and of itself, taken together they weave a rich tapestry of variabilities of pupils, teachers, curricula, as well as parents' and children's attitudes. The authors have utilized a range of appropriate data gathering procedures, including giving their own tests, which provide cultural consonance of tasks. They also interviewed parents, teachers, and children and observed teachers and pupils in the schoolroom. Sophisticated analyses of the data have been done and the results clearly stated. It is of interest that cognitive levels were virtually identical in all three cultures, although in first and fifth grades (the ones in which these studies were carried out) achievement varied greatly.

The purpose of the meeting of educators reported in *The New York Times,* and also of the findings reported in the two reprinted studies is to devise ways of improving the education of our American children. For any successful recommendations to emerge, it is necessary first to identify, as these papers do, the reasons for the differences in academic achievement in each of these three cultures as examined in kindergarten, first and fifth grades. Then, it will be necessary to ensure that suggested alterations not only be meaningful to the educational process, but also be essential that such changes be consonant with American cultural realities. When one considers the pride with which babies and toddlers work to master skills and ideas, it does seem to require special negative efforts to succeed in turning off such powerful learning drives during the grade school period.

PART III: COGNITION AND LEARNING

11

Inside Intelligence

Robert J. Sternberg
Yale University, New Haven, Connecticut

Cognitive science enables us to go beyond intelligence tests and understand how the human mind solves problems.

Just a decade ago, most of our understanding of human intelligence derived from the analysis of individual differences among people in their scores on various kinds of psychometric intelligence tests. Such understanding was not trivial, but neither did it enable scientists to get "inside intelligence": to understand the cognitive mechanisms that underlie the intelligent functioning observed not only in performance on tests but also in academic performance and in everyday life. During the past ten years, our understanding of these mechanisms has increased manyfold, the result of the application of the powerful methods of a newly emerging discipline often referred to as cognitive science.

Cognitive science is the study of the human mind as subjected to the scrutiny of the allied disciplines of psychology, computer science, philosophy, and linguistics. The goal of cognitive-scientific analysis of the mind is to understand the mechanisms that underlie phenomena as diverse as perception, learning, reasoning, and problem solving. Cognitive scientists are particularly interested in human intelligence, because intelligence represents, in some sense, the epitome of human functioning—that which makes us distinctively human.

Reprinted with permission from *American Scientist,* 1986, Vol. 74, 137–143. Copyright 1986 by the Scientific Research Society.

Preparation of this article was supported by a fellowship from the John Simon Guggenheim Foundation and by contracts from the Office of Naval Research and the Army Research Institute.

The purpose of this article is to survey the advances that have been made during the past decade in our understanding of human intelligence, and to present a consensual cognitive-scientific view of the nature of intelligence. Of course, there are disagreements among cognitive scientists, who, like other scientists, often emphasize the differences among their points of view in their exchanges. But these differences are dwarfed by the points of agreement, and many of the most striking developments in the field emerge in a shared view of intelligence. Thus, although individual cognitive scientists might not agree with everything said here, most of them would probably agree with the main points. A detailed analysis of the points of disagreement can be found elsewhere (e.g., Sternberg 1982, 1984; Kail and Pellegrino 1985; Sternberg 1985).

Before proceeding to the main part of this article, one caveat is in order. Intelligence is not wholly a cognitive phenomenon. At the level of behavior, what is considered to be intelligent can differ not only between cultures (Cole et al. 1971; Wober 1974; Laboratory of Comparative Human Cognition 1982) but also between individuals (Sternberg 1985). This article will be concerned, however, with the cognitive mechanisms underlying intelligence, which appear to be largely invariant across cultures, rather than with the manifestations of cognitive mechanisms in behavior, which are often culturally specific and in need of anthropological as well as cognitive-scientific analysis.

Getting inside human intelligence is even more difficult than getting inside a well-protected New York City apartment. One might imagine unlocking a door containing two locks, each requiring a different key. The two keys that provide access to intelligence represent two basic kinds of mental processes between which cognitive scientists often distinguish: cognitive, or nonexecutive, processes, and metacognitive, or executive, processes. Cognitive processes are used to solve problems of various kinds—whether they are problems as simple as interpreting just what it is that the individual is perceiving, or as complex as calculus—and to learn how to solve these problems in the first place. Metacognitive processes are used to plan, monitor, and evaluate the individual's performance (Brown 1978; Sternberg 1985).

COGNITIVE PROCESSES: PERFORMANCE

Performance processes are perhaps the most basic operations of intelligent functioning. They enable us to perceive the world and to make sense of our perceptions. Hunt and his colleagues (1975) were among the first to suggest that the abilities measured by conventional intelligence tests could be studied through the analysis of processes used in problem solving. Borrowing a task used by Posner and Mitchell (1967), they studied the nature of verbal ability. The task is quite simple, requiring only the matching of letters in terms of either their physical properties or their names. Subjects are presented with pairs of letters that either are or are not physical matches (e.g., "AA" and "bb" versus "Aa" and "Bb") and with pairs of letters that either are or are not name matches (e.g., "Aa," "BB," and "bB" versus "Ab," "ba," and "bA"). They must identify the letter pair either as a physical match (or mismatch) or as a name match (or mismatch) as rapidly as possible.

The typical finding in these experiments is that the difference between mean name match and mean physical match speed for each group of subjects is weakly to moderately correlated with scores on psychometric tests of verbal ability (e.g., vocabulary or reading comprehension). Physical match speed is subtracted from name match speed in order to control for sheer perceptual-motor speed in response. The correlation is used as evidence that speed of access to lexical information in long-term memory, as measured by name match minus physical match time, is related to level of verbal ability. The idea is that brighter individuals are able to retrieve information, and probably to store it, more rapidly than are less bright individuals. From this point of view, shared by others such as Jensen (1980), intelligent individuals are quick in their processing of information.

Whereas Hunt and his colleagues studied information processing by means of a very basic laboratory task originally used for another purpose (studying basic cognitive processes), one of my studies (1977) borrowed a more complex task commonly found on standard intelligence tests and considered to be one of the best measures of intelligence. This task is the analogy problem, which formed the cornerstone for one of the very first analyses of human intelligence, that of Charles Spearman (1923). I suggested that a better understanding of why analogies measure intelligence could be obtained by identifying the mental processes that underlie their solution.

Consider a verbal analogy problem, such as WASHINGTON is to ONE as LINCOLN is to (a) FIVE, (b) TEN, (c) FIFTEEN, (d) TWENTY. Just what mental processes enter into the solution of this problem? I suggested that five of the main processes are encoding, inference, mapping, application, and response. Encoding involves translating a stimulus into a mental representation. Here, for example, one might encode the information that Washington was a president, is on a bank note, and was a war leader. Inference involves finding a rule that relates the first term of an analogy to the second term. Some possible relations between WASH-INGTON and ONE are that Washington was the first president, that he appears on the $1 bill, and that he was a leader in the first major American war. Mapping involves finding a rule relating the two halves of the analogy—in the present case, finding the common features. Both Washington and Lincoln are presidents, faces on currency, and war leaders. Application involves applying the inferred relation of the first half to the second half to arrive at a solution. In this example, the answer is (a) FIVE, since Lincoln's portrait appears on the $5 bill as Washington's appears on the $1 bill. Response involves simply communicating one's response, whether through a pencil mark on an answer sheet, a verbal statement, or the push of a button on a computer console.

Using mathematical models to predict times to solve both verbal and nonverbal analogies, I was able to uncover some interesting aspects of human intelligence. First, higher scorers on standard tests of intelligence are faster at inferring, mapping, and applying relations, and at communicating their responses to analogy problems. This finding is consistent with the finding of Hunt and his colleagues that bright people are, in general, rapid processors of information. Second, however, the higher scorers were actually slower at encoding the information that they later manipulated than were the lower scorers. In other words, brighter individuals are not uniformly faster than duller ones. They appear to spend more time taking in information in order to assure that they have encoded the information richly and in detail. They thus avoid a situation in which they later have to go back and reencode the information, or change the way in which they encoded it. Third, people spend their time quite unevenly on the various mental operations. For example, in a typical verbal analogy, people spend roughly 54% of their time encoding the terms, 12% inferring relations, 10% mapping relations of a higher order, 7% applying relations, and 17% responding. Thus, if an analogy is solved in 5 seconds, as many as 2.7 of those seconds would be spent just in encoding the terms.

Perhaps the most important finding from this line of research emerged in a later, derivative study (Sternberg and Gardner 1983). We presented subjects not only with verbal and nonverbal analogies, but also with verbal and nonverbal series completions—e.g., what word comes next in the series SECOND: MINUTE: HOUR: DECADE: (a) TIME, (b) EON, (c) CENTURY, (d) YEAR?—and classifications—e.g., with which set of words does ITALY best fit: (a) VIETNAM, KOREA, (b) ROME, ATHENS, (c) MEXICO, GUATEMALA, (d) GERMANY, FRANCE? The critical finding from this study was that the performance processes used in solving analogies are essentially the same ones that are used in solving series completions and classifications. The results of the study suggest that the so-called general factor in human intelligence—that source of individual differences in test performance that accounts for the most variation in scores—can be understood largely in terms of differences in performance processes. In other words, it is possible to understand individual differences in test performances in terms of a relatively small set of general, basic cognitive processes.

COGNITIVE PROCESSES: LEARNING

The studies described above focused primarily on how people use what they know. But how do people acquire the information they are later able to use? My collaborators and I have been particularly interested in the processes underlying the learning of new information.

Consider for example, vocabulary, generally considered to be one of the best measures of individual differences in intelligence (Matarazzo 1972). Vocabulary tests are such good measures of intelligence because they indirectly measure the ability to acquire meanings of new words from natural contexts and thus reflect the ability to acquire new information (Jensen 1980; Sternberg and Powell 1983). In other words, highly verbal individuals are somehow better able to figure out meanings of previously unfamiliar words that they encounter in their everyday reading and listening. Consider an example of a passage Powell and I used. The subjects' task was to define the italicized words:

> Two ill-dressed people—one a tired woman of middle age and the other a tense young man—sat around a fire where the common meal was almost ready. The mother, Tanith, peered at her son through the *oam* of the bubbling stew. It had been a long time since his last *ceilidh,* and Tobar had changed greatly. Where once he had seemed all legs and clumsy joints, he now was well formed and in control of his lean, supple body. As they ate, Tobar told of his past year, recreating for Tanith how he had wandered long and far in his quest to gain the skills he would need to be permitted to rejoin the company. Then, their brief *ceilidh* over, Tobar walked over to touch his mother's arm and left.

How do people figure out the meanings of the unknown words, and thereby build up their vocabularies? According to our theory, there are three critical learning processes used in figuring out meanings. Selective encoding involves figuring out what information is relevant for learning the meaning of a new word. For example, relevant cues for figuring out the meaning of *oam* are that it emanates from a bubbling stew and that one can peer through it. Selective combination is used to put together in a meaningful way the information that is selectively encoded. It is not enough just to spot relevant cues. One must figure out how they fit into a coherent definition. Here, one has to combine selectively the information that *oam* is probably either transparent or translucent, and that it probably arises when a liquid substance is heated. Selective comparison is used to relate new to selected old information. What do we already know that can be useful in figuring out the meaning of a new word? One thing we know is that the bubbling of the stew probably means that it is boiling, and that boiling liquids often produce steam. *Oam* is thus identified as a synonym for steam.

This kind of analysis of verbal skills is complementary to that conducted by Hunt and his colleagues (1975), which focused on speed of information retrieval, what we here refer to as selective comparison. Our own studies focused on accuracy of information retrieval, as well as on the other aspects of information processing: could subjects retrieve the right information for figuring out the meanings of the new words?

The use of selective encoding, selective combination, and selective comparison is not limited to the acquisiton of vocabulary knowledge. These learning processes are also critical to less mundane forms of learning, and in particular to insightful learning. In analyzing such learning, Davidson and I concluded that insights seem to be of at least three kinds, corresponding to the processes of learning described above (Sternberg and Davidson 1982; Davidson and Sternberg 1984).

Alexander Fleming's discovery of penicillin is an example of a selective-encoding insight. Looking at a petri dish containing a culture that had become moldy and thus might have seemed to be a spoiled experiment, Fleming noticed that bacteria in the vicinity of the mold had been destroyed, presumably by the mold. Fleming zeroed in on that part of what he saw that was relevant to the discovery of an important antibiotic—penicillin. He selectively encoded the information in a way that many other scientists would have overlooked.

An example of a selective-combination insight would be Darwin's formulation of the theory of natural selection. The information needed to formulate this theory had been available to Darwin, and to others, for some time. What distinguished Darwin was his selectively combining this information so as to realize a plausible way in which species might evolve.

An example of a selective-comparison insight can be found in Kekulé's discovery of the structure of the benzene ring. Kekulé had been struggling with the question of this structure for some time, without success. Then one night he had a dream in which he imagined a snake curling back on itself and biting its tail. When Kekulé arose, he realized that the image of the curled snake formed a visual metaphor for the structure of the benzene ring. He was able to see the relation between two very disparate elements—the image of the snake and the structure of benzene. Selective comparison is largely the recognition of an analogy between old and new experience, as in Kekulé's discovery.

Davidson and I were not able to study insights like those of Fleming, Darwin, and Kekulé. Instead, we presented subjects—both children and adults—with problems of the kind found in books of puzzles:

If you have black socks and brown socks in your drawer, mixed in a ratio of 4 to 5, how many socks will you have to take out to make sure of having a pair of the same color?

Water lilies double in area every 24 hours. At the start of the summer, there is one water lily on a lake. It takes 60 days for the lake to be covered with water lilies. On what day is the lake half covered?

Both problems require insights, albeit of a fairly minor kind. Both require selective encoding—in the former case, recognition that the ratio is irrelevant, in the latter case, recognition that the fact of there being one water lily at the beginning of the summer is irrelevant. Both problems also require insights of selective combination—in the former case, figuring out that no matter how one draws socks from the drawer, one is guaranteed a match after three socks are drawn; in the latter case, recognizing that because the area coverage doubles each day, half of the lake is covered the day before the lake is fully covered (the 59th day). And both problems can be solved by selective comparison, just in case one has solved similar problems before, as might be the case for puzzle aficionados.

In our studies of children in grades 4 through 6, we compared children previously identified as gifted with children not so identified (Davidson and Sternberg 1984). Three major findings emerged. First, as we expected, the gifted children were better able to solve these problems than were the nongifted, and for the reasons we anticipated. The nongifted children, for example, tended to focus on the ratio in the socks problem, whereas the gifted children were more likely to ignore this information as irrelevant. Second, supplying the nongifted children with the insights needed to solve the problems substantially increased their performance, whereas supplying the gifted children with these insights had no effect. The reason was that the gifted children tended to have the insights spontaneously, and hence did not benefit from being given this information, whereas the nongifted children did not have the insights and thus benefited from being given them. Third, insight skills can be developed by training. In a five-week program for both the gifted and the nongifted children, we were able to effect significant improvement in their scores, relative to the scores of an untrained control group. Moreover, these gains were evident a year later, and transferred to solving problems of a kind that never appeared in the training program. Thus, it appears that insight skills differentiate the more from the less intelligent, but that they are trainable in both groups. The training did not eradicate individual differences: after both groups were trained, the differences remained, but with both groups performing at a higher level than they did initially.

Identification of the cognitive processes underlying intelligence can provide us with an understanding that is not supplied by global intelligence-test scores, in effect enabling us to make a start at getting inside intelligence. But it is not enough to identify cognitive processes. One must understand as well the metacognitive processes that drive the cognitive ones.

METACOGNITIVE PROCESSES

Used to plan, monitor, and evaluate one's performance of various kinds of tasks, the metacognitive processes, in essence, direct and receive feedback from the cognitive ones (Brown 1978; Sternberg 1985). The performance of tasks requires both kinds of processing: one could not get tasks done if one never left the planning stage; at the same time, one could get nothing done if one did not do some planning in the first place.

Various investigators have proposed different sets of metacognitive processes, which nevertheless overlap considerably. I include among such processes recognizing that a problem exists, defining the problem, selecting a set of cognitive processes to solve the problem, constructing a strategy for the solution of the problem, selecting a mental representation on which the processes and strategy will operate (e.g., a propositional representation or a spatial representation), allocating both internal and external resources to the problem, and monitoring one's solution of the problem.

Defining the nature of a problem is especially crucial to children's problem solving. Children are often unable to solve a problem if they cannot figure out its nature. Some theorists, such as Piaget (1972), have underestimated children's ability to solve problems because they have posed them in ways that children do not understand (Gelman and Baillargeon 1983).

A somewhat droll example of how important this understanding of the structure of problems is emerged in one of our studies of the development of analogical reasoning processes (Sternberg and Rifkin 1979). We presented children ranging from grade 2 through high school with two-choice picture analogies. The idea was for the children to select the better of the two possible answers. To our surprise, we found a number of second graders with scores of zero, which suggested that they could not reason analogically at all. We then went back to their test booklets and were astonished to find that rather than circling one of the possible answers, the children had circled one of the first two terms of the given analogy stem. We soon figured out what had happened: the children were students in a Jewish day school that normally had English-language instruction in the morning and Hebrew-language instruction in the afternoon. Having been tested in the afternoon, they had overgeneralized the right-to-left processing they normally did in the afternoon in reading Hebrew. They were well able to solve analogies, but they had misunderstood the nature of the task.

The ability to define a problem helps us distinguish between normally functioning and retarded individuals. A major feature separating the retarded from the normal individual is the retardate's need to be instructed explicitly and completely as to the nature of a particular task he is being asked to solve and the way it should be performed (Butterfield et al. 1973; Campione and Brown 1979). The importance of figuring out the nature of a problem is not limited to children and retarded persons. Indeed, Resnick and Glaser (1976) have argued that intelligence is largely the ability to learn in the absence of direct or complete instruction.

Older children differ from younger ones in ways other than defining problems. They often develop better strategies for solving problems than do the younger children. In our studies of analogical reasoning, for example, we have found qualitative differences between the strategies of younger children and those of older children and adults. For example, younger children tend to consider fewer features of a problem, encoding only part of it. This difference is crucial, because most of the errors our subjects make in analogical reasoning are due to premature termination of information processing (Sternberg 1977). Moreover, the difference is not limited to reasoning by analogy. Siegler (1978) studied children's performance on a wide variety of problem-solving tasks and found incomplete encoding to be a general characteristic of the younger children's information processing.

A second difference between younger and older children becomes particularly evident in the solution of verbal analogies. Younger children often attempt to solve the problems by word association, choosing as the correct answer the term that is most readily associated with the last given in the analogy (Achenbach 1970; Sternberg and Nigro 1980). In the analogy LAWYER is to CLIENT as DOCTOR is to (a) NURSE (b) PATIENT, (c) MEDICINE, (d) HOSPITAL, for example, younger children might select NURSE as the correct answer, because they associate a nurse more readily with a doctor than they do a patient.

Differences in strategies distinguish not only children from adults, but adults from other adults who vary in level of expertise within a given domain of problem solving. For example, Simon and Simon (1978) compared experts and novices in physics problem solving. Experts tended to use a "working forward" strategy, whereas novices tended to use a "working backward" strategy. The experts started from the givens in the problem and generated equations that could be solved from them. The novices started with an equation containing the unknown of the problem; if that equation did not work, they tried another, continuing with this procedure until they found an equation that contained the givens.

Another major difference between more and less intelligent problem solvers is the ways members of these two groups represent information. In a series of studies of cognitive development, for example, Smith and Kemler (1977) found that younger children are more apt to represent stimuli holistically, wheras older children and adults are more likely to represent stimuli analytically, decomposing them into their parts.

Expert and novice problem solvers have also been found to represent problems in qualitatively different ways. For example, Larkin (1979) found that expert physics problem solvers are more likely to construct some kind of analogue to a physical representation of a problem before they start solving the problem, whereas novices are more likely to proceed almost immediately to setting up equations. Chi and her colleagues (1982) found that novice problem solvers often organize their representation of a problem around dominant objects, such as an inclined plane, or around concepts, such as friction, that are mentioned explicitly in a problem. Experts, on the other hand, organize their representation around fundamental principles, such as conservation of energy, that derive from general knowledge only tacit in the problem statement. Representational differences extend to domains other than physics: they have been found

1. Suppose that all gem stones were made of foam rubber. Which of the following completions would then be correct for the analogy below?

WOOD : HARD :: DIAMOND ·

a. valuable; b. soft; c. brittle; d. hardest

2. Janet, Barbara, and Elaine are a housewife, lawyer, and physicist, although not necessarily in that order. Janet lives next door to the housewife. Barbara is the physicist's best friend. Elaine once wanted to be a lawyer but decided against it. Janet has seen Barbara within the last two days, but has not seen the physicist.

Janet, Barbara, and Elaine are, in that order, the

a. housewife, physicist, lawyer
b. physicist, lawyer, housewife
c. physicist, housewife, lawyer
d. lawyer, housewife, physicist

3. Josh and Sandy were discussing the Reds and the Blues, two baseball teams. Sandy asked Josh why he thought the Reds had a better chance of winning the pennant this year than did the Blues. Josh replied, "If every man on the Red team is better than every man on the Blue team, then the Reds must be the better team."

Josh is assuming that

a. inferences that apply to each part of a whole apply as well to the whole, and this assumption is true
b. inferences that apply to each part of a whole apply as well to the whole, and this assumption is false
c. inferences that apply to a whole apply as well to each part, and this assumption is true
d. inferences that apply to a whole apply as well to each part, and this assumption is false

4. The advertisement for the Sweet Life Savings Bank reads, "We guarantee the highest possible interest rates on all savings accounts." Professor Economos looked at the ad and immediately switched his money from the Drysdale Savings Bank to Sweet Life.

Assuming the Sweet Life Savings bank advertisement was honest, Professor Economos could be guaranteed to

a. earn higher interest at Sweet Life than at Drysdale
b. earn the same interest at Sweet Life as at Drysdale
c. earn at least as much at Sweet Life as at Drysdale
d. earn the same interest rate at Sweet Life as at any other bank making the same claim as Sweet Life

5. Select that answer option that represents either a necessary or forbidden property of the italicized word.

lion

a. fierce; b. white; c. mammalian; d. alive

in mathematics (e.g., Paige and Simon 1966) and political science (e.g., Voss et al. 1986).

One of the most elegant demonstrations of differences in representations among problem solvers was that of MacLeod and his colleagues (1978), who used a sentence-verification task devised by Clark and Chase (1972) to assess simple representational and problem-solving skills. In this task, the subject was shown a sentence such as "Star is above plus" and a picture such as "⁎" and had to indicate whether the picture correctly depicts the information in the sentence. Half the problems involved "true" answers, such as in the example, and half involved "false" answers (e.g., "Star is below plus" "⁎"). Moreover, half involved affirmative sentences, as in the two preceding examples, and half involved negative sentences (e.g., "Star is not below plus"). One of the most interesting findings in this study was that highly verbal subjects tended to adopt a verbal strategy and representation for information, wheras highly spatial subjects tended to adopt a spatial strategy and representation. The former group solved the problems through linguistic statements, whereas the latter group solved them by constructing a mental image of the picture.

Following up on this work, Hunt and Davidson (unpubl.) studied strategies for solving these problems as a function of age. Previous research had suggested that older individuals might have more difficulty than younger ones using a spatial representation of information (e.g., Horn 1968). Sure enough, older individuals were more likely to use a verbal strategy than were younger ones.

Differences in representations sometimes result from sheer amounts of knowledge available to members of different groups. For example, Chase and Simon (1973) compared expert and novice chess players, expecting to find that the experts differed somehow from novices in their mental processing of information. Instead, they found that the major difference between the two groups was the number of mental representations on which experts could draw in planning their subsequent moves. Experts had many thousands of chess patterns stored in long-term memory, whereas novices had relatively few. In essence, the expert must make the selective comparison between what he or she sees on the chess board and what is already stored in long-term memory. Subsequently, it has been found that the amount of knowledge makes a crucial difference to performance in a variety of fields, although in order for the knowledge to be used as needed, it must be represented in a way that makes it retrievable.

One of these fields is business management. Wagner and I (1985) studied what differentiates more successful from less successful business managers by giving executives tests of tacit knowledge—knowledge that one needs in a given field but that is not usually explicitly taught or even verbalized. In one problem, for example, the executives were presented with alternative criteria for choosing among various projects they might work on and were asked to rate how important each of the criteria was in the selection of a project. Such criteria would include how interesting the project might be, how noticeable performance on it would be to superiors, how difficult the project was likely to be, and so on. We found that more successful executives scored significantly higher on our measure of tacit knowledge than did less successful ones. However, when we gave the same test of tacit knowledge to college undergraduates, there was no correlation between the test and a standard psychometric measure of intelligence. This finding suggests that standard intelligence tests are incomplete as measures of business management ability because they fail to assess tacit knowledge important to the field.

Because people always have many demands upon their time, it is especially important that they allocate their resources in effective ways. No one is able to devote his or her full attention to every problem or every aspect of every problem, and so an important aspect of intelligence is deciding just how one's resources, and especially attentional resources, should be allocated.

The importance of how resources are allocated made itself particularly evident in two studies of intelligence. In one study, college students were asked to solve complex analogies (Sternberg 1981). In a standard analogy, only the fourth or last term is missing. In complex analogies, however, any one of the terms might be missing, or more than one term might be missing. For example, consider the analogy MAN is to SKIN as (a) DOG, (b) TREE is to (a) BARK, (b) CAT. In this particular analogy, the subject would have to recognize that the completions TREE and BARK form a sensible analogy (MAN is to SKIN as TREE is to BARK), whereas no other pair of completions does.

Our goal in this experiment was to isolate two levels of strategy planning. Global planning is the planning one does at a general level, whether for an entire set of test items, or for the day's tasks, or for one's career. Local planning is the planning one does at a specific level, whether for a single test item, or for a given task within a day, or for one stage of one's career. We were particularly interested in how better and poorer reasoners allocated their time between these two levels. By measuring and mathematically modeling the time subjects took to respond to various items, we were able to determine just how much time each subject spent on each of the two kinds of planning.

We found a qualitative difference in the ways in which better as opposed to poorer reasoners allocated their time between the two kinds of planning. Better reasoners tended to spend relatively more time on global planning than did poorer reasoners, but relatively less time on local planning. This finding is reminiscent of that mentioned earlier: better reasoners spend more time encoding terms of an analogy problem but less time operating on these encodings. Once again, the more intelligent problem solvers put more of their time "up front" in problem solving, in order to enable themselves to operate more efficiently once they get down to details. This finding regarding allocation of time is not limited to reasoning by analogy. A similar finding emerged in a study of physics problem solving by Larkin and her colleagues (1980).

In a second study, we extended this kind of analysis to reading comprehension (Wagner and Sternberg, in press). Although standard tests typically require examinees to read all of the passages with great care, in normal circumstances no one really has the time to read everything carefully. Rather, one allocates one's time on the basis of the kind of reading and its purpose. One does not read *American Scientist,* for example, in the way one reads *Newsweek,* nor does one read a scientific article vital to one's research in the way one reads an article of casual interest.

In our study, we asked college students to read eleven sets of four passages apiece, drawn equally from novels, newspapers, humanities texts, and science texts. Subjects were given free rein as to the order in which they read each of the sets of four passages and the amount of time they spent on each passage. They were told, however, to read one particular passage in each set for gist, a second for main ideas, a third for details, and a fourth for analysis of ideas. We then compared the allocation of time by the subjects, who were identified in advance as either good readers or poor readers. We found that good readers allocated their time according to their purpose, spending relatively more time on passages that needed to be read for details or analysis than those that were read for gist or main ideas. Poorer readers, however, showed a flat distribution of time across reading purposes; they spent equal amount of time on each of the four passages in a set, regardless of the purpose for which they were reading it. Again, the better performers showed a superior strategy for allocating time.

We have seen that cognitive scientists are attempting to unlock the doors to the mind by getting inside intelligence, seeking an understanding of the mental processes whereby people solve problems that challenge their intellectual abilities. Although more intelligent individuals perform many tasks more rapidly than do less intelligent ones, they perform certain cognitive operations relatively more slowly, because of a metacognitive strategy whereby they are able to allocate more time to global planning and encoding of stimuli and to speed up local planning and mental operations on the encoded stimuli. By studying both cognitive and metacognitive processes, we have a more complete view as to just when it pays to process information more rapidly, and when it pays to process it more slowly. Analyses of response times and patterns of errors in a wide variety of problems can provide the keys to unlock at least some of the mysteries of the mind. Through these techniques, cognitive scientists are increasing our understanding of the inner workings of intelligence.

REFERENCES

Achenbach, T.M. 1970. The children's associative responding test: A possible alternative to group IQ tests. *J. Educational Psychol.* 61:340–48.

Brown, A.L. 1978. Knowing when, where, and how to remember: A problem of metacognition. In *Advances in Instructional Psychology,* vol. 1, ed. R. Glaser, pp. 77–165. Erlbaum.

Butterfield, E.C., C. Wambold, and J. M. Belmont. 1973. On the theory and practice of improving short-term memory. *Am. J. Mental Deficiency* 77:654–69.

Campione, J.C., and A. L. Brown. 1979. Toward a theory of intelligence: Contributions from research with retarded children. In *Human Intelligence: Perspectives on Its Theory and Measurement,* ed. R.J. Sternberg and D.K. Detterman, pp. 139–64. Ablex.

Chase, W.G., and H.A. Simon. 1973. Perception in chess. *Cognitive Psychol.* 4:55–81.

Chi, M.T. H., R. Glaser, and R. Rees. 1982. Expertise in problem solving. In *Advances in the Psychology of Human Intelligence,* vol. 1, ed. R.J. Sternberg, pp. 7–75. Erlbaum.

Clark, H.H., and W.G. Chase. 1972. On the process of comparing sentences against pictures. *Cognitive Psychol.* 3:472–517.

Cole, M., J. Gay, J. Glick, and D. Sharp. 1971. *The Cultural Context of Learning and Thinking.* Basic Books.

Davidson, J.E., And R.J. Sternberg. 1984. The role of insight in intellectual giftedness. *Gifted Child Quart* 28:58–64.

Gelman, R., and R., Baillargeon. 1983. A review of some Piagetian concepts. In *Handbook of Child Psychology,* vol. 3, ed. J. Flavell and E. Markman, pp. 167–230. Wiley.

Horn, J.L. 1968. Organization of abilities and the development of intelligence. *Psychol. Rev.* 75:242–59.

Hunt, E.B., and J.E. Davidson, Unpubl. Age-related changes in strategies for sentence verification.

Hunt, E.B., C. Lunneborg, and J. Lewis. 1975. What does it mean to be high verbal? *Cognitive Psychol.* 7:194–227.

Jensen, A.R. 1980. *Bias in Mental Testing.* Free Press.

Kail, R.V., and J.W. Pellegrino. 1985. *Human Intelligence: Perspectives and Prospects.* Freeman.

Laboratory of Comparative Human Cognition. 1982. Culture and intelligence. In *Handbook of Human Intelligence,* ed. R.J. Sternberg, pp. 642–719. Cambridge Univ. Press.

Larkin, J. H. 1979. *Models of Competence in Solving Physics Problems.* Complex Information Processing working paper no. 408, Dept. of Psychol., Carnegie-Mellon Univ., Pitts-burgh, PA.

Larkin, J.H., J. McDermott, D.P. Simon, and H.A. Simon. 1980. Models of competence in solving physics problems. *Cognitive Sci.* 4:317–45.

MacLeod, C.M., E.B. Hunt, and N.N. Mathews. 1978. Individual differences in the verification of sentence-picture relationships. *J. Verbal Learning and Verbal Beh.* 17:493–507.

Matarazzo, J.D. 1972. *Wechsler's Measurement and Appraisal of Adult Intelligence.* Williams & Wilkins.

Paige, J.M., and H.A. Simon. 1966. Cognitive processes in solving algebra word problems. In *Problem Solving: Research, Method, and Theory,* ed. B. Kleinmuntz, pp. 51–148. Wiley.

Piaget, J. 1972. *The Psychology of Intelligence.* Littlefield, Adams.

Posner, M.I., and R.F. Mitchell. 1967. Chronometric analysis of classification. *Psychol. Rev.* 74:392–409.

Resnick, L.B., and R. Glaser, 1976. Problem solving and intelligence. In *The Nature of Intelligence,* ed. L.B. Resnick, pp. 205–30. Erlbaum.

Siegler, R.S. 1978. The origins of scientific reasoning. In *Children's Thinking: What Develops?* ed. R. Siegler, pp. 109–49. Erlbaum.

Simon, D.P., and H.A. Simon. 1978. Individual differences in solving physics problems. In *Children's Thinking; What Develops?* ed. R. Siegler, pp. 325–48. Erlbaum.

Smith, L.B., and D.G. Kemler, 1977. Developmental trends in free classification: Evidence for a new conceptualization of perceptual development. *J. Experimental Child Psychol.* 24:279–98.

Spearman, C. 1923. *The Nature of Intelligence and the Principles of Cognition.* Macmillan.

Sternberg, R.J. 1977. *Intelligence, Information Processing, and Analogical Reasoning: The Componential Analysis of Human Abilities.* Erlbaum.

———. 1981. Intelligence and nonentrenchment. *J. Educational Psychol.* 73:1–16.

———, ed. 1982. *Handbook of Human Intelligence.* Cambridge Univ. Press.

———, ed. 1984. *Human Abilities: An Information-Processing Approach.* Freeman.

———. 1985. *Beyond IQ: A Triarchic Theory of Human Intelligence.* Cambridge Univ. Press.

Sternberg, R.J., and J.E. Davidson, 1982. The mind of the puzzler. *Psychol. Today,* June, pp. 37–44.

Sternberg, R.J., and M.K. Gardner. 1983. Unities in inductive reasoning. *J. Experimental Psychol.: General* 112:80–116.

Sternberg, R.J., and G. Nigro. 1980. Developmental patterns in the solution of verbal analogies. *Child Devel.* 51:27–38.

Sternberg, R.J., and J.S. Powell. 1983. Comprehending verbal comprehension. *Am Psychol.* 38:878–93.

Sternberg, R.J., and B. Rifkin. 1979. The development of analogical reasoning processes. *J. Experimental Child Psychol.* 27:195–232.

Voss, J.F., R.H. Fincher-Keifer, T.R. Greene, and T.A. Post. 1986. Individual differences in performance: The contrastive approach to knowledge. In *Advances in the Psychology of Human Intelligence,* vol. 3, ed. R.J. Sternberg, pp. 297–334, Erlbaum.

Wagner, R.K., and R.J. Sternberg. 1985. Practical intelligence in real-world pursuits: The role of tacit knowledge. *J. Personality and Soc. Psychol.* 49:436–58.

———. In press. Executive processes in reading. In *Executive Processes in Reading,* ed. B. Britton. Erlbaum.

Wober, M. 1974. Towards an understanding of the Kiganda concept of intelligence. In *Culture and Cognition: Readings in Cross-cultural Psychology,* ed. J.W. Berry and P.R. Dasen, pp. 261–80. Methuen.

PART III: COGNITION AND LEARNING

12

Future of the LD Field:
Research and Practice

Barbara K. Keogh
University of California, Los Angeles

Barbara Keogh has long been concerned with the quality of research in the LD field. In looking to the future, she builds on the many issues and problems raised by the survey respondents and organizes the concerns under four major questions which she suggests can direct and guide our research and practice. Can LD be clearly and reliably differentiated from other mild handicaps? Can conceptual and relevant distinctions be identified within the broad LD category? Can treatment-condition links be demonstrated? What are the social and cultural influences on LD? Keogh presents a brief overview of the current state of the art to provide a context for considering each question and then offers her views on where we need to go from here and how we can get there. Among her conclusions, she sees as essential (a) the differentiation of LD from other problems, (b) identification of logical ways to organize the individual variations which characterize LD groups, (c) the gathering of data on such variations and on the specifics of intervention activity (in order to clarify treatment–condition links), and (d) recognition of social/cultural and social system influences on the nature of the child and institutional transactions and on LD identification and provision of services. Her suggestions for the immediate future stress the importance of temporarily separating the study of LD as a problem in development from concerns for service delivery, of thoroughly documenting program practices, and of rethinking our notions of defini-

Reprinted with permission from the *Journal of Learning Disabilities,* 1986, Vol. 19, No. 8, 455–460. Copyright 1986 by PRO-ED, Inc.

*tion and adopting a "shared attribute" approach. How shall the field ac-
complish all this? Keogh cautions it will be a slow and painful process and
explores why this is likely to be the case. At the same time, she sees the time
as being right for making sense out of LD.*

Predicting the future is, at best, a risky enterprise. Predicting the future
of something as ambiguous as learning disabilities (LD) is probably better
described as foolish. However, our rather brief history allows some
generalizations about problems and issues which no doubt affect where
we are going and what we will achieve. These issues are central to the field
and have implications for both research and practice. Indeed, they affect
the interactions between research and practice, often threatening the
validity of both. A number of problems have been identified and discussed by Adelman and Taylor (1985) in their introduction to this series
of articles, and their analysis receives strong consensual agreement from
most professionals in the field. Obvious topics of concern include the
definition of LD, treatment/intervention effectiveness, prevention, and
early identification, to name a few.

In my view, the many problems may be organized under four major
questions which can direct and guide our research and practice: Can LD
be clearly and reliably differentiated from other conditions of mild handicap? Can conceptual and relevant distinctions be identified within the
broad LD category? Can we demonstrate treatment-condition links?
What are social and cultural influences on LD? Answers to these questions may provide direction to the field by moving us out of our
seemingly endless preoccupation with "The Definition" and with our
often parochial professional or disciplinary perspectives. Answers may
also enhance our understanding of LD and what to do about it. A brief
overview of the current "state of the art" provides a context for considering these questions.

CURRENT STATUS OF THE FIELD

LD is the single largest category of special education services (*Sixth Annual Report to Congress,* prepared by the Office of Special Education Programs, 1984). LD is also the fastest growing category of special education
services, the numbers of LD identified pupils increasing from 757,213 in
1976–77 to 1,745,871 in 1982–83. The 1982–83 figure represents almost
4% of school children nationally and over 40% of children receiving special education services. Clearly, LD is an important component of
American education, yet it continues to be a service category charac-

terized by inconsistency and disagreement. Who and how many are identified reflect these inconsistencies. Examination of the prevalence of LD according to states (*Sixth Annual Report*) illustrates the point. In Rhode Island 63% of children ages 3 to 21 identified as handicapped were considered LD; comparable percentages for California, New Hampshire, and Texas were 55%, 58%, and 52%, respectively. In contrast, only 26% of handicapped children in Alabama were classified as LD, a prevalence figure similar to those reported in the states of Indiana (27%), Kentucky (27%), and South Carolina (29%). Apparently, identification of LD is, in part at least, related to geography as well as to pupils' characteristics.

Differences in identification as LD have also been shown to be related to disciplinary or professional perspectives and techniques, to the specific formula used for determining a discrepancy between ability and achievement, to the techniques and measures used in diagnosis, and to a variety of institutional or organizational constraints (Keogh, 1986). Included in the latter set of influences are such specifics as the number and availability of special programs, the administrative arrangements within school districts, the availability and work loads of school psychologists, and the legislative and political context in which schools function (Mehan, Meihls, Hertweck, & Crowdes, 1981). These influences become particularly powerful given the lack of an agreed–upon conceptual definition of LD. The consequences are inconsistent services and a confounded data base for study of LD. The four questions posed earlier address these confusions, and they provide direction for determining research and program priorities.

Can LD be differentiated from other mildly handicapping conditions? This question confronts directly the question of heterogeneity or homogeneity of similar but presumably different problem conditions. The question has particular pertinence to mild mental retardation and emotional disturbance, behavior disorders, and low achievement. Indeed, low achievement is often the single most common characteristic of many conditions of mild handicap. Importantly, it is sometimes difficult to make sound and reliable distinctions among subgroups. This point is well illustrated by the work of Ysseldyke and his colleagues (e.g., Ysseldyke, Algozzine, Shinn, & McGue, 1982), who have shown in a number of studies that school district classified LD pupils are often similar to pupils in other special education classifications or to unclassified pupils in regular education programs (see also the work of Shepard, 1983, and Shepard & Smith, 1983). Further, LD is often not just an academic learning or achievement problem, as documented in reports of the high number of behavioral, social, and affective problems in groups of LD pupils (Bryan & Bryan, 1981; Gresham, 1986).

On the surface the problems of delineation of differences among mildly handicapping conditions may be viewed primarily as a research issue (Keogh, 1986; Keogh & MacMillan, 1983). In fact, confounds across categories carry major consequences for the delivery of services. Who is served and under what conditions are practical questions which affect decisions about LD pupils and their families. The issue of differentiation of LD from other conditions, thus, must be considered by professionals who provide services to LD individuals as well as by reseachers who study the problem. The identification of conceptually defensible and operationally reliable criteria to delineate LD from other conditions is an important step in the future of the field. Without these distinctions, there is little basis for a separate classification or diagnostic category called LD.

Can conceptually and empirically meaningful distinctions be identified within the broad LD category? The first question was directed toward differences across or among special education categories, especially among conditions of mild handicap. The second question addresses the issue of within category heterogeneity. The single most accepted criterion of LD is an ability–achievement discrepancy. Reynolds (1984–85) points out that the ability–achievement discrepancy, a widely accepted criterion of LD, merely identifies a pool of potential LD individuals. The range of individual characteristics within this pool is broad (Keogh, Major–Kingsley, Omori–Gordon, & Reid, 1982). Clearly, there is no single prototypic LD pupil. LD pupils are characterized as much by their differences as by their similarity, and we deal with multiple disabilities, not a single unitary disability (McKinney, 1986). Yet, we continue to talk about programs and research subjects as if they represent a single condition. It is likely that both research and intervention would be furthered if we were to give up the search for "The Definition" and instead focus our attention on systematic description of the variations associated within LD.

As a start, I suggest that our efforts be directed toward a thorough documentation of the many expressions or characteristics of LD. Subsequent steps may involve delineation of coherent subgroups and the specification of relationships among groups and subgroups. The product of such effort would be taxonomy of learning disabilities which could encompass multiple definitions. A taxonomy would not reduce or diminish the interesting array of individual characteristics or variations now subsumed under the single category, LD. Rather, a taxonomy would bring order and rationality to the differences and would provide an organizational system which could advance our understanding of *learning disabilities* and how to treat them.

Acceptance of the notion that LD is not a single syndrome but rather is a set of related syndromes frees us from a number of constraints which currently limit our research and our intervention efforts. It should not surprise us that the results of many studies do not generalize or that interventions which work well in one school district are not effective in another. Pupil or subject characteristics interact with variations in programs and practices and make generalizations about LD limited at best. The task is to bring order to diversity. A number of efforts have already begun toward this goal. Torgesen (1982) has called for research with "rationally defined subgroups." Keogh and colleagues (1982) have argued for the use of a common set of marker variables for describing research samples and for testing intervention impact. A rapidly expanding research literature documents empirical efforts at subtyping (see Lyon, 1983, and McKinney, 1984, 1986, for discussion). Although implemented from somewhat different perspectives, these efforts appear promising as major steps toward a logical organization of the individual variations which characterize LD groups.

Can we demonstrate treatment-condition links? The search for aptitude-treatment-interactions (ATI) has a long and somewhat discouraging history (Cronbach, 1975; Cronbach & Snow, 1977). Yet, the notion that there are pupil-program links remains fundamental in our search for interventions with LD pupils. Some therapists argue for visual perceptual training on the assumption that LD is basically a visual perceptual problem. Others support the use of medication or psycholinguistic training or psychotherapy. While all might agree that a given treatment may not be appropriate for all LD individuals, the assumption is that the intervention of choice (or belief) is appropriate and effective for most. In fact, there is relatively little evidence to support the effectiveness of many intervention programs, and almost no solid evidence which allows a comparative test among programs.

At least two aspects of the problem must be addressed if we are to understand the interactions of LD pupils and the programs that are provided for them. The first set of issues relates to the characteristics of pupils served. This has already been addressed in questions one and two. The other part of the pupil-intervention equation has to do with the nature of the programs themselves. Programs, like pupils, may carry the same labels but may differ dramatically. Even where program philosophies or directives are clear and agreed upon, the accuracy of implementation may not be the same. Thus, two programs claiming to be perceptual-motor, or Piagetian, or psycholinguistic, may be operationalized in quite different ways. The specifics of implementation cannot be ignored. They represent important data in testing pupil-program interactions. Unfortunately, for the most part the assessment of program effectiveness has not included detailed and comprehensive descriptions of program practices. Such data are as necessary as information about pupils if we are to assess and analyze effective intervention practices.

While seemingly simple, accurate description is difficult to achieve. Clinicians and teachers are already burdened by considerable paperwork, and the process of accurate description may put additional demands on their time and energies. Further, professionals involved in the delivery of services may not be aware of inconsistencies or omissions in how a program is implemented. Finally, the documentation of program practices may be threatening to the individuals involved, as there may be unrecognized discrepancies between beliefs and reality. Clearly this is not a trivial matter which can be dealt with by administrative directive. Rather, comprehensive documentation of program practices, like the development of a taxonomy of pupil characteristics, requires commitment and support.

What are social/cultural and social systems influences on LD? The historical roots of LD were biological in that LD was equated with brain dysfunction or neurological impairment. From this perspective the diagnostic search was focused almost exclusively on the LD individual, and etiology and organically based symptoms were key criteria in clinical decisions. A number of professionals still hold this perspective and present reasonable arguments for diagnostic and treatment programs with a medical focus. It is likely that a subset of children within the LD category do, indeed, represent specific, neurologically based syndromes. However, as LD has assumed a more educational definition, diagnostic criteria and practices have changed and the focus has shifted so that both child and extrachild influences must be considered in identification and classification. This perspective receives support from developmental theorists who argue for the transactive nature of development (Sameroff, 1975; Sameroff & Chandler, 1975). It also receives support from psychologists and educators who approach problem development from a systems orientation (Ramey & MacPhee, 1986) or from a social-cultural perspective (Price-Williams & Gallimore, 1980). For the most part, however, the conduct of research and practice within the LD field has been carried out with an almost exclusive focus on the LD individual.

An extensive literature documents relationships between socio-economic status (SES) and problems in development (see Nichols & Chen, 1981; Werner & Smith, 1982). Children from economically disadvantaged homes have been shown to have a higher probability of developmental, social, and educational problems than do their more advantaged peers. It is likely also that they have a higher probability of developing learning disabilities. Yet, the exclusionary criteria in the definition of LD may lead to under-identification of LD pupils within this group. The social circumstances in which children find themselves influence the identification of LD in at least two ways: first, through the nature of the environment-child interactions and transactions; second, in the likelihood of identification and the availability and adequacy of services.

The latter point is well illustrated by the work of Mehan et al. (1981), who documented the effects of institutional constraints on referral and placement practices in special education. These researchers used qualitative, observational methods to describe the flow of special education decision making within schools, finding that progress through the special education system was not just a matter of pupil "symptoms," but rather was related directly to institutional characteristics of the school district; e.g., level of funding, availability of space in special programs, number and kind of alternative programs, etc. While from a scientific perspective we might like to think that decisions about LD are made exclusively on the basis of accepted and validated child attributes, from a social systems perspective it is clear that both child and institutional characteristics must be considered. This, of course, complicates the task for the researcher of LD, as it broadens the base of relevant data and implicates potentially complicated interactions between child and environment.

WHERE DO WE GO FROM HERE?

The material covered in this review has not really provided answers to the four questions posed. Yet the content may help define directions for our future activities. Many readers will not endorse the suggestions which follow as they may appear to go against conventional wisdom and long-held beliefs. However, these are issues which must be dealt with if the LD field is to be viable both scientifically and programmatically.

First, despite the appeal of the call for "relevant" research, for research which directly improves practice, it may be necessary to separate temporarily the study of LD as a problem in development from concerns for delivery of services to LD pupils. Our present research literature is for the most part derived from data in which child and social/institutional effects are hopelessly confounded, and this has diluted our understanding of both child conditions and program issues. For a time, at least, these need to be viewed as parallel but separate problems. The value of research which does not have immediate and direct application has been demonstrated in many scientific fields. There are a number of questions in LD which do not translate directly nor easily to direct services, e.g., the course of LD over time, the contribution of genetics, the power of specific information processing models, the organization and relationships among subtypes, the impact of different family accommodation patterns. Yet, these are important topics if we are to understand the nature of LD. Our understanding of them will in time lead to improved practices.

The call in the first suggestion was to free the study of LD from its programmatic ties, to separate issues of service delivery from investigation of LD conditions. The second recommendation is focused on the need for thorough and careful documentation of program practices, and for consideration of the comparative effectiveness of services. Despite the proliferation of programs for LD pupils, specifics and program practices vary dramatically in content, timing, intensity, and duration. Few data are available to document program practices or to evaluate relative effectiveness of specific components of programs. Few studies address social and institutional influences on referral, classification, and services. Such information is necessary if we are to make wise use of resources for a growing LD constituency. On the surface, the documentation of program practices seems a reasonable and relatively easy task. Yet, it is clear that a systematic effort requires support and involvement of both clinicians and administrators. It is also clear that the task requires commitment on an attitudinal level, as evaluation may challenge long-held beliefs.

Finally, the application of research to practice is contingent, in large part, on our willingness to rethink our notions of the definition of LD. From a multidefinitional perspective, we deal with many learning disabilities, not one learning disability. Thus, I have argued for a "shared attribute" definition (Keogh, 1986). From the starting point of an ability-achievement discrepancy, LD pupils branch out into a broad range of personal characteristics. Not all LD pupils have short-term memory problems, are hyperactive, or evidence visual perceptual problems. Many share some of these characteristics, however. Part of the research task is to identify consistencies and regularities within the symptom array, to bring order to a series of definitions of LD. Part of the programmatic task is to identify links between the conditions and interventions.

HOW DO WE GET THERE?

The truthful answer to this question is probably "slowly and painfully." Slowly, because the next steps involve more than just the accrual of information about LD individuals. Rather, progress depends on developing a meaningful conceptualization of LD. This will take time and likely will not occur in a neat, linear fashion. Painfully, because conceptual reorganization generates anxiety, controversy, and tension, sometimes even hostility. Yet the time seems right for making sense out of LD. We have gathered extensive information about LD individuals, this array reflecting many professional and disciplinary perspectives. We have implemented a range of intervention and treatment programs which serve LD individuals across an age range including preschool through young adulthood. We have active constituents and advocates who represent LD politically. Now the task for the professional community is to bring rationality, order, and meaningfulness to the field. This will require effort on a number of levels and from a number of different perspectives. In my view, it will necessarily involve at least three different groups: those who conduct research; those who collaborate and/or use research; and those who fund research.

Consider first the conduct of research. Although the volume of publication on LD has increased, this literature is fragmented, consisting primarily of unrelated single studies (unfortunately, sometimes of questionable quality) or of advocacy statements. There is limited generalization of findings across studies and many separate sets of data exist which are difficult to interpret. Part of the problem is that many studies stand alone as isolated efforts. Such studies often provide specific information about selected topics, but they provide only limited insight into major issues in LD. This is not to argue that single studies of LD should not be conducted or published. It does suggest, however, that our broader understanding of LD will derive from research which has a programmatic base, which builds over time, and which has focus and a coherent framework to guide individual studies.

The programmatic-single study issue is not a simple one, however. Programmatic research has many appeals but real limitations (see Keogh, 1983, and McKinney, 1983, for discussion). It requires a stable set of researchers and consistent funding. It may limit opportunities for other investigators, as resources are tied up in fewer but larger research efforts. It may lead to a restricted set of research topics, thus limiting our work on new and promising topics. Nevertheless, taken as a whole, the gains from organized programmatic research seem to outweigh the limitations. Our understanding of LD will likely be furthered as more investigators plan collaborative programs of research rather than relying on individual, single studies. One of the hows in how to get there, thus, is the recommendation for more programmatic research.

A closely related issue has to do with quality of research in LD. Improving quality is a problem which requires the attention and efforts of professionals in university training programs and journal editors alike. Although there are many doctoral training programs, a review of the research in LD suggests that we are producing many students with limited research skills. Many newly graduated PhDs have research experience restricted to their own dissertations. Yet, these graduates are expected to be productive researchers, to contribute to the scientific knowledge about LD, and to train other researchers in doctoral programs. Given the limitations of their own training, it should not surprise us that many university faculty are ill-prepared for these demanding tasks. An obvious direction for improving the quality of research, then, is to improve the quality of research training. This may mean advanced inservice training for university faculty, more collaborative research, graduate training which is focused on developing research skills, and research apprenticeships. Clearly, a research training emphasis is not one which is appropriate for all doctoral training programs in LD. The field needs quality training in a number of areas, e.g.,., curriculum, instruction, and policy—not just in research. As it is not reasonable to expect all programs to do all things, we may need to allow for more differentiated, yet focused, training programs. At the very least, those of us in university programs need to conduct critical self-evaluations of the adequacy of our training efforts and to implement ways to improve their quality.

Another path toward improving research in LD involves journal editors. Journal editors play a unique and important role in determining the direction and the quality of research which characterize a field. To the credit of the editors of the journals in LD and related fields, we have seen considerable improvement in the level of published research. However, even casual reading suggests that there is considerable room for improvement. If we are to upgrade the quality of both research and practice, we may well have to make the publication review and decision process more stringent. This may lead to slimmer volumes but better reading, a consequence most journal readers should appreciate.

Improving the quality of research and ultimately of practice is not just the responsibility of university researchers and journal editors, however. The conduct of research is also a matter of concern for professionals who provide direct services, for school and clinic personnel. If we are to develop a real understanding of LD, we must also study LD conditions within their natural contexts—the classroom, the clinic, and the recreation field. Yet, the conduct of research within service facilities places real burdens on service professionals. Researchers in classrooms may disrupt the regular program, may distract pupils, and may threaten teachers' peace of mind. The need for systematic and detailed information, collected in specific formats, may over-extend the time and energies of already overburdened clinicians or teachers. Arrangements of schedules and the freeing up of space for research may prove troublesome for school administrators. On a somewhat different level, research may seem unnecessary or unrelated to ongoing programs, thus may lack value or worth in the eyes of service professionals. Finally, research may threaten long-held beliefs and challenge well-established practices, thus eliciting anxiety and hostility. All of these represent very real barriers to the conduct of research in applied settings. The working relationships between research and service professionals have often been shaky, at best. Yet, understanding LD requires their cooperative and integrated efforts.

A final suggestion relates to governmental and private funding agencies. A coherent and consistent policy about research is necessary if we are to increase our understanding of LD. Two critical policy issues include the determination of research priorities and funding patterns. I suggested earlier in this paper that priority be given to programmatic research, and that understanding LD may require temporary separation of theoretical research from practice. These recommendations may not be popular in a field which has its roots in applied programs directed at individual pupils. Yet, our clinical history has not provided the conceptualization necessary to bring consensus to the field. If we are to achieve understanding of LD, we must have time and consistent support. The major support for research in LD rests with governmental agencies. Thus, federal policies and practices governing research in LD are central to the future of the field. Federal policy affects us in may ways: through support for training, for direct services, and for research. None of these can function well if support is uncertain, if priorities change frequently, or if funding schedules are disrupted. It is imperative that federal policy have coherence and continuity so that professionals involved in LD can get on with their work with confidence. Closely related, it should be emphasized that decisions about funding directly affect the direction of the field. The equity and quality of the review process, along with effective monitoring and evaluation of research efforts, contribute to the adequacy of research and, therefore, influence practice. The question of quality of project becomes especially important at a time when research funds are limited. Quality is not just the concern of researchers and journal editors; it is also of concern to funding agencies. Thus, it is imperative that review procedures and criteria are consistent and ensure quality.

I conclude by suggesting again that the future of the LD field relates directly to our willingness and ability to conceptualize and organize the many conditions subsumed by the LD label. Acceptance of the idea that there is not one learning disability but rather a number of different learning disabilities helps direct both research and practice. On a research level we need to provide a systematic way of organizing and describing the range of individual attributes which characterize LD individuals. On an applied level we need to determine which interventions or treatments are effective with which kinds of LD. On a research level we need to identify causes and correlates of various LD conditions, and to document the consequences over time. On an applied level we need to consider institutional arrangements for services, to develop and evaluate training programs for professionals, and to improve the quality and content of diagnosis and assessment. These are not easy goals to accomplish. They involve aspects of clinical decision making along with issues of research strategies and techniques. They require the expertise, commitment, and cooperation of researchers and program professionals. They also require coherent and consistent policy at local, state, and federal levels. Despite the problems, I am optimistic that these goals are attainable. We have made progress, but that progress underscores how far we have to go.

REFERENCES

Adelman, H.S., & Taylor, L. (1985). The future of the LD field: A survey of fundamental concerns. *Journal of Learning Disabilities, 18*(7), 423–427.

Bryan, T.H., & Bryan, J.H. (1981). Some personal and social experiences of learning disabled children. In B.K. Keogh (Ed.) *Advances in special education, Volume 4, Socialization influences on exceptionality.* Greenwich, CT: JAI Press.

Cronbach, L.J. (1975). Beyond the two disciplines of scientific psychology. *American Psychologist, 30*(2), 116–127.

Cronbach, L.J., & Snow, R.W. (1977). *Aptitudes and instructional methods.* New York: Irvington Press.

Gresham, F.M. (1986). Social competence and motivational characteristics of learning disabled students. In M. Wang, H. Walberg, & M. Reynolds (Eds.) *The handbook of special education: Research and Practice,* Vols. 1-3. Oxford, England: Pergamon Press.

Keogh, B.K. (1983). A lesson from Gestalt psychology. *Exceptional Education Quarterly, 4*(1), 115–128.

Keogh, B.K. (1986). Learning disabilities: Diversity in search of order. In M. Wang., H. Walberg, & M. Reynolds (Eds.), *The handbook of special education: research and practice.* Oxford, England: Pergamon Press.

Keogh, B.K. & MacMillan, D.L. (1983). The logic of sample selection: Who represents what? *Exceptional Education Quarterly, 4*(3), 84–96.

Keogh, B., Major-Kingsley, S., Omori-Gordon, & Reid, H.P. (1982). *A system of marker variables for the field of learning disabilities.* Syracuse, NY: Syracuse University Press.

Lyon, G.R. (1983). Subgroups of learning disabled readers: Clinical and empirical identification. In H. Myklebust, *Progress in learning disabilities* (Vol. V). New York: Grune and Stratton.

McKinney, J.D. (1983). Contributions of the institutes for research on learning disabilities. *Exceptional Education Quarterly, 4*(1), 129–144.

McKinney, J.D. (1984). The search for subtypes of specific learning disability. *Annual Review of Learning Disabilities, 2,* 19–26.

McKinney, J.D. (1986). Research on conceptually and empirically defined subtypes of learning disabilities. In M. Wang, H. Walberg, & M. Reynolds (Eds.), *The handbook of special education: Research and Practice.* Oxford, England: Pergamon Press.

Mehan, H., Meihls, J.L., Hertweck, A., & Crowdes, M. (1981). Identifying handicapped students. In S.B. Bacharach (Ed.), *Organizational behavior in school and school districts.* New York: Praeger Publications.

Nichols, P.L., & Chen, T.C. (1981). *Minimal brain dysfunction: A prospective study.* Hillsdale, NJ: Lawrence Erlbaum Associates.

Price-Williams, D., & Gallimore, R. (1980). The cultural perspective. In B.K. Keogh (Ed.), *Advances in special education, Volume 2: Perspectives on applications.* Greenwich, CT: JAI Press.

Ramey, C.T., & MacPhee, D. (1986). Developmental retardation: A systems theory perspective on risk and preventive intervention. In D.C. Farrah & J.D. McKinney (Eds.), *Risk in intellectual and psychosocial development.* New York: Academic Press.

Reynolds, C.R. (1984-85). Critical measurement issues in learning disabilities. *The Journal of Special Education, 18*(4), 451–476.

Sameroff, A. (1975). Transactional models in early social relations. *Human Development, 18,* 65–79.

Sameroff, A.J., & Chandler, M.J. (1975). Reproductive risk and the continuum of caretaking casualty. *Review of child development research,* Vol. 4. Chicago: University of Chicago Press.

Shepard, L. (1983). The role of measurement in educational policy: Lessons from the identification of learning disabilities. *Educational Measurement: Issues and Practice,* 4–8.

Shepard, L.A., & Smith, M.L. (1983). An evaluation of the identification of learning disabled students in Colorado. *Learning Disability Quarterly, 6,* 115–127.

Sixth Annual Report to Congress on the Implementation of Public Law 94–142: The Education for All Handicapped Children Act. (1984). Office of Special Education, U.S. Department of Education.

Torgesen, J.K. (1982). The use of rationally defined subgroups in research in reading disabilities. In J.P. Das, R.F. Mulcahey, & A.E. Wall (Eds.), *Theory and research in reading disabilities.* New York: Plenum Press.

Werner, E.F., & Smith, R.S. (1982). *Vulnerable but invincible: A longitudinal study of resilient children and youth.* New York: McGraw-Hill.

Ysseldyke, J.E., Algozzine, B., Shinn, M.R., & McGue, M. (1982). Similarities and differences between low achievers and students classified learning disabled. *The Journal of Special Education, 16*(1), 73–85.

13

Mathematics Achievement of Chinese, Japanese, and American Children

Harold W. Stevenson and Shin-ying Lee
University of Michigan, Ann Arbor
James W. Stigler
University of Chicago, Illinois

American kindergarten children lag behind Japanese children in their understanding of mathematics; by fifth grade they are surpassed by both Japanese and Chinese children. Efforts to isolate bases for these differences involved testing children on other achievement and cognitive tasks, interviewing mothers and teachers, and observing children in their classrooms. Cognitive abilities of children in the three countries are similar, but large differences exist in the children's life in school, the attitudes and beliefs of their mothers, and the involvement of both parents and children in schoolwork.

Poor scholastic performance by American children has focused attention on education, especially in mathematics and science. Funds for research on how to improve teaching have been allocated and commissions formed, such as a National Research Council committee exploring a research agenda for precollege education in mathematics, science, and technology. Recommendations to be made by this committee and others that have preceded it concentrate on the nation's secondary schools. The wisdom of this emphasis is questionable. Results emerging from a large cross-national study of elementary school children suggest that Americans should not focus solely on improving the performance of high school students. The problems arise earlier. American children appear to lag behind children in other countries in reading and mathematics as early as kindergarten and continue to perform less effectively during the years of elementary school. When differences in achievement arise so early in the child's formal education, more must be involved than inadequate formal educational practices. Improving secondary education is an important goal, but concentrating remedial efforts on secondary schools may come too late in the academic careers of most students to be effective.

Our research deals with the scholastic achievement of American, Chinese, and Japanese children in kindergarten and grades 1 and 5. Children were given achievement tests and a battery of cognitive tasks. The children and their mothers and teachers were interviewed and observations were made in the children's classrooms. These procedures have yielded an enormous array of information (1-5). In this article, we focus on the discussion of achievement in mathematics and factors that may contribute to the poor performance of American children in that area.

ACHIEVEMENT TESTS

Comparative studies of children's scholastic achievement are hindered by the lack of culturally fair, interesting, and psychometrically sound tests and research materials. It was necessary to construct material in order to test children in Taiwan, Japan, and the United States for our study. A team of bilingual researchers from each culture constructed tests and other research instruments with the aim of eliminating as much as possible any cultural bias (1,2).

Mathematics tests were based on the content of the textbooks used in the three cities in which we conducted our research. Analyses were made of each mathematical construct and operation and of the time that it was introduced in the textbook. The test for kindergarten children contained items assessing basic concepts and operations included in the curricula from kindergarten through the third grade. The mathematics test constructed for elementary school children contained 70 items derived from concepts and skills appearing in the mathematics curricula through grade 6. Some items required only computation, and others required application of mathematical principles to story problems.

Reading tests were based on analyses of the words, grammatical structures, and story content of the readers used in the three cities. There were separate tests for kindergarten and elementary school children. The kindergarten test tapped letter and word recognition and contained comprehension items of gradually increasing difficulty. The reading test for grades 1 through 6 consisted of three parts: sight reading of vocabulary, reading of meaningful text, and comprehension of text.

Tests were constructed for administration to one child at a time. The tests were not timed. The testing procedure required that the child continue in the test to the point where over a quarter of the items at a grade level were failed. The mathematics tests and the kindergarten reading test were given 6 months after the beginning of the school year. Reading tests were given 2 months earlier in grades 1 and 5. Carefully written instructions in all three languages and personal contact with the supervisors of the examiners helped produce testing procedures that were as comparable as possible in the three cities (7).

SELECTING THE CHILDREN

Children in only one city in each country were studied. In the United States, we selected children in the Minneapolis metropolitan area. Several factors led to this choice, the most important being that the residents of this area tend to come from native-born, English-speaking, economically sound families. Few are from a minority background. These factors, we assumed, would provide an advantageous cultural, economic, and linguistic environment for learning in school. If problems were found in Minneapolis, we assumed they would be compounded in other American cities where a greater proportion of the children speak English as a second language, come from economically disadvantaged homes, and have parents whose cultural backgrounds diverge from the typically middle-class milieu to which American elementary school curricula generally are addressed.

The Japanese city that we chose as being most comparable to Minneapolis was Sendai, which is located in the Tohoku region several hundred miles northeast of Tokyo. It, too, is a large, economically successful city, with little heavy industry and with an economic and cultural status in Japan similar to that of Minneapolis in the United States. Taipei was the Chinese city in which it was most feasible for us to conduct our research, in terms of language, size, colleagues, and other factors.

Ten schools in each city were selected to provide a representative sample of the city's elementary schools (6). Because we wanted to test children shortly after they entered elementary school and also near the end of their elementary education, we randomly chose two first-grade and two fifth-grade classrooms in each school. The age of school entrance is the same in all three countries and elementary school attendance is mandatory. From each classroom we randomly chose six boys and six girls. This procedure resulted in a sample of 240 first-graders and 240 fifth-graders from each city.

Kindergartens in Taiwan and Japan are mainly privately owned and attendance is not compulsory. Nevertheless, more than 98 percent of the 5-year-olds in Sendai and over 80 percent of the 5-year-olds in Taipei attend kindergarten for at least a full year. All Minneapolis children attend kindergarten. Children in the study came from 24 kindergarten classes in each city. In order to ensure that the samples of kindergarten and elementary school children in Taipei and Sendai would be comparable, the kindergartens chosen were among those attended by children from the ten elementary schools. Six boys and six girls were randomly chosen from each classroom, yielding a sample in each city of 288 children for study. A representative sample of 24 kindergarten classrooms was selected in the Minneapolis metropolitan area.

MATHEMATICS ACHIEVEMENT

The American children's scores were lower than those of the Japanese children in kindergarten and at grades 1 and 5, and lower than those of the Chinese children's at grades 1 and 5 (Table 1). Average scores for boys and girls did not show statistically significant differences from each other at any of the three grade levels.

Figure 1 shows graphically the result of transforming each child's score into a z score, which represents the departure in standard deviation units

Table 1. Mean scores ($\pm$SD) on the mathematics tests for kindergarten (K) and grades 1 and 5. Scheffé method contrasts: United States < Japan at kindergarten, grade 1, and grade 5 ($P < 0.001$); United States < Taiwan at grade 1 and grade 5 ($P < 0.01$). Sample sizes for United States, Taiwan, and Japan, respectively: kindergarten, 288, 286, and 280; grade 1, 237, 241, and 240; and grade 5, 238, 241, and 239.

Grade	United States	Taiwan	Japan
K	37.5 ± 5.6	37.8 ± 7.4	42.2 ± 5.1
1	17.1 ± 5.3	21.2 ± 5.5	20.1 ± 5.2
5	44.4 ± 6.2	50.8 ± 5.7	53.3 ± 7.5

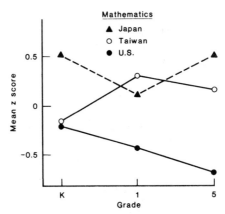

Figure 1. Children's performance on the mathematics test. (Standard deviations for kindergarten, grade 1, and grade 5 were as follows: Japan, 0.77, 0.93, and 1.00; Taiwan, 1.10, 0.98, and 0.76; United States, 0.83, 0.96, and 0.83).

from the mean of a distribution derived from the scores of the children in all three cities at each grade level. Scores were then recombined according to country, and the mean score of children in each country was determined. Consistently superior performance of the Japanese children and rapid improvement in the scores of the Chinese children from kindergarten through fifth grade are evident. Scores of the American children display a consistent decline compared to those of the Chinese and Japanese children.

Another way of considering the data is in terms of the performance in each classroom. Data for the first- and fifth-grade children are presented in Fig. 2. Each line represents one classroom. The height of the line represents the average score for the 12 children tested in each of the 20 classrooms in each city, and the width of the line represents the range of scores within each classroom. The z scores were obtained in a manner similar to that just described, except that the raw scores for both first- and fifth-graders were combined into a single distribution from which the z score for each child was computed. The z scores were then compiled for each classroom.

A high degree of overlap appears in the distributions of scores for the first-grade classrooms in the three cities. At the fifth-grade level there is a clear separation. The highest average score of an American fifth-grade classroom was below that of the Japanese fifth-grade classroom with the lowest average score. In addition, only one Chinese classroom showed an average score lower than the American classroom with the highest average score. Equally remarkable is the fact that the lowest average score

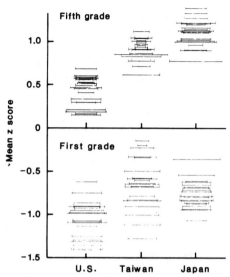

Figure 2. Performance in each classroom on the mathematics test.

for a fifth-grade American classroom was only slightly higher than the average score for the best first-grade Chinese classroom.

Viewed in still another way, the data indicate that among the 100 top scorers on the mathematics test at grade 1, there were only 15 American children. At grade 5, only one American child appeared among the 100 top scorers from the total sample of approximately 720 children. On the other hand, among the children receiving the 100 lowest scores at each grade, there were 58 American children at grade 1 and 67 at grade 5.

The low level of performance of American children was not due to a few exceptionally low-scoring classrooms nor to a particular area of weakness. They were as ineffective in calculating as in solving word problems. The search for an adequate explanation of these findings will be a long one, for many factors are involved in producing such large differences in performance. Some of the most obvious alternatives are discussed below, including the children's cognitive abilities and several factors related to school and home.

READING ACHIEVEMENT AND COGNITIVE ABILITIES

A look at results for the reading test helps clarify whether low levels of achievement generally characterized the academic performance of American children. Although reading scores show statistically significant differences among the three cities, the differences were less extreme than those in mathematics. Chinese children had the highest average scores and Japanese children the lowest. Average scores for the American children consistently were in the middle. Data presented in Fig. 3 from the vocabulary portion of the reading test illustrate these results.

Solving mathematics problems is one aspect of cognitive functioning. Perhaps differences in mathematics scores reflect differences in general intelligence among children in the three cultures. Although Lynn (8) has suggested that Japanese children display general cognitive superiority to American children, his study had numerous methodological problems, such as selective sampling of children in Japan (9). The cognitive tasks constructed especially for evaluating the intellectual functioning of Japanese, Chinese, and American children in this study offer data related to these cross-national comparisons. The tasks included performance tasks, such as perceptual speed, coding, and spatial abilities, and verbal tasks, such as vocabulary, verbal memory, and general information.

We found no evidence to support Lynn's suggestion; American children did not receive lower average scores than the Chinese and Japanese children during kindergarten or at grades 1 or 5. In fact, American children obtained the highest scores on many of the tasks during kindergarten and first grade. By the fifth grade there was no overall difference in the total scores received by the children in the three cities (3).

LIFE IN SCHOOL

Our information about the children's experiences in school is based on extensive observations made in each elementary school classroom.

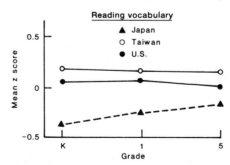

Figure 3. Children's performance on the vocabulary portion of the reading test. (Standard deviations for kindergarten, grade 1, and grade 5 were as follows: Taiwan, 0.99, 1.06, and 0.84; United States, 0.98; 1.12, and 1.07; Japan, 0.84, 0.72, and 1.05.)

Each classroom was visited according to a schedule in which the time of observation was randomized during a period of several weeks. The observer's attention was focused on the children for some of the observations and on the teacher for others. Behavior was coded according to an objective coding system (4). The number of hours of observaton was 1353 in Minneapolis, 1600 in Taipei, and 1200 in Sendai.

Learning depends, in part, on the amount of time spent in practicing the material to be learned. We therefore looked at the percentage of time devoted to academic activities, and especially to mathematics. American first-graders were engaged in academic activities a smaller percentage of time than the Chinese and Japanese children: 69.8 percent for the American children, 85.1 percent for the Chinese children, and 79.2 percent for the Japanese children.

By fifth grade, differences between the American and the Chinese and the Japanese children were greater than at the lower grades. American children spent 64.5 percent of their classroom time involved in academic activities. Chinese children spent 91.5 percent, and Japanese children, 87.4 percent. Assuming that our observations provide a representative picture of what went on in Minneapolis fifth-grade classrooms, we estimate that 19.6 hours per week (64.5 percent of the 30.4 hours the American children spend in school) were devoted to academic activities. This is less than half the estimate of 40.4 hours (91.5 percent of 44.1 hours that Chinese children attend school) devoted to academic activities in the fifth-grade Chinese classrooms, and not much less than half of the 32.6 hours (87.4 pecent of 37.3 hours that Japanese children attend school) in the Japanese classrooms.

In both grades 1 and 5, American children spent less than 20 percent of their time on the average studying mathematics in school. This was less than the percentage for either Chinese or Japanese children. At the fifth grade, language arts (including reading) and mathematics occupied approximately equal amounts of time for the Chinese and Japanese children, but the American children spent more than twice as much time on language arts (40 percent) as on mathematics (17 percent) (Fig. 4). In some of the American classrooms, no time was devoted to work in mathematics during the approximately 40 randomly selected hours when an observer was present. The high variability among American classrooms in the time allocated to the various academic subjects can be readily explained. There are precisely defined curricula in Taiwan and Japan, and teachers are expected to adhere closely to these curricula. American teachers are allowed to organize their classrooms much more according to their own desires; hence, there is greater variability among classrooms.

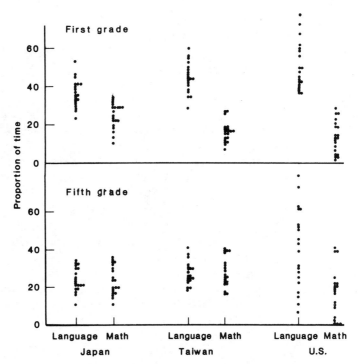

Figure 4. Proportion of time spent in each classroom on language arts and mathematics from classroom observations.

The leader of a classroom activity in which a child was engaged could be the teacher, another adult, such as a teacher's aide, or a child. Asian and American classrooms had strikingly different patterns of leadership. Children in Taipei were led by the teacher nearly 90 percent of the time; in Sendai, more than 70 percent of the time. Children in Minneapolis, in contrast, spent less than half their time in classrooms where they were led by the teacher. Children can learn without a teacher. Nevertheless, it seems likely that they could profit from having their teacher as a leader more than half of the time.

Moreover, American teachers spent proportionally much less time imparting information (21 percent) than did the Chinese (58 percent) or Japanese (33 percent) teachers. These are sobering results. American children were in school approximately 30 hours a week. This means that they were receiving information from the teacher for approximately 6 hours a week (0.21 times 30). Computing similar estimates for Chinese and Japanese classrooms gives values of 26 hours for Chinese children and 12 hours for Japanese children. American teachers actually spent somewhat more time giving directions than in imparting information (26 percent compared to 21 percent).

There were other interesting differences in the ways children spent their time in school. For example, we sometimes found that a child who was known to be at school was not present in the classroom. The child could be at the school office, on an errand for the teacher, in another classroom, or in the library. This occurred 18.4 percent of the time that an American fifth-grader was to be observed, but less than 0.2 percent of the time in Taipei and Sendai classrooms.

The comparatively low levels of achievement of the American children in mathematics appear to be attributable in part to the fact that they are not receiving amounts of instruction comparable to those received by children in Taiwan and Japan. These cross-national differences become even more profound when they are extended over the school year. Chinese and Japanese children spend half a day at school on Saturdays and have fewer holidays than do American children. As a result, American children attend school an average of 178 days a year; Chinese and Japanese children attend school for 240 days. In addition, Japanese fifth-graders were estimated by their mothers to spend an average of 1 hour more each day, and the Chinese children, 2 hours more each day at school than the American children. Taken together, these data point to enormous differences in the amounts of schooling young children receive in the three countries.

HOMEWORK

Learning occurs at home as well as at school. But our data indicate that neither American parents nor teachers of elementary school children tend to believe that homework is of much value. As a consequence, American children spend much less time on homework than do Japanese children, and both groups spend vastly less time on homework than do Chinese children. American mothers estimated that on weekdays their first-graders spent an average of 14 minutes a day on homework; the daily average for Chinese first-graders was 77 minutes, and for Japanese, 37 minutes. For fifth-graders, the estimate for the American children was 46 minutes a day; for the Chinese and Japanese fifth-graders the estimates were 114 and 57 minutes a day, respectively. On weekends, American children studied even less: an estimated 7 minutes on Saturday and 11 minutes on Sunday. The corresponding values for Chinese children were

83 and 73 minutes, and for the Japanese children, 37 and 29 minutes—and this was in addition to the half day in school on Saturday. American children also were given less help when they were doing their homework, according to their mothers' estimates. Someone, usually the mother, assisted the fifth-grade children with their homework an average of 14 minutes a day. The Chinese children were assisted by some family member an average of 27 minutes a day, and the Japanese children, 19 minutes a day.

Parental concern about a child's schoolwork was evident in another simple index, the possession of a desk. Only 63 percent of the American fifth-graders, but 98 percent of the Japanese and 95 percent of the Chinese fifth-graders had desks. When the Chinese and Japanese children were not occupied with homework, they were given other opportunities to practice by solving the problems appearing in the workbooks purchased for them by their parents. Only 28 percent of the parents of American fifth-graders, but 58 percent of the Japanese and 56 percent of the Chinese parents bought their children workbooks in mathematics. The discrepancy was even more pronounced in the purchase of workbooks in science, which were purchased by only 1 percent of the American parents, but 29 percent of the Japanese and 51 percent of the Chinese parents.

How did children in the three cities react to doing homework? Taipei children said they liked homework; children in Minneapolis said they did not like homework; and the attitudes of the Sendai children were somewhere in between. When asked to choose among an array of five frowning, neutral, or smiling faces to express their attitudes about homework, more than 60 percent of the Chinese fifth-graders chose a smiling face, more than 60 percent of the Japanese children chose a smiling or neutral face, and 60 percent of the American children chose a frowning face. Although 30 percent of the American children chose a smiling face at first grade, the percentage was half that among fifth-graders.

One indication of what teachers thought about homework appeared in their ratings of the value of homework and 15 other activities directed at helping children do well in school. Ratings given to the value of homework by American teachers placed it 15th among 16 items—lowest except for physical punishment. Chinese and Japanese teachers were much more positive; the average rating given by Chinese teachers on a 9-point scale was 7.3; by Japanese teachers, 5.8; and by American teachers, 4.4.

The small amounts of homework assigned to American children were not in conflict with the mothers' beliefs about how much schoolwork their child should be assigned. Among American mothers, 69 percent said that the amount of homework was "just right." Nor were the Chinese and Japanese mothers dissatisfied with the large amounts of homework assigned to their children; 82 percent of the Chinese mothers and 67 percent of the Japanese mothers thought the amount was "just right."

MOTHERS' EVALUATIONS

When asked to rate their child's achievement in mathematics, American mothers gave their children favorable evaluations. Ratings were made on nine-point scales, each anchored by five defining statements, ranging from "much below average" to "much above average." Although mothers were asked to compare their child with "other children of his or her age," the mean rating made by the American mothers for their child's ability in mathematics was 5.9, higher than the average rating 5.2 of the Chinese mothers and similar to the average of 5.8 of the Japanese mothers.

Mothers were also asked to rate children on several cognitive abilities, each defined by several words or a short phrase. Great care was taken to select words and phrases that express the same nuances of meaning in the three languages. American mothers consistently gave their children the highest average ratings and Japanese mothers gave their children the lowest. For example, on ratings of a child's intellectual ability, the average rating given by American mothers was 6.3, much above the 5.0 that would indicate an average level of ability. The average rating given by the Japanese mothers was 5.5, and by the Chinese mothers, 6.1.

Despite the positive bias of the American mothers, the rank order of their ratings was in line with the children's performance. The correlation between the mothers' ratings of the children's abilities in mathematics and the fifth-graders' scores on the mathematics test was 0.50 in Minneapolis, 0.37 in Taipei, and 0.54 in Sendai. The high ratings made by American mothers must be attributed to an excessively positive attitude, rather than to a failure to perceive a child's status in relation to other children. Conversely, the low ratings of Japanese mothers appear to reflect an effort to be more realistic in their evaluations.

The optimism of the American mothers was reflected in other ways. They were pleased with the job the schools were doing in educating their children: 91 percent judged that the school was doing an "excellent" or "good" job. Only 42 percent of the Chinese mothers and 39 percent of the Japanese mothers were this positive. Instead, the majority of the Chinese and Japanese mothers considered that the schools were doing a "fair" job.

The high esteem the American mothers had for their children's cognitive abilities extended to their satisfaction with their children's current academic performance. More than 40 percent of the American mothers described themselves as being "very satisfied" (Fig. 5). Fewer than 6 percent of the Chinese and Japanese mothers were this positive.

When asked if there were things about their children's education that could be improved, 45 percent of the American mothers of the fifth-graders who suggested improvements could be made emphasized improvement in academic subjects. The subject that they thought should get more emphasis was reading (48 percent of the suggestions). Mathematics and science were seldom mentioned (< 6 percent of the suggestions). The subjects mentioned most frequently by the Japanese mothers were reading and mathematics. Chinese mothers, on the other hand, believed that more emphasis should be given to music, art, and gym.

The positive attitudes of the mothers did not mean that American children liked school. In rating how well they liked school, 52 percent of the American children, compared to 86 percent of the Chinese fifth-graders, chose a smiling face. (The question was not asked in Japan).

Critics of Chinese and Japanese education often suggest that the high demands placed on children result in ambivalence or dislike of school. This does not seem to be the case in elementary schools. It is the American children who regard elementary school less positively. Expressing a dislike for school may be a socially acceptable reaction among American school children. Even young children in Taiwan and Japan are aware of the fact that education is highly prized in the Chinese and Japanese cultures. The emphasis on scholastic achievement may lead to the intense competition that is often said to characterize secondary schools in Taiwan and Japan, but negative consequences were not evident during the elementary school years. In fact, the children in all three cities appeared to be cheerful, enthusiastic, vigorous, and responsive.

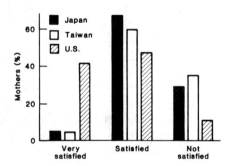

Figure 5. Mothers' attitudes toward children's academic performance.

Although some of these characteristics may be more vividly expressed in classrooms in Minneapolis, they are readily apparent to the observer who follows Chinese and Japanese children through their school day.

PARENTAL BELIEFS

Experiences that parents provide their children may be strongly influenced by their general beliefs about the components of success. For example, parents who emphasize ability as the most important requisite for success may be less disposed to stress the need to work hard than would parents who believe success is largely dependent on effort.

In exploring cultural differences in beliefs about the relative importance of factors leading to success in school, we asked the mothers to rank effort, natural ability, difficulty of the schoolwork, and luck or chance by importance in determining a child's performance in school. They were then asked to assign a total of ten points to the four factors. Japanese mothers assigned the most points to effort, and American mothers gave the largest number of points to ability (Fig. 6). The willingness of Japanese and Chinese children to work so hard in school may be due, in part, to the stronger belief on the part of their mothers in the value of hard work.

OUTSIDE ASSISTANCE

It has been suggested that the scholastic performance of young Chinese and Japanese children is due in part to outside tutoring. Articles about the *juku,* the cram schools of Japan, and the *buxiban,* the after-hours schools in Taiwan, have appeared in American newspapers. These seem to be phenomena associated with later years of schooling, for few mothers said that their elementary school children attended such classes.

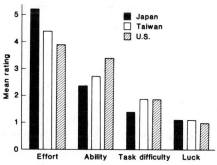

Figure 6. Mothers' ratings of factors contributing to academic success.

Children in all three of the cities that we studied were enrolled in after-school lessons or classes, but these were not necessarily ones that would help the children with their schoolwork. American children most frequently took lessons in various types of sports. Among Chinese children, the most popular lessons were in sports and calligraphy, and among Japanese children, the most popular lessons were in art and calligraphy. The percentage of children taking lessons in mathematics was higher in Sendai (7 percent) than in Taipei (2 percent), but not higher than the percentage in Minneapolis (8 percent).

THE TEACHERS

The number of hours teachers spent with the children each week did not show statistically significant differences among the three countries, despite the fact that the hours were spread out over 5.5 days a week in Taiwan and Japan, and only 5 days in the United States. American and Japanese teachers estimated that they spent 28 hours a week teaching, and the Chinese teachers, 30 hours. The amoung of time spent at school did differ greatly—an average of 51 hours for the Japanese teachers, 47 hours for the Chinese teachers, and 42 hours for the American teachers. This means that American teachers have little time when they are at school for activities other than those where they are directly responsible for the children in their classroom, a factor that may help explain the complaints of American teachers that they are overworked.

American teachers frequently said that if they could shed some of their nonacademic functions, they could spend more of their time actually teaching. A large amount of classroom time is spent in unproductive activities that can be attributed, in part, to the American teachers being asked to take on too many functions other than teaching, including the roles of counselor, family therapist, and surrogate parent. This diversion of energy is perhaps the most common problem of American elementary school teachers, and is one that was seldom mentioned by the teachers in Taipei and Sendai. Such problems are not due to there being a greater number of children in the American classrooms, for the average number of children in the Minneapolis elementary school classrooms was 21, whereas it was 47 in Tapei and 39 in Sendai.

Whether increased time for teaching would result in improved instruction in mathematics and science is questionable. When asked whether there were ways in which they would change the curriculum if they were free to do so, nearly a quarter of the American teachers had no suggestions. The two most frequent suggestions related to academic subjects involved placing more emphasis on "basics" (13 percent) and increasing the time available for reading, spelling, and language instruction (18 percent). Only one American teacher expressed a desire to spend more time on mathematics.

CURRENT DATA

The data for the elementary school children were collected in 1980, and for the kindergarten children in 1984. A follow-up study also was undertaken in 1984 of children who had been included in our first-grade sample, but now were in the fifth grade. Little change occurred in the children's performance during the four years. The mean score for the American children in 1984 on the mathematics test was 44.9, a score nearly identical to the average of 44.5 obtained by the fifth-graders 4 years earlier. The Japanese children remained ahead, with a mean score of 51.

Differences in the attitudes of mothers in the three countries were as strong as they had been 4 years earlier. In analyses of the 1984 data that have been completed, we have found, for example, that mothers of American fifth-graders were even more satisfied, and Chinese and Japanese mothers were just as dissatisfied with their child's performance in 1984 as mothers were in 1980. Nearly 60 percent of the American mothers, compared to 40 percent 4 years earlier, were "very satisfied" with their child's current academic performance. Fewer than 10 percent of the Chinese and Japanese mothers were "very satisfied."

CONCLUSIONS

Impetus for change often comes from dissatisfaction with the present state of affairs. Most American mothers interviewed in this study did not appear to be dissatisfied with their children's schools, and seem unlikely, therefore, to become advocates for reform. Moreover, the children, faced with parents who generally are satisfied and approving of what happens in school, must see little need to spend more time and effort on their schoolwork. The poor performance of American children in mathematics thus reflects a general failure to perceive that American elementary school children are performing ineffectively and that there is a need for improvement and change if the United States is to remain competitive with other countries in areas such as technology and science which require a solid foundation in mathematical skills.

The lack of time spent teaching mathematics may be a reflection of the view of American parents and teachers that education in elementary school is synonymous with learning to read. Large amounts of time are devoted to reading instruction, and if changes were to be made in the curriculum, both parents and teachers agreed that even greater proportions of time should be devoted to reading. Mathematics and science play a small role in Americans' conception of elementary education.

American mothers have unrealistically favorable evaluations of their children and what they are accomplishing in school. This optimism may lead to a sense of well-being but is unwarranted in the context of cross-national comparisons of children's scholastic achievement. When we look only within the United States, we may find cause to deplore the poor performance only of certain subgroups of our population. When we broaden our perspective to include children from other countries, we have cause for concern. Although a small proportion of American children perform superbly, the large majority appear to be falling behind their peers in other countries.

The data we have presented are from a single set of studies, conducted in particular locales and with particular methods. Nevertheless, the findings are directly in line with those from other cross-national studies of achievement in mathematics and science involving older children and adolescents (10-12). Preliminary results from the Second International Mathematics Study, for example, indicate that among eighth-graders from 20 countries, Japanese children received the highest scores in arithmetic, algebra, geometry, statistics, and measurement. The average scores of the American children on these tests ranged from 8th to 18th position. The poor performance of American children that begins in kindergarten is maintained through the later grades.

Regardless of the funds that may be allocated to the development and application of new methods of teaching, it seems obvious that children's success in mathematics and other subjects will depend on greater awareness and an increased willingness by American parents to be of direct assistance to their children. Schools may be improved, but the task of helping children reach higher levels of achievement cannot be accomplished without more cooperation and communication between the school and the home. Further, without greater acknowledgement of the importance of the elementary school years to children's education in mathematics and science, legislation to improve instruction in secondary schools may result in little more than exercises in remediation for most children.

REFERENCES AND NOTES

1. J. W. Stigler, S.Y. Lee, G. W. Lucker, H.W. Stevenson, *J. Educ. Psychol.* **74**, 315 (1982).
2. H.W. Stevenson et al., *Child Devel.* **53**, 1164 (1982).
3. H.W. Stevenson et al., ibid. **56**, 718 (1985).
4. H.W. Stevenson et al., in *Advances in Instructional Psychology*, R. Glaser, Ed. (Erlbaum, Hillside, NJ, in press).
5. H. W. Stevenson, H. Azuma, K. Hakuta, Eds., *Child Development and Education in Japan* (Freeman, New York, in press).
6. Care was taken to develop procedures that would result in the selection of representative samples of children within each city. Selection was made after we discussed our goals with educational authorities in each city. We obtained a list of schools stratified by region and socioeconomic status of the families. Schools in Taipei and Sendai were then selected at random so that the ten elementary schools would constitute a representative sample of schools within each city. In the Minneapolis metropolitan area, where there are many different school districts, we sought to adopt a procedure that was as comparable to that used in Sendai and Taipei as possible. All elementary schools in Sendai were public schools, but one private school was chosen in both Taipei and Minneapolis to represent the proportion of children in those cities that attend private schools. All children in each of the classrooms in Japan and Taiwan were included as potential subjects. In Minneapolis, parental permission had to be obtained before we could test a child. Parents were very cooperative; only 4.5 percent failed to return slips giving us permission to test their children. Children with IQ's below 70 were eliminated from the samples in all three cities.
7. Statistical analyses of the achievement tests indicated good reliability. Tests of the reliability of the mathematics test yielded values that ranged from 0.92 to 0.95 when the Cronbach α statistic was computed separately by grade and country. The coefficients of concordance for the three parts of the reading test ranged from 0.91 to 0.94 when computed separately for each country. Results for standardized tests of mathematics and reading were not obtained for purposes of comparison with our tests. The standardized achievement tests, if available, were not comparable among the three countries; the results often were not current; and they were group tests, rather than individually administered tests such as those used in this study.
8. R. Lynn, *Nature (London)* **297**, 222 (1982).
9. H.W. Stevenson and H. Azuma, ibid. **306**, 291 (1983).
10. T. Husén, *International Study of Achievement in Mathematics: A Comparison of Twelve Countries* (Wiley, New York, 1967).
11. L. C. Comber and J. Keeves, *Science Achievement in Nineteen Countries* (Wiley, New York, 1973).
12. "Preliminary report: Second International Mathematics Study" (University of Illinois, Urbana, 1984).
13. This article reports results from a collaborative study undertaken with S. Kitamura, S. Kimura, and T. Kato of Tohoku Fukushi College in Sendai, Japan, and C.C. Hsu of National Taiwan University in Taipei. Supported by NIMH grants MH 33259 and MH 30567.

Part IV

TEMPERAMENT STUDIES

The paper by Maziade and his associates reports additional findings from their longitudinal study of temperament in a large sample of French-speaking children in Quebec. (For the category of rhythmicity they prefer to use the term "predictability.") Their comparison of the ratings of the infancy and middle-childhood periods suggests that the temperamental cluster of difficult-to-manage children may vary somewhat in the two periods, at least in their culture. They also provide a review of the sex differences found in a large number of temperament studies and give additional data on SES correlations. Their point is well taken—it is important to keep sampling criteria and operational definitions constant if effective transcultural comparisons of different studies are to be made.

Reznick and his coworkers report a further follow-up study of their sample of inhibited and uninhibited children, which confirms their findings at earlier age periods. In a general way, their criteria for inhibition corresponds to our New York Longitudinal Study definition of withdrawal, and lack of inhibition corresponds to our rating of approach. The study by Reznick and his colleagues is of special interest in providing the first clear-cut correlation between a temperamental characteristic and specific psychophysiological findings. In the present study, when the children were five-and-a-half years old, the authors have also found differences in cognitive style. They offer a reasonable hypothesis as to the physiological mechanism that may be involved in the differences between the two groups of children.

Finally, Maziade and his coworkers examine the hypothesis that gentle delivery techniques, such as those proposed by Leboyer and others, will have a positive effect in child development by minimizing the stress and trauma of birth. However, when using infant temperament at four and eight months as the outcome variable, the study found no significant difference between the infants born with or without gentle delivery techniques. The authors emphasize that their findings must be interpreted

239

with caution, but the data do reaffirm the general principle that infant development is multidetermined, and that no single factor by itself will shape the nature of the child's psychological functioning.

PART IV: TEMPERAMENT STUDIES

14

Empirical Characteristics of the NYLS Temperament in Middle Childhood: Congruities and Incongruities with Other Studies

Michel Maziade, Pierrette Boutin, Robert Côté, and Jacques Thivierge

Hôtel-Dieu du Sacré Coeur de Jésus de Québec, Canada

Recent literature highlights the importance of studying the empirical qualities of the different models of temperament developed to date. The present paper deals specifically with the NYLS definition of temperament. The research data, gathered on a random sample (N = 647) from the Quebec City general population aged 8 and 12 years, do not replicate the main typology (similar to the NYLS "easy-difficult" cluster) previously identified in younger random samples of our population nor that found in other Swedish or American samples. The implications of the findings in terms of temperament main typology as well as in terms of SES and sex differences are discussed in the context of the other studies utilizing the NYLS definition of temperament. Developmental and methodological considerations are derived from the congruities and incongruities observed in the results of the various studies.

Reprinted with permission from *Child Psychiatry and Human Development,* 1986, Vol. 17, No. 1, 38–52. Copyright 1986 by Human Sciences Press.

We are thankful to the parents and teachers who have collaborated in this study. Thanks are also due to Chantal Mérette and Didier Leroux, and undergraduate students in statistics, for their participation in the data analysis, and to John R. Gallup, Ph.D., Laval University, for reviewing the English translation of this paper.

241

The corpus of published research on the New York Longitudinal Studies (NYLS) model of temperament has expanded considerably in the last two decades. Other important models, somewhat different from the NYLS categorization, have also been constructed [1,2,3]. However, the replication in diverse settings, age levels and cultures[4,5,6,7,8,9] of a main temperamental typology that appears quite similar to the Thomas and Chess "easy-difficult" cluster supports to some extent the theoretical construct of what they called the *behavioral style*. Even if there remain many questions about the concept and the best measuring devices to be used, the predictive validity of "difficult" temperament, as operationally defined by the current instruments, has also been further documented[10,11,12].

Scientifically, we never deal directly with the reality of things, but we work through models that we try to apply to the "observational reality" of nature in order to try to understand natural phenomena better, and ultimately we want to utilize our models for practical purposes. The fact that the NYLS construct of temperament appears to have some sound qualities does not mean that it is exclusive; it by no means rules out the possibility that other models of temperament may present important scientific qualities, either developmental or clinical. We feel that researchers ought to forego any inclination to maintain an attitude implying that they possess a unique model which would be the only right one; history proves that scientific conceptualizations of natural phenomena rarely last forever. Serious scientific effort should try to compare the forces and weaknesses of the different models in order to apply and use them according to their specific empirical meaningfulness and usefulness.

It is from such a perspective that this paper will deal with the NYLS operational definition of temperament. Wide-spread in child psychology and in other areas of psychiatric research, parental ratings are also much used in the field of child temperament. In testing the qualities of the different models, the various measuring devices are necessary intermediate points of contacts between the theoretical concepts and the behavioral results. The intermediary function of parental ratings, still a thorny issue, is worthy of our initial consideration. The pros and cons of ratings by parents have often been discussed [13,14,15]. Everyone now agrees that the debate must leave the ground of theoretical discussions and stick to the empirical findings derived from such measuring devices.

At the present time, it seems accepted that ratings of children's temperament by their parents can hardly ever tap only the intrinsic qualities within the child and that the measures we obtain contain contaminants from parental perception or from the child-parent transactional patterns[16]. But in the rating their children, it has been shown that parents do not seem to project onto the child as much as previously thought in terms of their personal temperamental traits[17], and that there is reasonably good concordance of parental ratings or interviews with direct observations[6,18,19].

Elsewhere we have already shown that the test-retest reliability usually obtained for parental ratings (r in the .70 to .80 range) leads to a 30% inconsistency in the results of the final comparisons, 3 to 4 weeks later, when the same large sample is reassessed[8]. But since parental ratings remain so far the only way to study large unbiased samples, we have to choose one of two possibilities: (1) to deal with this imperfect level of reliability that probably is inherent in such measurements and take it into account in discussing discrepancies in findings between studies or (2) to reject parental ratings as inefficient or unreliable. We believe that in the present state of research, the first choice is preferable, mainly because the second leaves us with no substitute solution for assessing properly selected large samples. In addition we have to consider that for temperament as well as for other experimental concepts in child development, the issue of reliability is intertwined with the issue of validity and meaningfulness[20].

Consequently, it seems to us that an appropriate and reasonable question in the present conjuncture is the following: Do we find coherence or chaos in results from ratings when comparing the findings of different studies in terms of the appearance of temperament clusters, sex differences, and demographic correlates? This question refers inevitably to the reliability of group measurements as well as to the consistency of relationships between temperament (i.e. similar operational definitions of temperament) and external parameters; the recurrent findings of such consistent relationships in different studies would help in enlightening the nature of what we assess as temperament as well as in further contributing to improve the quality of our measurements. Regarding the reliability for individuals in the group, which is also an important issue with respect to eventual clinical utilitization of temperament, the use of extremes on the temperamental continuum may provide at least a temporary solution for research and clinical purposes. The aspect of temporal stability of extreme measurements has already been demonstrated[21], and our own results show that extreme temperamental measurements from parental ratings show good predictive value in terms of behavior disorders[10] and an acceptable level of continuity in time[7,22].

This paper will present data on temperament gathered through parental ratings on a large population based sample aged 8 and 12 years. A review of the literature (see Table 4) shows that most studies report data in the first years of life but very few in middle childhood. The purposes of the present study were (1) to provide temperamental norms at this age level for our ongoing longitudinal studies; (2) to study the factorial structure, to look for temperamental clusters and make comparisons with our findings at other age levels in our French-speaking population in Quebec City; (3) to study other epidemiological characteristics of the NYLS model of temperament, especially regarding the association with demographic data and sex, and see if we might find consistency with previous studies.

SAMPLING AND PROCEDURE

We translated into French the Middle Childhood Temperament Questionnaire (MCTQ)[23] consisting of 99 items rated by parents on a 6 point Likert scale. The 99 items are spread among the nine temperament categories proposed by the New York Longitudinal Studies (NYLS)[4]. One of the NYLS categories, the rhythmicity of physiological functions, has been replaced in the MCTQ by behavioral predictability, which involves regularity in task performance and social behavior. The MCTQ is applicable to 8 to 12 year old children. We assessed the socioeconomic status (SES) according to the Hollingshead two-factor index of social position[24]. A random sample of 12 classes of grade three and 12 classes of grade six was selected according to the principle of proportional allocation within four schoolboards of Quebec City. The 24 classes consisted in all of 647 children (grade three: N = 313; grade six: N = 334); girls composed 52% of the sample. The mean age was 8.6 years for grade three and 11.7 years for grade six. In other words, this is a cross-sectional study of children partly in the third grade and partly in the sixth grade.

Each school director and teacher was met by a member of our research team in order to explain the purposes and the procedure of the study. Then the children received from the teacher the MCTQ, the socioeconomic status questionnaire and a letter of explanation which they took to their parents. The questionnaires were filled in and returned to the teacher. This procedure was performed a second time, three weeks later (retest). The rate of response was 82% at the test and 62% at the retest. The socioeconomic structure of the sample was: 11% Class I, 14% Class II, 16% Class III, 32% Class IV and 27% Class V; this repartition is very similar to the one obtained in two previous large samples in the general population[7,8].

RESULTS

In terms of reliability, Pearson correlations were calculated between the test and retest for each category and are reported in Table 1. In order to look at the structure of the MCTQ in our French-speaking population and to look for clustering of temperament traits, a principal component analysis (PCA) without rotation was performed on the nine category means for the whole sample, and separately for the two age groups and for the test and the retest measurements. We used a PCA without rotation because previous data showed that rotation introduces test-retest instability in the results[25,26]. Three factors explaining 66.8% of the variance were extracted; the loadings of each temperament category on the factors for the test are reported in Table 2. The first factor (F-1), composed mainly of adaptability, persistence, activity, mood, predictability and intensity, was found stable in the grade three and the grade six subsamples, at the test as well as at the retest. A Pearson correlation on the factor scores between the test and the retest yielded .84.

Sex Differences

The mean differences on each category for boys and girls were compared through a t-test (two-tailed): boys were found at the mean

Table 1. Pearson Test-Retest Correlations in Grade 3 and Grade 6 Subsamples and in Total Sample

	Grade 3 (N = 200)	Grade 6 (N = 155)	Total Sample (N = 355)
Activity	.82	.86	.84
Predictability	.73	.71	.72
Approach/Withdrawal	.80	.84	.82
Adaptability	.70	.72	.71
Intensity	.76	.72	.75
Mood	.80	.74	.77
Persistence	.79	.74	.77
Distractibility	.72	.68	.71
Threshold	.62	.58	.61

Table 2. Principal Component Analysis on the Temperament Categories at Age 9 (N = 254) and Age 12 (N = 264) (Test)

	F-1	F-2	F-3	Comm.
Adaptability	*.80*	−.15	.14	.69
	(*.79*)	(*−.24*)	(*.10*)	(*.69*)
Persistence	.75	−.36	−.22	.75
	(*.82*)	(*−.14*)	(*−.11*)	(*.71*)
Activity	.73	.30	−.22	.67
	(*.79*)	(*.15*)	(*−.19*)	(*.69*)
Mood	.73	−.19	.21	.62
	(*.81*)	(*−.15*)	(*.12*)	(*.69*)
Predictability	.69	−.30	−.34	.68
	(*.74*)	(*−.22*)	(*−.15*)	(*.61*)
Intensity	.57	.50	−.02	.58
	(*.63*)	(*.36*)	(*−.22*)	(*.58*)
Distractibility	.38	.59	.01	.50
	(*.34*)	(*.73*)	(*.09*)	(*.66*)
Threshold	.27	.52	.62	.73
	(*.17*)	(*.60*)	(*.65*)	(*.81*)
Approach/	.22	−.60	.62	.79
withdrawal	(*.23*)	(*−.49*)	(*.73*)	(*.82*)
Eigenvalue	3.35	1.60	1.04	
	(*3.72*)	(*1.44*)	(*1.10*)	
% Variance	37.3	17.9	11.6	
	(*41.4*)	(*16.0*)	(*12.2*)	

Loadings in parentheses correspond to age 12 (grade 6) sample.

significantly more active (p < .01), presented a higher sensory threshold (p < .01), were less predictable (p < .05) and somewhat less persistent (p = .06) than girls. We also studied the extremes (above 70th and under 30th centile) on each category through a test for comparing two population proportions and we obtained the same statistically significant differences for activity (p < .005) and threshold (p < .005); however, for the categories of predictability and persistence, we do not find at the extreme the significant difference that we find at the mean. This again brings up the necessity of choosing a multi-method approach in this type of group comparisons; some previous studies have already shown that the analysis at the extreme does not necessarily reflect what happens in the analysis at the mean when using such measuring instruments[7,8].

Social Class and Temperament

A one-way analysis of variance was performed on the test for each of the nine categories on the global sample and also for boys (N = 242) and girls (N = 266) separately and for the grade three sample and the grade six sample. We found no significant association between temperament and SES except for one category (predictability) that showed statistical significance in a consistent manner at the mean (Anova: F = 2.67, p = .03) and at the extreme (X^2 = 9.51, d.f. = 4, p = .05).

DISCUSSION

The MCTQ French version shows a level of test-retest reliability that is comparable to other such instruments. A principal component analysis identified a stable first factor (F-1) at test and retest and at the two age levels in our sample. Our present Factor I is mainly composed of the categories of adaptability, persistence, mood, activity, predictability and intensity. Thus, we do not replicate in the present sample aged 8 and 12 the same consistent typology that we clearly observed in our previous younger large samples drawn from the general population. Indeed, we had identified in infancy[7] and at age seven[8] a main typology (Factor I found through a principal component analysis) composed principally of adaptability, approach/withdrawal, mood, intensity and distractibility. A similar clustering of adaptability, approach, mood and intensity or distractibility has also been found elsewhere in several other studies on the first years of life[5,6,9,27].

We have previously discussed the similarity between our Factor I (F-1) found in younger samples, the Thomas and Chess' "easy-difficult" cluster and factor A[28] that they also identified through a PCA. We do not replicate this factor in the present middle childhood sample: many categories leading strongly on F-1 are now obviously different. While adaptability, mood and intensity are still present in the factor in this aged 8-12 sample, it is noteworthy that approach/withdrawal now loads weakly on F-1 (.22 test; .23 at retest) contrary to its strong loading at earlier ages in our population (.60 to .70)[7,8]. From a developmental point of view, this suggests that the reaction of approach or withdrawal in the first minutes following the appearance of a new stimulus is less important at age 8-12 that it can be in infancy and young childhood.

Interestingly, when we look at the categories that now load most strongly on F-1 in comparison to the F-1 found in infancy and at age seven in our population, we observe that approach/withdrawal gives way to persistence, activity and predictability which may indeed be of more importance than approach with respect to family and social adjustment in middle childhood. This is also indirectly suggested by the fact that the six categories now loading heavily on F-1 are also the ones that correlate significantly with the parental impression of difficulty to manage (Table 3). Table 3 also illustrates that these six categories correlated with this same parental impression in the Hegvik et al's American sample[23]. In other words, approach/withdrawal may be less significant in terms of what the parent expects or desires in a child's style in middle childhood, while the categories now loading strongly on F-1 may correspond more to the new standards of desirability.

Our data would also imply that the "difficult" temperament cluster, as described by Thomas and Chess, could be more significant in terms of risk in infancy and young childhood and less in later years. It is interesting to note that Chess and Thomas reported that their "difficult cluster" as measured at age three and five correlated with young adulthood adjustment[29,30]; since, unfortunately, they had no measurement of "difficultness" in middle childhood, it is impossible to institute a comparison with the effect of the "difficult" constellation as measured at that later age.

We cannot eliminate however the possibility that the above differences in findings on the PCA originate in part from differences in the

Table 3. Correlation Between Temperament Categories and Difficulty to Manage † †

Category	Correlation+	Hegvik et al's (1982) Correlation
Activity	0.39	0.34
Predictability	0.38	0.42
Approach/Withdrawal	0.12	0.25
Adaptability	0.52	0.63
Intensity	0.31	0.44
Mood	0.53	0.63
Persistence	0.45	0.44
Distractibility	0.14	0.13
Threshold	0.09	0.06

+Difficulty to manage correlates with high activity, low predictability, low adaptability, high intensity, negative mood and low persistence.

††The question to parents is: "How difficult is this child for you to manage or get along with?"

operational definitions of temperament at the items level between the MCTQ and the other instruments we previously used on younger samples: the Parent Temperament Questionnaire (PTQ) at age seven[8] and the Carey Infant Temperament Questionnaire (ITQ)[7]. One can notice indeed that there may be such differences especially for three categories: predictability replacing rhythmicity used at younger ages, persistence and distractibility. The concept of physiological rhythmicity present in the ITQ and the PTQ is replaced in the MCTQ by behavioral predictability.

With reference to persistence, all the MCTQ items refer more to longer attentional abilities (so that a very persistent child may be seen as having a more desirable style), while in the PTQ, four of the eight items referring to persistence may have a negative connotation when the child is very persistent (item 28: "When my child is promised something in the future, he/she keeps reminding parents constantly."). Similarly for distractibility, some items of the PTQ refer to the easiness or uneasiness through which a child can be switched to another activity if the parents interfere: in other words, it might partly refer to a soothability concept (for instance item 44: "If my child is upset, it is hard to comfort him."); conversely in the MCTQ, the distractibility items seem to refer more to the ability to pursue an activity in spite of noises or distractful events (item 32: "Reads a book without distraction while T.V. is on in same room"; item 12: "Looks up right away from play when telephone or door bell rings") which is closer to what is usually called "attention span and concentration." Differences in the operational definition of distractibility and persistence between MCTQ used at age 8-12 and the PTQ used at age seven may also be supported by our finding no continuity (r: .15 and .13) for these two categories between age seven and 12 in comparison to moderate or good continuity for the other NYLS temperament traits (r: .36 to .72)[22].

Another observation suggesting that the difference in findings regarding typologies at age 8-12 might come in part from differences in the instrument is the fact that through the PTQ on seven year old subjects, we still find the typology very close to the NYLS "easy-difficult" axis; whereas, when using the MCTQ on a eight year old sample, we do not find it. On one hand, it is not easy to explain developmentally such a temporal change in the main temperament profile derived from two large samples of our general population at only a year interval. On the other hand, however, many arguments would also support the view that there is a real change in typologies: for instance three categories (adaptability, mood and intensity) of the earlier "difficult" constellation remain in F-1 at age 8-12, which indicate that the change in the main typology is not full blown but rather partial or progressive. Moreover, operational differences are observable in the instruments used in the different studies at younger ages, and yet, they led to the recurrent identification of a similar main factor.

Our present results indicate a very slight or absent association between SES and temperament. This is consistent with our previous reports on large random samples in infancy[7] as well as at age seven[8]. This is also congruent with the NYLS report[4]. In Sweden, Persson-Blennow and McNeil[31] also found an absence of association with SES in a representative sample. Sameroff's study[32] reports a significant association between temperament and SES. However, our present findings again support the view previously discussed[8] that the difference in findings with Sameroff's study is probably to be found in their inadequate sampling for a research question concerning social class and temperament.

Interestingly, our present data again indicate that the only temperament trait that is associated with socioeconomic status is predictability. In our infants and seven year olds sample[7,8], only rhythmicity was also associated with SES in a consistent manner. Taken as a whole, the data derived from parental ratings in our three samples suggest that the measurement of the NYLS temperament is SES fair or, conversely, that SES does not influence temperament except for physiological rhythmicity or its MCTQ correspondence in middle childhood, predictability.

As regards sex differences, our present study reveals two differences found at the mean as well as in the extremes: boys are more active and present a higher sensory threshold. These two differences were also present in the Hegvik et al. sample[23], but these authors found many more differences between sexes. These discrepancies in findings might come from the difference in sampling; besides, Hegvik et al. did not report whether the differences they found on the groups means were also present in the extremes. Additionally, a review of the studies utilizing the NYLS model (Table 4) shows that more inconsistency than consistency exists in the comparison of sex differences in the studies. The only consistent trends that one may observe from the literature (Table 4) are: 1) that boys seem to appear in infancy more approaching or adaptable; 2) that there are more sex differences in later years than in infancy, a point already well shown by the review of the literature by Buss and Plomin[3] and 3) that in later years, boys seem more active and to have a higher sensory threshold.

This general lack of congruency in findings for sex differences in studies using the NYLS model raises the importance of considering the sampling and selection criteria as a possible source of bias and dis-

Table 4. Review of Sex Differences Found in Studies Utilizing the NYLS Model of Temperament

	Sampling	Rate of response	Age	Sex differences at the group mean:
Carey and McDevitt (1978)	Three private paediatric practices predominantly middle and upper middle class (N–203)	81%	4-8 months	Boys are more approaching.
Hsu, Soong, Stigler, Hong, Liang (1981)	Well-baby clinics from five hospitals of Taipi 37.6%–upper class 47.3%–middle class 14.1%–lower class (N–349 between 4 and 8 months)	100%	4-8 months	Boys are more approaching.
Sameroff, Seifer and Elias (1982)	Parents registered for pre-natal courses and parents suffering some form of psychopathology (N–386)	Not reported	4 months	Boys are more approaching.
Maziade et al (1984)	Birth cohort: (N–389) 4 months (N–741) 8 months	75.2% 78.2%	4 months 8 months	Boys are more approaching, more persistent, more distractible. Boys are more approaching.
Persson-Blennow and McNeil (1981)	Random sample (proportional allocation of infants under one year registered at 29 Well-Baby clinics of Malmo) (N–160)	94% 93%	6 months 1 year 2 years	Boys are more adaptable, more active, less distractible. Boys are more adaptable No difference.
NYLS (Chess and Thomas) (1984)	Sample gathered through personal contact; middle and upper-middle class (N–133)	94%	1 year 2 years 3 years 4 years	Boys are less active. Boys are more adaptable. Boys are less active, with lower threshold, more persistent. Boys are more adaptable, with lower threshold.

(continued)

Table 4. (*Continued*)

	Sampling	Rate of response	Age	Sex differences at the group mean:
Fullard, McDevitt and Carey (1984)	Two private paediatric clinics middle and upper-middle class (N–167 between 1 and 2 years) (N–142 between 2 and 3 years)	90%	1 year 2 years	Boys are more regular, more approaching and more active. Boys are more regular.
Matheny, Wilson and Nuss (1984)	Sampling of twins from a longitudinal study 30%–lower class 4%–upper class (N–89) 18 months (N–77) 24 months	Not reported	2 years 18 months	Boys are more adaptable. No difference.
Chen (1981)	Sampling method not reported (see Ciba symposium 89, tables p. 18) (N–1931)	Not reported	3-7 years	Boys are more active, more intense, with negative mood, more persistent. Boys are less distractible.
Maziade et al (1984)	Random sample (proportional allocation of classes in all school boards) (N–984)	94% (test) 84% (retest)	7 years 7 years	Boys are more active, with negative mood and higher threshold, less persistent. Boys are more active, with negative mood and higher threshold, more intense, less distractible.
Hegvik et al (1982)	Private paediatric practices (N–279); middle to upper-middle class District school (N–227)	93% 27%	8-12 years	Boys are more active, with higher threshold, less adaptable, with more negative mood, less predictable, less persistent.
Maziade et al (1985; present study)	Random sample (proportional allocation of classes in four school boards) (N–647)	82% (test) 62% (retest)	9-12 years 9-12 years	Boys are more active, with higher threshold, less predictable, less persistent. Boys are more active, with higher threshold, less predictable, less persistent.

sonance in findings for research questions concerning sex differences. Many studies do not appropriately report rates of response or sampling methods and very few studies use random sampling; also, we have little knowledge of the effect of a high non respondent rate on such characteristics as sex differences. In our opinion, this renders difficult any discussion of the discrepancies in finding between the studies. It is also possible that sex differences vary more transculturally than other comparisons involving, for instance, SES or temperament clusters.

SUMMARY

Temperament data gathered through parental ratings may generate consistent and interpretable findings, provided that one takes into account the sampling and the operational definition of temperament. Congruent results from various studies have been obtained with regard to the absence of association between SES and the NYLS temperament with the consistent exception of rhythmicity.

The literature supports consistency for the main temperament clusters up to age seven. However, our study did not reveal continued consistency between the ages of 8 and 12. In contrast with other studies, significant sex differences were only found in boys showing higher activity levels and higher sensory thresholds than girls. It is difficult to conceptualize why parental ratings in different studies would be less accurate or reliable for assessing sex differences when they are consistent for comparisons other than sex differences. It seems likely that either sampling or selection criteria may create undesirable distortions in the final comparison in different studies.

In addition, we must consider the effect on final comparisons of the imperfect test-retest reliability of the instrument currently in use, a point which has already been demonstrated[8]. Also, since more interest is now being paid to temperamental differences in children between cultures, it appears to us that sound transcultural comparisons depend upon researchers making every effort to keep constant their sampling methods and their operational definitions of temperament.

REFERENCES

1. Rothbart MK: Measurement of temperament in infancy. *Child Development,* 52:569–578, 1981.
2. Matheny AP: Bayley's infant behavior record: Behavioral components and twin analyses. *Child Development,* 51:1157–1167, 1980.

3. Buss AH and Plomin R (Eds): *A Temperament Theory of Personality Development.* New York: John Wiley & Sons, 1975.

4. Thomas A and Chess S (Eds): *Temperament and Development.* New York: Brunner/ Mazel, 1977.

5. Persson-Blennow I and McNeil TF: Factor analysis of temperament characteristics in children at 6 months, 1 year and 2 years of age. *British Journal of Educational Psychology, 52*:51–57, 1982.

6. Matheny AP, Wilson RS and Nuss SM: Toddler temperament: Stability across settings and over ages. *Child Development, 55*:1200–1211, 1984.

7. Maziade M, Boudreault M, Thivierge J, Capéraà P and Côté R: Infant temperament: SES and gender differences and reliability of measurement in a large Quebec sample. *Merrill-Palmer Quarterly, 30*:213–216, 1984.

8. Maziade M, Côté R, Boudreault M, Thivierge J and Capéraà P: The New York longitudinal studies model of temperament: Gender differences and demographic correlates in a French-speaking population. *Journal of the American Academy of Child Psychiatry, 23*:582–587, 1984.

9. Simonds JF and Simonds MP: Factor analysis of temperament category scores in a sample of nursery school children. *Journal of Clinical Psychology, 38*:359–366, 1981.

10. Maziade M, Capéraà P, Laplante B, Boudreault M, Thivierge J, Côté R and Boutin P: Value of difficult temperament among 7-year olds in the general population for predicting psychiatric diagnosis at age 12. *American Journal of Psychiatry, 142*:943–946, 1985.

11. Chess S and Thomas A (Eds): *Origins and Evolution of Behavior Disorders. From Infancy to Early Adult Life.* New York: Brunner/ Mazel, 1984.

12. Graham P, Rutter M and George S: Temperamental characteristics as predictors of behavior disorders in children. *American Journal of Orthopsychiatry, 43*:328–339, 1973.

13. Ciba Foundation Symposium 89 (Ed): General discussion I. In *Temperamental differences in infants and young children.* London: Pitman, 1982.

14. Hubert NC, Wachs TD, Peters-Martin P and Gandour MJ: The study of early temperament: Measurement and conceptual issues. *Child Development, 53*:571–600, 1982.

15. Vaughn BE, Taraldson BJ, Crichton L and Egeland B: The assessment of infant temperament: A critique of the Carey infant temperament questionnaire. *Infant Behavior and Development, 4*:1–17, 1981.

16. Rutter M: Temperament: Concepts, issues and problems. In Ciba Foundation Symposium 89 (Ed), *Temperamental differences in infants and young children.* London: Pitman, 1982, pp. 1–20.

17. Lyon ME and Plomin R: The measurement of temperament using parental ratings. *Journal of Child Psychology and Psychiatry, 22*:47–53, 1981.

18. Rothbart MK and Derryberry D: Development of individual differences in temperament. In Lamb ME and Brown AL (Eds) *Advances in developmental psychology, vol. 1.* Hillsdale: Lawrence Erlbaum, 1981.

19. Dunn J and Kendrick C: Studying temperament and parent-child interaction: Comparison of interview and direct observation. *Development Medicine and Child Neurology, 22*:484–496, 1980.

20. Rutter M: Chairman's closing remarks. In Ciba Foundation Symposium 89 (Ed), *Temperamental differences in infants and young children.* London: Pitman, 1982.

21. Rutter M: Epidemiological-longitudinal approaches to the study of development.

In Collins WA (Ed), *The concept of development. The Minnesota symposium of child psychology,* vol. 15. Hillsdale: Lawrence Erlbaum, 1982.

22. Maziade M, Côté R, Boudreault M, Thivierge J and Boutin P: Family correlates of temperament continuity and change across middle childhood. *American Journal of Orthopsychiatry,* 56:196–203, 1986.

23. Hegvik RL, McDevitt SC and Carey WB: The middle childhood temperament questionnaire. *Developmental and Behavioral Pediatrics,* 3:197–200, 1982.

24. Hollingshead AD (Ed): *Two-Factor Index of Social Position.* New Haven: Yale University Press, 1957.

25. Capéraà P, Côté R and Thivierge J: Hyperactivity: Comment on Trites' article. *Journal of Child Psychology and Psychiatry,* 26:485–486, 1985.

26. Thivierge J. Capéraà P, Boudreault M, Côté R and Maziade M: Reliability and Principal Component Analysis (PCA) of the Conners Teacher Questionnaire (CTQ). In Bloomingdale LM (Ed), *Attention deficit disorder: New treatments, psychopharmacology, attention research.* New York: Spectrum Publications, (in press), 1985.

27. Wilson RS and Matheny AP: Assessment of temperament in infant twins. *Developmental Psychology,* 19:172–183, 1983.

28. Thomas A, Chess S and Birch HG (Eds): *Temperament and Behavior Disorders in Children.* New York: New York University Press, 1968.

29. Chess S and Thomas A (Eds): Multiple regression analyses: Correlations between three-year ratings and early adult adaptation. In *Origins and evolution of behavior disorders. From infancy to early adult life.* New York: Brunner/Mazel, 1984.

30. Chess S and Thomas A (Eds): Set correlation analyses: Correlations between childhood and early adult ratings. In *Origins and evolution of behavior disorders. From infancy to early adult life.* New York: Brunner/Mazel, 1984.

31. Persson-Blennow I and McNeil TF: Temperament characteristics of children in relation to gender, birth order, and social class. *American Journal of Orthopsychiatry,* 51:710–714, 1981.

32. Sameroff AJ, Seifer R and Elias PK: Sociocultural variability in infant temperament ratings. *Child Development,* 53:164–173, 1982.

33. Carey WB and McDevitt SC: Revision of the infant temperament questionnaire. *Pediatrics,* 61:735–739, 1978.

34. Hsu CC, Soong WT, Stigler JW, Hong CC and Liang CC: The temperamental characteristics of Chinese babies. *Child Development,* 52:1337–1340, 1981.

35. Fullard W, McDevitt SC and Carey WB: Assessing temperament in one- to three-year old children. *Journal of Pediatric Psychology,* 9:205–217, 1984.

15

Inhibited and Uninhibited Children: A Follow-up Study

J. Steven Reznick, Jerome Kagan, Nancy Snidman, Michelle Gersten, Katherine Baak, and Allison Rosenberg

Harvard University, Cambridge, Massachusetts

A group of 46 children classified at 21 months as either behaviorally inhibited or uninhibited, and 18 children who were classified as falling at neither extreme, were observed at 5 ½ years of age in contexts designed to evaluate behavior in social situations and heart rate, heart rate variability, and pupillary dilation to cognitive tasks. Additionally, 43 of the 46 inhibited or uninhibited children had been evaluated in similar contexts when they were 4 years of age. At age 5 ½, the formerly inhibited children, compared with the uninhibited ones, were more inhibited with peers in both laboratory and school, as well as with an adult examiner in a testing situation, and more cautious in a situation of mild risk. As at the earlier ages, more inhibited children had a relatively high and stable heart rate. The inhibited children also had tonically larger pupillary dilations to cognitive stress, were either impulsive or reflective on a test with response uncertainty, and their mothers described them as shy with unfamiliar peers. It was suggested that one or more of the stress circuits that link the hypothalamus to the pituitary, reticular activating system and sym-

Reprinted with permission from *Child Development,* 1986, Vol. 57, 660–680. Copyright 1986 by the Society for Research in Child Development, Inc.

This research was supported by a grant from the John D. and Catherine T. MacArthur Foundation.

*pathetic chain are at a higher level of excitability among inhibited than
among uninhibited children.*

Two previous reports in this journal summarized longitudinal data
gathered on a group of Caucasian, middle-class children selected at 21
months of age to represent the extremes on one of two psychological
qualities we have called inhibition and lack of inhibition to the unfamiliar
(Garcia-Coll, Kagan, & Reznick, 1984; Kagan, Reznick, Clarke, Snidman,
& Garcia-Coll, 1984). The sample was selected from a larger group of 305
Caucasian children whose mothers, responding to questions in a telephone interview, described their children as tending to be either inhibited or uninhibited. On the basis of these interviews, 117 children
were invited to come to our laboratory, where their behavior to unfamiliar people and objects was quantified. The situations included: initial meeting with an unfamiliar examiner and subsequent encounters
with an unfamiliar set of toys, a woman model displaying a trio of acts that
were difficult to remember, a second female stranger, a large metal robot,
and temporary separation from the mother. The major behavioral signs
of inhibition were long latencies to interact with the unfamiliar adults,
retreat from an unfamiliar person or object, cessation of play or vocalization, clinging to the mother, and fretting or crying. The children who displayed these behaviors consistently across most of the incentives, as well
as those who did not, were selected to form groups of 28 extremely inhibited and 30 extremely uninhibited children. Each group represented
about 10% of the original sample. These 58 children returned to the
laboratory 1 month later to be observed in the same room with the same
incentives. There was reasonable stability of behavior across the 1-month
interval; the cross-episode correlation for a summary index of behavioral
inhibition was 0.6. Additionally, there was a positive association between
behavioral inhibition and absolute heart rate and a negative association
between behavioral inhibition and heart rate variability, defined as
the mean standard deviation of the heart period, while the children were
looking at unfamiliar pictures and listening to unfamiliar environmental
sounds and speech (for details, see Garcia-Coll et al., 1984).

Observations of 43 of these children at 4 years of age in both a peer play
and a testing context revealed that the behavioral differences between the
two extreme groups had been preserved to a significant degree. The
formerly inhibited children showed longer latencies to initiate play with
an unfamiliar child, made fewer approaches to the unfamiliar child, and
spent more time proximal to the mother and staring at the unfamiliar
child when observed in a laboratory playroom on two occasions that

lasted 40 min. In the individual testing situation the inhibited children showed higher and less variable (i.e., more stable) heart rates to a series of cognitive procedures, were more reluctant to guess on difficult cognitive items, and looked more often at the female examiner during the testing procedure. As at 21 months, there was a significant positive relation between inhibited behavior and a high and stable heart rate to moderately difficult cognitive tasks (average $r = 0.4$). There was slightly greater preservation of spontaneous behavior among the uninhibited children than preservation of restraint among the inhibited group, and the inhibited children who had a high and stable heart rate at 21 months remained more inhibited than did the inhibited children who had low and variable heart rates (Kagan et al., 1984). Similar results have emerged with a second cohort of Caucasian children who were selected to be extreme on one of these two behavioral qualities at 31 months of age and observed 1 year later when they were 43 months old (Snidman, 1984). The frequency of inhibited and uninhibited classifications did not correlate with sex or social class in either of these investigations.

The present report summarizes the results of an evaluation of the first cohort of children at 5½ years, 18 months after the last assessment. In addition to our interest in the stability of and relation between behavior and heart rate, the procedures were also designed to answer additional questions of theoretical relevance. One is a direct consequence of the hypothesis that inhibited children have a lower threshold for the generation of specific states of physiological arousal to unfamiliar, unexpected, or challenging events. Research during the past 2 decades has led physiologists to posit a set of separate neural circuits, originating in the hypothalamus (especially the paraventricular nucleus) and involving the pituitary and adrenal glands, the reticular activating system, and the sympathetic arm of the autonomic nervous system (Axelrod & Reisine, 1984; Reiser, 1984; Smith & DeVito, 1984). It is assumed that following encounter with unfamiliarity or challenge, discharge of the hypothalamus can lead to (*a*) secretion of ACTH by the pituitary, which results in production of cortisol by the adrenal cortex, (*b*) discharge of the reticular activating system and subsequent changes in muscle tone, or (*c*) discharge of the sympathetic nervous system and subsequent increases in heart rate, blood pressure, and pupillary dilation. Because pupillary dilation to mild cognitive stress is a potential index of sympathetic reactivity, we quantified this variable in order to add support to the hypothesis that the stress circuit is at a lower threshold among inhibited children.

Further, 5½-year-old children are mature enough to understand that in situations of choice they may become vulnerable to a state of uncertainty.

One such context is potential task failure; another is the possibility of physical harm. We observed the children in both classes of situations, one of which involved assessment of a reflective or an impulsive approach to a cognitive problem with response uncertainty. Finally, 5½-year-olds may have a symbolic representation of some of their salient psychological qualities. Inhibition and lack of inhibition are two such characteristics, and we wished to test the hypothesis that inhibited children would preferentially attend to a figure symbolic of fearfulness over one symbolizing boldness, while the uninhibited children would display the opposite profile.

METHOD

Subjects

The subjects were 24 children who had been classified as inhibited and 22 children classified as uninhibited when they were 21 months old. In addition, we evaluated 18 children whose behavior at 21 months fell between the two extremes. These control children had not been seen at 4 years of age and, for logistic reasons, were not observed in all of the procedural contexts to be described below. Two of the 24 inhibited and one of the 22 uninhibited children had not been evaluated at 4 years of age, and six children had incomplete data sets at age 5½ because of technical failures, refusal to take the heart rate electrodes, or parental unavailability for one of the sessions. There was a total of 27 boys and 37 girls, and the proportion of boys and girls in each of the three groups was similar.

Procedure

The inhibited and uninhibited children were observed in a laboratory on two occasions, and in their school setting during the first week of kindergarten in September and again in February of the same academic year. The first school visit occurred prior to the first laboratory session, and the second during the period when the laboratory sessions were being implemented. The procedures were designed to assess behavioral inhibition and lack of inhibition in unfamiliar social situations, avoidance of risk, and the tendency to show signs of sympathetic arousal and uncertainty to cognitive demands and potential failure in this relatively unfamiliar laboratory setting.

Laboratory Visit 1

Upon arriving at the laboratory, the child was greeted by a female examiner who was unfamiliar with the child and his or her prior classification. Most mothers remained with their child throughout the testing. Electrodes for recording heart rate and respiration were taped to the child's chest and back and the session began. The sequence of episodes follows.

Quiet period. The child was asked to sit quietly for a 30-sec period while heart rate was recorded.

Baseline 1. The child was asked to listen carefully while the examiner read a story supported by four pictures. (There were four 30-sec baseline periods throughout the session, and each baseline period involved a continuation of the story.) The purpose of the baseline period was to compare the child's heart rate while attending to a story, compared with a quiet period that had no special focus of attention.

Recognition memory: Prestress familiarization and test. The purpose of this procedure was to assess the child's baseline recognition memory prior to a series of cognitively difficult tasks. Later in the session we assessed the child's recognition memory in a parallel memory task to determine if the inhibited children showed a greater decrease in recognition memory performance than uninhibited children following the cognitive stress (Messer, 1968). After some practice trials to familiarize the child with the procedure, he or she was told to attend carefully to each of a series of slides presented on a screen and to try to remember each picture. The 24 chromatic slides were of familiar objects, representing many different categories, and were displayed for 5 sec.

After the 24 familiarization slides, each child was told that he or she would now see another set of slides, some of which were in the prior familiarization set, some of which were new. The child was to say "yes" if the picture had been seen before, and "no" if it had not. The child was then shown a second set of 24 slides, half of which had been in the previous set, half of which were new. The variables of interest were heart rate, heart rate variability, accuracy of performance, and response latency from the appearance of the picture to the child's decision. The child was then presented with four difficult cognitive tasks designed to increase task-related arousal.

Recall of words. The examiner first asked the child to repeat a series of words one at a time. The examiner then read the same words as part of a series containing two through six items, and the child was asked to remember all the words and to repeat them. The child was given an additional trial with a particular series if he or she failed to remember the words on the first attempt. The task was terminated when the child was successful on the six-word series or failed an easier series on two consecutive trials. A central purpose of this task was to record the child's voice under low (single word repetition) and high stress (recall of the series). Analyses of the fundamental frequency and variability of the pitch periods for each word will be part of a separate report.

Embedded figures test. In addition to producing cognitive stress, this procedure and the two that follow were administered in order to determine if inhibited and uninhibited children differed in their tendency to be reflective or impulsive on tests that contained response uncertainty. After practice trials to familiarize the child with the procedure, he or she was shown a series of six pictures of objects and test plates on which the object was disguised in a set of lines. The child was told to find the disguised figure in the test plate and was given feedback if correct or incorrect. The major variables were response latency to the first solution hypothesis, the number correct, and heart rate and heart rate variability.

Matching familiar figures. After familiarization trials to acquaint the child with the task, he or she was administered six matching familiar figure test items. Each item involved a standard picture of a familiar object and four variants. The child was shown the standard and a plate illustrating four alternatives, only one of which was identical with the standard. The child was asked to find the one variant that was identical with the standard. Response time to the first solution hypothesis, number correct, heart rate, and heart rate variability were the major variables coded.

Haptic procedure. The child was shown a three-dimensional object as a standard and told to place his or her hand behind a curtain and to explore haptically three different forms in order to determine which one of the three hidden forms was identical with the standard object to which the child had only visual access. The child was given practice trials in order to familiarize him or her with the task, followed by five test trials. On the first three test trials, the objects were familiar forms (dog, person, boat), but the last two trials involved unfamiliar geometric forms. A videocamera filmed the child's hand explorations of each form. The major variables coded were the number of forms explored, the time devoted to exploration of each form, latency to the first solution hypothesis, proportion of correct answers across the five items, and heart rate and heart rate variability.

Recognition memory: Poststress familiarization and test. The child was given a second test of recognition memory parallel to the first but involving a different set of 24 slides. The procedure was identical to the one described for prestress recognition memory, and the same variables were coded. As indicated earlier, the purpose of this procedure was to see if inhibited children showed a greater decrease in memory performance, compared with the earlier recognition memory score, than uninhibited children.

Baseline 2. The child was asked to sit quietly while the examiner read a second part of the baseline story and heart rate was recorded. After the second baseline, there was a break during which the child left the laboratory room and had some refreshment.

Baseline 3. After the break the child was asked to sit quietly and to listen to the third part of the story.

Empathy story. The child was told that he or she was going to see and hear a story consisting of slides and a simultaneous narration. The slides were 20 chromatic drawings of two children; female subjects saw girls, male subjects saw boys. The story was about two children; one was depicted as fearful, timid, and shy and the other as bold, fearless, and outgoing. The 20 slides described their adventures, which included being caught in a storm, trespassing on a man's property, and jumping across a large ravine. The examiner coded the child's duration of fixation of each figure by pressing one of two buttons corresponding to the right and left side of the screen. (Intercoder reliability for this variable in similar contexts is above .90). The left-right position of the two figures was counterbalanced. The examiner was unaware of the position of each of the figures during the coding. The primary variable of interest was the amount of attentiveness devoted to the fearful and the fearless child during the story, with the expectation that inhibited children would attend preferentially to the fearful child.

In addition to heart rate and heart rate variability, we also coded the occurrence of a heart rate acceleration to each of the 20 slides by examining the base heart rate during the 3 sec prior to the picture and comparing that rate with the initial direction of heart rate following the appearance of the slide. If the heart rate began to ascend, and the mean of the two highest heart rates at the top of that ascent was higher than the mean heart rate during the base period, an acceleration was coded. If the heart rate began to decelerate upon the presentation of the slides, and the mean of the two lowest beats at the trough was lower than the mean during the base period, a deceleration was coded. Neither an acceleration nor a deceleration was coded if there was no change in heart rate.

Active-passive pictures. The child was asked to describe a series of chromatic slides presented on a screen. A set of 13 pictures was presented, 11 of which had an active and a passive member of a dyad (e.g., one animal approaching an animal lying down; one adult pointing a finger at another; an animal chasing a child). The right-left positions of the active and passive agents were counterbalanced. The examiner coded the duration of fixation of each picture. Preference for attending to the active or the passive figure was based on percent fixation to that picture relative to the preference for that side of the screen across all pictures, with the expectation that inhibited children would attend preferentially to the passive figure. Heart rate and heart variability were also recorded.

Baseline 4. The examiner finished the story by reading the narration that accompanied the last set of four pictures.

Quiet period. The session ended with a 30-sec quiet period in which the child was asked to sit quietly.

In addition to the variables described above, we also coded a small number of variables from the videotape of the child's behavior during the testing session. Coders unfamiliar with the child's prior classification tallied the following behaviors: number of times the child glanced up at the examiner, number of spontaneous comments to the examiner that were unprovoked and not demanded by the examiner's question, and gross motor movements of trunk and limbs. Our observations at age 4 led us to expect that the inhibited children would look at the examiner more often but would speak and show gross motor movement less often. Intercoder reliability for the variables was established by having a second person code these responses, trial by trial, for nine randomly selected children. The reliability coefficient for "look examiner" was 0.99. Because the remaining two variables were relatively infrequent, we computed a percent agreement between the two coders, eliminating trials when both coders reported absence of the response. For spontaneous comments, the percent agreement was 93%; for gross motor movement it was 99%. Intercorrelation of the three variables revealed the expected significant, positive correlation for spontaneous comments and gross motor movement ($r = .34$, $p < .05$). However, looking at the examiner was independent of both variables. Thus, we created an average standard score for the two correlated variables. Because most of the derived variables indexed behavioral inhibition, we reversed the standard score for this variable and called it *laboratory inhibition*. We retained "look examiner" as a separate variable because it had previously differentiated between inhibited and uninhibited children at 4 years of age, and because individual differences in this response were preserved from 4 to 5½ years ($r = .61$, $p < .01$).

Laboratory Visit 2

Risk room. When the child and mother arrived for the second laboratory visit, they were taken to a room that contained three novel objects that invited exploration: a beam set at an angle of 30° to the floor, a large black box with a circular hole and a handle which, if pressed, produced an unusual noise, and a set of bars mounted so that the child's feet would have to leave the floor in order to play on them. The examiner left the room, saying she would return in a few minutes; the child and mother were in the room for 5 min. The purpose of the procedure was to determine if inhibited children would be more reluctant than uninhibited ones to play with the novel objects, and we coded the following variables from videotape: latency to perform each of the four actions (i.e., latency to walk on the beam, to pull down the handle of the box, to put a hand into the hole, and to leave the floor while holding onto the bars), total time that the child remained proximal to the mother, and total time not playing with any of the objects in the room. Reliability was established by having seven randomly selected subjects recoded by another observer. The intercoder reliability for each of the variables was extremely high (in the upper nineties). Because these six variables were positively correlated (correlations ranged from .47 to .91), we created a derived variable, called *risk avoidance,* that represented the mean standard score for: latency to initiate play with any toy, number of novel acts not initiated, total time proximal to the mother, and total time not playing.

After 5 min, an unfamiliar woman entered the room and invited the child to initiate each of the four novel acts, and most children performed them. The woman then asked the child to go to a mattress that lay on the floor under the bars and to fall backward onto the mattress. This procedure was implemented because observations of the children at earlier ages suggested that inhibited children had greater postural tension. The variable coded was whether the child fell in an uninterrupted movement so that the back of the head touched the mattress, or whether the child fell first to a sitting position. The variable, called *inhibited fall,* was coded 1 if the child fell in an uninterrupted movement, 2 if the child first sat and then fell so that its head touched the mattress, or 3 if the child fell to a sitting position only and never fell back on the mattress.

Finally, the woman invited the child to play a game. She brought in a box about 12 inches on each side and a ball the size of a volleyball and told the child that he or she was to throw the ball so that it went into the basket. The child was asked to decide how near or far the basket should be placed. The child could choose to put the basket near (less than 12 inches), moderately far (about 3 feet away), or very far (6 feet away). The child was given three trials, and the variable analyzed was the number of trials (out of three) that the child chose to place the basket close (called *task caution*). The expectation was that inhibited children would behave more cautiously and choose the near position more frequently than uninhibited children.

Peer play. A pair of children of the same sex, one inhibited and one uninhibited, based on the 21-month classification, was observed in the same playroom in which each child had been on four prior occasions. The two mothers sat on a couch reading magazines or conversing while the two children played for 30 min. The variables coded included latency to play with the first toy, latency to approach the other child, latency to first vocalization, total time looking at the other child while not in social interaction, and total time proximal to the mother while not playing. We also coded frequency of toy seizures, aggressive acts, and number of times the child ran across the room, but these three responses were so infrequent (median < 1.0) that we eliminated them from further analyses. The intercoder reliabilities for the first five variables ranged from .83 to .99. A factor analysis revealed a first factor of four positively correlated variables: latency to play, latency to make first approach, time proximal to mother, and time staring at the other child. Latency to vocalization was not significantly related to any of the variables; hence, it was eliminated. A mean standard score for the four correlated variables was computed, and this derived variable was called *peer play inhibition*. (The control children were not observed in the peer play situation).

Pupillary dilation. Each child was then taken to a laboratory that contained a Gulf and Western Pupillometer System. Pupillary dilation was recorded during an initial baseline period, and a subsequent series of cognitive procedures: listening to a story; recalling lists of three, four, five, and six words read by the examiner; inferring an object from an oral description of some of its characteristics (e.g., the examiner said, "I am thinking of something that is white, round, and cold"); deciding which of two objects was larger (e.g., a watch or a dime); digit span; listening to a second story; and a final baseline period. Pupillary diameters during the 15-min battery were sampled at 10 Hz. All diameter values were stored on tape for each phase of each trial. In order to eliminate artifacts due to eye blinks, the criterion for inclusion of a value in the analysis was three consecutive identical values. The primary variable was the mean of the nine largest pupillary dilation values for each of the trials of each task, as well as the mean of the nine largest values for the interval before each trial.

Mother Interview

Several weeks later, the examiner interviewed each mother over the telephone. The mother was asked about the child's illnesses, current fears, typical reactions to people, adjustment to school, and the presence of particular symptoms such as excessive perspiration, constipation, and sleeplessness. The mother's rating of the child's degree of shyness with other people was quantified on a three-point scale, where 1 designated outgoing, 2 represented a little shy, and 3 represented the mother's belief that the child was extremely shy.

School Observations

The children were observed in their kindergarten classroom twice, once during the first week of school and once in February, by an observer who had no knowledge of the child's prior behavior or classification. The control children were not observed in the school setting. Fourteen observers were trained to do spot observations for a small set of behavioral variables. Each observer carried a small device that issued a signal via earphone every 15 sec for the first observations in September, and every 10 sec for the observations in February. At the signal the observer looked at the child and noted on a prepared scoring form whether (a) the child was alone, with one or more peers, or with a teacher, and (b) what activity the child was engaged in at that time. The variables included: inactive, involved in play, offers help, requests aid, laughs, cries, approaches another person, talks, looks at another person. These data were gathered for approximately 90 min of free play during the first week of kindergarten and again for an additional 90 min of free play 6 months later. The data from periods when the teacher structured the activities of the classroom were not analyzed because they provided minimal opportunity for variability in behavior among the children.

Interobserver reliability for the fall observations was determined by treating one of the authors (M.G.) as the criterion and having each of the other observers independently code videotapes of several different children in a classroom setting. The percent agreement between each of the 13 observers and the criterion coder ranged from 86% to 93%. The February visits to the school were made by only four observers, two of whom had visited in the fall. However, these two coders watched different children on their winter visit. Interobserver reliabilities for the February visit were computed by having each observer code behavior in a natural school setting. Percentage agreement between each of the three coders and M.G. ranged from 93% to 99%. The denominator for computing percent agreement did not include instances in which no behavior was coded by either observer.

Many of the variables coded were infrequent, with median values less than 1.0. A factor analysis of the remaining variables revealed a first factor with three correlated variables for the September observation: number of observations in which the child was alone, looking at a peer, or in social interaction (this variable was negatively correlated with the first two). The cluster of three correlated variables from the February observation included: number of observations in which the child was alone and looking at another peer, in social interaction, or talking with another person (the latter two were negatively correlated with frequency of looking at the peer). Because the fall and winter factors were positively correlated ($r = .42$, $p < .01$), we computed an average score for the two clusters (reversing, of course, the values for social interaction and talking to a peer so that a high score on the derived variable reflects behavioral inhibition). This derived variable was called *school inhibition*.

RESULTS AND DISCUSSION

Presentation of the results is organized around the following three questions: (*a*) the organization of contemporaneous variables presumed to index inhibition and lack of inhibition, (*b*) the contemporaneous data on heart rate and heart rate variability and its relation to inhibited and uninhibited behavior, and (*c*) the predictive relations between behavioral and heart rate data gathered at 21 and 48 months, on the one hand, and the major behavioral and autonomic variables evaluated at 5½ years of age.

Behavior at 5½ Years

The preceding section described the major variables selected for analysis. Because we believe each of the major situations (testing, risk room, peer play, and school) provides a different set of incentives for the display of inhibited or uninhibited behavior, we decided to retain the separateness of the contexts in the analyses that follow. However, because each of the situations reveals different opportunities to express a deeper disposition toward inhibition, we also computed an aggregate index of inhibition by averaging the standard scores for the five major variables: peer play inhibition, laboratory inhibition, school inhibition, risk avoidance, and look at examiner. We did not include in the aggregate index inhibited fall and task caution because they were based on a much smaller sample of behavior, but we shall describe the correlations between these and the other variables in the text.

Table 1 presents the intercorrelations among the five major indexes of inhibition, along with the aggregate index. The aggregate index of inhibition was significantly correlated with each of the five separate variables (r ranged from .37 to .73), and with inhibited fall ($r = .33$, $p < .05$), but not with task caution ($r = .22$). The tendency to be vocally quiet and motorically still in the testing situation (laboratory inhibition) was positively related to inhibition in school ($r = .45$, $p < .01$) and to risk avoidance ($r = .41$, $p < .01$). Finally, peer play inhibition was significantly related to glances at the examiner ($r = .30$, $p < .05$). At 4 years of age, the comparable correlation was .35. There were no significant relations between contemporary indexes of inhibited or uninhibited behavior and quality of performance on the recognition memory, word recall, embedded figures, matching familiar figures, or haptic tests. This result, which is consonant with earlier findings, suggests that inhibited and uninhibited children perform similarly on many cognitive tests.

Heart Period and Heart Period Variability

The heart period and heart period variability values (smaller heart periods reflect higher heart rates) were highly correlated across the separate episodes (correlations ranged between 0.8 and 0.9 for both period and variability), and the correlation between mean heart period and variability averaged 0.7. Despite the high intertask correlations, we retained separate, derived scores for three classes of episodes: mean of

Table 1. Correlations Among the Major Behavioral Indexes of Inhibition at 5½ Years of Age

Variable	1	2	3	4	5	6
1. Peer play inhibition...	...	.21	.04	.26	.30*	.63***
2. Laboratory inhibition .		...	.45**	.41**	−.09	.64***
3. School inhibition			...	.22	−.31	.37**
4. Risk avoidance				....	.21	.73***
5. Look examiner					...	.51***
6. Aggregate inhibition ..						...

* = $p < .05$.
** = $p < .01$.
*** = $p < .001$.

the two quiet periods and the four baselines, called *baseline heart rate*; mean for tasks where the child did not have to talk or move (familiarization phases of recognition memory, listening to words, and empathy story), called *quiet tasks*; and mean for those tasks requiring the child to speak or to move (embedded figures, matching familiar figures, haptic visual matching, test phases of recognition memory, and active-passive pictures), called *active tasks*. Although the correlations for either heart period or variability within the separate episodes of the three classes of tasks were very high, the correlations were even higher when cognitive stress was imposed during the quiet and active cognitive procedures, as compared with the correlations across the six baseline values.

Relation Between Heart Period and Behavior

Table 2 contains the correlations between heart period and variability to the quiet tasks, and the five major contemporaneous indexes of inhibited behavior at 5½ years of age. The magnitude and pattern of the correlations with behavior were very similar when we used heart period values during baseline or the active tasks.

A high heart rate (i.e., a low heart period) and low variability were both significantly related to the aggregate index of inhibition as well as look at examiner. A high heart rate was also significantly related to peer play inhibition and risk avoidance but not to school inhibition, task caution, or inhibited fall. In general, a high and stable heart rate was more closely related to the responses that reflect an initial restraint rather than lack of social spontaneity. When we created a derived restraint variable based on

Table 2. Correlations Between Heart Period and Heart Period Variability to the Quiet Tasks and Selected Behavioral Variables at 5½ Years of Age

Behavioral Variables	Heart Period Quiet Tasks	Variability Quiet Tasks
Peer play inhibition	−.34*	−.26
Laboratory inhibition	−.06	−.06
School inhibition	−.21	−.21
Risk avoidance	−.34*	−.26
Look examiner	−.34*	−.33*
Aggregate inhibition	−.46***	−.42**

* = $p < .05$.
** = $p < .01$.
*** = $p < .001$.

staring at the peer in the school situation, peer play inhibition cluster, look at examiner, and risk avoidance, we found a significant negative correlation with heart period and variability ($r = -.49$, $p < .01$; $r = -.42$, $p < .01$). But a derived spontaneity variable based on frequency of social interaction in the school and talking to the examiner and gross motor movement during the testing session was independent of both heart rate and variability ($r = .06, .06$). Thus, even though there is a significant correlation between the behaviors reflecting initial restraint in an unfamiliar situation and those reflecting lack of social spontaneity, the former is more closely tied to a high and stable heart rate than is the latter. The magnitudes of the correlations between heart rate and behavior at 5½ years are very similar to those found at 4 years of age. For example, the 4-year correlations between the index of inhibited behavior in a peer play situation and heart rate and variability were $-.33$ and $-.39$.

Prediction of Profiles at 5½ Years

We now consider the predictive relations between inhibited or uninhibited behavior and the heart rate profiles at 21 and 48 months and the major variables assessed at 5½ years: the six behavioral indexes, task caution, inhibited fall, maternal report, heart rate and heart rate variability, pupillary dilation, conceptualization of self, and reflection-impulsivity. Unless noted otherwise, the adjective inhibited or uninhibited always refers to the initial classification of the child at 21 months of age.

Prediction of inhibited behavior. Table 3 presents the correlations between the major behavioral and heart rate indexes gathered at 21 and 48 months and the behavioral variables evaluated at 5½ years. The index of inhibition at age 4 represented the mean standard score for four variables: latency to approach the peer, latency to enter a plastic tunnel in the playroom, time proximal to mother while not playing, and frequency of glances at the unfamiliar peer. The index of uninhibited behavior at age 4 represented the mean standard score for frequency of running across the room and approaches to the other child across two different play sessions with different pairs of children. The indexes of inhibited and uninhibited behavior were treated separately because the correlation between the two indexes was only $-.41$, and we believe each is measuring different psychological qualities.

There was good preservation of differences in behavior from 21 and 48 months, with the differences better preserved from age 4 to 5½ than from 21 months to 5½ years. The aggregate index of inhibition at 5½ years was

Table 3. Prediction of Behavior at 5½ Years from Earlier Data

Variable at Age 5½	Index of Inhibition at 21 Months	Heart Period at 21 Months	Variability at 21 Months	Index of Inhibition at Age 4	Uninhibited Index at Age 4	Heart Period Quiet Tasks at Age 4	Variability Quiet Tasks at Age 4
Peer play inhibition	.43**	-.09	-.14	.76***	-.38**	-.21	-.18
Laboratory inhibition	.38**	.09	.02	.27	-.44**	-.15	-.18
School inhibition	.34*	.16	-.01	.12	-.35*	-.20	-.17
Risk avoidance	.19	.04	-.01	.35*	-.32*	-.38**	-.32*
Look examiner	.22	-.06	-.02	.41**	-.03	-.21	-.28
Aggregate index of inhibition	.52***	.03	-.06	.67***	-.49***	-.39**	-.39**
Task caution	.35*	-.11	-.01	.25	-.51***	-.38**	-.21
Inhibited fall	.40**	.05	.19	.32*	-.24	-.29	-.12
Maternal report: shy	.55***	-.01	.10	.36**	-.49***	-.28	-.13

significantly related to behavior at both 21 months and 4 years. When the aggregate index of inhibition at 5½ was the criterion, 78% of the children fell into their expected category, based on their initial classification at 21 months (inhibited children falling above the median and uninhibited children falling below the median on the aggregate index). As might be expected, the most robust relation involved similar contexts—inhibited behavior with the unfamiliar peer in the play situation at age 4 and 5½ years ($r = .76$, $p < .001$). Table 3 reveals the wisdom of keeping the indexes of inhibited and uninhibited behavior at age 4 separate. Restrained behavior with the peer and frequent looks at the examiner were more clearly related to the 4-year-old index of inhibited behavior, while behavior at school was more clearly related to the earlier index of uninhibited behavior. The inhibited children also glanced more often at the examiner when they were seen at 4 years of age; the stability coefficient for this variable from 4 to 5½ years was .61 ($p < .01$). The index of inhibition at 21 months predicted inhibition at school and in the testing situation, as well as task caution and a restrained fall on the mattress. Further, a high and stable heart rate at age 4 predicted the aggregate index of inhibition at age 5.

Maternal interview at 20 months and 5½ years. The initial selection of children for the laboratory assessment at 21 months was based on the mother's answers to eight questions posed in a brief telephone interview several weeks earlier. The mother had to decide whether it was usual or unusual for her child to show timidity, shyness, or fear in each of the following situations: visit to the doctor, new babysitter, unfamiliar pets, unfamiliar child, unfamiliar adult, unfamiliar place, and an unfamiliar visitor to the home. The final question asked whether the child required more than 10 min to feel at ease in a new place. An index of inhibition was computed representing the sum of the answers indicative of timidity (actual scores ranged from 0 to 7). The answers to these eight questions were predictive of the children's behavior several weeks later when they came to the laboratory for the initial behavioral assessment at 21 months ($r = .41, p < .01$). Eighty percent of the children with scores of 4 or more who were included in the longitudinal study were subsequently classified as inhibited, while 80% of the children with scores of less than 4 were classified as uninhibited at that early age. Additionally, each child's inhibition score based on this brief interview predicted the index of inhibited behavior at age 4 ($r = .53$, $p < .001$), the aggregate index of inhibition at 5½ years of age ($r = .53, p < .001$), as well as a higher and more stable heart rate at 4 years of age ($r = .41, p < .01; r = .40, p < .01$), and at age 5½ ($r = .40$, $p < .01; r = .34$, $p < .05$).

At 5½ years the interviewer asked the mother to classify her child as either outgoing, a little shy, or extremely shy. This three-point scale was positively correlated with the index of inhibition taken from the telephone interview at 21 months ($r = .33, p < .05$) as well as with the indexes of behavioral inhibition at 21 months ($r = .55, p < .01$), 4 years ($r = .36, p < .05$), and the aggregate index of inhibition at 5½ years ($r = .33, p < .05$). Although these data indicate some agreement between the mother's conception of her child's degree of timidity and the more objective observations, it must be noted that these children were selected to be extreme on these qualities. Equivalently robust relations might not occur for a random sample of children.

Prediction of Heart Rate and Variability

Figures 1 and 2 illustrate the heart period and heart period variability values for the children who had been classified as inhibited or un-

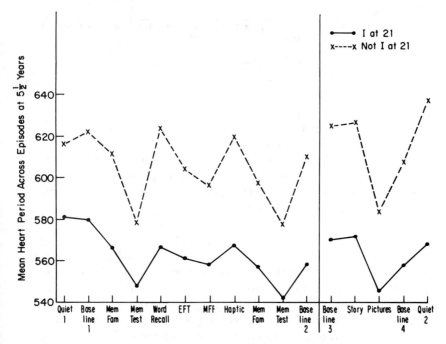

Figure 1. Mean heart period at 5½ years for children classified as inhibited and not inhibited at 21 months.

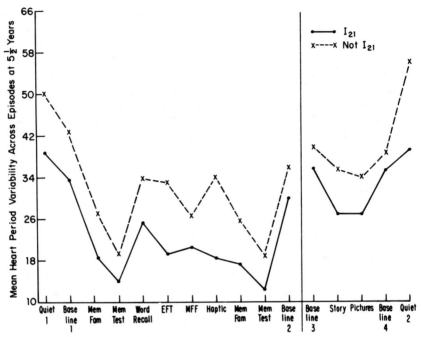

Figure 2. Mean heart period variability at 5½ years for children classified as inhibited and not inhibited at 21 months.

inhibited at 21 months. Even though the form of the function was identical for the two groups—most children showed their highest heart rates and lowest variabilities to the test phases of recognition memory—the inhibited children had higher and more stable heart rates on every episode. A repeated-measures analysis of variance across the episodes, comparing inhibited and uninhibited children, showed a main effect of group for both heart period and variability, $F(1,42) = 6.36, p < .01; F(1,42) = 3.95, p < .05$. Thus, for the third time—at 21 and 48 months, and now at 5½ years—inhibited children had higher and more stable heart rates to cognitive demands than did uninhibited children. Comparison of the mean heart period values (across all tasks) for inhibited, uninhibited, and control children also revealed a significant effect of group, $F(2,59) = 5.07, p < .01$, for heart period, $F(2,59) = 4.65, p < .01$ for variability. Post-hoc Duncan tests revealed that the inhibited children had significantly higher heart rates and lower variabilities than both the uninhibited and the control children. The mean heart period values across all episodes for inhibited, uninhibited, and controls were 561, 611, and 617 msec; for variability, the comparable values were 26, 36, and 41 msec. This pattern suggests that it is the inhibited children who have a distinctive profile of heart rate reactivity. As we shall see, a similar result emerged for pupillary dilation.

This is the first time that inhibited children had higher and more stable heart rates to the initial quiet and baseline periods when no cognitive demand was being made on them. This finding suggests that at the more mature age the inhibited children may have been thinking about the test battery before it began, either on their way to the laboratory or when the electrodes were being placed on their chest. It appears that, with age, uncertainty becomes anticipatory.

Table 4 contains the correlations between behavioral and heart rate variables at 21 and 48 months and the two heart rate variables at 5½ years. The 21-month cardiac data were gathered while the children were looking at slides and listening to speech and sounds.* The 4-year data were gathered over the course of a 1-hour battery, similar to the one administered at 5½ years, that included baseline periods, a memory task, listening to two short stories and a longer story about a fearful and a fearless child, and describing a series of pictures. The heart rate values to the quiet tasks referred to the mean rate and variability values obtained on those tasks where the child sat quietly and listened to the three stories.

Heart rate variability at 21 and 48 months predicted variability at 5½, with the relation stronger from age 4 than from 21 months. Differences in heart rate were preserved from 4 to 5½ years, but not from the first assessment. Further, behavioral inhibition at 21 and 48 months predicted both a higher and more stable heart rate at 5½ years.

Acceleratory trends. The frequency of cardiac accelerations to each of the 20 pictures comprising the story about the fearful and fearless children was an especially sensitive dependent variable. Inhibited children had an average of 6.2 accelerations, while uninhibited children had a mean of 3.7 accelerations, $t(42) = 2.62$, $p < .01$; the correlation between the aggregate index of inhibition at 5½ years and number of accelerations was .35 ($p < .01$). The best contemporary correlate of number of accelerations was the mother's rating of shyness ($r = .42$, $p < .01$). As

---

*The cardiac data at 21 months, which were recorded on FM tape and subsequently digitized and timed, had more missing data points than the cardiac signals at 4 and 5½ years of age, which were timed on-line by a microprocessor. Therefore, we regard the later data as more reliable.

Table 4. Prediction of Heart Rate and Pupillary Dilation at 5½ Years from Earlier Data

Variable at Age 5½	Index of Inhibition at 21 Months	Heart Period at 21 Months	Variability at 21 Months	Index of Inhibition at Age 4	Uninhibited Index at Age 4	Heart Period Quiet Tasks at Age 4	Variability Quiet Tasks at Age 4
Heart:							
Heart period: quiet tasks	−.44**	.15	.19	−.46**	.40*	.58***	.54***
Variability: quiet tasks	−.39**	.11	.39**	−.44**	.27	.44**	.64***
Number of accelerations: story	.47**	−.41**	−.37**	.42**	−.40**	−.24	−.33*
Pupil:							
Baseline	.22	−.06	.16	.36*	−.43**	−.18	−.05
Mean size: pretrial	.25	−.01	.25	.27	−.37*	−.13	−.01
Mean size: all trials	.17	.00	.27	.26	−.37*	−.08	.05

revealed in Table 4, the best early predictor of number of accelerations was inhibition at 21 months. A high rate and low variability at both 21 and 48 months also predicted frequent acceleratory reactions. Surprisingly, mean heart rate at 21 months was a better predictor of number of accelerations at age 5½ than heart rate or heart rate variability at 5½ years.

The same pattern emerged to a very similar story administered to these children when they were 4 years old. The index of inhibition at 21 months also predicted number of accelerations at age 4 ($r = .59$, $p < .01$). Further, half of the inhibited, but only 10% of the uninhibited, children were above the median in number of accelerations to the stories administered at both ages, while only 12% of the inhibited, but 50% of the uninhibited, children were below the median on number of accelerations at both ages ($\chi^2 = 9.0$, $p < .01$).

In addition, more inhibited than uninhibited children had a higher and less variable heart rate on the final quiet period at the end of the battery than on the first quiet period 90 min earlier ($\chi^2 = 5.7$, $p < .01$), although there was not a significant interaction between behavioral group and the magnitude of change in heart rate, based on an analysis of variance. Further, more inhibited children showed a cardiac acceleratory trend during the two familiarization and two test phases of recognition memory; 56% of the inhibited, versus 25% of the uninhibited, children showed a rise in heart rate on three or all four of these episodes ($\chi^2 = 4.6$, $p < .05$).

A similar result emerged at 4 years of age. Thirty-seven children had good heart rate records at both 4 and 5½ years (19 inhibited and 18 uninhibited). When the heart rate values for the first and last cognitive tasks at both ages were compared, 13 of 19 inhibited children showed an acceleratory trend across the battery at both ages; only three showed a deceleratory trend, and six showed no clear trend. Among the uninhibited children only three displayed an acceleratory trend and eight showed a deceleratory trend at both ages ($\chi^2 = 7.2$, $p < .01$). With one exception, every one of the children who was inhibited on all three assessments showed an acceleratory trend at both 4 and 5½ years. In sum, the consistently inhibited children were more likely to show higher tonic heart rates at rest, more frequent accelerations to specific cognitive trials, and acceleration over the course of an entire episode.

The combination of behavior and heart rate. In order to evaluate the relative predictive power of behavior and heart rate, we computed a regression analysis using the aggregate index at 5½ years as the criterion and the major behavioral and heart rate variables at the earlier ages as separate predictors. Although heart rate and heart rate variability are significant correlates of behavioral inhibition, there was no significant unique variance associated with heart rate or heart rate variability over and above the variance attributable to behavioral inhibition at 21 months and 4 years.

However, in an alternative analysis, we combined behavior and heart rate and classified children into one of four groups based on their data at both 21 and 48 months: children who were both inhibited and had a high and stable heart rate at the two earlier ages, children who were inhibited but had a low and variable heart rate at both ages, children who were un-inhibited but had a high and stable heart rate, and, finally, uninhibited children with a low and variable heart rate. These divisions were based on median splits for heart period and heart period variability. The maximal sample sizes for the four groups were 13, 9, 5, and 16, respectively.

Analyses of variance and post hoc Duncan tests revealed that the 13 inhibited children with high and stable heart rates at the two early ages were significantly different at 5½ years from each of the other three groups for the following variables: total time staring at the unfamiliar peer, $F(3,37) = 6.50, p < .01$; time proximal to the mother while not playing, $F(3,37) = 4.26, p < .01$; and risk avoidance, $F(3,37) = 3.61, p < .05$. Additionally, the telephone interview revealed that the inhibited children with high and stable heart rates had more unusual, contemporaneous fears (excluding the two common fears of large animals and the dark). These fears included elevators, heights, a strong wind, ice machines, bugs, and fires $(\chi^2 = 9.5, 3\ df, p < .05)$. Further, 10 of the 13 inhibited children with a high and stable heart rate had one or more of the following symptoms during the first year of life: chronic constipation, allergy, extreme irritability, frequent sleeplessness, together with one or more unusual contemporary fears. Among the remaining three groups, the frequencies were one, two, and one child $(\chi^2 = 10.7, 3\ df, p < .05)$. Thus, although heart rate did not add significant variance in a regression analysis with the aggregate index as the criterion, it did aid the prediction of contemporary fears and behavior in the peer play and risk situations.

Prediction of Pupillary Dilation

The individual test items on each episode produced a reliable increase in pupil size of about 0.3 mm, or 5%–6% of the average pupil size, on over 90% of the trials. This magnitude of increase in pupil size to a test item is comparable to the magnitude of change seen in adults given similar cognitive tests (Beatty, 1982; Stanners, Coulter, Sweet, & Murphy, 1979).

Although the children classified as inhibited or uninhibited at 21 months did not differ in the frequency or the magnitude of the increase in pupil size to a test item, the two groups did differ in average pupil size on both pretrial and trial periods, with inhibited children having larger pupillary dilations (see Fig. 3).

A repeated-measures analysis of variance on mean pupil size for inhibited and uninhibited children across each of the episodes revealed a significant group difference for both the trial and pretrial values, $F(1,269) = 20.9$, $p < .001$, for trial; $F(1,154) = 17.3$, $p < .001$, for pretrial. There was a significant effect of episode for the trial values, $F(6,269) = 2.8$, $p < .01$, but no group $\times$ episode interaction, with pupil sizes significantly larger to the initial baseline and first cognitive task than to the final baseline period. A repeated-measures analysis of variance comparing inhibited, uninhibited, and control children for each episode revealed a significant effect for behavioral group, $F(2,352) = 11.77$,

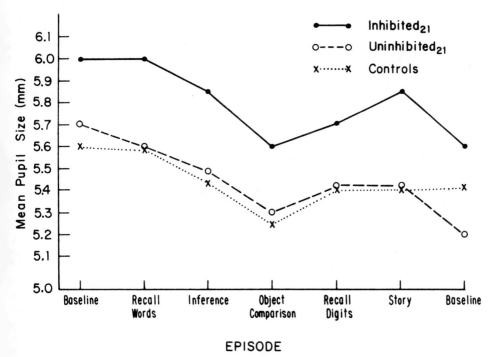

Figure 3. Mean pupil size at 5½ years for children classified as inhibited, not inhibited, or neither at 21 months.

$p < .01$, and task, $F(6,352) = 2.23$, $p < .05$. The inhibited children had significantly larger pupils than either the uninhibited or control children, and pupil size to the initial baseline in the first task was larger than pupil size to the remaining tasks. This pattern is similar to that noted for heart rate.

Table 4 presents the predictive correlations between behavior and heart rate at 21 and 48 months and three pupil measurements at 5½ years. Behavioral inhibition at age 4 predicted larger pupil sizes during the baseline, and uninhibited behavior at age 4 predicted smaller pupil sizes for baseline and tasks. However, with one exception, pupil size was not significantly related to any of the contemporary indexes of inhibited behavior at 5 ½ years of age nor to the earlier indexes of heart rate or heart rate variability. The one exception was a modest but positive relation between mean pupil size, across all trials, and the mother's rating of the child's current degree of shyness ($r = .30$, $p < .05$). These facts suggest that the peer play assessment at age 4 was especially sensitive in capturing a psychological quality shared by inhibited children. We suggest that this quality might be called uncertainty in unfamiliar situations.

In addition to an absolutely larger pupil, a majority of the inhibited children (67%) either maintained or increased their pupil size over the course of the episodes; only 36% of the uninhibited children did so ($\chi^2 = 3.8$, $p < .05$). The control children were more similar to the inhibited in their tendency to maintain pupil size (75% did so) but more similar to the uninhibited children in displaying absolutely smaller pupils. The minimal habituation of pupil size among inhibited children is analogous to maintaining a high and stable heart rate over the course of cognitive testing. Hence, the significant relation between magnitude of change in pupil (from first to second baseline of the pupil battery) and magnitude of change in heart period from the first to the second memory test ($r = .55$, $p < .001$) is not surprising. Although more inhibited children maintained larger pupils over the course of the battery, some uninhibited children also displayed large pupil sizes, suggesting that other psychological factors, especially the degree of mental effort associated with problem solving, make a large contribution to pupil size. For example, six children with large pupils were uninhibited boys with low heart rates. It is likely that these boys had large pupils because they were motivated to solve the tasks, not because they possessed the special state of uncertainty we have assumed is characteristic of many inhibited children. This conclusion is in accord with Beatty's (1982) statement that individual differences in psychological arousal can affect tonic pupillary diameter, but not the brief phasic response to a cognitive demand that "reflects the momentary level of processing load" (p. 289). Stanners et al. (1979) agree: "There may be a hierarchy of control for the pupillary response such that cognitive demands take first priority and arousal effects show up only if cognitive demands are minimal" (p. 329).

In sum, although there was a significant correlation between behavioral inhibition at the early ages and absolute pupil size, the increase in pupil size to a problem was less sensitive than the combination of heart rate and heart rate variability in distinguishing inhibited from uninhibited children. The radial muscles of the iris responsible for pupillary dilation have alpha adrenergic receptors, while the heart contains beta adrenergic receptors. This difference in receptor type implies that the psychological conditions that promote a maximal response from the pupil are different from the conditions that lead to a rise in heart rate and a decrease in variability. In a study of adults, the modal response to viewing pictorial stimuli was pupillary dilation and cardiac deceleration (the latter is parasympathetically mediated), and there was no relation between magnitude of heart rate acceleration and pupillary dilation (Libby, Lacey, & Lacey, 1973). The relative independence of the responsiveness of pupil and heart when cognitive demands are imposed is in accord with the suggestion (Williams, in press) that contexts provoking only mental effort lead to increases in epinephrine, while contexts that provoke both mental effort and psychological uncertainty, or distress lead to increases in both epinephrine and cortisol. The total corpus of data supports those investigators , and especially the Laceys (Lacey & Lacey, 1974), who have contended that there is no general syndrome of sympathetic activation, especially in mildly stressful situations.

Preferential Attention to Passive and Fearful Figures

There was no significant relation between an attentional preference for the passive or the fearful versus active or fearless figures, on the one hand, and behavioral inhibition at 5½ years. However, the children who were consistently inhibited or uninhibited on all three assessments (based on median splits for the behavioral index at 21 months, the mean standard scores for the inhibited and uninhibited behavioral clusters at age 4, and the aggregate index at 5½ years) did look preferentially at the fearful and fearless figures in the story in the predicted manner. Significantly more of the consistently inhibited children showed a preference for the fearful figure, while more of the consistently uninhibited children looked longer at the fearless figure ($\chi^2 = 6.5$, $p < .01$).

Further, a suggestive relation emerged when we examined the pattern of attentional preferences to the active-passive figures administered at both age 4 and age 5½, and the fearless or fearful figures administered at age 5½. Twelve of the 15 inhibited children administered all three tasks showed a preference for the passive or fearful figure on two or all three of the procedures; only three children showed a preference for the active or the fearless figure on at least two occasions. However, among the uninhibited children, only five showed a preference for the passive or fearful figure on two or all three procedures and seven displayed a preference for the active or fearless figure ($\chi^2 = 4.1$, $p < .05$).

Reflection-Impulsivity

The three tasks designed to index a reflective or an impulsive approach to cognitive tasks with response uncertainty were embedded figures, matching familiar figures, and the haptic visual test. We also coded reaction time to the child's yes/no answers during the two recognition memory tests. There were, therefore, five separate occasions on which we gathered latency data to a decision in a cognitive context.

Although there was intraindividual consistency for response time on the two memory tasks ($r = .61$), there was a less hardy relation between response times to the two memory tests and response times to embedded figures, matching familiar figures, or the haptic tests. Further, the correlations for response times among the three tests were only .27, .40, and .54.

To our surprise, more inhibited than uninhibited children had reaction times that were either very fast or very slow on the haptic and matching familiar figures tests. This trend was seen most clearly on the haptic procedure. The videotapes were coded for the number of forms the child explored before offering his or her first solution hypothesis, and the time devoted to each exploration of a form. Selection of these two variables was based on the hypothesis that exploring many forms and devoting a long time to at least two explorations indicated a reflective approach to the tasks. Examination of the distributions of the major scores led us to adopt the following criteria: A child was classified as reflective if, across all five test items, he or she explored at least 13 or more forms, and two or more of those explorations lasted at least 5 sec. A child was classified as impulsive if he or she had 12 or fewer explorations and one or fewer trials with a 5-sec exploration. Most of the inhibited children were either reflective (35%) or impulsive (40%), while most of the uninhibited children were neither reflective nor impulsive (85%) ($\chi^2 = 13.2$, 2 *df*, $p < .01$).

GENERAL DISCUSSION

These data affirm earlier evidence for moderate stability of inhibited and uninhibited behavior, preservation of the two heart rate parameters, and a positive relation between a high and stable heart rate and behavioral inhibition. Although the control children were not observed in the peer play or school contexts, their reactions to the remaining tasks formed a unique profile that differed from that of both the inhibited and uninhibited groups. Tonic heart rate and pupillary values for the controls were more similar to those of the uninhibited children, but their behavioral responses in the risk room and with the examiner in the testing situation were intermediate between the two extreme groups. In the testing situation, the controls looked at the examiner more often and talked less often than the uninhibited children. In the risk room, the controls were a little more cautious than the uninhibited children.

The stability of inhibited and uninhibited behavior in this sample is supported by several independent, short- and long-term, longitudinal studies of young children. For example, in an earlier study of Chinese and Caucasian infants who were followed from 3 to 29 months of age (half raised at home and half attending a day-care center), the Chinese children were consistently more inhibited with unfamiliar people, less spontaneously vocal, more upset at separation from their mother, and also displayed more stable heart rates across the period of study. Further, the mothers of the Chinese infants reported that a salient characteristic of their infant was a tendency to stay very close to them (Kagan, Kearsley, & Zelazo, 1978). Other investigators have also reported preservation of individual differences in qualities such as fearfulness or timidity and its opposite (G. W. Bronson, 1970; Bronson & Pankey, 1977; W. Bronson, 1981; Hinde, Stevenson-Hinde, & Tamplin, 1985; Kagan & Moss, 1962), and a recent study of the preservation of extremely shy and withdrawn behavior over a 3-year period in elementary school children revealed high stability coefficients ($r = .06$) (Moskowitz, Schwartzman, & Ledingham, 1985). Although stability of a class of behavior is enhanced when socializing agents support and encourage the behavior, it is important to note that a majority of the mothers of inhibited children told the interviewer they were worried about their child's shyness and timidity and were implementing practices that would discourage this class of behavior. In some cases, these parental practices were successful.

The coherence of all the information enhances the credibility of the hypothesis, suggested in the introduction, that a proportion of the inhibited children have a lower threshold for arousal of one or more of the neural circuits that involve the hypothalamic link to the pituitary-adrenal axis, reticular activating system, and the sympathetic nervous system (Axelrod & Reisine, 1984). The preservation of the differences in heart rate and variability, and the relation of these two variables, along with maintenance of a large pupil, to inhibited behavior represent important sources of support for that hypothesis, but they do not prove it. A lower threshold in any of these circuits could be the result of: (1) structural elements in the hypothalamus, pituitary, autonomic nervous system, or peripheral target organs, (2) higher levels of central catecholamines, especially norepinephrine, or (3) lower levels of those endogenous chemicals, especially the opioids, that have the capacity to dampen the arousal of parts of these stress circuits. Although existing evidence does not permit elimination of any of these explanations, research on genetically mediated influences on other classes of behavior often implicate endogenous differences in biochemistry. There is clear evidence that the catecholamine system in the brain is under genetic control (Ciarenello, 1979) and good evidence for genetic influences on inhibited and uninhibited behavior (Buss & Plomin, 1984; Daniels & Plomin, 1985). Further, there is a relation among 1-year-olds between intensity of crying following separation from the mother in the home and higher levels of urinary cortisol, as well as preservation of individual differences in cortisol levels from 1 to 3 years of age ($r = .55$) (Tennes, 1984). The stability coefficient for cortisol is similar in magnitude to the longitudinal correlations we have reported for both inhibited and uninhibited behavior and heart rate variability.*

A reasonable, albeit hypothetical, argument holds that the locus coeruleus, a brain stem structure that is the main source of central norepinephrine, produces more of this neurotransmitter in some of the inhibited children. If this were true, the stress circuits would be at a higher level of excitability and prone to discharge to slight increases in uncertainty or challenge (Charney & Redmond, 1983). Reiser (1984) suggests that the locus coeruleus functions as a gating system that differentially adjusts the gain of both excitatory and inhibitory systems and, as a result, "the system renders ordinarily neutral innocuous stimuli anxiety provoking" (p. 150). Kopin (1984) argues that genetic differences in the amount of norepinephrine secreted to anticipated stress among different

---

*Analyses of cortisol levels from saliva samples obtained during the early morning at home as well as prior to the first laboratory testing session reveal significantly higher levels of cortisol for inhibited children on both occasions. These data are summarized in Lutz's (1985) honors research project at Radcliffe College.

animal strains may be analogous to differences in proneness to anxiety among humans, and Charney, Heninger, and Breier (1984) believe that increases in central norepinephrine are causally related to attacks of panic anxiety in human patients. The histories of adult panic patients suggest that many were inhibited during early childhood (Gittelman & Klein, 1984). The higher levels of norepinephrine could be due to more secretory cells, higher levels of the regulating enzymes, or the responsiveness of these enzymes to stimulation. Although this hypothesis remains extremely speculative, these data and those of others are supportive of this mechanism (Ciarenello, 1983). After finding major individual differences among adults in the heart rate and norepinephrine response to cognitive stress, McCubbin, Richardson, Langer, Kizer, and Obrist (1983) conclude that "plasma catecholamine responses to stress reflect an underlying sympathetic neuronal mechanism which is an important correlate of individual differences in the hemodynamic response to behavioral stress" (p. 109).

Comparative psychologists and physiologists have reported comparable results among strains of mice, rats, and monkeys who are differentially prone to sympathetic activation of the heart and other target organs of the autonomic nervous system (Blizard, Hansen, & Freedman, 1982; McCarty, 1983; Suomi, Kraemer, Baysinger, & DeLizio, 1981). Because selective breeding for defecation in an open field test or high blood pressure (two criteria used in work with rodents) is likely to be accompanied by special morphological and/or physiological consequences, it is unlikely that there is complete identity between the differences found in the pedigreed animal strains and the differences we have found between inhibited and uninhibited children. But, on the other hand, the similarities in vulnerability to discharge of one or more of the stress circuits provide an initial basis for the interpretations we have proposed. We emphasize the separateness of the circuits because we believe it is more useful theoretically to assume a family of related arousal states than to posit a general state of arousal with different empirical measures treated as indexing that state with differential accuracy.

This interpretation of the differences between inhibited an uninhibited children bears some resemblance to Pavlov's (1941) distinction between weak and strong nervous systems (inhibited children have a weak nervous system; uninhibited children a strong nervous system), Gellhorn's (1967) later distinction between ergotropic and trophotropic functions of the autonomic nervous system, and Jung's (1959) description of the differences between introverts and extroverts. It is of interest that scores on the introversion-extroversion scale of most personality questionnaires show heritability (Scarr & Kidd, 1983), are correlated with the same autonomic variables that characterize inhibited and uninhibited children (Hinton & Craske, 1977), and are stable over long periods of time (Buss & Plomin, 1984). In one study these scores were preserved over a 45-year period from young adulthood to old age (Conley, 1984). The complete corpus of empirical data renders these speculative ideas a bit more reasonable than they were when they were originally formulated. However, because the first assessment of these children occurred at 21 months of age, it is possible that the physiological differences between the two groups are simply consequences of the socialization practices that produced these two behavioral groups. Future research will have to determine the differential validity of these two interpretations.

The data imply that an unfamiliar or challenging event that is minimally stressful for most children is treated as more stressful by a majority of the children we have called inhibited. There are at least two different psychological, as opposed to physiological, mechanisms that might produce this difference in level of uncertainty. One argument claims that inhibited children in a novel or challenging context generate more cognitive representations of possible events that might occur in the future and, being unable to resolve them, become uncertain. This hypothesis might explain the higher heart rate to the quiet cognitive tasks, but will not explain why inhibited children also show a rise in heart rate while watching the pictures and listening to the narration about the fearful and fearless children. During this episode the child's attentional system is captured by the processing of information, and it is unlikely that the child is also generating thoughts about the future.

A second possibility is that the inhibited children perceive the assessment contexts as more discrepant than uninhibited children do. This explanation is reasonable for the testing and peer play situations, but is not appropriate for the data gathered on the February visit to the child's classroom. It is unlikely that, after 6 months in the same school, the inhibited child continues to perceive the room, the teacher, and classmates as unfamiliar. That is why we favor an interpretation that relies on the idea that one of the important differences between inhibited and uninhibited children is the presence in the former of higher levels of central norepinephrine that amplify uncertainty and the excitability of the stress circuit as a result of unfamiliarity, unpredictability, or challenge.*

---

*Analyses of norepinephrine and MHPG, a derivative of norepinephrine, taken from urine samples after the first laboratory session, reveal significantly higher levels of both compounds among the inhibited children. These analyses were performed by Richard J. Wyatt and Farouk Karoum of Saint Elizabeth's Hospital, Washington, DC.

This suggestion leads one to regard some of the behaviors of inhibited children as acts that are released by the combination of their particular states of psychological uncertainty and physiological arousal and the presence of specific targets, rather than as instrumentally conditioned behaviors. For example, the inhibited children, at both 4 and 5½ years, looked more often at the peer in the play situation, as well as at school, and at the examiner in the testing context. One traditional explanation, which relies on a past history of encounters with adults and peers, would claim that these experiences taught the child to expect criticism or attack from these agents. Hence, the frequent glances are treated as a category of conditioned response. But we favor an explanation that is similar to the one proposed by Valenstein, Cox, and Kakolewski (1970), who studied the effects of hypothalamic stimulation on the behavior of rats. The specific behaviors displayed by the animal following stimulation varied appropriately with the objects that were present in the cage, whether food, water, or wood chips.

The higher level of arousal in one or more of the stress circuits may lower the threshold for context-appropriate reactions. Because the most relevant source of uncertainty in the testing situation is the examiner, the inhibited child looks at her frequently. Similarly, because peers are a relevant source of uncertainty in the school setting, the inhibited child glances often at the other children. Inhibited children do not look at the examiner or a peer only because they have learned that this response provides desirable information, or because it lowers their level of uncertainty or arousal. Rather, the examiner and the peer are appropriate targets for the "looking response" when the child is uncertain and physiologically aroused, just as pulling at one's hair, biting one's nails, or drumming one's fingers on a desk are responses released while sitting outside a surgeon's office. Variations in degree of arousal of the stress circuits as well as psychological uncertainty lead each child or adult to issue actions at available targets, even though those targets may not be the historical origins of those behaviors.

It is not clear whether the stress circuits of inhibited children are always under higher arousal or only when the children encounter unfamiliar events, task challenge, possible harm, or potential rejection. Perhaps the differences between inhibited and uninhibited children are best viewed as manifestations of a differential potential for excitability and subsequent discharge of one or more of the stress circuits. We suggest that if an adult who had been an inhibited child with the correlated physiological signs finds a vocation and a set of friends that keep uncertainty low, he or she will probably avoid regular rises in arousal of the stress circuits and will not necessarily appear to be shy or cautious with friends and family. Further, the modal incentives for uncertainty change with development. An unfamiliar child is a more potent incentive for a 3-year-old than for a 15-year-old. On the other hand, possible failure at a school task or job interview is a more salient incentive for the adolescent than for the toddler. The changing profile of incentives for uncertainty means that chance and conscious selection of environmental contexts affect the probability that uncertainty will be generated. Thus, the degree of preservation of inhibited or uninhibited behavior within a person will necessarily change with development. Hence, the possibility of a biological contribution to these behaviors does not guarantee indefinite stability of these profiles.

REFERENCES

Axelrod, J., & Reisine, T. D. (1984). Stress hormones: Their interaction and regulations. *Science, 224,* 452–459.

Beatty, J. (1982). Task-evoked pupillary responses, processing load, and the structure of processing resources. *Psychological Bulletin, 91,* 276–292.

Blizard, D. A., Hansen, C. T., & Freedman, L. S. (1982). Open field behavior in the MR/N and MNR/N rat strains. *Behavior Genetics, 12,* 459–466.

Bronson, G. W. (1970). Fear of visual novelty. *Developmental Psychology, 2,* 33–40.

Bronson, G. W., & Pankey, W. B. (1977). On the distinction between fear and wariness. *Child Development, 48,* 1167–1183.

Bronson, W. (1981). *Toddlers' behavior with agemates.* Norwood, NJ: Ablex.

Buss, A. H., & Plomin, R. (1984). *Temperament: Early developing personality traits.* Hillsdale, NJ: Erlbaum.

Charney, D. S., Heninger, G. R., & Breier, A. (1984). Noradrenergic function in panic anxiety. *Archives of General Psychiatry, 41,* 751–763.

Charney, D. S., & Redmond, D. E. (1983). Neurobiological mechanisms in human anxiety. *Neuropharmacology, 22,* 1531–1536.

Ciarenello, R. D. (1979). Genetic control of the catecholamine biosynthetic enzymes. In J. Shire (Ed.), *Genetic variation in hormone systems* (pp. 49–62). Boca Raton, FL: CRL Press.

Ciarenello, R. D. (1983). Neurochemical aspects of stress. In N. Garmezy & M. Rutter (Eds.), *Stress, coping, and development in children* (pp. 85–105). New York: McGraw Hill.

Conley, J. J. (1984). Longitudinal consistency of adult personality. *Journal of Personality and Social Psychology, 47,* 1325–1337.

Daniels, D., & Plomin, R. (1985). Origins of individual differences in shyness. *Developmental Psychology, 21,* 118–121.

Garcia-Coll, C., Kagan, J., & Reznick, J. S. (1984). Behavioral inhibition in young children. *Child Development, 55,* 1005–1019.

Gellhorn, E. (1967). *Principles of autonomic-somatic integrations.* Minneapolis: University of Minnesota Press.

Gittelman, R., & Klein, D. F. (1984). Relationship between separation anxiety and panic and agoraphobic disorders. *Psychopathology,* **17,** (Suppl. 1), 56–65.

Hinde, R. A., Stevenson-Hinde, J., & Tamplin, A. (1985). Characteristics of three- to four-year-olds assessed at home and their interactions in preschool. *Developmental Psychology,* **21,** 130–140.

Hinton, J. W., & Craske, B. (1977). Differential effects of test stress on the heart rates of extroverts and introverts. *Biological Psychology,* **5,** 23–28.

Jung, C. J. (1959). *Collected works of C.J. Jung.* Princeton, NJ: Princeton University Press.

Kagan, J., Kearsley, R. B., & Zelazo, P. R. (1978). *Infancy: Its place in human development.* Cambridge, MA: Harvard University Press.

Kagan, J., & Moss, H. A. (1962). *Birth to maturity.* New York: Wiley.

Kagan, J., Reznick, J. S., Clarke, C., Snidman, N., & Garcia-Coll, C. (1984). Behavioral inhibition to the unfamiliar. *Child Development,* **55,** 2212–2225.

Kopin, I. J. (1984). Avenues of investigation for the role of catecholamines in anxiety. *Psychopathology,* **17,** 83–97.

Lacey, J. I., & Lacey, B. C. (1974). Heart rate responses and behavior. *Journal of Personality and Social Psychology,* **30,** 1–39.

Libby, W. L, Lacey, B. C., & Lacey, J. I. (1973). Pupillary and cardiac activity during visual attention. *Psychophysiology,* **10,** 270–294.

Lutz, P. D. (1985). *Behavioral predictors of stress response.* Unpublished honors thesis, Radcliffe College.

McCarty, R. (1983). Stress behavior and the sympathetic-adrenomedullary system. In L. A. Pohorecky & J. Brick (Eds.), *Stress and alcohol use* (pp. 7–22). New York: Elsevier.

McCubbin, J. A., Richardson, J. E., Langer, A. W., Kizer, J. S., & Obrist, P. A. (1983). Sympathetic neuronal function and left ventricular performance during behavioral stress in humans. *Psychophysiology,* **20,** 102–110.

Messer, S. B. (1968). *The effect of anxiety over intellectual performance on reflective and impulsive children.* Unpublished doctoral dissertation, Harvard University.

Moskowitz, D. S., Schwartzman, A. E., & Ledingham, J. E. (1985). Stability and change in aggression and withdrawal in middle childhood and early adolescence. *Journal of Abnormal Psychology,* **94,** 30–41.

Pavlov, I. P. (1941). *Lectures on conditioned reflexes: Vol. 2. Conditioned reflexes and psychiatry* (W. H. Gantt, Trans.). New York: International Publishers.

Porges, S. W., & Coles, M. G. H. (1982). Individual differences in respiratory-heart period coupling and heart and heart period responses during two attention demanding tasks. *Physiological Psychology,* **10,** 215–220.

Reiser, M. F. (1984). *Mind, brain, body.* New York: Basic.

Scarr, S., & Kidd, K. K. (1983). Developmental behavior genetics. In M.M. Haith & J.J. Campos (Eds.), P.H. Mussen (Series Ed.), *Handbook of child psychology: Vol 2. Infancy and developmental psychobiology* (pp. 345–433). New York: Wiley.

Smith, O. A., & DeVito, J. L. (1984). Central neural integration for the control of autonomic responses associated with emotion. In W. M. Cowan, E. M. Shooter, C. F. Stevens, & R. F. Thompson (Eds.), *Annual review of neurosciences* (Vol. 7, pp. 43–65). Palo Alto, CA: Annual Reviews.

Snidman, N. (1984). *Behavioral restraint and the central nervous system.* Unpublished doctoral dissertation, University of California, Los Angeles.

Stanners, R. F., Coulter, M., Sweet, A. W., & Murphy, P. (1979). The pupillary response as an indicator of arousal in cognition. *Motivation and Emotion,* **3,** 319–340.

Suomi, S. J., Kraemer, G. W., Baysinger, C. M., & DeLizio, R. D. (1981). Inherited and experiential factors associated with individual differences in anxious behavior displayed by rhesus monkeys. In D. F. Kline & J. Rabkin (Eds.), *Anxiety: New research and changing concepts* (pp. 179–199). New York: Raven.

Tennes, K. (1982). The role of hormones in mother-infant transactions. In R. N. Emde & R. J. Harmon (Eds.), *The development of attachment and affiliative systems* (pp. 75–80). New York: Plenum.

Valenstein, E. S., Cox, V. C., & Kakolewski, J. W. (1970). Reexamination of the role of the hypothalamus in motivation. *Psychological Review, 77,* 16–31.

Williams, R. B. (in press). Neuroendocrine response patterns and stress: Biobehavioral mechanisms of disease. In R. B. Williams (Eds.), *Perspectives on behavioral medicine: Neuroendrocrine control and behavior.* New York: Academic Press.

16

Influence of Gentle Birth Delivery Procedures and Other Perinatal Circumstances on Infant Temperament: Developmental and Social Implications

Michel Maziade, Maurice Boudreault,
Robert Côté, and Jacques Thivierge
Laval University, Sainte Foy, Québec

Gentle delivery techniques (GDT) such as those proposed by Leboyer[1] and by Rappoport[2] have been said to have a positive effect on child development through minimizing the stress and trauma of birth. However, very little controlled research has studied the effect of such techniques on later human development, personality, or temperament.[3]

A type of GDT strongly inspired by the Leboyer approach has been available to our population. Thus, in the framework of another study on infant temperament,[4] we systematically gathered data about delivery techniques and other perinatal circumstances and attempted to relate them to infant temperament as subsequently measured by the Carey Infant Temperament Questionnaire (ITQ).[5] This paper concerns two

Reprinted with permission from *The Journal of Pediatrics,* 1986, Vol. 108, No. 1, 134–136. Copyright 1986 by the C.V. Mosby Company.

Supported by Grant RS-422 from Le Conseil Québécois de la Recherche Sociale and by Grant 80-21 from the Hospital for Sick Children Foundation.

We thank Dr. Philippe Capéraà, Ph.D., professor of statistics, Laval University, for collaboration in analyzing the data, and Mrs. Chantal Mérette, undergraduate student in statistics, for help with the study; and the Community Health Department of the Hôpital Saint-Sacrement de Québec for collaboration in gathering the data.

research questions: First, are temperamentally "easy" infants overrepresented in the GDT group in the first year of life in our general population? Second, are perinatal procedures, such as rooming-in, type of anaesthesia, or cesarean birth, associated with temperament in infancy?

METHODS

We used a birth cohort previously set up for other research purposes; this sample has been described.[4] Because of the availability of data about the delivery, only the visited half of our sample, consisting of all babies born during a 7-month period in the catchment area (population 170,000) of the Community Health Department of the Hôpital Saint-Sacrement de Québec, was used for this study. Of the 358 infants, 49% were boys. Socioeconomic status of the sample according to the Hollingshead index was 8.5% class I, 10.5% class II, 18.5% class III, 34% class IV, and 28.5% class V.

We divided the GDT used in Quebec City (and inspired by Leboyer) into seven operational points according to current obstetrical practice in this city: (1) minimum sound, (2) dimmed lighting in the delivery room, (3) delay in clamping the cord, (4) baby skin-to-skin contact to the mother's abdomen, (5) warm-water bathing of the infant in the delivery room, (6) no use of forceps, and (7) no or local anesthetic. A GDT birth was defined by at least five of these seven characteristics; 53 (15%) births met the criteria. Most of this information was gathered from the medical charts in the neonatal unit or, when not available, was requested from the parents. The sample included 37 (10%) babies delivered by cesarean section and 50 (14%) whose mothers had rooming-in. General anesthetics were administered to 19 (5%) mothers, regional anesthetics to 255 (71%); 84 (24%) received no anesthetic.

Temperament was assessed at 4 and 8 months by means of a French translation of the revised ITQ,[5] a widely used parental rating scale based on the New York Longitudinal Studies (NYLS) model of temperament.[6] The reliability, factor structure, and continuity of temperament measurement have been described elsewhere.[4]

RESULTS

Study infants were grouped according to factor score on our bipolar factor I, determined by principal component analysis. This factor was very similar to the NYLS "easy"-"difficult" axis.[7] The mean of the factor scores of the GDT group (n = 53) at 4 months and at 8 months was compared with the mean of the non-GDT group (n = 225) by two tailed t test; no statistically significant difference was found (P = 0.62, P = 0.66). In addition, each infant was assigned a percentile according to position on the distribution of the temperament factor scores (from "easy" to "difficult"). We compared the difference in proportion of infants with easy vs difficult temperament in the GDT groups with the rest of the sample. Easy temperament was defined as between percentiles 0 and 30, difficult as between 70 and 100. By means of a two-sided proportion test, we again found no difference between easy and difficult infants in the two groups (Table), nor was there any difference with more extreme cut-off points on easy-difficult factor I or when analyzing boys and girls separately. We then studied the relationship between GDT and non-GDT and each of the nine NYLS temperament categories; the Wilcoxon rank sum test showed only one significant difference (persistence at 8 months, P = 0.02) among 18 comparisons. An analysis of the infants at the extremes of each temperament category led to comparable conclusions. We obtained the same results with and without "no use of forceps" or "no anesthetic" as necessary criteria of a GDT birth.

We compared infants with 2 to 4 days of rooming-in (n = 50) with those without rooming-in. By the same method described above, t test analysis of easy-difficult factor scores showed no significant difference at 4 months (P = 0.67) or at 8 months (P = 0.76). A comparison of infants at the extremes, as for GDT birth, yielded no significant difference. For the nine temperament categories, the Wilcoxon rank sum test identified only one statistically significant difference that was consistent from 4 to 8 months. An examination of the association between general anaesthetics (n = 19) and temperament revealed no significant or substantial dif-

Table. Temperamentally easy and difficult infants in GDT and non-GDT groups

	Age 4 mo				Age 8 mo			
	GDT	Non-GDT ††	Total	P*	GDT	Non-GDT	Total	P*
Easy	11	81	92		12	80	92	
Others	38	182	220		41	181	222	
	49†	263	312	0.23	53	261	314	0.45
Difficult	14	79	93		13	50	63	
Others	35	184	219		40	211	251	
	49	263	312	0.83	53	261	314	0.84

Easy and difficult infants are defined, respectively, as those with scores < 30th and > 70th percentiles.
*Two-sided test; all differences not significant.
†Information incomplete for four subjects.
††Non-GDT are defined as those having no more than 1 of the 7 operational criteria of GDT.

ference; however, the small number of subjects must be considered in these latter analyses. Cesarean birth (n = 37) was associated with no significant difference, either on the easy and difficult factors or on each of the nine temperament categories.

DISCUSSION

Our results suggest very little or no influence of gentle delivery techniques, as inspired by Leboyer, on the NYLS model of temperament in the first year of life. This method of delivery does not appear to lead to "easier" temperament or more favorable characteristics during that period. This is to some extent congruent with the findings of a controlled study by Nelson et al.[3] They compared 28 infants assigned to the Leboyer technique with 26 control subjects and found no difference on the Bayley Scales of Infant Development at 8 months and no difference on the Carey ITQ. For the ITQ, however, no details were reported on the method of analysis and the norms used. Nelson et al. raised the possibility that the absence of difference resulted from the fact that only minimal differences existed between the two methods of delivery that they used or because of their small sample size. We arrived at a similar conclusion using a large population-based sample and comparing GDT with other deliveries. Nelson et al. also underscored the possibility that their selection of mothers attuned to the Leboyer delivery (who were then randomly assigned to the control or the study group) might also have diminished the differences in the comparisons. We simply compared those subjects of our birth cohort who experienced GDT with others who had not.

Nevertheless, our findings must be interpreted with prudence. Even if the obstetrical practices are very much influenced by Leboyer in certain hospitals of Quebec City, Leboyer would probably argue, and to some extent rightly so, that obstetricians and nurses do not apply his approach and philosophy fully. In addition, we cannot eliminate the possibility that our temperament measurement method is not sensitive enough and might not detect other aspects of development or personality that GDT could influence.

In any case, our results and those of Nelson et al.[3] suggest that mothers need not choose painful natural delivery because of scientific evidence that it favors more positive infant development. Conversely, our findings must not be interpreted as encouragement of a return to "hard" obstetrical procedures. If there is no danger to the physical health of the baby and the mother, GDT may certainly be defended on the basis of humanitarian considerations while waiting for more scientific and controlled studies on the possible effects on infant development.

Our data also indicate that other perinatal experiences assessed have no or very little influence on temperament; many questions remain regarding the possible influence of environmental or biologic factors on temperament.[8-10]

REFERENCES

1. Leboyer F. Pour une naissance sans violence. Paris: Editions du Seuil, 1974.
2. Rappoport D. Pour une naissance sans violence: résultats d'une première enquête. Bull Psychol 1976;29:552.
3. Nelson NM, Murray WE, Saigal S, et al. A randomized clinical trial of the Leboyer approach to childbirth. N. Engl J Med 1980;302:655.
4. Maziade M, Boudreault M, Thivierge J, Capéraà P, Côté R. Infant temperament: SES and gender differences and reliability of measurement in a large Quebec sample. Merrill-Palmer Q 1984;30:213.
5. Carey WB, McDevitt SC. Revision of the infant temperament questionnaire. Pediatrics 1978;61:735.
6. Thomas A, Chess S. Temperament and development. New York: Brunner/Mazel, 1977.
7. Maziade M, Côté R, Boudreault M, et al. The New York Longitudinal Studies model of temperament: gender differences and demographic correlates in a French-speaking population. J Am Acad Child Psychiatry 1984;23:582.
8. Torgersen AM. Influence of genetic factors on temperament development in early childhood. Ciba Foundation Symposium. Temperamental differences in infants and young children. 1982;89:141–154.
9. Wilson RS. Intrinsic determinants of temperament. Ciba Foundation Symposium. Temperamental differences in infants and young children. 1982;89:121–140.
10. Matheny AP. Twin similarity in the developmental transformations of infant temperament as measured in a multimethod, longitudinal study. Acta Genet Med Gemellol (Roma) 1984;33:181.

Part V

SPECIAL STRESS AND COPING

This year's section takes up a number of special stresses to which children can be subjected, and the coping mechanisms they, their families, and mental health professionals can utilize to help these youngsters cope with their difficulties. Sadly, the issues covered, as varied as they are, represent only a small fraction of the stresses and disasters that befall millions of children in this world, whether from within or from outside the family, or both. The image of the happy idyllic period of childhood is a stereotype that only a minority of children is fortunate to experience.

Pynoos and Eth describe in detail a very sensitive and helpful approach with a child who has to deal with the acute shock and overwhelming stress that occur after witnessing an extreme episode of violence committed against a member of the family. The authors report that their intervention gives a sense of immediate relief to the child and reestablishes human relatedness. The one limitation of the study is that no long-term follow-up of their treatment approach is reported.

Children are appearing more and more frequently as court witnesses by court order. Such an appearance, especially for young children, presents the child with a strange, confusing, and all too often highly stressful situation. Terr documents the many complex issues that are involved and emphasizes thoughtfully the responsibility of the child psychiatrist in dealing with these questions. As she puts it graphically, "the child witness is a solitary traveler wandering through a strange maze of institutions, people and customs. He will need a guide—a professional one. The child psychiatrist can fill this role."

Galante and Foa report a study of the psychological trauma and treatment effectiveness for a larger group of children who experienced a devastating earthquake in a rugged rural mountain region of central Italy. The immediate death toll was high, and many narrow streets were inundated with tons of rubble which blocked all escape routes. Rescue efforts were slow and many children were witnesses to the pathetic cries of trapped victims, many of whom did not survive. The authors describe their methods of pretesting the children for symptoms of disturbance six months after the tragedy, their treatment methods, and their reevaluation of the children a year after the first testing. Their findings as to the factors most likely to induce chronic stress reactions, and their follow-up on the effectiveness of their treatment procedures provide us with a valuable addition to the literature on special stresses and coping in children.

The paper by Rigamer describes the politically motivated disasters encountered by the American communities in Afghanistan and Pakistan in 1978–79. The host governments in these countries could not be relied on to provide protection, and the American families were gripped with a realistic, substantial, and sustained level of apprehension. The author concentrates on the effect of this special stress on the children and the effectiveness of the specific therapeutic measures undertaken. Of special interest was the pervasive attitude of denial by the adults that the children needed attention and the necessity of breaking through this denial before effective counseling and treatment of the children could be institutional.

Though these papers describe very different types of special stress, they do reiterate several themes common to all such events: Children can suffer chronic symptoms caused by severely acute traumatic events; time alone will not necessarily eliminate the symptoms; and prompt and sensitive therapeutic intervention, which helps the child face and cope with the *specific* trauma he or she has experienced, in addition to general supportive efforts by family and community, can be effective in helping the youngster in mastering the destructive results of the event.

PART V: SPECIAL STRESS AND COPING

17

Witness to Violence:
The Child Interview

Robert S. Pynoos and Spencer Eth
University of California, Los Angeles

*In this paper, we present a widely applicable technique of interviewing
the traumatized child who has recently witnessed an extreme act of
violence. This technique has been used with over 200 children in a variety
of clinical settings including homicide, suicide, rape, aggravated assault,
accidental death, kidnapping, school and community violence. The easily
learned, three-stage approach allows for proper exploration, support and
closure within a 90-minute initial interview. The format proceeds from a
projective drawing and story telling, to discussion of the actual traumatic
situation and the perceptual impact, to issues centered on the aftermath
and its consequences for the child. Our interview format is conceptualized
as an acute consultation service available to assist the child, the child's
family, and the larger social network in functioning more effectively
following the child's psychic trauma.*

Although there has been a growing awareness of the importance of
work with traumatized children such as victims of physical or sexual
abuse and kidnapping, there is a larger population of children who have
been witness to violence, and suffer from the aftereffects of that psychic

Reprinted with permission from the *Journal of the American Academy of Child Psychiatry,*
1986, Vol. 25, No. 3, 306–319. Copyright 1986 by the American Academy of Child
and Adolescent Psychiatry.

The authors wish to thank Drs. Theodore Shapiro, Robert Michels and E. James
Anthony for their thoughtful comments on our work, and Janice Berman for her editorial
and secretarial support.

trauma (Pynoos and Eth, 1985). For example, the Sheriff's Homicide Division of Los Angeles County estimates that dependent children witness between 10 and 20% of the approximately 2,000 annual homicides in their jurisdiction.

It is difficult to imagine a more harrowing experience than for a child to witness a parent's murder, suicide or rape. Anyone who has attempted to assist children who have recently been so traumatized will understand the difficulty in knowing how to proceed. The child may exhibit many of the characteristics of an acute posttraumatic stress response. As a result, he or she can present as numb or mute. Direct inquiry about the traumatic event may be unproductive, leaving the interviewer feeling stymied and the child further entrenched in detachment. In addition, the child will frequently be in a state of mourning for the lost parent, further complicating the clinical interview.

In this paper, we describe an initial interview technique that has proven successful in helping a psychiatric consultant to engage young children in conversation shortly after witnessing a traumatic or violent event. It is intended for use with children from 3 to 16 years of age. This technique enables the interviewer to gain insight into the child's understanding of the event and to characterize the behavioral and emotional responses in order to provide specific professional support to the child soon after the trauma. The interview technique has undergone a series of revisions as our experience has grown, and particularly as we have learned from the children's own comments about the interview. The interview has proven to be a generic technique applicable for use with children who have witnessed murder, suicide, rape, accidental death, aggravated assault, kidnapping, and school or community violence. To date, we have employed it with over 200 children. In addition, the interview format has been readily taught to other mental health professionals who have themselves successfully used it in a variety of clinical settings.

INTERVIEW FORMAT

This specialized interview technique is designed for use in the initial meeting with a recently traumatized child. It is presented here as a coherent three-stage process: opening, trauma, and closure. The format begins by permitting the child first to express the impact of the trauma in play and fantasy, and through metaphor, by use of a projective free drawing and story telling task. This opening enables the consultant to appreciate the child's preliminary means of coping and defensive maneuvers. Second, the interviewer shifts attention to the actual traumatic episode. In order to foster mastery of the traumatic anxiety, he overcomes the efforts of the child to avoid and deny, and supports a thorough exploration of the child's experience. Finally, the consultant can then assist the child in addressing his or her current life concerns with an increased sense of security, competence and mastery. As with any clinical interview, the suggested order may be modified somewhat as a function of the child's particular responses, but it is important to adhere to the general format. Each major step in the interview process may be depicted through a series of drawings. In our experience, the entire interview requires approximately 90 minutes.

Prior to the interview, it is important to have obtained from the family, police or other sources some description of the family circumstances, the violent event, and the child's subsequent behavior or responses. The interviewer can then be alert to important references or omissions in the child's account.

FIRST STAGE: OPENING

Establishing the focus. After greeting the child in our usual way, we share that we have had experience in talking to other children who have "gone through what you have gone through." Others can say that they are interested in understanding with the child what it was like to go through what he or she has been through. By making that statement, we establish a focus for the interview, inform the child that he or she is not alone in the predicament, and offer some ego support to the child by our willingness to look together at what has occurred. After these preliminary comments, we do not find it necessary or helpful to have other persons, e.g., family, relatives, or guardians present. We see each child alone in a quiet room.

Free drawing and story telling. Upon being seated, the child is given pencil and paper, and asked to "draw whatever you'd like but something you can tell a story about." The child is reassured that the quality of the drawing is of no concern, and allowed to approach the task without distraction or interference. By stepping aside, the interviewer may encourage the child to attend fully to the creative work. All the children have applied themselves to this task, although there may be an initial period of hesitance. The youngest children, those under 4 years of age, are engaged in play along with their scribbling and are asked similarly "to make up a story." Our emphasis is for the children to begin in whatever manner is most acceptable to them. This approach allows for the child's imagination to be temporarily relieved from reality and superego constraints

(Waelder, 1933). The children we have seen have energetically taken to this activity even hours after witnessing a violent event. The drawings and stories vary considerably in their projective style and content, from examples of nearly direct accounts, to richly endowed works of fiction.

Children appear to be more comfortable with this manner of therapeutic engagement than the alternative style of direct inquiry. This opening is seen ultimately to facilitate a later open discussion of the traumatic occurrence. The interviewer hopes by his expression of interest, level of enthusiasm, and occasional playfulness, to encourage the child to regain more spontaneity. This step begins the process of countering the passive, detached stance of the traumatized witness. The interviewer encourages the child to elaborate further on both the drawing and story. This can be done by general questions, i.e., "What happens next?" or by inquiring about some section or detail. Elaboration usually allows the interviewer to gain an initial appreciation of the child's life circumstances.

Traumatic reference. The key concept in this opening stage is that the violent event remains intrusive on the child's mind and will be represented somewhere in the drawing or story. The interviewer's task is to identify the traumatic references. These may be obvious or obscure, but are invariably present and recognizable.

While telling the story, the child is seen to struggle with unacceptable, painful or frightening feelings which may disguise the traumatic reference. The drawing and story provide clues to the sources of the child's anxiety and means of coping.

We have found four common psychological methods in the preadolescent group to limit or regulate their anxiety within the first weeks after the event. "Denial-in-fantasy" allows the child to mitigate painful reality by imaginatively reversing the violent outcome. The child may provide a more acceptable ending. For example, one 5-year-old whose father, a stunt man, was fatally shot in a family feud, suddenly introduced a safety net after a clown in her story has been maliciously pushed off a high wire. Another group of children avoid reminding themselves of the event by inhibiting spontaneous thought. For instance, an 8-year-old failed to mention the prominent television set he placed in the picture. When asked, he animatedly told of a program in which Bugs Bunny is shot at but safely outruns the attacker's blasts. These children display momentary interruptions of their fantasy elaboration in order to avoid associations to the trauma. A third group cannot at first engage in fantasy. They remain fixed to the trauma and only draw the actual scene. They will without request begin to give an unemotional journalistic but incomplete account of the event. For instance, one 8-year-old introduced himself by saying, "I'm Tommy, my father killed my mother." A fourth group remains in a constant state of anxious arousal, as if to prepare for future danger. In his story, one child emphasized his lack of personal security after his father's murder. This 7-year-old boy told in his story of a kidnapping from a front yard that was once safe to play in. These children will keep themselves preoccupied with thoughts of further harm in lieu of discussing the real event.

SECOND STAGE: TRAUMA

Reliving the Experience

Emotional release. The transition in the interview from the child's drawing and story telling to the explicit discussion of the violent event is a critical moment for the clinician and child alike. We have found it timely and practical to link some aspect of the drawing or story directly to the trauma. For example, we might say: "I'll bet you wish that:" 1) "Your father could have been saved at the end like the clown," or 2) "Your babysitter could have gotten away from the man who was about to stab her," or, 3) "By saying what happened over and over again, you would get used to it," or, 4) "Your father were still here to protect you." What often follows is a profound emotional outcry from the child. Now the child needs to feel the interviewer's willingness to be a supportive presence and to protect the child from being overwhelmed by the intensity or prolongation of the emotional release. The interviewer must be prepared to share in the grief and horror and to offer the child physical comfort.

Reconstruction

Catharis does not adequately describe the goal of emotional release. Before the child proceeds to "relive the experience," he first must attain a state in which he does not feel too threatened by his emotional responses, a state in which he has the hope, at least, of being able to begin to cope with them. If this is adequately achieved, the child will appear ready to provide a verbal description of the event. The interviewer can then direct the child by suggesting that "Now is a good time to tell what happened and what you saw." The child will recreate the traumatic milieu through various devices. He may first choose to reenact in action or draw the violent scene, but the interviewer must encourage the child to translate the actions or pictorial depiction into words. Props—dolls, puppets, toys, weapons, etc.—are made available. The child may become engrossed in the reenactment play, so that the interviewer must be willing to participate—for instance, acting as the assailant, victim, police or paramedic.

The child should then be supported in his focus on the central action the child witnessed when physical harm was inflicted: the push to the floor, the blow with the fist, the plunge with the knife, the blast of a shotgun, the moment of forced sexual penetration. It may require firm support by the interviewer for the child to draw the particular moment of violence. Although a marked increase in anxiety may precede the child's doing so, afterward the child appears strengthened in his or her mastery of the trauma.

Occasionally, it is not until this step that the pain of the reality is experienced. Again, the interviewer may tactfully facilitate the emotional release by stating, for instance, "I bet you wish the gun had been pointed as you drew it, away from your father, so it would have gone off harmlessly."

Perceptual experience. We follow this description of the action by addressing the child's sensory experience of the episode: the sight and sound of the gunfire, the screams or sudden silence of the victim, the first sight of blood, the splash of blood on the child's own clothes, the death agony of the victim, and the sirens of the police arrival. This recall can be elicited by a comment such as "Boy, you must have gotten blood on you." In several cases we have been surprised to have the child add that he or she was wearing the very pants which had been stained with blood during the violent episode. In addition, whenever a child describes an intense feeling state, we ask him about the concomitant physical sensation. For example, after a child said "It felt awful," we asked where he felt it. He replied, "My heart hurt, it was beating so fast."

Throughout this account of the traumatic event, the child's selection will be influenced by cognitive development and style, previous history of trauma, violence or loss, and the actual circumstances. The child is also continually attempting to cope with the accompanying affects: helplessness, passivity, fear, rage, confusion, guilt, and even excitement.

The role of the interviewer is to function as a holding environment in order to provide a safe and protected setting so that the child can further work at mastery despite the rising anxiety level. The interviewer does not allow the child to digress from this all-important task. He may need to question the child to ensure that the circumstances and aftermath are fully reviewed. Following completion of the child's account, the interviewer must be sensitive to how physically exhausted and emotionally spent the child may be in contrast to the usual psychiatric session. Relaxation time and snacks should be offered. The child needs to feel that he or she is being adequately cared for during this emotionally challenging time.

Special detailing. The child may imbue a particular detail with special traumatic meaning (Freud, 1965). These details are of psychodynamic importance and often provide clues to the child's initial identification, for example, with the aggressor, the victim or, we may add, the protector, including the police. One adolescent girl became preoccupied because her mother had been shot while wearing a dress the daughter had lent the mother that morning. A 5-year-old dwelled on whether his deceased mother's legs were broken, in part because he had worn leg casts as a toddler and wished to have her fixed up in that way, too. Another boy painfully recalled having been immediately made to wear the belt used by his father to beat his mother to death in order to hide the evidence. While recognizing the unconscious significance of these details, the immediate goal of the interviewer is to help the child distinguish himself from either the victim or the assailant.

Worst moment. The interviewer can then proceed to ask about the worst moment for the child. It may not be what an adult would assume, nor even something as yet mentioned. Even young children have sufficient observing ego to reflect on the event and then movingly describe a uniquely painful moment. This may include a memory from earlier in the day or from the violent occurrence or from afterward. One 8-year-old broke down in tears as he told of the moment when he found a razor blade under his suicidal mother's bleeding arm. He had been sent out that day to buy the razor blades, he thought, to make paper mache objects. He cried in total disillusionment. One 7-year-old girl painfully related that her father had called out her nickname as he died from a gunshot wound. A 14-year-old girl described a moment of intolerable anger when in passing her father at the police station he said, "I'm sorry," having just shot-gunned her mother to death. A 5-year-old expressed his intense disappointment that on Christmas Eve Santa Claus had not arrived but a bad man, a killer, instead. This exchange is a particularly empathic moment for the child as he feels especially understood and close to the interviewer.

Violence/physical mutilation. The interviewer must now be willing to guide the child to approach the impact of the violence and physical mutilation. Children may be haunted by an unforgettable visual image and may struggle to unburden themselves of the sight. Certain children may insist on drawing a picture of the mutilated or wounded parent. Other children may be more reluctant, but with proper support will draw the horrifying and painful sight.

We have been impressed with the child's need to restore an image of the parent as physically intact or undamaged. In cases of parental death, the funeral offers an opportunity to view the parent as once again restored. Inquiries about this ceremony are especially fruitful. We will also ask if the children have a photograph of their parent and, if one is available, we will look at it with the child during the interview. In addition to aiding the grief process, this step helps the child to invoke earlier, happier images of the parent to counteract the more recent, gruesome sight. However, the validation of external reality and physical death or injury needs to be confirmed and, especially, for the younger child to be concretely represented in play or drawing. Only when children are secure in the belief of their parent's physical death have we seen children speak openly of their grief (Furman, 1974).

Coping with the Experience

Issues of human accountability.. These are acts of human violence, not of natural disasters. Struggles over human accountability add considerably to the child's difficulty in achieving mastery. As recognized with adults, posttraumatic stress disorder is made more severe and longer lasting when the stressor is of human design, especially human-induced violence (DMS-III; Frederick, 1980; West and Coburn, 1984). As one 12-year-old said, "I'm mad at the way she did go. Because that hurt. I just wanted her to die naturally, not die because someone shot her." The child must confront his awareness and conflicts over who is responsible. He may wish at first to avoid the issue by calling the event an accident, but this provides only superficial relief.

The interviewer explores the issue of whom the child holds accountable for the act, his own understanding of the motive, and the child's conjecture about ways it could have been prevented. For example, we ask "How come it happened?" And then, "What would make someone do something like that?" If the assailant is a stranger, it may be easy for the child to assign blame. However, family violence can throw the child into an intense conflict of loyalty and he may suppress certain thoughts as unacceptable to other family members. The child might have already expressed his view in the story telling. A 7-year-old saw her mother shoot her father as he scuffled with her two brothers, who were trying to protect the mother from further physical assault. Everyone else held the abusive, alcoholic father at fault. However, in her story, this child assigned blame to two young, evil boys who unexpectedly appear and are intent on murderous troublemaking. She clearly missed her father and would not add blame to her memory of him, but neither could she accuse her mother. So she silently held her brothers responsible for the death.

The assignment of responsibility is not always fixed and may be seen to vary during the course of the interview. The child may be most disturbed by thoughts about the victim's actions, for instance, in wondering why the mother would be so provocative as to have yelled at her estranged husband the following: "Go ahead, shoot me. Show the kids what a big man you are."

Inner plans of action. We have been particularly impressed by the children's immediate efforts to reverse their helplessness by formulating a plan of action that would have remedied the situation. Lifton (1979) has referred to these cognitive reappraisals after catastrophic loss of life as "inner plans of action" and suggests they are repeatedly used to contend with the "death imprint." As we have observed, the inner plans of action may seek to alter the precipitating events, to undo the violent act, to reverse the lethal consequences, or to gain safe retaliation. Their content and time frame are developmentally influenced (Eth and Pynoos, 1984).

Because of their limited cognitive skills, the preschool children do not appear to imagine alternate actions they might have taken on their own to prevent or alter the episode. It is they, therefore, who feel the most helpless. They may choose to flee or stay, look or turn away, be attentive, or try to sleep, but all of these are the choices of a passive witness, not a participant. The preschool child may fantasize about outside help having provided needed third party intervention, and, in his play, look to the interviewer to fill this role.

In contrast, school age children do not act as mere witnesses. They can participate, if only in fantasy. They can imagine having called the police, locking the doors, grabbing a weapon away from the assailant, even capturing the assailant, before finally offering aid to the victim. Not surprisingly, these inner plans of action are nearly always confined to the day of the event. For example, with the interviewer playing the role of the assailant, one 10-year-old boy acted out how he imagined surprising the murderer, kicking the gun out of his hand, and tossing it to his unarmed father.

Adolescents can imagine alternative actions over a much longer period of time. They do not merely fantasize participation, but can implicate their own action or inaction in a more realistic fashion. One 14-year-old bitterly regretted her failure to unload her father's gun when she had had the chance 2 weeks before. A 17-year-old boy, in trying to stop the rape of his mother, was overpowered by the assailant in a hand-to-hand knife fight, and, afterward, continued to imagine ways he could kill the man if he ever faced him again.

Especially important are ways the child imagines the parent could have been "fixed up" or aided after the injuries were sustained. For example, the young boy who was concerned with the thought that his mother's legs were broken also had the opportunity to ask a doctor for help during his story play. With the interviewer's aid, he then fixed up the broken legs of his fictional injured race car driver. Furthermore, expression of these particular fantasies may provide enough emotional relief that certain children, who had been reluctant to describe the mutilation, will now do so. One 8-year-old boy enacted a sequence in which he imagined his father is taken by ambulance to the hospital, operated on, the bullet removed, and the wound stitched closed. With encouragement, he then readily drew the view of the bleeding chest wound that continued to intrude on his mind.

We carefully explore all these cognitive reappraisals (Folkman and Lazarus, 1984) for they are the best indication of the ways the child is troubled by feelings of self-blame for not doing more. Enactment of these "inner plans of action" can offset lingering feelings of personal responsibility.

Punishment or retaliation. This discussion of blame can raise the question of punishment or retaliation. It may prove difficult for the child because it can reveal unbearable feelings of guilt in some children and frightening fantasies or dreams of revenge in others. In part, these feelings serve to counter the true helplessness at the moment of the violent act. We will allow the children to give full expression to these feelings before reminding them of the realistic limitations to what they could have done at the time. The children often look relieved by permission to imagine the tortures, mutilations, or execution they have reserved for the assailant, and readily draw a picture of "What you'd like to see happen to him." Afterward we will respond, "I see it feels good to imagine getting back at the bad man who stabbed your father," adding "I mean, to be able to do something to him now, when you really couldn't have stopped him at the time."

Counterretaliation. Themes of revenge may be associated with fears of counterretaliation by the assailant. The child may be afraid of the assailant's return and confused over what has actually happened to the suspect. If the assailant is already arrested, the child may be fearful over the future release of the suspect. We are concerned about how rarely the child is reassured about these matters by the police or the local district attorney.

Child's impulse control. If the child attributes the assailant's action to anger, hate, rejection, or craziness, etc., it is pertinent to ask, for example, "What do you do when you get angry?" and to explore the challenge to the child's own impulse control. Viewing an open display of violence may not only cause the child to lose trust in adult restraint, but he or she may acutely fear his or her own capability, especially in light of conscious revenge fantasies, and be concerned about the lack of proper external support.

Previous trauma. After this discussion, it is common for a child spontaneously to mention past traumatic experiences. We have learned from children of further instances of child abuse, violent family deaths, unreported suicidal behavior, physical injuries, or accidents.

Traumatic dreams. At this point, we inquire about recent dreams that may be remembered. Often a child reports anxiety dreams directly related to the traumatic event. The child may be fearful that the dream represents a portent of the future, not only of being victim of a violent assault, but sometimes becoming an avenging killer, too.

Future orientation. It is now appropriate to ask the child about his or her concerns for the future, specifically as they relate to the potential dangers in interpersonal relationships. The child may have immediately after the trauma crystallized a vivid and restricted view of his or her own future. One child described how when he grows up he intends to live in an unaccessible fortress surrounded by many guard dogs. Many children stated that they never intend to marry or have children for fear of a similar violent outcome. Even school age children sometimes described changes in career plans for when they got older. For example, one 7-year-old, within days of her father's killing, reported she suddenly decided on a new life ambition, to become a stand-up comic who dressed in rags and made others laugh.

Similarly, the child feels burdened with an awareness of his or her unfortunate legacy. Children will complain about the novelty and stigma of being the heir of a parent who died by murder or suicide. For instance, one 11-year-old girl bitterly lamented her fate as a daughter of a "man who burned himself to death."

Current stresses. When sufficient mastery of the traumatic anxiety has been achieved, the child can more actively address the life stresses engendered as a consequence of the traumatic event. He or she may spontaneously and pointedly inquire about placement, or schooling, or be easily encouraged to do so.

We survey a number of the common, easily overlooked issues that may add to the child's distress. These include contacts with the police and legal system, changes in living situation or schooling, awareness of media coverage, and concerns about social stigmata. We offer to help redress any oversights in the child's care. For example, in going to stay with her grandparents after her mother's murder, a 14-year-old had to abruptly change schools and lost the companionship of her established circle of friends. We were able to arrange to have her old friends visit her at her new home. Exploration of these posttraumatic consequences enables the child to consider the impact of the event on his current life circumstances.

THIRD STAGE: CLOSURE

Recapitulation. The sensitive process of terminating the interview is now begun. The first step is to elicit the child's cooperation in reviewing and summarizing the session. We attempt to make the child's responses seem more acceptable by emphasizing how understandable, realistic, and universal they are. By doing so, we also hope to have the child feel less alone and alienated, and more ready to receive further support from others. The interviewer returns to the initial drawing and story. The link to the trauma may be more clearly indicated perhaps by pointing out a similarity to the child's later reenactment or recounting.

Realistic fears. It is important to repeat that it is all right to have felt helpless or afraid at the time and then sad or angry. We also make reference to what other children have told us after being in similar circumstances. The threat to the parent is so overwhelming at the time of the violence that many children do not entertain a realistic appraisal of their own personal jeopardy. Afterward, they may ignore, leave unacknowledged, or suppress any fear they might have experienced for their own safety. In one case, we could point out how far away from the shooting the child placed himself in his drawing when in fact he was so close as to have easily been shot himself. This intervention alleviated rather than aggravated the child's anxiety, perhaps by unburdening the child of the need to suppress his fears.

Expectable course. We share with the children the expectable course for them as they pass through the course of their traumatic reactions. For example, we might say, "There will be times at school when you think about your mom, and feel sad." Or, "You may feel frightened to see a knife at home." Or, "You may jump at the sound of a loud noise," or "You may have some bad dreams but they'll happen less and less with time." We suggest they share these reactions with trusted adults to gain further assistance at these difficult moments.

Child's courage. The child's beleaguered self-esteem needs support. We may be able to acknowledge the child's bravery. For instance, in one case a 5-year-old scampered out a window and down a fire escape to seek help for her wounded mother. One convenient method is to reflect on the child's performance during the interview, not only telling him what a good job he did but, more important, complimenting him on his courage to engage in such difficult talk. We will actually say, "You are very brave." Children invariably swell with pride upon hearing these words.

Child's critique. The child is then asked to describe what has been helpful or disturbing about the interview. The children are usually quite candid. They will describe what issue had been "toughest" to talk about, what had been unhelpful, and what made them feel better. In fact, they have been our best teachers. Before we understood the role of suppressed fear, one child turned to one of us and exclaimed, "Boy, was it good to say how afraid I was."

Leave-taking. As we end the interview, we give expression of our respect for the child and the privilege of having shared the interview experience with him. We then emphasize our availability to be called on in the future. We generally give the child, however young, our professional card with our telephone number. It is important to leave open the opportunity for contact, as often the trauma will be reactivated—on its anniversary date, for instance. At such times many children have sought us out despite the brevity of this initial contact. In those cases where the child has been referred for further treatment we have observed that this consultation with proper closure has facilitated the child's adaptation to the treatment situation.

CASE ILLUSTRATION

Lisa, who is 11 years old, was interviewed 5 days after her mother had been fatally shot by the mother's estranged boyfriend, Jim. On the day of the murder Lisa and her mother were at home babysitting for a neighbor's infant, while Lisa's younger sister was at school. When interviewed, Lisa and her sister were temporarily residing with a cousin and her young children.

The consultant began the interview by inviting Lisa to draw a picture and make up a story about it (Fig.1).

Lisa: We woke up in the morning and we were packing. Then we get into our car and the moving truck. We're loading everything onto the truck and we're moving so that if Jim came back he

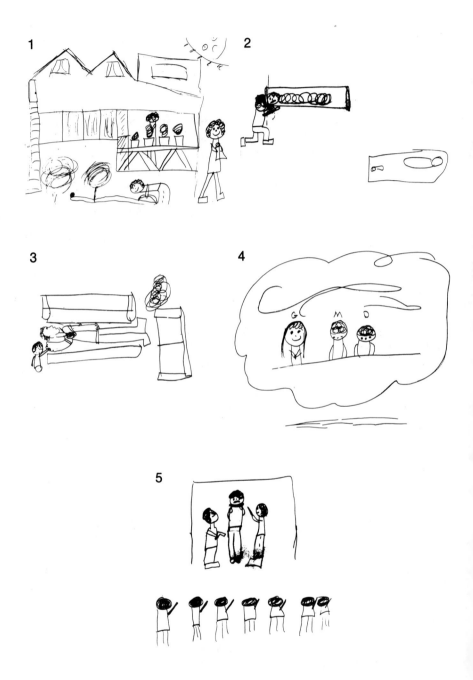

Figures 1–5. Patient's drawings of traumatic event.

wouldn't find us, so he can't shoot my mother. That's my mother who is moving the plant. My sister is watering the grass and I'm helping to take the plants off the porch. And everyone is feeling happy.

My mother loves plants. She had house plants and all kinds of plants. I don't really know the name of them but she had lots of plants around the house. She took good care of them. She didn't really like us helping with the plants because we might do something wrong and they might die. She wanted to take care of them herself.

Right afterward the plants were all given to neighbors except two. These were ones Mother especially grew for me and my sister and cut into the shape of a lion and a hippo. I'm going to make sure to keep watering them.

Consultant (C): This is the kind of story you would have liked to have happen instead of what did.

Lisa: Yes (she begins to cry and is comforted by the interviewer). She had just been offered a job a couple of days before the accident happened. She never had a chance to take it. We could then have afforded to move. Now she's moved to heaven and we're going to have to move somewhere else (she continues to cry and accepts physical consolation).

C: I know it's going to make you sad to talk about some of this.

Lisa: I don't care.

C: Maybe this is a good time to tell what happened (she then begins to describe the actual murder scene and was encouraged to draw a picture of it (Fig. 2).

Lisa: This is my mother bundled up on the couch. She's just waking up. The man is right here, talking in front of her face. At first I was just taking a nap and the baby was just in the bedroom. When I came out and saw him with the gun I was so scared, I just stood there looking. He was flicking the gun in her face. He then shot her. He kept shooting her until he got to the door, and then he ran out somewhere.

I waited until I heard our screen door shut, 'cause I didn't want to get shot. Then I ran up to my mother, who was rolling off the couch and she fell on her side. I rolled her over and was talking to her. I was crying and I was mad because I didn't know what to do. I grabbed the phone to call the police but I think they'd already been called by the neighbors. Before the police came I was on the floor with her. Her eyes were down, her eyelids were like half-closed, and her hair was kind of messed up, sticking out. Blood was everywhere. I was trying to open her eyes. I was trying to wake her up—you know, by shaking her face. I thought maybe if I did something wrong she would do something. I tried to listen to her heart and to take her pulse. I couldn't find anything. I'd seen that on a soap opera I watched with my mother when somebody got shot. Also, you know how when you can't breathe how you press their stomach or something, I was trying to do that so she could breathe, but she wasn't breathing right, and when she took a breath then blood started to come onto the floor. I kept talking to her but she wouldn't talk. I thought if only she could talk then everything could be all right. I just took her hand in mine, and kept shaking it while telling her to hang on. I was crying and I asked God to save my Mommy and I'd be a good girl, but he took her (Fig. 3). Afterward I went and locked all the doors.

C: You tried your best to help her if you could. I'm sure you couldn't stop the bleeding. You worry you could have done more.

Lisa: There was too much blood.

C: Did you get blood on you, too?

Lisa: It was on these pants. These were the pants I was wearing. But they've been washed. I guess I had some right here 'cause I was listening to her heart. Her shirt was full of blood, and when she tried to breathe she made a sound like this (she inhales in a gasping manner) and she did it for a long time. Sometimes I remember how the gun sounded, how loud it was.

C: It's really something to go through.

Lisa: I am not really mad at the fact that she's dead because you know everybody has to go, but I am mad at the way she did go. Because that hurt. I just wanted her to die naturally, not to die of a shooting or stabbing or strangling or something like that.

It just doesn't feel right. Oh, how she died. Like that, horrible. She should have died natural, and maybe I could have been grown because that way I wouldn't have lost a mother truly. I was scared when the police came because first they knocked on the door real loud. But I saw the fire truck and it had a siren on. So I knew it was the police. They didn't barge in as I thought they might have. When the police came I wanted to stay with my mother but they moved me to the next room for awhile.

That's bad that he's not been found yet. I was thinking that my mother would be looking for him and tell me, so then I could tell the police and they'd find him (she draws her mother in heaven (Fig. 4)).

She is in heaven with God. He has long hair. Jesus had long hair. She's looking down on us. When she sees us cry she cries too. She'll make sure we've all left so if Jim comes back he'll have a big surprise because nobody will be there.

C: Do you get scared?

Lisa: I got scared this morning. I didn't want to go outside because Jim could be somewhere outside. I asked my uncle to get his gun and scare away the man I saw across the street. Maybe we could catch Jim, get him to drop his gun and bring him to the police station.

C: You called it an accident, not murder.

Lisa: Just a name I picked for it. But a man really did it. Murder sounds like when somebody chokes or strangles somebody. I guess I'd say he killed her because that doesn't mean so much physical contact. Maybe if I hadn't woke up she wouldn't be dead. He probably got scared when I saw him with the gun.

C: And he did something terrible to your mother. What makes a person do something like that?

Lisa: I guess hate and anger. He wasn't our friend and she told him she didn't want to see him. I guess he got angry at that.

C: What would you like to see happen to him?

Lisa: I was dreaming that all my cousins and our relatives were dressed, you know, how they put you up against the wall and blindfold you and shoot you. I had the same knife he used to stab my mother and the same gun that he shot her with. Then I went up to him and said, "Do you remember this, now you can feel it." And I stabbed him right where he stabbed my mother. Then I said, "I guess you remember this, too," and then I shot him. Then I moved, and everybody started shooting him (she comments on how good a picture that is to draw (Fig. 5)). It felt good like I was getting back at him. The hands are behind his back. He's tied up and the scarf is around his neck because we took it off so he could see what happens.

C: Do you know what will happen if he's arrested?

Lisa: He'll go to jail. But I want him to stay in jail for the rest of his life, since he took a life from somebody he ought to get his life down to nothing.

C: There must be times when you get angry at somebody.

Lisa: When I get angry I don't like to show my feelings. I just keep them in. I hold my breath and just don't think about it. But since my mother's death I can't really control it all because the way people treat us it seems like it's all our fault she was dead. The way they're telling us to change so quickly. They want us to do things their way. It's kind of hard for us because we just lost a mother. He must have had a hot temper. When I get mad at my sister now I get afraid I might hit or hurt her. I don't like that.

C: Do you ever think about her relationship with men and what it will be like for you when you get older?

Lisa: I said I'd never get married and have kids, 'cause if me and him fight, something might happen to me where I have to die. Then I will leave my kids just like my mother had to leave. And I don't want to do that to my kids. I had that thought the same day she died. I was thinking about when I have grown kids she'll never be able to see her grandkids in person.

(Toward the end of the interview Lisa began to address some of her current concerns.) We might have to go to an orphanage. I don't want to. Nobody is there like relatives or anything. One reason I don't want to go to a foster home is because they might separate me and my sister. It's bad enough we lost our mother.

C: Remember you told me how well your mother looked after her plants. I think you want somebody to look after you with that much care. You must feel that God is being very unkind in letting this kind of thing happen in your life.

Lisa: Yeah. That sure isn't fair because I understand He wanted her to leave us in this way but why did it have to happen? Or, the least He could have done was wait until a certain age when we could have been on our own.

C: How has it been to talk with me?

Lisa: It made me feel hurt and stuff, but it also made me feel good.

DISCUSSION

Overview

We have described a complete interview format designed to assist children who have witnessed a violent act. The helpless, passive experience of watching the moment or moments of a violent act and its injurious consequences constitutes an immediate psychic trauma for the child (Pynoos and Eth, 1985). The viewing is painful, frightening, and distressing. Our work has been with the most traumatic cases: a parent's suicide, murder, or rape (Eth and Pynoos, 1983; Pynoos and Eth, 1985; Pynoos et al., 1981). We think the "hammer effect" of examining catastrophic violence has brought to light more visibly the processes needed to work with children in many other clinical settings.

Although the technique we have described may appear rigidly structured, in fact, the sessions generally follow the child's lead and are rarely experienced as arbitrary or stifling. It would seem that there is an underlying logic to the interview proceeding in this way. We have been impressed that some child psychiatrists intuitively conduct their initial interviews with traumatized children in exactly this way without consciously recognizing the unique format. Most other clinicians will miss the child's cues and lose the opportunity for ready exploration of the traumatic material. There have been occasions where we have tacitly colluded with the child's avoidance and omitted some component of the interview, only to learn afterward that incomplete mastery of the trauma-related anxiety had been achieved. We caution child therapists who feel inclined to avoid the traumatic material to be aware of counter-transference identification with the affected child.

Particular attention must be paid to the final phase of the interview as incomplete closure threatens the effectiveness of the session. Without proper closure the child will be left struggling with traumatic material without adequate enhancement of ego function with which to bind his anxiety. In that situation, the interview can be experienced as unsettling.

This technique has been readily learned by a number of child therapists and applied to their work with a variety of traumatized children. We have noted that some of our colleagues have voiced concern that the interview's focus on the traumatic event could unduly upset an already victimized child. Our extensive experience, supported by the work of several other investigators (Ayalon, 1983; Frederick, 1985) confirms that open discussion of the trauma offers immediate relief and *not* further distress to the child. Recent adult investigators have suggested that there may be an optimum time to provide intervention beyond which it is more difficult to achieve ego restoration and improved affective tolerance (Horowitz and Kaltreider, 1979; Van Der Kolk and Ducey, 1984).

Childhood Trauma

Recent reviews have discussed the significant psychological impact for children of a wide variety of traumatic experiences (Eth and Pynoos,

1985; Terr, 1984). There is better recognition of the intrapsychic, behavioral and physiologic changes that can occur. There may be prominent intrusive and avoidant phenomena, increased states of arousal and incident specific new behaviors. Reports of long-term effects have included pessimistic life attitudes, alterations in personality, diminished self-esteem and disturbances in interpersonal relationships. Because these traumatic sequelae do not necessarily pass with time, there is an obvious need to develop effective methods of early intervention.

The landmark paper on the treatment of trauma in childhood was written by Levy (1938). "Release therapy" was specifically devised as a psychotherapeutic technique to resolve symptoms arising from a "definitely known traumatic episode." The child's traumatic anxieties, especially those related to aggressive behaviors inhibited by fear were discharged through directed play. Levy's technique has not received further exploration, in part because of its limited scope.

Analogous Model

In searching for an analogous model of therapeutic trauma consultation, we have been impressed with the resemblance between our technique and that adopted by military psychiatrists for the treatment of soldiers who have viewed a buddy killed or maimed in combat (Fox, 1974; Glass, 1947, 1954; Grinker and Spiegel, 1943; Hendin et al., 1981; Kardiner, 1941; Kolb and Mutalipassi, 1982; Lifton, 1982; Smith, 1982; Teicher, 1953; U.S. Public Health Service, 1943). The principles we share include: 1) the witnessing of extreme violence constitutes a unique, severe, psychic trauma; 2) the importance of "front-line intervention" before maladaptive ego resolution is organized; 3) since "ego contraction" is a primary consequence of the trauma, major efforts are directed at ego restitution and coping enhancement; 4) mastery required an affectively experienced "reliving," including a comprehensive review of the traumatic event; 5) aggressive themes, especially of retaliation, threaten ego restoration and must be fully explored; 6) an "outraged superego" responds to the passivity of the trauma experience by insisting that more should have been done to save the victim, and its demands must be relived by the interview; 7) absent or pathologic grief results from efforts to avoid re-evoking traumatic anxiety; and 8) sustained mastery can only be achieved through reintegration into the group, family, or community.

Similar interview methods follow from these principles. We remain flexible: at times insisting the child continue, at other times participating theatrically in the reliving of the episode, and occasionally assuming the role of an interested bystander. Whenever stifled grief emerges, we offer open consolation and physical comfort. We underscore the realistic fears associated with a danger, and normalize the anxiety in reexperiencing the event in session. However, the two techniques differ in handling the opening phase of the interview. Since soldiers display traumatic amnesia or disavowal, narcosynthesis or hypnosis were often necessary adjuncts to penetrating these defenses. On the other hand, we have found that children remain consciously aware of the traumatic event, though diminishing its pain through the use of denial-in-fantasy or avoidance.

The Interview

Our interview format is conceptualized as an acute consultation service available to assist the child, the child's family, and the larger social network in functioning more effectively in the aftermath of the child's psychological trauma. The explicit goal is to identify the immediate effects of the trauma, with the child's attention and energy reserved exclusively for this task. The role of the consultant is to serve as an auxiliary ego to provide the encouragement needed to complete the assignment. In this regard, the technique is not unlike Winnicott's (1971) use of the squiggle in his single session consultations.

The choice of a free drawing maneuver is advantageous for several different reasons (Gardner, 1979). Coincidentally, in 1918 on the battlefront at La Fauche, France, drawings were successfully employed to provide access to repressed memories of traumatic scenes (U.S. Public Health Service, 1943). As described, this opening offers a comfortable play activity for the child. His or her own creation then serves as a stimulus for verbalization at a time otherwise known for stony silence. The drawing is referred to often during the remainder of the interview, and as a product of the child's own mind represents an acceptable link to the traumatic situation. As a projective device, the drawing invariably signifies the child's unconscious preoccupation with the traumatic memory. Lifton (1982) has termed this "the indelible image." Since the mode of witnessing the violence was visual, it is appropriate and desirable that the drawing employ that sensory apparatus as well (Horowitz, 1970). According to Piaget and Inhelder (1969): "Drawing . . . should be considered as being halfway between symbolic play and the mental image" (p. 54). By confronting the violent scene on paper, the child begins to distance him or herself from the traumatic memory. Importantly, the child also initiates motor and verbal activities which counteract the passivity of the traumatic experience. This action helps reverse the sense of helplessness and establish an interpersonal connection, fostering trauma mastery.

Denial in fantasy is one way the child can psychologically avert "objective pain" and danger without disrupting reality testing (Freud, 1937). In tactfully addressing the child's idiosyncratic use of this means of coping, we have been impressed by the immediate restoration of affect heralded by what Horowitz and Kaltreider (1979) termed an emotional "outcry." With the ego more tolerant of the painful reality, the child is able, at his or her own pace and manner, to describe the traumatic events.

Sharing the traumatic memories with the consultant begins the process of mastering the traumatic experience. By speaking and playing, the child can partially correct the passive helplessness of the witness role. The session also bolsters the child's observing ego and reality testing functions, which tend to dispel cognitive confusion and encourage active coping (Caplan, 1981). In so doing, the child is assisted to identify traumatic reminders that elicit psychophysiologic reactions, intrusive imagery, and intense affective responses. The goal is to increase the child's sense of being able to anticipate or, at least, manage their recurrence.

Whatever his outward behavior or mood may suggest, the mind of even the young child is preoccupied with inner plans of action in the acute aftermath of a violent trauma. They provide important clues to the child's earliest efforts to master the trauma. Attention to these conscious fantasies enhances the child's understanding of the ways he or she is trying to overcome the helplessness he experienced and is essential to working through of the trauma. It is important to assist the child in distinguishing his or her own aggressive impulses from those of the assailant.

Our child interview is not designed simply to elicit a journalistic recounting of the episode but rather to recapture the child's affective experience of the traumatic events. Exploration of the "worst moment," special detailing and affectively charged interpersonal exchanges, all assist in this task. Consistent with modern views of autobiographical memory, this form of recall is understood to be subjective reconstruction (Bartlett, 1932; Kris, 1956; Paul, 1967). Rather than dampen all feelings, the child must retain confidence that he or she is not helpless in the face of his or her emotions—that is, neither to fear a loss of impulse control nor a flood of unbearable emotion (Krystal, 1978).

Exploration of the child's revenge fantasies is a key step in this process. It is often followed by a perceivable increase in spontaneity and affective range. In the critique of the interview, children frequently chose the depiction of their revenge fantasy when asked to "point to the drawing that helped the most." We have observed continued affective constriction in children where this step in the interview has not been successful.

Probably the best gauge of the effectiveness of the trauma exploration is the enhanced desire of the child to discuss the subsequent life stresses brought on by the event, and, to be actively involved in decisions about his care. Early intervention may therefore be all important to prevent the traumatized child from passively accepting a series of imposed changes in his life. The child may have constructive ideas about ways in which some things can be done to minimize the continued upset in his or her life. We would especially caution the child expert in regard to custody issues. We have observed that child therapists too often become involved in evaluating a child to render an opinion regarding custody while the child remains untreated for prominent signs of severe posttraumatic stress.

Modifying Factors

There are factors besides the violent event itself which contribute to the child's individual response to the psychic trauma. Age and level of ego development influence his or her experience of the event, initial efforts to cope, and later understanding of responsibility. The preschooler is particularly helpless and passive in the face of danger. He or she will make repeated use of denial in fantasy to restore the parent unharmed after the trauma without imagining ways to prevent or intervene during the episode. Reparative and retaliatory actions must be carried out by adults in their name. Latency age children have expanded their role as witness to include participation, if only in fantasy. They can imagine taking the gun, chasing the assailant, and healing the injured parent. As a consequence, they begin to feel some degree of responsibility and frequently fantasize about personal revenge. The adolescent shows not only preoccupation with the violent act but is also concerned with the interplay of assailant, victim, themselves, and others. They are likely in the interview to emphasize their own behavior during the traumatic episode. Motive, circumstance, and justice emerge as complex issues.

Another consideration is the child's previous experience with psychological trauma. Sadly, many of the children we have interviewed are suffering from the cumulative effect of multiple traumas. Although we begin by focusing on the most recent event, we soon come to discover the preceding series of incidents which never have been previously explored. These children may have come to speak in a manner to lessen the impact of the terror. However, we have not observed them to be immunized or injured by their past exposure to abuse or violence. The recurrence of intrusive memories of these prior experiences may hamper their recovery from the current trauma, and needs to be addressed. However, the recent event which the child has witnessed is startlingly novel. No observation of previous violence can prepare a child for the sight of a mother's murder. Even the youngest child can identify it as "the beating where Mommy didn't get up and talk again." The interview begins the painful process of opening the child to his or her memories and offering relief through therapeutic contact.

The presence of preexisting psychological conflicts or frank psychopathology handicaps the child in his or her efforts to cope with the impact of the traumatic event and is readily apparent in the session. For example, the presence of an untreated attention deficit disorder interfered by distracting one child from being able to maintain the needed sustained attention even within the therapeutic consultation. Disturbed children are priority candidates for this technique, although further psychiatric intervention is generally indicated.

We would recommend deferring this interview procedure for those children who have themselves been the direct victim of physical injury. Although these children may have also experienced considerable psychological trauma as a consequence of witnessing violence, attention to their own injuries must take precedence. We suggest postponing consideration of the observational insult while the child's ego resources are rightfully centered on his or her bodily damage. As recovery proceeds, the child will then become available to participate actively in this specialized interview technique. This further step is necessary before the child can fully overcome both of these traumas, the physical and psychological.

Benefits

The interview can be helpful for the child in several different ways. After addressing the actual trauma, the child is in a position to more freely concentrate on the grief work and on other critical issues confronting the child in the wake of a family tragedy. We have met with children whose grieving was interrupted by an intrusive memory of the traumatic event, such as the sight of a physically mutilated parent. The interview session relieves the burden of those recollections and the mourning process can be resumed (Eth and Pynoos, 1985).

Following the consultation, many children appear noticeably less alienated and detached. In part, this clinical improvement derives directly from the detailed exploration of the traumatic situation and its consequences. The single session provides immediate relief for the child, at a time when the child is otherwise feeling very badly. As the child begins to feel better in the presence of the trusted consultant, the child re-establishes the capacity to engage in interpersonal relationships. The child's receptivity to human contact, which was nurtured during the session, can then be transferred to others in the child's support network. In effect, the interview functions as a bridge to those caretaking adults available to the child. By so doing, the technique opens the child to therapeutic influences in his or her environment.

Short-term benefits for the child arise from the consultant assuming the role of child advocate. With permission and in the child's presence, we share with the parent or guardian dominant themes of the session and identified traumatic reminders. We also discuss the natural course of traumatic reactions to prepare them to assist the child at home. We might also confer with school and social service personnel. It is especially useful to develop a close affiliation with the judicial authorities, as the child witness to criminal violence can be forced to play a prominent role in criminal proceedings. We have commented on this subject at length elsewhere (Pynoos and Eth, 1984).

Unfortunately, the traumatized child is in a particularly precarious position. Whatever gains may have accrued during the interview process are jeopardized by external factors in the child's social nexus. For instance, placement in the home of a psychotic relative sabotaged the tenuous progress of one orphaned preschool girl. But if the social system is supportive and understanding, then the ego restitution initiated during the session can be consolidated, expanded, and offered as a model for other family members (Polak et al., 1975).

We hesitate to predict that our interview technique will prove to be preventive. Although therapeutic consultations may have long-term benefits, both desired and unanticipated, not enough controlled long-term observations of results have not yet been conducted. However, there are initial reports of long-term deleterious consequences arising from childhood trauma (Gislason and Call, 1982) suggesting this to be an important area for in-depth study. In the meanwhile, we can draw upon the psychiatric experience with war neuroses to recommend prompt intervention and full exploration of the trauma. Investigators of adult posttraumatic stress disorders have also argued that there may be an optimum time for intervention, when the intrusive phenomena are most apparent and the associated affect most readily available (Horowitz, 1970); Van Der Kolk and Ducey, 1984). With promising results reported for adults (Horowitz and Kaltreider, 1979), there is need to investigate the technique and efficacy of brief therapy with children exposed to violence. However, these methods will need modification to take into account important developmental considerations.

The interview technique, though not explicitly diagnostic, does allow the consultant to assess the child's adaptation to crisis. Gross indicators of psychopathology are readily apparent, whether they be products of chronic disability or acute decompensation. Hence, the interview serves the purpose of screening the child for the need for a formal referral psychiatric evaluation or treatment. In addition, the technique specifically examines for the presence or severity of a posttraumatic stress disorder, a common finding in this population of traumatized children. Those children who require further psychiatric assistance will be able to draw on the positive experience of the interview to prepare for and accept future therapeutic contacts.

CONCLUSION

We have presented a method of interviewing children who have recently suffered a personal disaster. It is our contention that the witnessing of extreme violence constitutes a psychological trauma for the child. The immediate consequences often include ego contraction, affective intolerance, and estrangement, as well as grief. Despite prominent posttraumatic stress reactions, children have the capacity and in fact the desire to collaborate with an adult in directly confronting the traumatic incident soon after its occurrence. Unfortunately, the child's family is often struggling with its own avoidance of traumatic anxiety. It is therefore essential that the child have the opportunity to explore the traumatic episode in the reassuring presence of an unaffected adult (Pynoos and Eth, 1986). Through the use of free drawings and story telling, the consultant is able to engage the child in an exploration of the events associated with the experience of overwhelming anxiety. The response is a sense of immediate relief and a reestablishment of human relatedness. We hope that this easily learned technique becomes widely available to assist the many traumatized children at a time of great need.

REFERENCES

Ayalon, O. (1982), Children as hostage. *Practitioner,* 226:1773–1781.
Bartlett, F.C. (1932), *Remembering.* Cambridge, Mass: Cambridge University Press.
Caplan, G. (1981), Mastery of stress: psychological aspects. *J. Amer. Psychiat.,* 138:413–420.

Eth, S. & Pynoos, R. (1983), Children who witness the homicide of a parent. Presented at the 1983 annual meeting of the American Academy of Child Psychiatry.

_____ (1984), Developmental perspectives on psychic trauma in childhood. In: *Trauma and Its Wake,* ed. C.R. Figley. New York: Brunner/Mazel.

_____ (1985), Interaction of trauma and grief in childhood. In: *Posttraumatic Stress Disorder in Children,* Chap 8, ed. S. Eth and R. Pynoos. Washington, D.C.: American Psychiatric Press.

Folkman, S. & Lazarus, R. (1984), Personal control and stress and coping processes. *J. Pers. Soc. Psychol.,* 46:839–852.

Fox, R.P. (1974), Narcissistic rage and the problem of combat aggression. *Arch. Gen. Psychiat.,* 31:807–811.

Frederick, C. (1980), Effects of natural v. human induced violence upon victims. *Evaluation and Change,* Special Issue, 71–75.

_____ (1985), Children traumatized by catastrophic situations. In: *Posttraumatic Stress Disorder in Children,* Chap 4, ed. S. Eth & R. Pynoos. Washington, D.C.: American Psychiatric Press.

Freud, A. (1937), *The Ego and Mechanisms of Defense.* London: Hogarth Press.

_____ (1965), *Normality and Pathology in Childhood.* New York: International Universities Press.

Furman, E (1974), *A Child's Parent Dies.* New Haven, Conn.: Yale University Press.

Gardner, R. (1979), Helping children cooperate in therapy. In: *Basic Handbook of Child Psychiatry,* Vol. 4, ed. J.D. Noshpitz et al. New York: Basic Books.

Gislason, I.L. & Call, J. (1982), Dog bite in infancy: trauma and personality development. *This Journal,* 21:203–207.

Glass, A.J. (1947), Effectiveness of forward treatment. *Bull. U.S. Army Med. Dept.,* 7:1034–1041.

_____ (1954), Psychotherapy in the combat zone. *Amer. J. Psychiat.,* 110:725–731.

Grinker, R. R. & Spiegel, J.P. (1943), War Neuroses in North Africa: the Tunisian campaign. The Air Surgeon, Army Air Forces, September, New York: Josiah Macy, Jr. Foundation.

Hendin, H., Pollinger, A., Singer, P. & Ulman, R.B. (1981), Meanings of combat and the development of post-traumatic stress disorder. *Amer. J. Psychiat.,* 138:1490–1493.

Horowitz, J. (1970), *Image Formation and Cognition.* New York: Appleton-Century-Crofts.

Horowitz, M. & Kaltreider, N. (1979), Brief therapy of the stress response syndrome. *Psychiat. Clin. N. Amer.* 2, No. 2, August.

Kardiner, A. (1941), The traumatic neuroses of war. In: *Psychosomatic Medical Monograph.* New York: Paul Hoeber, pp. 11–111.

Kolb, L. & Mutalipassi, L. (1982), The conditioned emotional response: a subclass of the chronic and delayed post-traumatic stress disorder. *Psychiat. Ann.,* 12:979–987.

Kris, E. (1956), The recovery of childhood memories in psychoanalysis. *The Psychoanalytic Study of the Child,* 11:54–88.

Krystal, J. (1978), Trauma and affects. *The Psychoanalytic Study of the Child,* 33:81–116.

Levy, D.M. (1938), Release therapy in young children. *Psychiatry,* 1:387–390.

Lifton, R.J. (1979), *The Broken Connection.* New York: Simon & Schuster.

_____ (1982), The psychology of the survivor and the death imprint. *Psychiat. Ann.,* 12:1011–1020.

Paul, I.H. (1967), The concept of schema in memory theory. *Psychol. Issues,* 18/19:218–258.

Piaget, T. & Inhelder, B. (1969), *The Psychology of the Child.* New York: Basic Books.

Polak, P.R., Egan, D., Vanderberg, R., et al. (1975), Prevention in mental health: a controlled study. *Amer. J. Psychiat.,* 132:146–149.

Pynoos, R. & Eth, S. (1984), The child as witness to homicide. *J. Soc. Issues,* 40:87–108.

———— (1985), Children traumatized by witnessing of personal violence. In: *Posttraumatic Stress Disorder in Children,* Chap. 2, ed. S. Eth & R. Pynoos. Washington, D.C.: American Psychiatric Press.

———— (1986), Witnessing violence: special interventions with children. In: *The Violent Home,* ed. M. Lystad. New York: Brunner/Mazel.

———— Gilman, K. & Shapiro, T. (1981), Children's response to parental suicidal behavior. Presented at the 1981 annual meeting of the American Academy of Child Psychiatry.

Smith, J.R. (1982), Personal responsibility in traumatic stress reactions. *Psychiat. Ann.,* 12:1021–1030.

Teicher, J.D. (1953), "Combat fatigue" or "death anxiety neurosis." *J. Nerv. Ment. Dis.,* 117:232–242.

Terr, L. (1984), Children at risk. In: *Psychiatry Update,* Vol III, ed. L. Grinspoon. Washington, D.C.: American Psychiatric Press.

U.S. Public Health Service. (1943), Proceedings of Conference on Traumatic War Neuroses in Merchant Seamen, New York Academy of Medicine (January 28).

Van Der Kolk, B. & Ducey, C. (1984), Clinical implication of the Rorschach in posttraumatic stress disorder. In: *Traumatic Stress Disorder: Psychological and Biological Sequelae,* ed. B. Van Der Kolk. Washington, D.C.: American Psychiatric Press.

Waelder, R. (1933), The psychoanalytic theory of play. *Psychoanal. Quart.,* 11:208–224.

Winnicott, D.W. (1971), *Therapeutic Consultations in Child Psychiatry.* New York: Basic Books.

West, L. J. & Coburn, K. (1984), Posttraumatic anxiety. In: *Diagnosis and Treatment of Anxiety Disorders,* ed. R.O. Pasnau. Washington, D.C.: American Psychiatric Press.

18

The Child Psychiatrist and the Child Witness: Traveling Companions by Necessity, if Not by Design

Lenore C. Terr

University of California, San Francisco

Children are appearing as courtroom witnesses with increasing frequency. Although no one has yet systematically studied the effect of trials upon children, there is considerable controversy about the effect of children upon trials. Some of the relevant issues include suggestibility, memory retention, the effect of psychic trauma upon children's thinking, and the relative developmental abilities of children. Because there are child psychiatric issues, child psychiatrists will be expected to participate in legal processes involving children as witnesses. The author of this article cites what is currently known about children in the courtroom and outlines how a child psychiatrist can most effectively participate—in the consulting room, at trial, and in the arena of public policy.

Not every child psychiatrist wishes to accompany the child who has been an eyewitness or who has been abused, disputed, injured, stolen, or traumatized through the vast reaches of the legal system. Many of us, in fact, avoid the courts the very same way the rushed worker out on a lunch break ignores the confused tourist asking for directions. But the well-set

Reprinted with permission from the *Journal of the American Academy of Child Psychiatry,* 1986, Vol. 25, No. 4, 462–472. Copyright 1986 by the American Academy of Child and Adolescent Psychiatry.
All names of patients and facilities are disguised.

look away may not be enough at this point in our history. Children are
coming forward so often with hideous tales of personal terror, sexual misuse, neglect, and untenable conducts forced upon them by others—let
alone stories of "alleged" murder and mayhem they say they have
witnessed—that we child psychiatrists are increasingly being sought by
courts to help sort out what is "real" versus childhood fantasy; what is
"actual" versus suggested; and if, whether, and why a child is lying.

Here is an example of our professional dilemma: Not so very long ago,
a well-trained child psychiatrist, the only one in a certain small community, refused to treat a 6-year-old boy who, at 4, had been stuck for
about 20 hours in his ghetto project elevator. The child psychiatrist
denied the little boy treatment for his severe post-traumatic stress disorder because the child was involved in litigation against a national elevator
manufacturer and against the housing authority of the large urban center
from which he had moved. After his ordeal, the small lad refused to be
confined in schoolrooms, panicked in the dark, dreamed repeated
nightmares of his own death, and often could not find his own toys
because he had "stuck" them away somewhere. He liked the small town
psychiatrist, and he did not know or care about any pending lawsuits. His
parents, underprivileged and uneducated as they were, understood
without doubt that little William was "different" from the moment he
emerged from that elevator, and they, indeed, wanted recompense for
William from "the system." Even more than that, though, they needed
help for their little boy. But the local child psychiatrist had developed a
policy—no treatment while a lawsuit was pending—a hard and fast rule.
The psychiatrist wished to avoid "the law."

There were at least three places where our legal system might not go
along with this child psychiatrist's "policy:" (1) William was a crucial
eyewitness, not just a victim. His word was being pitted against that of a
national expert on elevators, of the two local repairmen who had fixed the
elevator after William was confined for 18 hours (they said they had seen
William skip about a bit), and of the urban housing authorities who knew
for years that William's family had been problematic. Some "expert" in
the field of child development would have to come to court to help
qualify the young child to be allowed to testify—for if William were not
accepted as a witness, the adult experts hired by the defense would stand
entirely unopposed. The best possible explainer of his qualifications as a
potential witness would be the one who knew William the best—the treating child psychiatrist; (2) without treatment certain aspects of William's
post-traumatic stress disorder were worsening, as do many such symptoms and signs of this condition in both childhood (Terr, 1983a) and
adulthood (Archibald and Tuddenham, 1965; Leopold and Dillon, 1963;

Ploeger, 1972). Law officials would look at the child's failure to arrange for any treatment as bad faith, as an attempt on his part to "milk" the system for more money. The child psychiatrist who had refused William treatment would, therefore, have to explain—in court—why the case had been turned down; and (3) the psychiatrist would be deposed and come to court if any preliminary child psychiatric evaluation whatsoever had been undertaken. Since the child was a crucial witness to the elevator scene—and the only on-the-spot witness for at least 18 hours—confirmatory legal evidence from the psychiatric evaluation would be demanded whether or not the child had undergone treatment.

The statute of limitations for personal injury lawsuits in childhood is age 18 + 1—thus William theoretically runs the chance of receiving no treatment through his entire childhood, that is, *if* every child psychiatrist takes the same "hard and fast" position that this one did. As it turned out, William's evaluating child psychiatrist was unable to avoid several pretrial subpoenas for delivery of the records and for deposition. The psychiatrist, when trial time comes, will probably have to take the witness stand—a reluctant, and sad to say, sorry "expert."

TREND TO PUT MORE CHILDREN ON THE WITNESS STAND

In the daily papers and the newscasts we are catching more and more glimpses of children who have "witnessed" something real and frightening. With the trends toward two-working-parent households, "latchkey" arrangements after school, and a burgeoning day care, nursery school, and babysitting industry, youngsters are being increasingly exposed to a wider range of individuals and greater independence and circulation within rban environments, while they simultaneously experience less vigilance from their schools. The states do not always license child care facilities with suitable thoroughness, nor do they consistently check on the relatives of the person being licensed. Regardless of the state's care or lack thereof, some parents put their children into day care facilities entirely disregarding the issues of licensing. Furthermore, working parents are often afraid to investigate the references or to employ probing interviews with those about to provide care for their youngsters for fear that the potential "arrangements" will fall through. The crux of the problem lies in the tremendous demand for inexpensive child care and the attraction to this field of some unqualified persons.

Equally important to the increased negligence and the pseudo-independence being foisted upon today's youngsters, we are hearing more—probably greater actual numbers—of child abuse, incest, child snatching, and witnessed violence cases *within* families. Investigators first became interested in this kind of problem in the early 1960s, so it is still a relatively "new" field, but it has already been clinically demonstrated that violence breeds violence (Silver et al., 1969; Steele and Pollock, 1974), and thus, violence may spread whenever an abusive family reproduces. Furthermore, breaking the incest taboo for the child certainly grays the absolute qualities of this sexual taboo for the man, to whom the child, after all, is, "father." Suicide is also contagious within families (Cain and Fast, 1972; Farberow and Simon, 1969), as are the effects of psychic trauma (Terr, 1979).

Mental indoctrination of youngsters is becoming more prevalent, too, in our society—a current, although probably not as quantitatively impressive trend as are the aforementioned. *The Manchurian Candidate,* a widely read book and popular 1960s movie (Condon, 1959), the effect of "the big lie," highly publicized statements from returning Korean War prisoners, George Romney's famous confession "I've been brainwashed," and science and pseudo-science from the aerospace lab, the sleep lab, and the sensory deprivation unit have provided the lay public over the years with the general idea that telling a false story repeatedly enough to those who depend on you for food, sleep, shelter, and approval will eventually create a belief. This "technique" is being used, as a matter of fact, with more and more devastating effects, upon child witnesses in divorce cases (Benedek and Schetky, 1985). An increasing number of youngsters are being offered or are offering themselves as witnesses to policemen and family courts in instances where all visitation with one parent stands to be cut off.

We went through a different, but related, trend to this in the late 1970s, which fortunately has begun to reverse itself. The testimony of youngsters garnered under hypnosis by the police or their representatives had been increasingly used in the 1970s and early 1980s to convict supposed felons. The efforts of a few forensic psychiatrists (see particularly Orne (1979) and Diamond (1980)) drastically curtailed this practice. Misuse of police interrogation techniques with children, particularly involving suggestion, and inadvertently suggestive comments from therapists to their charges, however, still present serious problems. Whenever we consider the general topic of child witnesses, the problem of suggestion must be strongly taken into account (Goodman, 1984a; Loftus, 1980; Loftus and Davies, 1984).

The subject of the child as legal witness, therefore, is of growing, pressing, and current concern. Several investigators have already found that sending children out into the hands of the legal system does not necessarily work to the children's benefit (Goldstein et al., 1973; Terr and

Watson, 1968; Wald, 1975). But no studies have yet been done on the actual effects of courtroom witnessing on a child. In this regard, however, Pynoos and Eth (1984) give an account of a 5-year-old child witness to homicide, who, after long delays in the beginning of the murder trial, developed an irrational fear of the cross-examining attorney. In the course of the Chowchilla kidnapping studies, two kidnapped girls (Terrie and Rachel) revealed that they had become so upset while testifying at the 1977 criminal trial, that the proceedings had to be delayed until they could compose themselves. A third Chowchilla kidnap victim (Barbara) panicked when the courtroom elevator that she rode temporarily went out of order. These accounts, though anecdotal, indicate that there would be value in a systematic study of the psychological effect of courtroom experiences upon children who testify. The legal profession awaits the results of such research (Parker, 1982).

The current movement in U.S. law is to bring as much evidence as possible into the courtroom, even if that means letting small children over age 4 testify (Goodman, 1984b). Trial judges who might, at an earlier time, have summarily dismissed on "voir dire" examination many youngsters (Terr, 1980) because they did not understand the oath or they showed insufficient "understanding" of the procedures or of their roles as witnesses, or because they were under 10 (the common law age of competency to testify), find themselves doing very little now (except in juvenile and family courts) to protect youthful witnesses from coming to court and then from experiencing overbearing cross examinations, confusing or tricky questions, or flagrant misinterpretations of their developmental abilities (Parker, 1982). Despite a cautionary law review article published in 1969 warning courts to protect child witnesses from shock, fright, and embarrassment (Libai, 1969), the judges hearing civil suits and criminal cases have not done much to help or to understand the increasing numbers of youngsters whom they are requiring to appear.

Current psychological studies, indicating that school-age children's ability to separate fantasies from memories of real events are almost as good as those of adults, give teeth to the law's current tendency to allow more youngsters to testify (Johnson and Foley, 1984). Furthermore, experimental psychological research into suggestibility and perception show that children, although less efficient at remembering than are adults, are sometimes better at picking out seemingly irrelevant details that would actually help in the courtroom (Neisser, 1979). Youngsters fail to respond to the kinds of prejudices that interfere with adult perceptions (Allport and Postman, 1947) and they may entirely ignore verbal suggestions that rely on subtle differences between words—a pitfall to the adult witness (Dale et al., 1978). On the other hand, children do fall prey, more easily than adults, to suggestions they *do* understand (Loftus and Davies, 1984). Experimental psychologists have not been able—under the simulation of life circumstances—to differentiate the accuracy of children's perceptions and memories from those of adults (Marin et al., 1979). With two exceptions (Dent and Stephenson, 1979; Marin et al., 1979), however, the relevant psychological studies of children's perceptions and memories have been made, not from simulated events, but from movie watching, game playing, or test-taking exercises. The role of severe stress or psychic trauma has not, for obvious reasons, been studied experimentally.

Role of the Child Psychiatrist

What do we child psychiatrists do about this fast growing problem? Certainly we must frame and investigate research questions regarding child witnesses. But that is not enough. We are currently being asked—pressed, actually—to do some immediate things that previously we might never have considered doing. We must evaluate the memories (Timnick, 1985) and treat the psychiatric conditions of an ever increasing number of youngsters who say that they were abused, sexually misused, terrified, or terrorized by someone—and at the same time we must come in person to the courts to help qualify these youngsters to testify and to testify ourselves about them (Terr, 1980). Just as importantly, we must prepare children to take the witness stand. How do we proceed? I propose that we do this on three fronts—in our own consulting room, at court, and in the arena of public policy. These three places in which the child psychiatrist functions with and for the child witness will provide the framework for the remainder of this article.

OFFICE EVALUATION AND TREATMENT OF CHILD WITNESSES

If a child is alleged to have been an eyewitness to someone else's violence or is him or herself the victim of abuse, sex, or neglect, four general principles may help the psychiatrist evaluating this little "witness." (Pynoos and Eth (1986) have prepared a 90-minute format for the more specific evaluation of child witnesses to homicide).

1. Look for corroborating psychiatric findings. If the child or his or her parent states that certain things happened, the youngster should show confirmatory symptoms and signs related to his or her "trauma," or at least, to the profound stress endured. These would include—for fully verbal children at the time of the experience—a remembered detailed story in child language, varying over time in the wording but consistent in its major thrust (Terr, 1980); problems with constriction of range of emotions in those youngsters exposed to chronic, repeated abuses (Green, 1983); persistent sadness in youngsters who have witnessed a death (Pynoos et al., 1985); compulsive repetition of parts of the shock in post-traumatic dreams, play and art, and behavioral or psychophysiologic reenactment (Terr 1979, 1983a); a sense of futurelessness (Terr, 1983a, 1983b, 1983c); ongoing misperceptions or distorted memories of originally traumatic perceptions (Terr, 1983a, 1985a); and fears (Terr, 1981a, 1983a). For children who were not yet verbal (up to age 2-3) at the time of their "witnessed" experiences, the psychiatric findings will be any or all of the above except, in certain instances, for a fully remembered and articulated "story" of the event (Terr, 1985b). (Gislason and Call (1982), however, found full recall of the traumatic event in 3 youngsters under age 36 months at the time they were attacked by dogs.) Without some or all of the findings of post-traumatic stress disorder in a child who says he or she has witnessed a terrifying event, the child psychiatrist must consider the possibility that falsehood, mental indoctrination, and/or suggestion underlie the child's tale.

A brief, but dramatic case vignette may shed some light on the need for corroborating findings. A superior court in the state of Nevada requested a psychiatric evaluation of 8-year-old Loretta because her mother had committed suicide 6 months earlier, "willing" the child to the mother's married sister. A living father, divorced from the mother when the child was 2 years old, came forward in Nevada, demanding the child. He had been out of contact with the child by California court order from the time Loretta was 3 years old because the preschooler had accused him of sexually abusing her on their visitations. A California judge, reading the vivid description of oral sex that Loretta, at 3, had given to a policewoman, had permanently stopped all visits between Loretta and her father. The mother moved to Nevada, never telling the father where she lived. When Loretta's mother killed herself, her family hid the mother's death from the father. The mother's will—although not at all binding to family courts when they consider "the best interests of the child"—had already gone into effect.

By the time the 8-year-old child came for her first psychiatric session, she had already begun admiring and liking her father (the Nevada court had assigned them weekend visitations). Loretta showed no current symptoms of a sexual nature, nor did she show the fears, rage, and withdrawal that incest victims are said to exhibit years after their experience (Herman, 1981). The little girl could produce no memories of sex with her father, nor did she give a history of compulsive masturbation or engagement in reenactive sexual conducts with other children. She was, however, overwhelmed by the suicide of her mother, and she showed several definite findings related to this trauma: persistent sadness, an omen, survivor's guilt, repetitive metaphoric, poetic thoughts about death, and terrible nightmares about her mother.

Old police reports were available. The 3-year-old Loretta had talked in detail about whitish, sticky fluids coming from her father's penis which, she said, had been hard and big. The wording was simple and convincing, but Loretta had been interviewed by a policewoman only once. No child psychiatric examination had ever been done. On the basis of the child "witness's" accusation, she had lost her father—permanently as a matter of fact—if not for her mother's final act.

On examination in the child psychiatrist's office, Loretta could remember nothing about going to the California police when she was 3. But she did remember, however, coming forward once to the police in Nevada "to get rid of Mom's boyfriend." That time, she said, she had told the police a story about white stuff and the man's penis. The tale had "worked well," Loretta explained. "Me and Mommy never saw Frank again."

"Why did you tell that story to the police, Loretta?"

"Because," the child replied, "Mommy had a big imagination. I didn't want her to kill herself, and I always knew that she might. Frank never really did any stuff to me, but I needed to take care of Mommy. So I told the stuff she told me."

The child was given back permanently by the State of Nevada to her father.

2. In order to avoid suggestion to a potential witness, mentally and verbally separate the psychiatric evaluation process from treatment. (McDonald, 1965). Strive not to "suggest" anything to the child witness during the evaluation sessions, and do not use "leading questions." Avoid putting new, more adult words to a child's account. Consider carefully whether to give a child "anatomically correct dolls" that may prematurely suggest sexuality to a youngster who has not yet remembered, told, or played-out in more general fashion a sexual trauma. (Children play "sex" with cars, blocks, Alice-in-Wonderland, Little Bo-Peep, dollhouse furniture, etc., so why use such specific dolls early in the course of a general psychiatric observation?) Do not "preset" a child's play for him or her in the course of evaluation, even though this is an excellent treatment technique (Shapiro, 1973; Terr, 1983d). Avoid overinterpretation or overeducation.

Do not use hypnosis or sodium amytal techniques during evaluation—the child psychiatrist who does this may inadvertently entirely "disqualify" the child as a witness (Diamond, 1980). Avoid group evaluations in order to minimize contagion, spread, or suggestion of symptoms from one child to another (Terr, 1985b).

A certain amount of education, clarification, and interpretation, obviously, is necessary to psychodynamic treatment. If a great deal of this will be utilized in the evaluation of a future witness, however, one might consider asking a second child psychiatrist to evaluate the youngster before starting psychotherapy.

3. Remember the case. Keep good word-for-word notes. These are simply self-reminders. Write a report, if requested, of the child's evaluation, and then keep brief notes on those treatment sessions in which the child makes important comments, indulges in significant behaviors and play, or reports and associates to dreams. Note any new findings that come to light.

4. Collect sufficient data. See all persons in the child's family or those willing to participate in the evaluation process. Siblings may offer confirmatory observations and/or findings that are entirely unknown to the parents. Sisters and brothers, themselves, may be unrecognized "witnesses." The allegedly offending parent, be he snatcher or abuser, should be seen, if not by the child psychiatrist, then by another psychiatrist. Psychiatric observation of the child *with* this person is quite illuminating. Put all requests to evaluate siblings, parents, housekeepers, and others in writing and keep a copy in the files.

Talk to the police, lawyers, court workers or judges. Ask them to supply pertinent medical records, crime reports, autopsies, eyewitness statements, and other relevant documents. Confirmatory information and any and all conflicting information should be understood by the child psychiatrist within the context of the child witness's history, mental examination, and developmental phase.

Under extreme stress and afterwards, some children exhibit perceptual and cognitive mistakes (Terr, 1985a) and fantasy elaborations (Terr, 1985b). These errors depend, in part, upon the suddenness and severity of the trauma, the child's developmental immaturities, and whether or not the youngster previously knew the perpetrator. A child's contradiction of police and eye witness reports, therefore, does not indicate, in and of itself, lying or suggestion.

Watch police and other reports for evidences of "leading" young children. Fear is highly contagious. Panic, play, and other traumatic effects can be imparted vicariously (Terr, 1981b).

In the context of suggestion and vicarious traumatization, the following letter, sent by a police department to the parents of young children who had been clients years earlier at the "Della Stone Day Care Center," illustrates how easy it is to alarm an entire community.

Dear Parent:

This Department is conducting a criminal investigation involving child molestation (288 P.C.). Cal Smith, an employee of Della Stone's Day Care Center, was arrested yesterday by this Department.

The following procedure is obviously an unpleasant one, but to protect the rights of your children as well as the rights of the accused, this inquiry is necessary for a complete investigation.

Records indicate that your child has been or is currently a student at the center. We are asking your assistance in this continuing investigation. Please question your child to see if he or she has been a witness to any crime or if he or she has been a victim. Our investigation indicates that possible criminal acts include: oral sex, fondling of genitals, buttock or chest area, and sodomy, possibly committed under the pretense of "taking the child's temperature." Also, photos may have been taken of children without their clothing. Any information from your child regarding having ever observed Cal Smith leave a classroom alone with a child during any nap period, or if they ever observed Cal Smith tie up a child is important.

Please complete the enclosed information form and return it to this Department in the enclosed stamped return envelope as soon as possible. We will contact you if circumstances dictate same.

We ask you to please keep this investigation strictly confidential because of the nature of the charges and the highly emotional effect it could have on our community. Please do not discuss this investigation with anyone outside your immediate family. Do not contact or discuss this investigation with Cal Smith, any member of the accused defendant's family, or employees connected with Della Stone's Day Care Center.

THERE IS NO EVIDENCE TO INDICATE THAT THE MANAGEMENT OF DELLA STONE'S PRESCHOOL HAD ANY KNOWLEDGE OF THIS SITUATION AND NO DETRIMENTAL INFORMATION CONCERNING THE OPERATION OF

THE SCHOOL HAS BEEN DISCOVERED DURING THIS INVESTIGATION. ALOS (sic), NO OTHER EMPLOYEE IN THE SCHOOL IS UNDER INVESTIGATION FOR ANY CRIMINAL ACT.

Your prompt attention to this matter and reply no later than [1 week from the date of the letter] will be appreciated.

> Unsigned, typed name of the Chief of Police
> Signed name of a Police Captain, Investigative Division.

What spun out from this flamingly suggestive letter was one of the most massive child sex abuse scandals ever heard in a U.S. court. It will probably take years to unwind the, perhaps, impossibly tangled skein of children's "stories" that followed—what must have seemed to be to the shocked parents reading it—a "standard" police inquiry.

HELPING THE CHILD TO COPE WITH COURT (AND HELPING THE COURT TO COPE WITH A CHILD WITNESS)

Psychiatrist Helps in Cases of Intrafamilial Abuse

There are certain things that at times are far worse for a child than continuing personally to endure terrible events—these "worse things" have to do with the permanent loss of a family member, with responsibility for sending a loved one to jail, with loss of economic support, with disloyalty to someone close, and with being killed or mutilated by a family member (Terr, 1980). Thus the risks of loss of the object (of care and protection), of death, of loss of love, of castration, and of conscience—the classic Freudian risks with the exception of death—may impede a child's eventual usefulness or cooperation as a legal witness (Pynoos and Eth, 1984; Rosenfeld, 1979; Terr, 1980).

When a child comes under threat of testifying against a parent, the first fears listed strongly outweigh the later ones. The common experience of workers in the sexual abuse field, for instance, is that children will consistently tell an incest story until the eve of the trial, and then withdraw the story. Why? Largely because the child realizes that he or she will lose a parent—a loved or needed person. The child's fear of loss of the object may far outweigh his or her need for revenge, sexual fears, or the tugs of his or her own conscience.

The basis for youthful refusal to testify or for last minute disavowal from the witness stand often lies in society's insistence on handling intrafamilial abuses within the criminal justice system (DeFrancis, 1969; Terr and Watson, 1968; Wald, 1975). As long as a child senses that his parent must go to jail for incest, neglect, or abuse, there is a good chance that the youngster will ultimately back off as a witness, saying that he had been imagining things or that the doctors and social workers were wrong.

In instances of homicide within the family, fear of death or serious injury may preclude the child from being willing to testify. There may be peculiar twists if the child does appear in court. In the case of "Sarah" (Terr, 1980), for instance, the child testified willingly against her father, who, she said, had murdered her mother. There was insufficient evidence supporting this youthful testimony to convince the jury, however, and the father was eventually acquitted. After the trial, the child automatically went off to live with her allegedly murderous father, the person about whom Sarah had just willingly given damning testimony—a dilemma, certainly, for this young lady.

What, then, is the answer to the loyalty conflicts inherent in child testimony? There are a few "answers," though none of them complete solutions. First, cases of intrafamilial abuse, sex, and neglect (other than homicide or attempted homicide) should be handled inside the juvenile or family court systems, not within the criminal courts. Second, in those criminal cases involving murder or other serious crimes attributed to a parent, the child should be given the option not to testify on the basis of a child-parent, "privilege." There was one successful claim of this privilege in 1983, when in Nevada, a U.S. District Court ruled that a 32-year-old man, Charles Agosto, did not have to testify before a grand jury regarding the alleged organized-crime activities of his father, Joseph Agosto (*San Francisco Chronicle,* 1983). Minor children, however, have not yet begun to find any significant shelter behind the shield of a protective privilege.

The third "answer" is a psychiatric one. The child psychiatrist, taking great care to maintain objectivity, may, on occasion, have the opportunity to testify instead of the child—bypassing the conflicted youngster's testimony about his or her family (Terr, 1980, 1984). It is important that the psychiatrist not be put into the position of gathering hearsay evidence for the police. But if confirmatory medical or psychiatric findings regarding a child's malnutrition, sexual injury, or physical misuse are already known because of medical and psychiatric examinations, the child psychiatrist can go to court instead of the child, bringing with him this "evidence."

Psychiatrist Helps in Cases in Which the Child Must Testify

In civil or criminal matters in which a child, as a crucial witness or as the only witness, must take the witness stand, the psychiatrist may fill several functions, professionally assessing the nature of the child's experience and preparing for its presentation at court. As part of the assessment, the psychiatrist may look into the interrogatory techniques used by the police in order to determine if the child witness was the victim of misunderstanding, suggestion, or veiled threat. He may help to arrange for the gathering of medical and psychiatric data from the child. This can include anatomical specimens, still photographs, and any other materials corroborating or refuting the child's alleged experience (Terr, 1984). The psychiatrist may videotape the child "playing-out" what he says he "saw," reenacting or otherwise telling about the ordeal. The psychiatrist may also make tapes of the child interacting with an alleged abuser (Terr, 1984, 1985c). These tapes may serve to buttress expert testimony. Any objective data collected, saved, and eventually presented should be far more convincing to the court than would be a description given by the child alone. The psychiatrist may see the child for several sessions over time, checking out the basic consistency of the youngster's story, the youngster's use of colloquial language, and the variability of his wording (Terr, 1980). He also evaluates and explains to the court any developmental factors that bear upon the child's potential usefulness or "truthfulness" as a legal witness.

On occasion, a child psychiatrist may be allowed to testify *for* a very young child or for a retarded youngster who is a crucial witness (Terr, 1985c). If the data collected by the child psychiatrist are complete enough, the toddler, preschooler, or developmentally disabled child may be entirely excused from the court. Of course, the psychiatrist, then, will have to "take the heat," but this type of expert participation may save the most immature child witnesses from having to endure the confusion, embarrassment, and harrassment of appearing as witnesses. One principle behind the possibility of appearing for the child is "res gestae," a hearsay exception which allows the spontaneous declaration of a person suddenly excited by an event to be reported in court by another (Parker, 1982). A second principle allowing psychiatric testimony to bypass the child's testimony is the permission, granted to the expert witness, to give the basis for his opinion (Wigmore, 1976). A psychiatric appearance in lieu of the child should be particularly acceptable to courts hearing cases in which a child witness cannot qualify to testify. Courts generally acknowledge their unease with those below the age at which language is acquired (*Wheeler* v. *United States,* 1895).

Older children may need psychiatric expert testimony, not to bypass, but to buttress their own. One boy, Harold, 14, said to his psychiatrist immediately after stepping out of the judge's chambers in his father's and mother's divorce custody case, "I didn't tell the judge a thing that I wanted to. And he didn't ask." Harold urged the psychiatrist, "I'm counting on *you* to tell my story. **OK**?" That "telling it for the child" is an important function of the child psychiatrist in court. No matter how well prepared or how "old" he may be, a child witness may panic at his moment of truth.

A subgroup of the American Bar Association, the National Legal Resource Center for Child Advocacy and Protection (1984), has taken the strong position that expert testimony of mental health professionals be allowed into court "to explain the dynamics of child sexual abuse." Certainly, the explaining of underlying psychological, developmental, and brain mechanisms is an important function of any child psychiatric expert witness, but not only in sex cases.

One novel approach that the child psychiatrist might consider, along with attorneys, of course, is to arrange for a judge to observe a preverbal child "witness" in chambers—with or without the parents (Terr, 1984, 1985c). If the case speaks for itself, the judge, as an educated lay person with regard to children, will see the "repetition compulsion"—and thus, will be able to judge, himself. This could be risky because the youngster might choose this very moment to act atypically, but in the vast majority of instances, the infant or young toddler can be counted on repeatedly to demonstrate his disturbances. Of course, the child psychiatrist must provide explanations.

The child psychiatrist can help prepare an older youngster to face the courtroom experience alone. Pynoos and Eth (1984) have led the profession in this regard. These two authors suggest that, circumstances permitting, in advance of the trial the mental health professional take the child to look over the courtroom and hear about the procedures. They advise preparing the youngster for cross examination as well as for the fact that the alleged criminal will be in court, perhaps, strongly disagreeing. Just as in preparing a child for surgery, the readying procedure can be run-through either on-site or in the psychiatrist's office. Certainly, too, as in surgery, something unexpected, unanticipated, and untold may happen anyway. We know, however, that covering most bases beforehand is better than covering none at all (Levy, 1945).

"Debriefing" the child witness after the trial would be helpful. No one on the legal side of the case usually wants to speak with witnesses after they are "finished." Whenever possible, therefore, the child psychiatrist should ask the young witness to come in for a psychiatric session after the trial is over. Children make interesting observations at this time, and since a crisis point has just passed, some misconceptions, misperceptions, and fears can effectively be approached in such a session, perhaps with significant relief for the child.

THE CHILD PSYCHIATRIST AND PUBLIC POLICY REGARDING CHILD WITNESSES

There are several immediate questions of interest to the public that child psychiatrists are being called upon to answer—and some other questions that will take considerable time and effort to work out, let alone even to frame.

Closed Circuit Television Testimony

The "hot" topic right now is whether children, especially those who have been sexually abused, should be excused entirely from the courtroom to appear, instead, as witnesses on closed-circuit television (Pynoos and Eth, 1984). This topic assumes that testifying in open court is, in and of itself, "bad" for children. Certainly when one sees the cross-examining abuses to which youngsters are exposed by unscrupulous lawyers (such as the recent instance in Los Angeles, when the attorney, after the child held up fingers for his age, complained to the court that this preschooler was unable to *say* how old he was and therefore unqualified to be a witness), one wonders whether children should participate in trials at all. But television would not protect the youngster against child-ignorant or tricky cross examination. All it would really do is keep the child—in certain instances—from seeing the defendant(s). One wonders if closed-circuit television is really worth all this fuss. It will, perhaps, lull courts into thinking that sexually abused children will automatically tell the truth on television, when, in fact there are far deeper reasons (besides embarrassment and fear about telling a story to all of those people, including the perpetrator, in the open courtroom) that may interfere with a child's forthrightness.

In certain instances, it actually *helps* a child to "stand up" in court and, thereby, take societally approved revenge on the person who harmed him. The Chowchilla youngsters who testified against their abductors felt it might have helped them to do so. This benefit, however, could not be proven from any objective findings at Chowchilla (the study was not designed to pick this up).

The child, by taking the witness stand, may give up a trauma-inspired identification. In the case of Jonathan Scott, 11, for instance, who was held hostage by an escaped killer for 11 hours, the young boy was able to spontaneously work out his "Stockholm syndrome" (Ochberg, 1983) by facing his abductor from the witness stand. The accused man vigorously wagged his head "no" when the young lad claimed, under oath, that the man had tried to fondle his penis. Jonathan suddenly realized that his abductor was a hardened liar. That headshake "no" in the open court did far more to help the young boy give up his begrudging admiration for the convict than had two earlier psychiatric sessions.

Fully participating in the courtroom process may help some previously overwhelmed children to feel more potent. Laws mandating closed-circuit television for every single child witness might, therefore, backfire in certain instances. Television could better be used as a legally defined option available to the child witness on request by the youngster, the child psychiatrist, or the child's legal representative (see Parker (1982) for the suggestion that every child witness be assigned a specialized lawyer). Closed-circuit television testimony, on the other hand, may eventually be found to interfere with the defendant's sixth amendment rights to confront and cross examine his accusers (Parker, 1982), and for this reason, this practice may never reach the wide usage currently being demanded (*California SB46, Torres,* 1985).

Monitored Investigatory Procedures

We are leaning that grueling police questioning of children without parents at hand does take place. (This author interviewed one early adolescent child witness to homicide who had been grilled 8–10 hours without any access to her mother.) Leading questions further distort the stories that children eventually tell. One exploratory session between child and police or protective service workers may, in effect, serve to convict a "criminal" or to remove a child from his parent(s), perhaps for an entire childhood. Perhaps the United States should consider taking the paths cleared by Germany and Israel (Goodman, 1984b) allowing allegedly abused children to be interviewed by mental health professionals rather than by the police. There is no question, however, that such trained behavioral scientists may themselves slip into the suggestive mode. Certainly, if we continue in this country to leave the interviewing of children to the police, then we must train our law enforcement personnel in open-ended questioning techniques. And they must be watched.

Because of the serious effects of police or "therapists" interviews upon children's lives, psychiatrists must insist upon monitoring police investigations of youthful witnesses. It would be preferable if a child psychiatrist, directly observing a police session on closed circuit television or through a one-way screen, could interrupt and say "Enough! This child is becoming confused—anxious—too angry." But we might also accept the idea of full television taping of all police interrogations of child witnesses so that the interviews could be reviewed after the fact by a child psychiatrist. Random psychiatric on-site checking of police and protective service agents could probably accomplish the same end as on-the-spot viewing or tape reviewing. The goal would be to achieve more objective and benign investigations of child witnesses. Letters announcing police investigations, such as the one quoted earlier in this article, should be checked first with a child psychiatrist before "papering" a community and unleashing generalized hysteria.

Constraints Against the Mental Indoctrination of Child Witnesses

Difficult as these cases are to prove, the adult indoctrination of children for the purposes of legal witnessing must be made unlawful. Parental "setting-up" of youngsters to testify falsely is bad for our courts and worse for our children. It is naive to conclude on the basis of reports from the sex abuse field, rather than upon those that come from the divorce courts, that false reports do not often happen (Berliner and Barbieri, 1984). Benedek and Schetky (1985) have reviewed 18 custody cases in which sexual abuse was alleged by one parent. Of these, only 8 cases could be confirmed through corroborating findings in the child's psychology, in the child-parent relationship, or from outside medical or police reports. One false report by a child has appeared earlier in this paper. This kind of adult-instigated offense, when proven, should be considered a misdemeanor, perhaps a felony, punishable with stiff fines. False accusations from youngsters, the real stuff of the 17th century witch trials at Salem, but for a few centuries now, almost exclusively the domain of fiction writers such as Arthur Miller (*The Crucible*) or Lillian Hellman (*The Children's Hour*), are becoming a problem. Unless we effectively punish (hopefully *not* by jailing them) those adults who put children up to false denunciations, the number of child-parent relationships tragically torn apart on this basis will steadily increase.

Child-Parent Privilege

A child should not have to testify against his or her parent. That children are ordered to do so now violates the privacy of communications within families as well as the possible future health and well-being of youngsters.

At present, no state allows for a legal child-parent privilege. It appears that "the law" considers it more important to gather and hear full evidence against possibly criminal parents than to excuse youngsters from having to testify against their own families. However, the potential mental health benefits of giving youngsters an option to use the child-parent privilege far outweigh the risks. By taking the privilege, children would not be put in the impossible psychological bind of testifying against loved ones or against those upon whom they rely for sustenance, nor would they be forced to lie on the witness stand or to back off as witnesses at the very last minute. If such a privilege were granted, we would be spared a number of court-originated mental problems ("iurogenic" would be a proposed word for the ill health brought on or worsened by the legal profession). The Solano County, California Superior Court case, in which a 12-year-old girl was kept in solitary confinement for over a week by a criminal court judge who had ordered that the resistant young lady testify against her stepfather in a felonious incest trial, reads like a cautionary tale in this regard (*New York Times,* 1984). This type of ugly situation is preventable.

Letting children take a child-parent privilege would require that our police investigators do better—they would have to collect more supporting data, interview more secondary witnesses, and use more pediatric and psychiatric examinations. The option of taking this privilege would also require that child witnesses consistently be given the opportunity to work with their own court-appointed legal representatives (Parker, 1982). The extra expenses incurred would be well-worth the investment.

Some Thoughts for the Future

It would be a happy day, indeed, if children rarely had to appear in court. Currently, however, more and more youngsters are being ordered to do so. What can be done over the long run about the problems that are leading children in ever-increasing numbers onto the witness chair? One might consider a few of these, only partial, solutions: (1) better licensing of day care, babysitting, foster home, and nursery programs. This would include interviews of all workers and immediate family members of the licensee and subsequent interviews with any newly hired workers. Frequent, random checking by state agents of all child care homes and institutions would also help to prevent abuse and neglect; (2) investment of government and business into solo or shared child care programs aimed at furtherance of child mental health; (3) a return to "in loco parentis" obligations of schools—this would include adequate supervision of school buses, playgrounds, and after school or nighttime programs; (4) an attempt to move intrafamilial sex, neglect, or violence out of the criminal courts into the family court system, with ongoing vigorous attempts to work out therapeutic programs that would allow for treatment of the majority of child victims inside their own homes and within their own families; (5) shared computer lists among states and long-term parole or probation "tracking" of persons who have been convicted of criminal acts against children or who have lost childcare licenses; and (6) collection of social security numbers and drivers' permit numbers from all parents initially registering their babies in pediatric practices (Terr, 1983c). These numbers would enable most parentally snatched youngsters to be tracked down and returned quickly.

SUMMARY

This paper has reviewed and critiqued much of what we presently know about children as legal witnesses. It is apparent that almost every child psychiatrist will occasionally be called upon to work with a young victim or bystander. These unfortunate cases are becoming far more prevalent. The legal system is demanding that child witnesses appear in court.

Not all children tell the "truth"—some falsify because of loyalty conflicts or because they are mentally indoctrinated, and some fall inadvertent victims to suggestion. A child psychiatrist may, therefore, not only have to help "qualify" a child as a witness, testify instead of—or along with him, explain his testimony to the court, prepare him for the witness chair, but also assess the veracity of the child's story. The psychiatrist must be careful to separate the evaluation process from treatment in his own mind and in the child's and family's understanding. He may proceed with psychotherapy in legal cases, but safeguards will be needed.

Closed-circuit television, on request, appears helpful for some child witnesses. Furthermore, if police interrogations of children were monitored (either consistently or at random) by child psychiatrists, suggestive and leading questions might eventually become less of a problem. Our legislators should consider employing legal constraints against those who would mentally indoctrinate children. Judges and lawmakers would be well advised, also, to look into the possibility of a child-parent privilege.

The child witness is a solitary traveler wandering through a strange maze of institutions, people, and customs. He will need a guide—a professional one. The child psychiatrist can fill this role. Not only is the psychiatrist able to look ahead to make sure that the routes are safe, and that the traveler knows what is coming next—but he will translate, as well. He must watch his small charge, assessing him for weariness, confusion, and even oddly enough, for an occasional forged passport. The land of legalities is too complex and too brutal for the young person to take on alone. The psychiatrist must prepare him or herself. The little travelers are coming!

REFERENCES

Allport, G. & Postman, L. (1947), *The Psychology of Rumor.* New York: Henry Holt.

Archibald, H. & Tuddenham, R. (1965), Persistent stress reaction after combat. *Arch. Gen. Psychiat.,* 12:475–481.

Benedek, E. & Schetky, D. (1985), Allegations of sexual abuse in child custody and visitation disputes. In: *Emerging Issues in Child Psychiatry and the Law,* ed. D. Schetky & E. Benedek, New York: Brunner/Mazel, pp. 145–156.

Berliner, L. & Barbieri, M.K. (1984), The testimony of the child victim of sexual assault. *J. Soc. Issues,* 40:125–137.

Cain, A. & Fast, I. (1972), Children's disturbed reactions to parent suicide: distortions of guilt, communication, and identification. In: *Survivors of Suicide,* ed. A. Cain & I. Fast. Springfield, Ill.: Charles C Thomas, pp. 93–111.

California SB 46, *Torres,* 1985.

Condon, R. (1959), *The Manchurian Candidate.* New York: McGraw-Hill.

Dale, P.S., Loftus, E.F. & Rathbun, L. (1978), The influence of the form of the question on the eyewitness testimony of preschool children. J. *Psycholing. Res.,* 7:269–277.

DeFrancis, V. (1969), *Protecting the Child Victims of Sex Crimes Committed by Adults.* Denver: The American Humane Association.

Dent, H. & Stephenson, G.M. (1979), Identification evidence: experimental investigations of factors affecting the reliability of juvenile and adult witnesses. In: *Psychology, Law and Legal Processes,* ed. D.P. Farrington, K. Hawkins & S.M. Loyd-Bostock, Atlantic Highlands, N.J.: Humanities Press, pp. 195–206.

Diamond, B. (1980), Inherent problems in the use of pretrial hypnosis on a prospective witness. *Calif. Law Rev.,* 68:313–349.

Farberow, N. & Simon, M. (1969), Suicide in Los Angeles and Vienna: an intercultural report. *U.S. Pub. Hlth. Rep.,* 84:389–403.

Gislason, L. & Call, J. (1982), Dog bite in infancy: trauma and personality development. *This Journal,* 21:203–207.

Goldstein, J. Freud, A. & Solnit, A. (1973), *Beyond the Best Interests of the Child.* New York: Free Press.

Goodman, G. (1984a), Children's testimony in historical perspective. *J. Soc. Issues,* 40:9–31.

_____ (1984b), The child witness: conclusions and future directions for research and legal practice. *J. Soc. Issues,* 40:157–175.

Green, A. (1983), Dimension of psychological trauma in abused children. *This Journal,* 22:231–237.

Herman, J.L. (1981), *Father Daughter Incest.* Cambridge: Harvard University Press.

Johnson, M. & Foley, M.A. (1984), Differentiating fact from fantasy: the reliability of children's memory. *J. Soc. Issues,* 40:33–50.

Leopold, R. & Dillon, H. (1963), The psycho-anatomy of a disaster: a longtime study of post-traumatic neuroses in survivors of a maritime explosion. *Amer. J. Psychiat.,* 119:913–921.

Libai, D. (1969), The protection of the child victim of a sexual offense in the criminal justice system. *Wayne Law Rev.,* 15:977–984.

Levy, D. (1945), Psychic trauma of operations in children and a note on combat neurosis. *Amer. J. Dis. Child.,* 69:7–25.

Loftus, E. (1980), *Memory.* Reading Mass.: Addison Wesley.

_____ & Davies, G. (1984), Distortions in the memory of children. *J. Soc. Issues,* 40:51–67.

Marin, B.V., Holmes, D.L., Guth, M. & Kovac, P. (1979), The potential of children as eyewitnesses: a comparison of children and adults on eyewitness tasks. *Law Hum. Behav.,* 3:295–305.

McDonald, M. (1965), The psychiatric evaluation of children. *This Journal,* 4:569–612.

National Legal Resource Center for Child Advocacy and Protection, New American Bar Association Child Sexual Abuse Law Reform Project (1984).

Neisser, U. (1979), The control of information pickup in selective looking. In: *Perception and Its Development: A Tribute to Eleanor Gibson,* ed. A.D. Pick. Hillsdale, N.J.: Erlbaum, pp. 201–219.

New York Times (1984), Girl in California held in contempt, January 8, p. 19.

Ochberg, F. (1983), Hostage victims. In: *Terrorism,* ed.B. Eichelman, D. Soskis, & W. Reid. Washington, D.C.: American Psychiatric Association, pp. 83–88.

Orne, M.T. (1979), The use and misuse of hypnosis in court. *Int. J. Clin. Exp. Hypnosis,* 27:311–341.

Parker, J. (1982), The rights of child witnesses: is the court a protector or perpetrator? *New Eng. Law Rev.,* 17:643–717.

Ploeger, A. (1972), A ten-year follow-up of miners trapped for two weeks under threatening circumstances. In: *Stress and Anxiety,* ed. C. Spielberger & J. Sarason. Washington, D.C.: Hemisphere, pp. 23–28.

Pynoos, R. & Eth, S. (1984), The child as witness to homicide. *J. Soc. Issues,* 40:2:87–108.

_____ (1986), Witness to violence: the child interview. *This Journal,* 25:306–319.

_____ Frederick, C., Arroyo, W., Nader, K., Eth, S., Lyon-Levine, M., Silverstein, S. & Nunez, W. (1985), Post-traumatic stress in school age children. Presented at the annual meeting of the American Psychiatric Association, Dallas (May).

Rosenfeld, A.A. (1979), Endogamic incest and the victim-perpetrator model. *Amer. J. Dis. Child.,* 133:406–410.

San Francisco Chronicle (1983), Court says kids can't be forced to testify against parents, January 18, p. 12.

Shapiro, S. (1973), Preventive analysis following a trauma: a 4½ year old girl witnesses a stillbirth. *The Psychoanalytic Study of the Child,* 28:249–285.

Silver, L., Dublin, C. & Lourie, R. (1969), Does violence breed violence? Contribution from a study of the child abuse syndrome. *Amer. J. Psychiat.,* 126:404–407.

Steele, B. & Pollock, C. (1974), A psychiatric study of parents who abuse infants and small children. In: *The battered child,* Ed. 2, ed. R.E. Helfer & C.H. Kempe. Chicago: University of Chicago, pp. 80–133.

Terr, L. (1979), Children of Chowchilla: a study of psychic trauma. *The Psychoanalytic Study of the Child,* 34:547–623.

—————— (1980), The child as a witness. In: *Child Psychiatry and the Law,* ed. D. Schetky & E. Benedek, New York: Brunner/Mazel, pp. 207–221.

—————— (1981a), Psychic trauma in children: observations following the Chowchilla schoolbus kidnapping. *Amer. J. Psychiat.,* 138:14–19.

—————— (1981b), "Forbidden games": post-traumatic child's play. *This Journal,* 20:741–760.

—————— (1983a), Chowchilla revisited: the effects of psychic trauma four years after a schoolbus kidnapping. *Amer. J. Psychiat.,* 140:1543–1550.

—————— (1983b), Time sense following psychic trauma: a clinical study of ten adults and twenty children. *Amer. J. Orthopsychiat.,* 53:244–261.

—————— (1983c), Life attitudes, dreams, and psychic trauma in a group of "normal" children. *This Journal,* 22:221–230.

—————— (1983d), Play therapy and psychic trauma: a preliminary report. In: *Handbook of Play Therapy,* ed. C. Schaefer & K. O'Connor. New York: Wiley-Interscience, pp. 308–319.

—————— (1983e), Child snatching: a new epidemic of an ancient malady. *J. Pediat.,* 103:151–156.

—————— (1984), The baby in court. In: *Frontiers of Infant Psychiatry,* Vol. 2, ed. J.D. Call, E. Galenson & R. Tyson. New York: Basic Books, pp. 490–494.

—————— (1985a), Remembered images in psychic trauma: one explanation for the supernatural. *The Psychoanalytic Study of the Child,* 40:493–533.

—————— (1985b), Children traumatized in small groups. In: *Post-traumatic Stress Disorder in Children,* ed. S. Eth & R. Pynoos. Washington, D.C.: American Psychiatric Press, pp. 45–70.

—————— (1985c), The baby as a witness. In: *Emerging Issues in Child Psychiatry and the Law,* ed. D. Schetky & E. Benedek. New York: Basic Books, pp. 313–323.

—————— & Watson, A. (1968), The battered child rebrutalized: ten cases of medical/legal confusion. *Amer. J. Psychiat.,* 124:126–133.

Timnick, L. (1985), Court: how reliable? *Los Angeles Times,* April 18, p. 32.

Wald, M. (1975), State intervention on behalf of "neglected" children: a search for realistic standards. *Stanford Law Rev.,* 17:985–1040.

Wheeler v. *United States* (1895), 159 U.S. 523, 40 L Ed 244, 16 SCt 93.

Wigmore, J.H. (1976), *Evidence in Trials at Common Law.* Boston: Little, Brown.

PART V: SPECIAL STRESS AND COPING

19

An Epidemiological Study of Psychic Trauma and Treatment Effectiveness for Children After a Natural Disaster

Rosemarie Galante and Dario Foa
University of Milan, Italy

Approximately 300 Italian elementary school children who were victims of a devastating earthquake were surveyed in an epidemiological study. The measure used was the Rutter Behavioral Questionnaire for Completion by Teachers. In one village a treatment program was developed and implemented. A frequency count of the expressed earthquake-related fears and anxieties was taken during every treatment session. Treatment consisted of a gradual series of steps that led to a replaying of the earthquake. It was hypothesized that the number of children shown to be at risk for developing neurotic or antisocial problems would be positively correlated with the amount of destruction in a village. This was not verified. It was also hypothesized that treatment would reduce earthquake fears and the number of children at risk. This was verified. The village where treatment was carried out for 1 academic year showed a significant drop in the at-risk scores. Conclusions were that treatment alleviates symptoms but that

Reprinted with permission from the *Journal of the American Academy of Child Psychiatry,* 1986, Vol. 25, No. 3, 357–363. Copyright 1986 by the American Academy of Child and Adolescent Psychiatry.

The authors acknowledge the assistance of Professor Cesa-Bianchi, Director of the Medical Psychology Department, University of Milan; and Antonio Caruso, Sebastiano Maugeri, Anna Petroccioni, and Laura Jessen for their assistance.

An early version of this paper was presented at the American Academy of Child Psychiatry Annual Meeting, Washington, D.C., Oct. 20, 1981.

the number of children at risk seems to be more related to the length of time
needed for the community to reorganize after the disaster.

On November 23, 1980, a devastating earthquake struck the rugged rural mountain region of central Italy. The death toll in this sparsely populated area was surprisingly high. Over 4000 people lost their lives and tens of thousands lost their homes in the 116 villages damaged by the earthquake. Particularly affected by the tragedy were the children of these communities. They were affected not only by the earthquake but also by the unfortunate circumstances that surrounded the tragedy and augmented the number of fatalities and psychic trauma. The children's memories of those events were to dominate their lives long after the seismic shocks that had destroyed their world subsided.

Those charming mountain-top medieval villages with their narrow, steep, and winding streets became instant and horrendous death traps as the mortar and stone structures collapsed. The streets were immediately inundated with tons of rubble which blocked all escape routes. This nightmare "no-escape" situation was one of the themes that plagued the children. Another disturbing aspect was related to the rescue efforts.

Due to their isolation, the destruction of communication lines, and Italy's small emergency relief resources, there were at times delays of 2 and 3 days before help arrived. In the long wait the survivors made vain efforts to dig out the victims, who pleaded for rescue for days before dying. The children, who were witnesses to these pathetic scenes, later recalled with precision the time when each victim was last heard from. They later made constant references to those moments.

This additional loss of life, attributed by the earthquake victims to the failure of emergency assistance, provoked a bitterness and hostility that made the disaster relief even more difficult. The children were affected by their own reactions to these scenes as well as by the angry responses of their families and communities.

In an attempt to make up for this initial delay in response and to supplement the relief forces, there was a great deal of volunteering from public and private sectors. Each regional government took responsibility for a part of the disaster area. The region of Lombardy (which includes Milan) assisted the six villages at the epicenter. Disaster relief teams were formed consisting of health, sanitation, education, and mental health professionals. The University of Milan participated in this effort. We at the medical psychology department were given the task of working with the children.

It was deceptively easy sitting in an office at the University to project our part of the relief services. One of our team (D.F.) was to handle the problems with the local personnel in reopening the schools and the other (M.G.) was to work with the traumatized children of the six villages. Although eventually implemented, this plan almost did not survive the first impact with the chaotic reality of the situation. After a somber reassessment of the problems involved we realized that our prior experience was not an adequate preparation to enable us to respond to the needs of these children.

In the first days after the earthquake the children displayed a wide range of disturbed behaviors. They were apathetic, aggressive, and even at times assaultive. Behaviors were extreme and exaggerated. Their reactions were certainly understandable since they had been subjected to scenes of sudden and prolonged death, had lost their homes and all their belongings, and lived in the unrecognizable remnants of their community. Helping the children seemed an immense and impossible task. In spite of the urgency of the situation we decided it was imperative to research what others had done in working with disaster-related traumas in order to have an idea about what we might expect to accomplish.

In the event of a disaster, children have been identified as being among the more susceptible elements of the population to suffer from posttraumatic stress syndrome (PTSS) (Frederick, 1982). In a summary of the findings of different disasters, it was found that, in three-quarters of the children, symptoms were still evident 2 years after the traumatizing event. A review of the psychiatric literature that relates to the general phenomena of psychic trauma in children provides some understanding of why children are particularly vulnerable.

Bowlby (1973), in his well-known work on loss in children, states that any unwilling separation from the caretakers of a child gives rise to emotional distress, and personality disturbances. He also pointed out that children's problems are often overlooked while others in the family respond to a loss. The children's rebuffed feelings often fuel problems that emerge long after. Since the family's response is such an important (though obvious) factor, it is often cited in the literature.

Caplan (1964) also considered the family reaction to be a deciding factor in how well the members cope with and recover from their trauma. He predicted the onset of disorganized behaviors when normal defense mechanisms (individual or collective) fail to cope with a hazardous situation. Without normal support systems (as when all family members are subject to danger), recovery becomes more difficult.

The Buffalo Creek children, who suffered traumas after a devastating flood, showed no improvement with the passage of time (Newman,

1976). All children were found to be affected (including children born after the event). Newman found a correlation between the family's reaction, developmental level of the child, the amount of exposure to the trauma, and the degree of psychic trauma. Treatment was recommended to counteract the negative effects.

There are few studies that describe follow-up or treatment after a traumatic event. Most studies describe the crisis interventions that are made at the time. One of the few to deal with treatment after the events is that of Terr.

Terr (1981), in her work with psychic trauma of kidnap victims, speaks of the long-lasting effects of the trauma. She found that symptoms may not be observed by the parents for up to a year after the trauma. Among the symptoms were: fears of recurrence, fears of other trauma, repetitive relating of the trauma, and "playing" the trauma. She reported a reduction in symptoms in many cases after brief counseling.

Another study describes counseling in a traumatic situation with children involved in an earthquake. Howard and Gordon (1972) after the San Fernando earthquake found that counseling coupled with community outreach was important in making contact with the large numbers of children manifesting symptoms. Although brief counseling was effective in most cases, 1-year follow-ups showed that some children still had symptoms.

In summary, there seems to be agreement on a few basic points. Children can be expected to develop symptoms of stress and trauma after a disaster. These symptoms are more likely to occur when the family is also involved. These symptoms tend to be long lasting and do not necessarily disappear with the passage of time. Children suffering loss may be particularly susceptible even though their problems may not emerge for years. Given that some children do not show outward signs of disturbance they tend to be overlooked by the adults around them after a loss. Brief counseling, though useful, is not completely effective in relieving long-lasting symptoms.

It seemed that our Italian children met every criteria for being susceptible to developing long-lasting psychic trauma. We therefore decided that we should broaden the length and the scope of our planned intervention in the area.

Our revised project for our six villages consisted of three phases:

Phase 1. Pretesting. Six months after the earthquake all the children were tested to discover the numbers and location of children at "risk." We were fortunate in finding a screening instrument that had been validated on an Italian population sample, the Rutter Children's Behavior Questionnaire for Completion by Teachers. A score of nine or more on the Rutter scale indicates that the child is at "risk" of developing neurotic or antisocial disturbances (Zimmerman-Tansella et al., 1978).

Phase 2. Treatment. The treatment program was implemented in the village with the highest number of children at "risk."

Phase 3. Posttesting. Eighteen months after the earthquake all children were retested (a year after pretesting).

Realizing that in such chaotic field conditions we could not hope to conduct a rigorous investigation we nevertheless attempted to answer a few basic questions that could enable us to fulfill our commitments in a meaningful manner.

We were interested in knowing if: (1) there would be a higher percentage of children at risk in the villages that had suffered the most destruction; (2) children who had suffered deaths in the family would have a higher number of at risk scores than those who did not; and (3) children who had been part of the treatment program would have a greater reduction in the number of at risk scores than those who had not.

PHASE 1

Method

Subjects

The questionnaire has been completed for all the first through fourth graders in the six villages studied (total 300).

Procedure

Six months after the earthquake the questionnaire was distributed to the elementary school teachers by research assistants (psychology interns). At the same time the children were asked to draw a house, a tree, and a person (by the research assistants).

A chi square (χ^2) analysis was peformed on the at risk scores in relationship to deaths in the family. A χ^2 analysis was also used to determine the appropriateness of the Rutter scale used on the earthquake children by comparing them with the Verona sample of the first through fourth graders (data from an unpublished manuscript, Zimmerman (1977)). The overall death, damage, and destruction in the individual communities and at risk scores were compared.

Results

A significant correlation between deaths in the family and at-risk scores occurred only in Calabritto and in the total scores (Table 1).

Although there were great differences in the proportion of at-risk scores between the villages, these differences were not always related to the amount of damage, destruction, and death in that community (Table 2).

An analysis of the totaled scores of Verona and the earthquake area revealed no significant differences in the two populations ($\chi^2, p < 0.10$). (All three phases of the project will be discussed together at the conclusion of this report.)

PHASE 2

Method

Subjects

Subjects included all of the first through fourth grade elementary school children of Calabritto (this village was selected for treatment because there were the largest number of children at risk).

Procedure

For 1 academic year at approximately monthly intervals one of the investigators (M.G.) conducted a week long series of group sessions. Each group of four met for 1 hour, once, during each series of sessions. The

Table 1. Death and Risk Scores[a]

Village	6 Months after	18 Months after
Calabritto	0.001	NS
Caposele	NS	NS
Conza	NS	NS
Laviano	NS	NS
Pesco Pagano	NS	NS
Teora	NS	NS
Total	0.000	NS

[a] NS = not significant.

Table 2. Damage and At-Risk Scores

| Village | Total Damages | | | Rutter Scores 1–4 Grades | |
| | Damaged homes (%) | Destroyed homes (%) | Deaths (%) | Assessed after 6 months | |
				Total no.	Percent risk
Calabritto	95	80	8	62	47
Caposele	85	60	1	40	8
Conza	100	100	25	41	20
Laviano	100	100	37	35	43
Pesco Pagano	80	60	8	77	9
Teora	95	65	3	45	9

first introductory session was held in the classroom; all others were held in a separate room. The treatment program was the same for all grades (first to fourth) with adjustments made in language to keep the treatment age-appropriate. Notes were taken on each child, for each session, and a frequency count of all earthquake-related behaviors was taken and compared with other behaviors on a checklist.

Treatment program

Session 1. Objective: To give permission to communicate openly, particularly about the earthquake. Activity: Drawing while listening to stories about San Francisco's recovery from earthquakes and its seismic proof constructions.

Session 2. Objective: To openly discuss fears and to demonstrate that being afraid was a common shared reaction. Activity: Children drawing while listening to a story about a child who is afraid but too timid to ask for help. This was followed by a discussion of their drawings and their feelings. (They told what they did when they were afraid.)

Session 3. Objective: To discuss myths and erroneous beliefs about earthquakes. Activity: Children drawing while listening to a story about a child being afraid of earthquakes recurring because he did not understand how they occurred. This was followed by the children's talking about their beliefs and a "lesson" on earthquakes.

Session 4. Objective: To involve the children in an active discharge of feelings about the earthquake and place the earthquake in the past. The activity consisted of making a large joint drawing of Calabritto and furnishing it with small toys (cars, dolls, and furniture). This inevitably stimulated a spontaneous "acting out" of the earthquake. The focus was on what they did *after* the earthquake to resume a normal life.

Session 5. Objective: To release the power of the images of the deaths and focus on building the future. Activity: Role-playing (with a drawing of Calabritto that included the cemetery) and funeral rituals. The future of the "New Calabritto" was then planned.

Session 6. Objective: To develop the idea that one is not a "victim of the fates" but could take an active part in one's own survival. Activity: Role-playing being parents, teaching children to survive in various emergency situations, i.e., floods, earthquakes, and accidents.

Session 7. Objective: To give the children an opportunity to bring up whatever they chose to in "closing." The activity was a free drawing and discussion.

Analysis of data

Clinical observations were made of each child for each session. From the notes taken a frequency count was made of all fears mentioned and of all earthquake related issues (Fig. 1).

Results

During the first session the children interacted with each other rather than with the investigator. They were either extremely aggressive (active fighting) or silent and apprehensive. In spite of their disruptive or distracted behavior they were attentive to the story.

The drawings were full of menacing features and the environment tended to be threatening. The children did not draw the earthquake or their destroyed village. Some of the children began to speak about the earthquake. A third grade boy said, "My uncle called for help during the

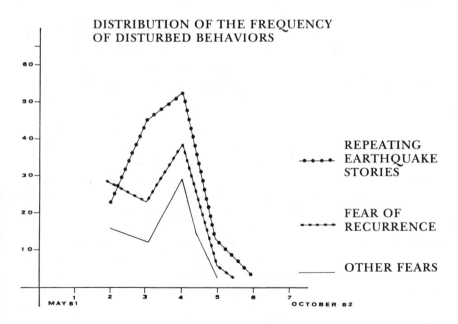

Figure 1. Comparison of frequency count of behaviors with participation in treatment.

night. He talked until 3 in the morning, then he died. When he was dug out he was cut in half." This and other accounts were repeated in a hurried matter-of-fact tone of voice.

In Session 2 many of the children spoke about the earthquake. There was a repetitious, monotonous, well-rehearsed air to all these earthquake stories. Some spoke of omens. A second-grade boy said, "Ten days before the earthquake my uncle said that we would all die together. He died with my aunt and cousins." Others had anniversary fears. Many stated calmly, "On Nov. 23, there will be another one." There were also fears of all kinds of impending doom. A second-grader said, "Every night when I go to bed I think that the world will split in half at Calabritto and I will fall to the center. Will I get burned?" The children seemed to be trying to prepare and protect themselves against their fears of recurrence of a disaster.

Session 3 was characterized by a sharp increase in expression of fears and retelling of the earthquake stories. Comments ranged from open expressions of fears to complete denial: a 7-year-old girl said, "Sometimes I just suddenly start screaming." Another stated, "Sometimes I just start yelling 'Earthquake!' 'Earthquake!'" A third, reflecting denial, said, "It's no use to be afraid or cry. I never cry." There were strange comments that were interjected as their defenses began to break down: "Even the dogs cried after the earthquake. The end of the world is coming in 19 years." This statement was spoken in a hushed tone by a second-grade boy (whose dog had died in the earthquake). A third-grade girl seemed to reassure herself when she said, "The old should die. The young should live." Session four was the high point of repetition of earthquake stories and the relaying of all types of fears.

By Session 4 the children had moved into the prefabricated schools and homes. Instead of taking a step forward with the attainment of these eargerly awaited developments, they regressed to the earlier exaggerated ways of behaving. Consistent with those exaggerated emotions their attachment to the investigator became intense. Their drawings (which were done in addition to the group project) began to have symbolic references to their actual losses. A seemingly cheerful 8-year-old girl drew two figures and omitted the lower half of their bodies. Her mother had remained paralyzed from the waist down as the result of earthquake injuries. A typical comment on the playing of "earthquake" by an 8-year-old demonstrated how his attempts to limit the disaster were quickly overcome by his fears: "I don't want any wars. No one dies or gets hurt. Maybe I get hurt, but not in a war, in an accident. Killers arrive and kill everyone. We send for the police. Then there is a big earthquake and we take everyone to the cemetery. Then we have a big party and forget about it."

By Session 5, the children had developed a passionate and possessive attachment to the investigator. They were also strongly involved in the session. They seemed to want to put order in the untidy and capricious disaster by killing off everyone in the "earthquake" game. A fourth-grade girl comments, "First there is a volcanic eruption and that family all dies. The people are left sorry. Then there is an earthquake and everyone dies. Well, maybe three people lived. They went to another valley but they wished they died because they had no one left. So they killed themselves." This was accompanied by shaking of the table, a simulation of the rumble of the earthquake, and gleeful laughter. The children were delighted to fit the disaster into a more comprehensible scheme; everyone has the same fate. At this point the first open reference to their losses was made in their drawings. For instance, one 7-year-old drew a picture of his friends in a mausoleum.

Session 6 was much less intense than the preceding sessions. The children continued to participate in the role-playing but in a much more relaxed mood. There was almost no talk of fears in spite of the stimulating disaster scenes. The children planned the future with some skepticism but the doubts were related to realistic issues rather than apocalyptic fears.

Session 7 was the closure session. The children drew and chatted about everyday issues. There was no mention of earthquake-related themes.

The frequency count on the behavioral checklist showed a dramatic drop in all earthquake-related fears and other fears after the role-playing of the earthquake.

PHASE 3

Method

Subjects

The first through fourth grade elementary school children who were present at the pretest.

Procedure

Eighteen months after the earthquake (1 year after the pretesting) the questionnaire was redistributed to the same teachers by different research assistants (psychology interns).

Analysis of data

A χ^2 analysis was performed on the correlations between pre- and posttest scores in the different villages and of the correlation between the posttest score and the deaths in the family.

Results

There was a significant difference in the pre- and posttest test scores in three villages. In Calabritto and Teora there was a decrease in at risk scores. In Caposele there was an increase (Table 3). In the posttest scores there was no significant correlation between deaths and at risk scores.

DISCUSSION

Our hypothesis that there would be a greater reduction of at-risk scores in the children who had been in the treatment program was confirmed. Not only the at-risk scores but also the "frequency of expressed fears" dropped significantly.

The children themselves made it clear that they had a strong need of the sessions. They fought to be the first to enter and had to be evicted at the end. On more than one occasion irate children bombarded the pre-fab treatment room with stones, attempting to storm their way back in after their turn was over. This could not be explained as a need for art and drama. These activities were already offered by the school and were poorly attended. The children seemed to want to work through the feelings that were not expressed in routine retelling of the earthquake stories.

Many of the same reactions reported by Terr (1981) were present in these children. The children spoke of an infinite variety of real and fantastic fears. They spoke of omens and had fears of a recurrence around the anniversary of the earthquake. There were also instances of reenactment behaviors as when the children would absentmindedly break into the sound of the earthquake rumble. All of this came to an abrupt halt after the dramatizations of the earthquake.

The children seemed to need an oppportunity to master the earthquake experience as well as discharge feelings. The acting out of the disaster appeared to give them a chance to regain a feeling of control over their environment. After the dramatizations they were able to respond to an implicit suggestion to put the earthquake in the past by actively planning

Table 3. Correlation Between At-Risk Scores Before and After Interventions (1–4th Grades)[a]

Village	6 Months after		18 Months after		p	Risk
	Total no.	Percent at risk	Total no.	Percent at risk		
Calabrito	62	47	62	34	0.01	–
Caposele	40	8	40	20	0.05	+
Conza	41	20	41	20	0.01	–
Laviano	35	43	35	43	NS	
Pesco Pagano	77	9	77	24	NS	
Teora	45	9	45	7	0.01	–

[a] NS = not significant.

their future. The children needed a structured experience in order to begin to master and overcome their traumatic fears.

Our hypothesis that there would be more children at risk among those who had suffered a death in the family was not confirmed. Although there were differences in the pretesting at the time the posttesting was done (18 months after the earthquake) these differences had disappeared.

Either the children are more resilient than previously expected or community loss may be less traumatizing than individual loss. Another possibility is that this screening instrument is not sensitive to the kinds of problems that may have been generated. Other measures of the Calabritto children have been taken and are waiting analysis. This further exploration could provide more definitive answers to this question.

Another hypothesis that was not confirmed was the hypothesis that related to the amount of destruction being correlated with at-risk scores. It is interesting to explore why this hypothesis was not confirmed.

In considering why there were inconsistent results in the communities, we can eliminate pre-disaster differences. The communities share a common historical and cultural background that goes back approximately a thousand years. Therefore, an examination of the differences in the response to the event itself and the aftermath of the disaster is in order.

In all of the villages the experiences were essentially the same, with the exception of Laviano and Calabritto. The differences in these two communities were that they lacked coordination since the community leaders were either absent or missing. The effect was to delay many essential services including the resumption of regular school service.

The schools were particularly needed to keep the children occupied. The parents spent most their time beseiging the relief headquarters demanding better services. This not only absorbed their time and energy but also provoked a state of anger that was constant. Their bitterness was augmented by their awareness that the "others" (other villages) were "doing better." The families were strained and infuriated. Since the importance of the effect of the families has already been discussed, this in great part could explain the poor performance of these children.

A community that did surprisingly well was Conza. Just as the lack of coordinated leadership in the emergency situation was deleterious at Calabritto and Laviano, so the presence of effective support systems was positive in the case of Conza. In spite of the fact that the village had been rebuilt in a new location (as in Laviano) the children were doing very well. The school principal informed us with pride that in the first days after the earthquake the children were gathered (first under a tree and then under a tent) to enable them to express their feelings. It appears that as in the treatment program in Calabritto the opportunity to openly work through the fear and grief is critical.

The only other village where there was a significant decrease in at-risk scores is Teora. Once again we have evidence that instead of neglecting or attempting to avoid earthquake issues in Teora they were frequently brought out. They even self-published a book entitled *Teora Before and After*.

Open treatment of earthquake issues is important. It is still open for discussion if it is important that this be handled by specially trained personnel.

CONCLUSIONS

Children seem to be more resilient than they might be expected to be in the event of a disaster if a few basic needs are met: (1) most important is the availability of their family support systems. If the family is in a position to respond to the child instead of being absorbed by other issues the child seems to do better; (2) it appears to be helpful if the daily routine is quickly reestablished. Rapid resumption of school services is important; and (3) children are able to profit by a structured opportunity to discuss and work through their fears and disaster experiences.

The working through of their fears could be handled by local trained personnel and would not necessarily require a specially trained professional. This would permit a larger number of children to benefit by the treatment program.

The example of Conza and Teora confirms our conclusions. With or without a treatment program, given the minimum of these conditions, children can begin the long process of overcoming the negative effects of their tragic experience.

REFERENCES

Bowlby, J. (1973), *Attachment and Loss,* Vol. 2. New York: Basic Books.
Caplan, G. (1964), *Principles of Preventive Psychiatry.* New York: Basic Books.
Fredrick, C.J. (1982), Children of disaster. Paper read at the International Association of Child and Adolescent Psychiatry and Allied Professions, Dublin, Ireland.
Howard, S.J & Gordon, N.S. (1972), Mental health intervention in a major disaster. NIMH research grant MH 21649-09. Child Guidance Clinic, San Fernando, Calif.
Newman, C.J. (1976), Children of disaster: clinical observations at Buffalo Creek. *Amer. J. Psychiat.,* 133:306–312.

Terr, L.C. (1981), Psychic trauma in children: observations following the Chowchilla
    school-bus kidnapping. *Amer. J. Psychiat.,* 138:14–19.
Zimmerman, C. (1977), Unpublished manuscript.
Zimmerman-Tansella, CH., Minghetti, S., Tacconi, A. & Tansella, M. (1978), The
    children's behavioral questionnaire for completion by teachers in an Italian sample.
    Preliminary results. *J. Child Psychol. Psychiat.,* 19:167–173.

20

Psychological Management of Children in a National Crisis

Elmore F. Rigamer
United States State Department—Vienna, Washington, D.C.

This paper describes the psychological reactions of children in a national disaster and the intervention program which was developed through work with parents and teachers. The children studied are members of the American diplomatic communities in Afghanistan and Pakistan. The adults' initial response to the effect of the trauma on the children was denial, and this dynamic had to be addressed before the management suggestions of the consultant could be utilized. The majority of the children mastered the psychological effects of the trauma through repetitive narrations, drawings, and play. These activities seemed necessary to restore their emotional equilibrium. There was a small number of children, however, who appeared to adapt by shutting out all stimuli emanating from the event.

What follows is a description of the psychological management of children in a national disaster. The children and their families were members of the United States diplomatic community living in Afghanistan and Pakistan during the politically turbulent years of 1978 and 1979. During this period, I was assigned as a psychiatrist to the American Embassy in Kabul to develop a community mental health program for the American Foreign Service people serving there and in the neighboring

Reprinted with permission from the *Journal of the American Academy of Child Psychiatry*, 1986, Vol. 25. No. 3, 364–369. Copyright 1986 by the American Academy of Child and Adolescent Psychiatry.

countries of Pakistan, India, Nepal and Bangladesh. This brief presentation focuses on the children; although, of course, the intervention program necessarily involved all members of the resident American Community.

From April 1978 through November 1979 the American Community in Kabul experienced a threat from the Palestinian Liberation Organization, a Soviet sponsored political coup, and the assassination of the American Ambassador. Within the same period, the razing of the United States Embassy in the neighboring country of Pakistan forced the abrupt return home of American women and children for 10 months. In none of these occurrences could the host country government be relied upon to provide protection to diplomats and their families. These events, coupled with the hostage crisis in Iran, provided a substantial basis for a sustained level of apprehension and fear among Americans residing in these countries in 1978 and 1979.

INTERVENTION PROGRAM

The intervention program was developed in response to parents' request for assistance in managing their children's reactions to the political revolution which occurred in Afghanistan in April 1978. The individual and community approaches which evolved during the course of this work were to be used in the subsequent crisis situations in the region; the two most threatening to Americans were the assassination of the American Ambassador to Afghanistan and the destruction of the American Embassy in Pakistan. The examples presented here are taken from these three occurrences.

Living in the United State, it may be difficult to realize the impact such events have on Americans residing in a foreign country. The assassination in particular had a devastating effect on the American people stationed in Kabul at that time. People were dazed, finding it impossible to believe that such a horrifying act actually took place. True, other American ambassadors had been assassinated. But in this country there had been no suggestion that there was any significant anti-American sentiment among Afghans. In fact, Afghans looked then and still look to Americans for help in persuading the Russians to leave their country. The presumed sense of acceptance and security made the event all the more shocking and impossible to understand. Moreover, after the assassination one could not be sure that a new wave of terrorist activities against Americans would not be underway.

The entire community went into mourning. Families consoled each other and patiently listened to one another's emotional responses to the tragedy. Everyone attended the funeral services and accompanied the ambassador's body to the airport where it was then taken home to the United States. There was an intense admixture of sadness, anger, and fear. After the immediate shock of the event had passed, the next issue that had to be faced was the one of personal security and the possibility of having to leave the country if the situation deteriorated. People dealt with these emotions through the supportive network which a community of exiles in a foreign land usually forms in more normal times and almost always establishes in a crisis.

The adults for the most part seemed to be handling their own anxieties fairly well; when faced with the children and their responses to what was taking place, however, their resiliency and coping abilities foundered. Initially, parents and teachers were puzzled as to how to respond to questions the children were asking. "Will we be bombed too?" a child asked after passing an area strafed during an air attack of the revolution. "Can we get out of here or do we have to stay like the Afghans?" Or, another child asked after the death of the ambassador, "Are they going to kill more Americans?" and "Could Daddy be killed because he has an important job too?"

Reassurance was not enough; young ones repeated their questions while older ones tested answers and voiced more fears. Anxiety and its behavioral manifestations were not responding to the usual approaches parents adopt when their children are worried. When a situation like this develops one has the constituents of a crisis—the continued failure of problem-solving efforts when faced with a conflict. As has eloquently been explained by Caplan (1981), there is cognitive blunting and confusion with the result that one's problem-solving capacities are handicapped. An easy solution seemed to be to advise the parents to allow the children to talk and to encourage tolerance of the temporary regressive responses. But in a crisis that affects an entire community, such as a national disaster, everyone's coping abilities are put to test; so that for most of the adults their natural intuitive responses to the child's anxieties were simply not forthcoming (Block et al., 1956).

Intervention Approaches

Intervention was made in four areas: group discussions with parents, meetings and minilectures on relevant areas of child development with teachers, classroom observations and group discussions with children, and, finally, consultations with Embassy officials on the management of groups under stress. This last aspect is not treated in this paper.

Intervention with Parents

Foreign Service communities in developing countries have relationships and interactions very much like those in a small American town. In fact many families choose posts where the sense of community is known to be good. Group dynamics are pronounced and, in times of trouble, support as well as anxiety by contagion are both readily available. Apart from the unifying effect a shared disaster promotes, there already exists a disposition for foreigners to band together in an alien land. In Kabul the group already existed, and it provided an effective milieu in which to formulate community programs as well as to provide assistance and direction to individuals. It was very easy to marshall the resources of its members for uses in the approaches described in this paper. Direction, support, and information were given with the purpose of making the adults more effectively available to the children. But to accomplish this, specific suggestions on how to manage a frightened child were not enough. Parents needed help in understanding their initial, and what proved to be unhelpful, responses to the children's reactions to the disasters.

In the aftermath of the Afghan revolution when people met, there could be no topic of conversation other than who was doing what when the event took place, what else could have happened, what more was to come, and so on. Narratives were repeated innumerable times with the driven quality that so regularly characterizes responses to trauma, psychological or physical (Freud, 1914; Furst, 1967). Yet the adults' first responses to the children's repetitious talk were based on denial. When a child voiced a worry, adults were inclined to rush in with reassurance before the child could finish talking. In the classroom a teacher might listen at first and then, without much comment, would attempt to return the children to the tasks of the day. The distortions which were resulting from young children's fantasies were quickly silenced. There was a distinct tendency on the part of adults to hurry the child on in his talk, to challenge his perceptions prematurely, and to encourage him to go out and play, because nothing else bad would happen again. (If the child had not finished what he had to say, when he did go out to play war games seemed to be the play of choice). The process of mastering the trauma through verbalization and repetitious play was being unwittingly aborted.

There are individual as well institutional explanations for the use of denial in such situations. In a disaster everyone wants to believe that the event will not repeat itself; the occurrence is regarded as an aberration that will not take place again. With the abrupt and forced realization that one is not above the natural event of death, repression and denial come quickly back into play. Living in a hostile region and having to remain there, one naturally wants to recapture the belief that everything will be fine once again. Contributing to this righting mechanism is the occasional institutional pressure for diplomats to carry on and strive to report the hopeful or positive developments in the local political scene. For a parent to take the position that the child was not bothered by what took place, even when the child's behavior pointed to the contrary, reflected a denial not only of the effects of trauma on the child but also served to discount to the parent the seriousness of the event. Often the child's happy mood was cited as justification that he or she had not really been troubled or adversely affected.

It seemed therefore that the adults needed to deny the impact of trauma on the children; they used denial much more than the children did. With the child's relative lack of suppression and repression, his or her voicing of fears and raising other dreaded possibilities challenged the adults' defensive posture. The first request made of the consultant was for help in responding to questions the children were raising. Parents did not know whether to admit to the child that they were afraid. There was less trouble admitting sadness, but the concern about admitting fear was that the child would panic or become further upset if the parent acknowledged that he or she too was worried about what would happen next. To what extent does one admit one's fears?

While driving through Kabul, a mother reassured her child the worse was over. As soon as she said this, she came to a check point and panicked when a soldier pushed his machine gun into the car window mistakenly thinking she was not going to stop.

It is not right to belie feelings which are obvious to the child, but at the same time parents feel obliged to rid the child of unpleasant emotions. Through group discussions parents concluded that there was something to be gained if they admitted that they were afraid, and at the same time they assured the child that they were managing. The goal became not to dispel the feelings but to provide the child with a model of how to cope with them for the time.

Children from 5 through 7 years asked questions about the bombing such as, "Will this happen to us?" "Will we have to go home?" "Will you have to go home while I am at school?" Parents could better answer these questions once they recognized that, for a child in this age group, separation anxiety was a primary concern and was often beneath his or her repeated questioning and clinging. In answering the question if they were also able to speak to this concern, they were more successful in reassuring the child. Once the phenomenon of separation anxiety was understood and accepted, the community also made the decision actually to have the children remain closer to home by holding school temporarily in two sites instead of one. With this change there would be less risk of a child being unable to reach his parents should a new outbreak of fighting make it impossible to cross town.

Children from ages 7 to 11 tended to press further with such questions as, "What if we are killed?" "What if they attack us and our arms or legs are shot off?" The issue with them was one more concerned with bodily integrity and fear of injury than merely with separation, although this too was an issue. Understanding this, parents were in a much better position to respond effectively to the child's anxious and sometimes persistent queries.

Adolescents carried questions still further and, therefore, were told more. It was helpful to acknowledge their maturity by having various embassy officials meet with them for briefings. (This, incidentally, was also an important part of the intervention with the adult community.) When one adolescent pushed to the ultimate and asked, "Could a condition arise here where it would be impossible for us to get out?" an honest response was given. At the same time it was made clear what was being done, and which additional steps would be taken should the situation deteriorate further. I was impressed with the level of sophistication evidenced by these high school students. I believe that their coping abilities were enhanced when the measures taken spoke not only to their immediate needs but also addressed, as well, the developmental concerns characteristic for their age. Managed with the implicit assumption that they could handle more information than their younger peers, they responded accordingly.

Intervention in the School

School consultation had already been a part of the community mental health program for the embassy communities in Kabul and Islamabad. The faculty was accustomed to the idea of using a consultant, so that after the first crisis it naturally followed that we would discuss the matter in our weekly meeting. For the 2 weeks following the Afghan revolution, I met with groups of teachers two to three times a week. We shared our observations of the children and discussed management techniques for the classroom. The teachers were grouped according to the ages of the children they taught. I myself observed children in the classroom and on the playground. The small size of the school (122 students distributed approximately evenly in kindergarten through grade 12) made it possible for me to meet with each class. For an example of one such classroom conversation see Appendix I.

As with the parents, the teachers had to be reassured that it was necessary to allow the children to go over repeatedly their perception of what had taken place. Once their hesitation in allowing this was overcome, little else had to be done in the way of advising technique. As with the parents, the teachers wanted to know how to answer. Their tendency was to clarify distortions and offer reassurance at the child's first expression of fear. The timing of a comment on the part of a teacher was especially important. In the immediate aftermath of a crisis the net effect of a teacher's untimely comment, however positive, was to interrupt the conversational flow. Teachers of younger children were more apt to do this than were those who taught children in the middle grades and high school.

Adults mired in the crises themselves may have a harder time tolerating the frequency and intensity of an anxious child's verbalizations. Their protective instincts come into play, perhaps in response to the helplessness their own victim state creates. Adults feel better if they can make things better for the children. The recommendation was not that the conversation should go unmonitored; when verbalizations became progressively bizarre, as they did with a particularly anxious youngster, the group discussion was redirected. The teachers had to be reassured that going over the event would not make things worse, but was necessary and helpful.

Children from 6 through 9 years retold the events of the revolution and the assassination with a mixture of fantasy and fact; several focused their observations on their parents whose status of functioning was obviously very important to them. The younger ones, who were not verbal, were assisted to express what they felt through drawings and play.

In the middle school there was the expected insistence on the facts of these events, with conflict among students who could not agree on what actually took place. In the high school, there were more true discussions. Intellectualization was a well utilized method of dealing with frightening possibilities, and, given their age, the possibilities and alternatives they focused on were realistic and plausible.

With each of the incidents referred to here the majority of children age 10 or under almost uniformly became afraid of the host country's people.

Separation anxieties developed in 6 children (ages 5–7) when they were away from their parents. For all but 2, this response was not difficult to resolve and had disappeared by the second week after the event. For older children, hostile and suspicious feelings lingered and had not been resolved by the time they departed from the country; these reactions were more characteristic of children 11 through 15. Where mobs were involved in the violence, fears of groups of men made it impossible for these children to go anywhere in the city without American adults. The fear was generalized and most intense when they were in the street traveling from place to place.

After the assassination of the ambassador in Kabul, children spoke angrily about Afghans and showed an interesting response to the non-American students. Fights broke out on the school bus with the American children roughing up their non-American peers. We were perplexed as to why this was happening, especially to non-Afghans. In our discussion with the children, the focus had been on distinguishing the few Afghans responsible for the tragedy from the majority of the people in the country who had always been and still were gracious hosts. The explanations came when an 11-year-old boy volunteered, "Well they're foreigners too. These foreigners killed our ambassador and we hate them too." This brings up the interrelationship of cognitive operations and affective states in the young. Younger children and older ones under stress utilized almost exclusively inductive reasoning, generalizing from the particular to the general, in forming conclusions about strangers. This thinking in turn worsened their anxieties and fears. In the discussions we held, children spoke readily about all Pakistanis or all Afghans being suspect.

When the second grade class in Kabul returned to school after the coup and discovered that the pet rabbits were dead, they announced almost in unison, "The Afghans did this." In Foreign Service children up to late adolescence, one observes almost a uniform rejection of the host country culture, but these reactions were intensified when there was an objective basis for the antipathy.

First, second and third graders voiced fears that their fathers would be killed as the ambassador was since they were Americans and had important jobs too: "If it could happen to the ambassador, it could happen to Daddy." One youngster, 9 years old, knew the countries and names of the American ambassadors who had been assassinated over the last 10 years, and he brought this up in the discussion to show that it happened all the time. Dealing with such fears is difficult when events which justify them continue to occur. Although the children from Kabul had moved on by the time of the Iranian hostage crisis, one mother wrote to tell me that her young son was affected by the news of the hostages. He was now demanding they leave their new post and return home for fear that something else would happen.

In Kabul, there were two children who had been in therapy earlier in their lives, one 5 years ago at age 6, another for 2 years just prior to coming to the post at age 13. These children did not show any unusual responses until the second major event, the assassination of the ambassador which followed the coup by 9 months. The girl returned to the symptoms of hoarding food and compulsive lying, while the young adolescent boy became depressed and felt as he had when his parents divorced. He was able to say that he felt the same way now as he had then; he gave as a reason that nothing mattered so why should he be bothered with anything. These two children and a third adolescent not reported here were overwhelmed by the occurrences and have required continued treatment.

DISCUSSION

The children in this study were trying to come to grips with a crisis in a manner consistent with their age, level of development, and previous experiences. They showed more distress when the adults who dealt with them resorted to denial as a coping mechanism.

One group of children, however, favored denial as a means of accommodating to each traumatic event. This group, smaller in number, did not deal with stress in the active manner used by their peers, but rather remained on the periphery of discussions at school and did not feel compelled to go over the events repeatedly with their parents at home. Unlike those who were not talking but were expressing symptoms, this group showed no impairment of functioning either by their own account or by their parents' and teachers.' They walled off or shut out horrifying stimuli, stating that they did not feel much and especially did not feel fear. Though these children were not followed for longer than 6 months, the assumption is that they may be like the adolescents, described by Wallerstein and Kelly (1974), who get through their parents' divorce by not participating on any level in the trauma as it unfolds. They posed no problem provided their defenses were respected.

With the other groups, those for whom denial was ineffective or where the repetition compulsion was unwittingly disrupted, their reactions to the stress were compounded as the adults persisted with habitual problem-solving measures even when they were proving ineffective. These are the factors that create a psychological crisis (Caplan, 1981; Ewing, 1978).

In such occurrences the outcome can be easily influenced by the intervention of others. While the person in the crisis may not be operating at an optimum level, he very often is receptive to outside help. This calls for the therapist to assume an explicit, directive, and encouraging role. He guides the individual to an accurate cognitive appraisal of the situation knowing that the more that is understood about internal and external events, the more likely an adaptive resolution can be reached. In the work with parents and teachers discussed here, this entailed group discussions of how children respond to stress and the responses adults could make to help them to adapt. The use of the group served to encourage people to develop patterns of accepting help from interpersonal resources within the community, and this became an integral part of the intervention program for subsequent crises.

APPENDIX I: CLASSROOM DISCUSSION

This conversation took place in a third grade classroom during the week following the assassination of the American ambassador in Kabul. The teacher began the discussion by asking what had happened during the weekend. A class member responded by saying he had visited so and so's house and played baseball or had gone to the commissary.

The teacher repeated, "Well, what else happened?"

Jane: "I was going to take a balloon to school today, but the worst thing that happened to me was that my mother would not let me take a balloon."

"Yes, we were going to take balloons too," said another, "but my mother would not allow me to either." A feature of the conversation was that when the children were not talking about what had affected them, their talk became increasingly meaningless or nonsensical. The child continued, "Only babies carry balloons to school; that is why my mother would not let me carry them."

"No, our mothers will not let us carry balloons to school, because the balloons will pop and that will sound like a gun shot," Eileen corrected.

The teacher repeated for the third time, "What else happened this weekend?"

Harry: "Well, I don't know about these other kids; I think they are all lying. We all stayed home this weekend because the ambassador died this weekend. We stayed home this weekend because it was a sad time; we went out to see him go; we went to his funeral."

Eileen: "Yes, he was sent back to America. A whole lot of people were at the airport, but no Afghans were there. They killed him and they did not even come to the airport."

This was something that was noticeable. The Afghan authorities did not attend the funeral services, and their absence caused comments which filtered down to the children. Harry continues, "They did not even come to the airport after they shot him all through the head and the heart and the chest and the legs. This was something really stupid and really mean. He was really a nice guy. When he was at my house, he played baseball with me and when we went to visit him, he asked my mother, 'Do you want tea or coffee?'"

Lisa: "And his poor wife came all the way here and they had her turn around and go right back without being able to go shopping on Chicken Street." Here we see expressed the peculiar mixture or coexistence of opposing feelings, the blend of the tragic with day to day life events. The wide fluctuations in the child's emotional and cognitive states explain these seeming paradoxes. This is one explanation of why the diagnosis of childhood depression is often missed in children, particularly if the therapist expects to find a sustained depressive mood.

Mary: "My mommy saw what happened. She saw everything; she knows more than anybody knows and she knows someone who saw even more than she saw. But she won't tell who it is—it is a big secret. No one else knows." Whereupon a little girl popped up and gave the name of the person who knew the big secret and she was quite right, children being as they are notorious enemies of conspiracy.

The following part of the conversation continued on for several minutes. One child said, "Then his arm came off, then his leg was shot, then there was blood everywhere and his eyes came out and there were five bullets in his head."

"No, there were four bullets in his head."

"No, there were five bullets in his head."

There was a need to go over these gruesome details. It was uncomfortable to hear but they could not stop talking about this.

Harry adds: "There were several people in the room and there were lots of problems about how many people really were in that room." Amazing, for this was indeed one of the controversies that surrounded the bizarre incidents of the assassination, but one which was supposedly discussed privately. He continued, "Now we can't go on the streets ever again. My daddy cannot go on the streets;

he will be killed because he has an important job too. But my daddy said they are not going to take him because he is not going to stop for policeman any more." (The ambassador was taken when he willingly stopped at the request of a terrorist posing as a policeman.)

"The Ambassador was killed because the Afghan Government would not wait; they just would not wait. President Carter was on the phone; the U.S. Government said to wait but the Afghans said to shoot and they shot. And my mother said that these people are really stubborn; nobody expected that they would wait; they don't do what you tell them anyway."

James: "We are really going to kick them; the American Government has Marines in Peshawar and marines and soldiers are going to come over right now."

Sean: "No, the Marines can't come any more; people will really get very mad at us if we let the Marines come."

Patrick: "But we are mad at them anyway; we don't care if the world or other people are mad at us; they killed our ambassador."

"People say that tourists did this."

Mary: "Yes, my mother said that tourists did this and that there are a lot of bad tourists here. They always come here to take drugs." They were confusing the word "terrorist" with "tourist" but generalized from this assumption to all the hippie-looking folks in town at that time.

"These hippie people that come through," she continues, "they not only take drugs which are bad for you, but maybe one of them even killed the ambassador."

Harry: "No you dummy, not *tourist, terrorist.* Terrorists are people who kill other people to get something that they want."

Lisa: "You know this government really likes the Russians, the ones who killed Daoud are the same ones who killed the ambassador."

Patrick, very excited, shouts, "No, no, they are not the same ones; that is not so; my mother said that Teraki tried to help us here. Teraki killed Daoud and the Russians helped Teraki do this, but he did not want this to happen, so it is not the same people who killed Daoud."

The little boy who initiated the conversation said, "I want to talk about the bullets going through his veins." Mary names the people who were there when the Ambassador was killed and says that they told her everything that took place.

Lisa: "My mom has been crying all weekend. Whenever I go into her room, she tells me to go back into my room or to go outside and play."

Harry: "Well, my mother lets me see her cry; she thinks it upsets me, but it really doesn't. After I saw her cry, I went outside and I played ball."

Mary: "I knew that they would kill him as soon as they got him; they wouldn't let him go; he wouldn't tell any secrets and they wanted secrets."

Harry, who kept calling kids dummy, said, "No, you dummy, they didn't want secrets, they wanted money."

Lisa: "No, you are both wrong. You both are dummies; they did not want money; they wanted people released who were taken by the coup." This was the alleged reason.

Sean: "If they take us all because we are Americans and put us in that hotel and blow up the hotel then the American Army will come from Peshawar."

Harry: "No they still wouldn't come." So the teacher says, "Do you think that they will take all of us and put us in that hotel?"

Patrick: "No, the ambassador was the easiest one to get to, and they really don't want to do this to all of us. He had an important job; we are not in danger."

The teacher explains, "That's right. He was important and that was what happened to him." Whereupon Lisa interrupts, "Well I think that he could have gotten out of the room. If he had pretended that he was on their team, when they were asleep, he could have gotten out."

Alice: "Why didn't they take the Afghan President instead of taking our ambassador?"

Lisa: "Don't you understand why they didn't take the Afghan President? They didn't take him because they wanted prisoners released, and if they had taken him there would be no one there to release the prisoners. He wouldn't be there to go open the door to let the prisoners out."

REFERENCES

Block, D., Silber, E. & Perry, S.E. (1956), Some factors in the emotional reactions of children to disaster. *Amer. J. Psychiat.,* 113:416–420.

Caplan, G. (1981), Mastery of stress: psychosocial aspects. *Amer. J. Psychiat.,* 138:413–420.

Ewing, C.P. (1978), *Crisis Intervention as Psychotherapy.* New York: Oxford University Press.

Freud, S. (1914), Remembering, Repeating, and Working Through. *Standard Edition,* 12:147–156. London: Hogarth Press, 1962.

Furst, S. (1967), *Psychic Trauma.* New York: Basic Books.

Wallerstein, J.S. & Kelly, J.B. (1974), The effects of parental divorce: the adolescent experience. In: *The Child in His Family: Children at Psychiatric Risk,* ed. E.J. Anthony & C. Koupernik. New York: John Wiley & Sons.

Part VI
SPECIFIC CLINICAL SYNDROMES

The paper by Voeller, "Right-Hemisphere Deficit Syndrome in Children," examines the possible relationships between right-brain hemisphere dysfunctions in children and their behavioral deviations. It is a clear exploration of a possible clinical syndrome, which merits a great deal of investigation. The author lists seven issues suggested by the findings, which require further study. We would add an eighth issue, namely the need to compare these findings with a comparison group with left-hemisphere dysfunction.

Clearly, this paper leaves much to be done. Its virtue is the clarity with which it opens the question of relationship between right-hemisphere lesions in children and their concurrent behavior disorders. Part of its value is also the specificity of the additional research that the author's findings highlight.

There has already been considerable documentation that a characteristic constellation of behavior disorders tends to be found in girls with Turner's syndrome after puberty. It is not clear, however, whether this behavioral syndrome of social immaturity, low emotional arousal, and need for outside structure, amongst others, is due entirely to biologic brain features, to small stature, to delayed puberty, and/or to the other noticeable negative physical features of Turner's syndrome, such as webbed neck and digital and nail defects.

In the present study by McCauley and his associates, two groups were compared: (1) Turner's syndrome; and (2) short-statured girls matched for age, height, verbal IQ, and family SES. Well-selected questionnaires tapped both mothers' and teachers' views of these girls' significant differences in social functioning, and acceptance of the Turner's girls in contrast with the control group was found. The authors discuss these differences in terms of the various factors that contribute to the findings.

An excellent critique, "An Examination of the Borderline Diagnosis in Children," by Greenman and her coworkers searches out the similarities and dissimilarities of the diagnosis of adult borderline syndrome in the childhood and adolescent years. Using a sample of hospitalized children divided into those fulfilling the borderline criteria of Bemporad's group and the control children who did not, the results of the Greenman study were both in disagreement with the authors' own hypothesis and with prior data arising from studies of borderline children by other authors. Their results raise doubts, at least with regard to their own sample of nonpsychotic children, that there is a syndrome of borderline personality in children.

The authors mention their plan to follow up these subjects. Such a follow-up could give us valuable data as to the *predictive* significance of how predictable are these childrens' patterns of behavior with respect to further performance, and whether current vulnerability to reality testing loss will, over time, remain at the same level, heal, or move toward frank psychosis.

Anorexia nervosa has long been a puzzle to the layperson and professional alike. The fact of an otherwise physically normal person, usually a female, starving herself to the point of malnutrition while believing herself to be fat is hard to understand. Most previous reports have focused upon possible etiologies, clinical descriptions associations in some cases with additional clinical diagnoses, and the relative value of various therapeutic approaches. As has been pointed out by Steinhausen and Glanville in a review article, "Follow-up Studies of Anorexia Nervosa: A Review of Research Findings," which was published in the 1984 volume of this series, previous follow-up studies have been of limited value as they have failed to utilize assessment instruments that could supply comparability between studies. In the present article, "Long-Term Follow-up of Anorexia Nervosa," by Toner and her group, these methodological inadequacies have been remedied. We have, therefore, a detailed, thorough, long-term follow-up study of anorexic and bulimic cases, along with a control group utilizing a number of measures that can be replicated by other investigators.

While there have been a number of studies of obsessive-compulsive neuroses in children, this paper by Rapoport, "Childhood Obsessive Compulsive Disorder," has brought together the available information in a concise and clear review and has also reported the data of her own extensive NIMH study. It is of interest that the onset of obsessive-compulsive behavior is discontinuous with the children's premorbid personality. There is enough of a hint of possible association with Tourette's syndrome, with conduct disorder, and with neurological findings to supply leads for future exploration. To date, no one medication has proven to be of particular helpfulness in diminishing or eliminating symptoms.

PART VI: SPECIFIC CLINICAL SYNDROMES

21

Right-Hemisphere Deficit Syndrome in Children

Kytja K.S. Voeller
Medical College of Ohio, Toledo

The author describes 15 children with behavioral disturbances, a characteristic neuropsychological profile, and neurological findings consistent with right-hemisphere damage or dysfunction. Almost all of the children had attention deficit disorder. Some were obtuse or unable to interpret social cues, others could not express their feelings but appeared to be sensitive and aware of the emotions of others. The older children were generally in psychotherapy or counseling but responded poorly, suggesting that a different approach to treatment may be indicated.

It is generally accepted that the right hemisphere of the human brain has a special role in maintaining attention, processing visuospatial information, and expressing and interpreting emotional information (1-3). Although the behavioral sequelae of right-hemisphere lesions in adults have been well described, there have been few descriptions of a similar syndrome in children. Denckla (4) noted that children with left-sided neurological signs (therefore, right cerebral dysfunction) manifested so-

Reprinted with permission from the *American Journal of Psychiatry*, 1986, Vol. 143, No. 8, 1004–1009. Copyright 1986 by the American Psychiatric Association.

Presented at the 138th annual meeting of the American Psychiatric Association, Dallas, May 18–24, 1985.

Supported in part by Biomedical Research Support grant RR-05700 from the National Institutes of Health.

The author thanks Dr. V.R. Fitzgerald for his comments and Drs. M. Denckla, A. Galaburda, and J. Kemph for their critical reading of the manuscript.

cial failure with their peers. Weintraub and Mesulam (5) described 14 adolescents and adults with right-hemisphere deficits who had a pervasive disturbance of their capacity to interact with other human beings. From a psychiatric perspective, Horton (6) hypothesized a relationship between nondominant parietal lobe dysfunction, inability to develop relationships, and personality disorder. The psychiatrist who treats children should be aware that disturbed function of the right hemisphere can produce a characteristic syndrome that may require special therapeutic strategies.

In this report I describe the behavioral, neurological, and neuropsychological characteristics of 15 children with evidence of right-hemisphere dysfunction.

METHOD

Fifteen patients, 10 boys and five girls ranging in age from 5 to 13 years, were selected out of some 600 children referred for a pediatric neurological evaluation for behavior and learning problems. Criteria for selection were evidence of a right-hemisphere lesion or dysfunction (on the basis of a neurological examination and/or a CAT scan), age between 5 and 13 years, and a verbal or performance IQ of 90 or more. Patients were excluded if there was evidence of bilateral brain involvement or if they had been adopted and pertinent information was missing. A detailed history was compiled from hospital and school records as well as from interviews with parents, teachers, and therapists. Information regarding prenatal or perinatal encephalopathic events, neonatal behavior, development, school performance, learning problems, behavior, and family history was recorded. The standard neurological examination was supplemented by a fine motor battery (Denckla's fine motor tests [7] and the Purdue Pegboard [8]). Each child was tested using the WISC-R or the Wechsler Preschool and Primary Scale of Intelligence. Also used was a neuropsychological battery consisting of a variety of language tasks including the Oldfield Naming Test (9,10), the Rey-Osterrieth Complex Figure (11) or a simpler figure developed for younger children, and the Wide Range Achievement Test (12) supplemented by other academic measures, the Woodcock Reading Mastery Test (13) and the Key Math test (14).

Two tests, the Affect Recognition Test (15, 16) and the Auditory Affect Recognition Test (17; Tallman et al., unpublished paper), which were developed to assess a child's ability to interpret the affective states of others, were administered. Norms for the Affect Recognition Test are based on Hanson's (15) study of 95 normal girls and 113 boys age 5–9 years. The Auditory Affect Recognition Test norms are derived from Tallman's study (17) of 80 normal girls and 80 normal boys age 5–12 years. In the 24-item Affect Recognition Test the child selects the appropriate stimulus out of a set of five pictures; e.g., "Show me the child who is happy" (or sad, angry, or frightened). The Auditory Affect Recognition Test involves matching 30 samples of a 20-word segment of speech, filtered so that only the intonational pattern remains, to five stick figures that are happy, sad, angry, frightened, or loving. Raw scores on these tasks were converted into z scores, using the norms developed by Hanson (15) and Tallman (17), thus removing age as a variable. The results of CAT scans performed using a third-generation scanner and EEGs were available for all patients except one.

RESULTS

Seven patients had abnormal obstetrical histories: patients 2, 5, and 7 were premature; patient 3 was a 46-week, postmature infant who had had a traumatic delivery and neonatal seizures; patients 4 and 8 sustained hypoxic insults; and patient 15 had been exposed to multiple problems during the pregnancy. Four patients had suffered postnatal injuries: patient 15 had had a hypoxic episode in infancy; patient 10 had developed a left hemiparesis and seizures following an episode of dehydration with a high fever at the age of 4; and patients 11 and 12 had had right-sided skull fractures at the age of 4 and 5 years, respectively. Eight families (those of patients 1, 3, 5, 6, 8, 9, 13, 14) reported that close relatives had emotional problems and difficulty in interpersonal relationships. For instance, the mother of patient 9 described her husband as having "no emotions. He is always laid back and nothing seems to bother him or make him take something seriously."

Seven subjects were reported to have preferred the right hand before 1 year of age, which suggests an early left hemiparesis.

As shown in table 1, two subjects were left-handed. Patient 3, who had no family history of sinistrality, was said to have had a bilateral brachial plexus palsy at birth, which may account for the atypical hand preference. However, on several fine motor tasks, his left-handed performance was considerably poorer than his right-handed. Patient 4, whose mother was left-handed, also preferred the left hand despite left-sided motor and parietal signs. Nine subjects (patients 2, 3, 6, 7, 8, 9, 13, 14, 15) had left-sided motor signs—asymmetry of the face, posturing of the left upper extremity on toe-walking, left hyperreflexia, left Babinski signs and/or poor

Table 1. Characteristics of 15 Children with Behavioral Disturbances

Patient	Sex	Age (years)	Abnormal History		Family History of Emotional Problems	Age Hand Preference Manifested (years)	Presence of Neurological Impairment			CAT Scan Findings[b]
			Obstetrical	Postnatal			Asymmetrical Opticokinetic Nystagmus	Motor Signs[a]	Parietal Deficit	
1	M	5			Yes	<1	Yes	Yes	Yes	Atypical R<L asymmetry
2	M	6	Yes			<1		Yes		Dilated R lateral ventricle
3c	M	7	Yes		Yes	>5		Yes		Normal
4c	M	7	Yes			>2	Yes	Yes		Dilated R lateral ventricle
5	F	7	Yes		Yes	<1	Yes	Yes		Hypodensity R temporal lobe
6	F	7			Yes	2		Yes		Normal
7	F	8	Yes			<1		Yes		Dilated R lateral ventricle
8	M	8	Yes		Yes	<1		Yes		—
9	M	9			Yes	2	Yes	Yes		Atypical R<L asymmetry
10	M	9		Yes		>4		Yes	Yes	R parietal lesion
11	M	10		Yes		>5		Yes	Yes	Enlarged R sylvian fissure
12	M	10		Yes		—	Yes	Yes	Yes	R parietal lesion
13	F	11			Yes	<1		Yes		Normal
14	M	11			Yes	2		Yes		Atypical R<L asymmetry
15	F	13	Yes	Yes		<1		Yes		Normal

aLeft-sided motor signs, manifested by gait asymmetry, decreased left arm swing, left hyperreflexia, left Babinski sign, flattening of left nasolabial fold, poorer left-handed performance on fine motor battery than in normal population.

bAtypical R<L asymmetry refers to marked underdevelopment of right hemisphere, without obvious atrophy, to a degree that exceeds normal cerebral asymmetry.

cLeft-handed.

left-handed performance on the fine motor battery. They did not have asymmetric opticokinetic nystagmus or parietal sensory signs (a deficit in graphesthesia, asterognosis, or extinction of left-sided stimuli on double simultaneous stimulation). Five subjects (patients 4, 5, 10, 11, 12) had motor signs in combination with asymmetrical opticokinetic nystagmus and/or parietal sensory signs. Patient 11 was the only one to manifest left-sided neglect. Patient 1, who had no motor signs, had asymmetrical opticokinetic nystagmus and a left parietal sensory deficit. Although he did not manifest left-sided neglect when he was examined at age 5 years, his mother had reported him as having a pronounced right-sided gaze preference as a newborn.

As shown in table 1, four types of CAT scan abnormality were noted: large right parietal lesions (patients 10 and 12), mild degrees of focal atrophy or attenuation (patients 5 and 11), a dilated right lateral ventricle (patients 2, 4, and 7), and a striking asymmetry in size of the hemispheres (right smaller than left) that exceeded the normal cerebral asymmetry seen in right-handed individuals (patients 1, 9, and 14). Patients 3, 6, 13, and 15 had normal CAT scan results.

EEGs revealed right parietal spikes in patients 4 and 10, a right anterior temporal spike focus in patient 3, and decreased voltage over the right parietal area in patient 11. The remaining subjects had normal EEG results.

The mean±SD verbal IQ (108.7 ± 18.2) was significantly higher than the mean±SD performance IQ (91.2 ± 16.1) (t = 3.48, df = 14, $p <$ .005, paired sample t test, one-tailed). Nine of 14 subjects (64%) had a verbal-performance gap that exceeded 15 points; a verbal-performance gap of 15 points is significant at the $p <$ .01 level (18). Testing the sample proportion of 64%, we found the gap to be significant (binomial distribution, N = 15, r = 9, $p <$ .0001). Only patient 2 had a performance IQ that was 10 points higher than his verbal IQ (see table 2).

The subjects performed significantly better in reading than arithmetic on the Wide Range Achievement Test (t = 3.48, df = 14, p < .005, paired sample t test, one-tailed). This pattern of scores was corroborated through testing with the Woodcock Reading Mastery Test and the Key Math test.

All subjects except patients 2 and 10 were either in small special education settings or in private schools. Their behavior was hard to manage at home and in the classroom. As shown in table 3, 14, of the 15 children (93%) were extremely distractible and inattentive and met the criteria for the *DSM-III* classification of attention deficit disorder. Eight were also hyperactive. (The subjects had been selected without regard to the issues

Table 2. IQs and Wide Range Achievement Test Scores of 15 Children with Behavioral Disturbances

Patient	IQ[a]			Wide Range Achievement Test Standard Score		
	Verbal	Performance	Verbal Minus Performance	Reading	Spelling	Arithmetic
1	126	76	50	95	95	105
2	75	91	−16	108	108	98
3	126	99	27	92	95	80
4	95	69	26	85	99	92
5	135	86	49	105	107	96
6	90	58	32	129	108	89
7	108	102	6	108	89	96
8	129	106	23	109	87	99
9	91	91	0	109	94	80
10	94	91	3	92	86	92
11	97	81	16	109	100	92
12	105	86	19	89	95	81
13	124	102	22	100	97	98
14	127	114	13	106	108	92
15	109	116	−17	94	95	77

[a]The Wechsler Preschool and Primary Scale of Intelligence was administered to subjects 1 and 3; the WISC-R to all others.

Table 3. Hyperactivity and Behavior Problems in 15 Children with Behavioral Disturbances[a]

Patient	Hyperactivity		Drug Treatment	Atypical Prosody	Gesturing Deficit	Shyness, Withdrawal	Insensitivity	Poor Peer Relations
	Age at Onset	Attention Deficit						
1	Neonate	Yes	Yes	Yes		No	Yes	Yes
2	Neonate	Yes	Yes	Yes			Yes	Yes
3	3 years	Yes	Yes	Yes	Yes	Yes		Yes
4	3 years	Yes		Yes	Yes	Yes		Yes
5	5 years	Yes	Yes			Yes		Yes
6	1 year	Yes		Yes	Yes		Yes	Yes
7	Infancy	Yes					Yes	Yes
8	4–5 years	Yes	Yes			Yes		Yes
9	Infancy	Yes		Yes	Yes	Yes		—
10	—					Yes		Yes
11	4 years	Yes		Yes	Yes	Yes		—[b]
12	5 years	Yes	Yes	Yes	Yes		Yes	Yes
13	Neonate	Yes	Yes	Yes			Yes	Yes
14	2–3 years	Yes		Yes	Yes		Yes	Yes
15	Neonate	Yes		Yes	Yes	Yes		Yes

[a]Onset of hyperactivity and drug treatment was determined from parental history and medical records. Information regarding attention deficit, withdrawal, obtuseness, and peer relationships is based on history from parents, school officials, and therapists. Data on shyness, attention deficit, interpersonal skills, deficient prosody, and gesturing are based on direct observation.

[b]Patient 11 had a bone disease and was often in a cast. There were few complaints about his peer relationships, but his mobility was limited, and he spent much of his time under adult supervision.

of attention deficit disorder or hyperactivity.) The probability of encountering 93% of children with attention deficit disorder in a sample is significant (binomial distribution, N = 15, r = 14, $p < .0001$), and stands in sharp contrast to the prevalence of 3%–10% for attention deficit disorder in the population of school-age children. Seven patients had been treated with pemoline or methylphenidate. The only child who was neither distractible nor hyperactive was a shy, withdrawn boy (patient 10) who had been left-handed (his mother was also left-handed) before the acute onset of a left hemiparesis at age 5 years. It is possible that there was atypical cerebral asymmetry. As to age at onset of hyperactivity, four children (patients 1, 2, 13, and 15) were described as irritable, active, inconsolable neonates, which suggests either a preceding encephalopathic event or congenital predisposition. In contrast, patient 6 was described by her mother as a very "good" newborn who was extremely quiet and "did not need affection."

Eight of the children were withdrawn and isolated. Other children avoided them and considered them "weird." Although some of the subjects could play with one other child, particularly a younger child who could be "bossed," they could not play with groups of children. Seven children were obtuse and behaved inappropriately and often were involved in fights—they pushed and crowded their classmates, who then would hit them. They could not maintain friendships. One mother noted that her daughter "can make friends but loses them just as fast as she makes them." The children were also on a different "wavelength" than their peers. The mother of patient 4 reported that when she was driving her son in a car with other boys, "they were talking about ball games and he was talking about the way train signals worked." They often could not grasp the nuances of social situations. Patient 1 had no fear of strangers and did not know when an adult was furious with him. When testing patient 2, an examiner noted, "He was a most difficult child . . . he was unusually unaware of such things as being timed, so that he would stop and . . . talk to me during a timed task." This child's father stated flatly that he "could not get along with him at all." The unawareness and lack of concern about the consequences of antisocial acts contributed to the arrest of a 13-year-old girl (patient 15) for shoplifting. The girl had been assured by another child that "nothing would happen" if she took the purse.

The components of emotional expression—prosody, facial expression, and gesture—have not been defined for the pediatric age group. Nonetheless, half of the patients appeared to have atypical prosody: patients 1, 2, and 4 had the high-pitched rapid rates of speech that have been described by adults with left hemiplegia (19). Patient 15 had a very soft, low-pitched voice; patients 3 and 9 had monotonous, robot-like intonations. Patients 3, 4, 6, and 12 seemed "deadpan" and had a limited repertoire of expressions. Patient 9 made inappropriate facial expressions and rocked rhythmically. Eye contact was deficient in most of the patients and was of particular concern to teachers. For instance, the teacher of patient 1 complained that it was very difficult to get his attention ("It is necessary to first establish eye contact").

The mean±SD z scores were −1.13 ± 1.5 for the Affect Recognition Test and −2.14 ± 1.12 for the Auditory Affect Recognition Test (see table 4). Since by definition the mean z score of the control subjects is 0.0, the subjects as a group performed below the level expected for their normal peers. In order to test the hypothesis that subjects with parietal lesions would perform more poorly on these tasks than would subjects without parietal lesions, I compared the performance of the subjects with parietal lesions (alone, or in combination with anterior lesions) to that of subjects who did not have evidence of parietal lesions, i.e., who had only motor signs. Although there was a sizable difference between the mean±SD group z scores of the parietal and anterior lesion groups on the Affect Recognition Test (parietal group = −1.4 ± 1.96; nonparietal =

Table 4. Affect Recognition Scores in 15 Children with Behavioral Disturbances

Patient	Affect Recognition Test (15, 16) z Score[a]	Auditory Affect Recognition Test (17) z Score[a]
1	−3.0	−2.3
2	−0.9	−1.8
3	0.8	−0.2
4	−3.6	−3.2
5	−1.4	−2.2
6	−0.5	−2.6
7	−1.1	−1.2
8	—	—
9	−0.4	—
10	1.0	−3.6
11	−2.3	−2.0
12	—	−2.9
13	—	−0.4
14	—	−3.3
15	—	—

[a]Patient's raw score minus mean of age-matched control subjects divided by the standard deviation of age-matched control subjects.

-0.4 ± 0.9), this difference did not reach statistical significance (t = -0.94, df = 8, p = .37, independent sample t test, one-tailed). However, on the Auditory Affect Recognition Test, the groups' mean±SD z scores were significantly different: parietal group = -2.7 ± 0.63; non-parietal = 1.6 ± 1.22 (t = -1.99, df = 10, p = .038, independent sample t test, one-tailed).

Patients 3, 7, 8, 9, and 15 were receiving some form of psychotherapy or counseling. The patients did not respond well to therapy, as their behavior and interpersonal interactions were hard to modify. The parents of patient 15, who was seeing a psychologist, reported that some of her disruptive behaviors at home had improved. The parents of patient 9 left group therapy after a few months, feeling that there had been little change.

DISCUSSION

It appears that right-hemisphere dysfunction has a profound impact on a child's capacity to develop the ability to behave in an effectively appropriate fashion and to perceive the emotional states of other human beings. Left-sided neurological findings, better verbal than visuospatial abilities, and higher reading and spelling than arithmetic achievement test scores seem to characterize this group of children.

Some of the subjects performed better than one might expect on the facial Affect Recognition Test. There are several reasons for this. First, one often finds considerable variability in the severity with which adults respond to right-hemisphere lesions, and children are no different. Second, the ability to interpret facial affective cues appears to develop earlier than does the ability to interpret intonational patterns, and the normal child learns to recognize certain emotions earlier than others. Gates (20) showed that by the age of 3 years, 70% of her subjects could recognize the facial expression "happy," but only 30% could recognize "angry" and none recognized "fear" or "anguish." Thus, the Affect Recognition Test is an "easy" test for the 9-year-old because it deals primarily with the recognition of affective states that are mastered early in development. There is need for a more sensitive instrument for testing the older child. Finally, Ross (2) observed that in adults, frontal lesions impair the expression of emotion (i.e., produce atypical prosody and gesturing), whereas lesions affecting the parietal area interfere with the perception and interpretation of the emotional states of others. In the children described here, the subgroup with parietal lesions, performed more poorly than did those who did not have evidence of parietal lesions, which suggests that there is a similar localization operating. However, this is obviously a preliminary study and needs to be expanded.

An equally intriguing finding, worthy of further study, is the remarkably high percentage of children in this group with right-hemisphere deficits who also manifested attention deficit disorder with or without hyperactivity. Brumback and Staton (21) have suggested that such a relationship between right-hemisphere involvement, attention deficit disorder, and depression might exist. Certainly, studies on adults indicate that right-hemisphere lesions have profound effects on attentional mechanisms (22).

The child's interpersonal and behavior problems should not be attributed purely to the associated attention deficit disorder. There are many children with attention deficit disorder who do not have the profound disturbances in interpretation and expression of affect manifested by the subjects in this study. Moreover, drug treatment improved the attention deficit but did not change the other behavioral or learning problems.

Several other issues require further study:

1. Although studies in progress would support the idea that the right hemisphere has a special role in the processing of affect in children (Voeller, unpublished paper), more rigorously controlled studies of the impact of brain lesions in childhood on the perception of affect need to be carried out. The different roles of the right and left hemispheres and of the effect of cortical and subcortical lesions need to be further elucidated.

2. Does the timing of the brain insult affect the outcome? Do children with prenatal or perinatal lesions respond in the same fashion as do children who sustain lesions later in childhood? On the basis of this study, it appears that both early and late lesions have an impact on the acquisition of the expression and interpretation of emotion, but this still remains speculative.

3. Is there a genetic form of this syndrome? Several patients had family members with similar atypical behaviors. In the series of older subjects reported on by Weintraub and Mesulam (5) there also appeared to be a genetic component.

4. What are normal prosody, eye contact, and gesture in children? Although a physician can describe adult behavior in a meaningful way using terms such as "flat affect," "diminished eye contact," and "atypical prosody," it is hard to know what is abnormal and what is not in children. A well-designed study of the expression of affect in children would make it possible to define atypical behaviors in a more rigorous manner.

5. What is the relationship of this syndrome to alexithymia (23)? The constricted emotional functioning and lack of expression of these patients and the possible hereditary component suggest a similarity between the two syndromes.

6. Is there an overlap between the children described here and the depressed children with left-sided neurological signs (therefore, having right-hemisphere involvement) who were described by Brumback and Staton (21)?

7. How well will these children respond to traditional psychotherapy? They need to learn how to interpret the social cues that occur in everyday interpersonal interactions. Therapy may be more successful if it is focused on teaching the child to *express* emotion appropriately ("When you feel that way, you are sad and you look like this") or on how to *interpret* the significance of facial expression in others ("When Johnny looks like that, he is very angry with you"). Minskoff (24) has suggested an approach for teaching children to learn to make such discriminations. Identification with the therapist may also provide a mechanism for learning about appropriate expression and interpretation of affect. However, as Ross and Rush (25) noted in adults, one cannot conclude that because a patient does not express affect he or she does not feel it. It remains to be seen if children with these deficits will be able to learn to discriminate between the subtle nuances of the communication of affect sufficiently well to maintain normal peer relationships.

REFERENCES

1. Heilman KM, Bowers D, Valenstein E: Emotional disorders associated with neurological diseases, in Neuropsychology. Edited by Heilman KM, Valenstein E. New York, Oxford University Press, 1985
2. Ross ED: The aprosodias: functional-anatomic organization of the affect components of language in the right hemisphere. Arch Neurol 38:561–569, 1981
3. Mesulam M-M: A cortical network for directed attention and unilateral neglect. Ann Neurol 10:309–325, 1981
4. Denckla MB: Minimal brain dysfunction, in Education and the Brain. Edited by Chall J, Mirsky A. Chicago, University of Chicago Press, 1978
5. Weintraub S, Mesulam M-M: Developmental learning disabilities and the right hemisphere: emotional, interpersonal and cognitive components. Arch Neurol 40:463–468, 1983
6. Horton PC: Personality disorder and parietal lobe dysfunction. Am J. Psychiatry 133:782–785, 1976
7. Denckla MB: Development of speed in repetitive and successive finger movements in normal children. Dev Med Child Neurol 16:729–741, 1973
8. Costa LD, Scarola LM, Rapin I: Purdue Pegboard scores for normal grammar school children. Percept Mot Skills 18:748–750, 1964

9. Oldfield RC, Wingfield A: A series of Pictures for Use in Object-Naming. Medical Research Council Psycholinguistic Research Unit Special Report Plu/65/19. London, Medical Research Council, 1965

10. Denckla M, Rudel R: Naming of object-drawings by dyslexic and other learning disabled children. Brain Lang 3:1-15, 1976

11. Rey A. Lexamen psychologique dans les cas d'encephalopathie traumatique. Arch Psychol 28:286-340, 1942

12. Jastak JF, Jastak SR: The Wide Range Achievement Test Manual. Wilmington, Del, Guidance Associates, 1978

13. Woodcock RW: Woodcock Reading Mastery Test. Circle Pines, Minn, American Guidance Service, 1973

14. Connolly AM, Nachtman W, Pritchett EM: Key Math, Diagnostic Arithmetic Test. Circle Pines, Minn, American Guidance Service, 1976

15. Hanson J: The effects of localized right cerebral dysfunction on affect recognition skills of primary school aged children (doctoral dissertation). Toledo, Ohio, University of Toledo, College of Education, 1982

16. Voeller K, Hanson J: The effect of right hemisphere deficit on affect recognition in children (abstract). Ann Neurol 14:360, 1983

17. Tallman JH: The identification of emotional meanings in electronically filtered speech: a study of right brain injured and normal children (doctoral dissertation). Toledo, Ohio, University of Toledo, College of Education, 1984

18. Kaufman AS: Intelligent Testing with the WISC-R. New York, John Wiley & Sons, 1979, p 24

19. Dordain M, Degos J-D, Dordain G: Troubles de la voix dans les hemiplegies gauches. Rev Laryngol Otol Rhinol (Bord) 92:178-186, 1971

20. Gates GS: An experimental study of the growth of social perception. J. Educational Psychol 14:449-461, 1923

21. Brumback RA, Staton RD: An hypothesis regarding the commonality of right hemisphere involvement in learning disability attentional disorder, and childhood major depressive disorder. Percept Mot Skills 55:1091-1097, 1982

22. Heilman KM, Watson RT, Valenstein E: Neglect and related disorders, in Clinical Neuropsychology. Edited by Heilman KM, Valenstein E. New York, Oxford University Press, 1985

23. Taylor GJ: Alexithymia: concept, measurement, and implications for treatment. Am J Psychiatry 141:725-732, 1984

24. Minskoff EH: A teaching approach for developing nonverbal communication skills in students with social perception deficits. J Learning Disability 13:118-124, 1980

25. Ross ED, Rush EJ: Diagnostic issues and neuroanatomical correlates of depression in brain-damaged patients: implications for a neurology of depression. Arch Gen Psychiatry 38:1344-1354, 1981

PART VI: SPECIFIC CLINICAL SYNDROMES

22

Psychosocial Functioning in Girls with Turner's Syndrome and Short Stature: Social Skills, Behavior Problems, and Self-Concept

Elizabeth McCauley
University of Washington School of Medicine, Seattle
Joanne Ito
University of Washington, Seattle
Thomas Kay
New York University Medical Center, New York

The social relationships and behavioral characteristics of 17 preadolescent and adolescent girls with Turner's syndrome were assessed in comparison to a control group of 16 short stature girls of comparable age, height, verbal IQ and family socioeconomic status. The assessment included parent and teacher ratings of social and behavioral functioning as well as subjective self-report data. The results depict the Turner's syndrome subjects as doing more poorly in terms of peer relationships and having more behavioral problems than short stature controls. The Turner's syndrome subjects were described by parents and teachers as having

Reprinted from the *Journal of the American Academy of Child Psychiatry*, 1986, Vol. 25, No. 1, 105–112. Copyright 1986 by the American Academy of Child and Adolescent Psychiatry.
    This investigation was supported in part by Biomedical Research Funds from the Children's Orthopedic Hospital and Medical Center. The authors thank Drs. V. Sybert, R. Pagon, R. Mauseth, V. Kelley, and V. Lewis, R. N., Melanie Pepin, M.S. and J. Johnson, M.S. for their help in subject recruitment. We also thank Ms. Marianne Bischell for her help in data collection and Ms. Marge Ferris for her preparation of the manuscript.

fewer friends, needing more structure to socialize and to complete tasks, and having more difficulty understanding social cues. Behavioral problems were endorsed on all subscales of the Child Behavior Checklist with most problems in the area of immature, socially isolated behavior. The results are discussed in relation to the role of delayed sexual maturation, other physical anomalies, and brain maturation.

Individuals with Turner's syndrome are phenotypic females with an absent or structurally abnormal second sex chromosome. These patients have been the focus of research efforts aimed at evaluating the impact of sex chromosomal anomalies on subsequent growth and development. Research efforts looking at the psychological development of these patients have identified cognitive impairment in the area of visual-spatial problem solving (Alexander et al., 1966; Money, 1963; Money and Alexander, 1966; Money and Granoff, 1965; Shaffer, 1962; Silbert et al., 1977). Other studies have focused on identifying the incidence of gender identity related problems and major psychiatric disorders in this patient group.

Investigations of issues related to gender identity formation (Ehrhardt et al., 1970; Garron and Vander Stoep, 1969; Money and Mittenthal, 1970) have consistently found strong female gender identification in women with Turner's syndrome. For example Ehrhardt et al. (1970) found that, in contrast to a control group matched for age and socio-economic level, patients with Turner's syndrome showed patterns of conventional or stereotyped female behavior with a significantly lower incidence of tomboyism during childhood. Sexual orientation is consistently reported as heterosexual, but sexual drive in adult patients has been described as low (Garron and Vander Stoep, 1969; Hampson et al., 1955).

In the area of psychopathology, occasional case reports detail serious psychopathology (Raft et al., 1976; Sabbath et al., 1961), and an increased frequency of anorexia nervosa has been noted (Halmi and DeBault, 1974; Kron et al., 1977). However, studies of groups of women with Turner's syndrome do not describe a consistent pattern of psychiatric symptoms or a markedly increased prevalence of major psychiatric problems (Garron and Vander Stoep, 1969; Hampson et al., 1955; Money and Mittenthal, 1970; Shaffer, 1962). These studies do describe similarities in personality patterns within their samples of Turner's syndrome patients. Money and Mittenthal (1970) describe the predominant personality feature as "inertia of emotional arousal" further characterized by unassertiveness, compliance and ready acceptance of misfortune.

In a more recent study, Nielsen et al. (1977) contrasted the social and psychological adjustment of 45 Turner's syndrome patients 7–39 years of age with that of two control groups. One control group was the natural sisters of the patients and the second was a group of short stature women with primary amenorrhea but no chromosomal anomaly. They found a low frequency of psychopathology in all three groups, and no differences in academic or occupational achievement. The Turner's syndrome sample was seen as less socially mature than their sibs as measured by factors such as extent of peer relationships, independence from parents, and marrying or living with a partner. However, they did not differ significantly from the other short stature women in this regard. As an additional aspect of the study, Baekgaard et al. (1978) looked at the performance of 31 of the Turner's syndrome women on the Maudsley Personality Inventory in contrast to that of 16 sisters, 9 control women, and an additional control group of female nurses. The Turner's syndrome patient sample scored significantly lower than any of the control groups on the Neuroticism Scale. Their scores on this scale were unusually low, which suggests individuals who are not easily aroused and have a high tolerance for stress. Baekgaard and colleagues (1978) interpret these results as stemming from the impact the loss or anomalous formation of one X chromosome has on early central nervous system development and later cerebral integration.

In a study focusing on child and adolescent patients Sonis et al. (1983) compared the socialization and behavioral profiles as measured by the Child Behavior Checklist (Achenbach, 1978, Achenbach and Edlebrock, 1979) of 16 girls with Turner's syndrome compared to a control group of girls matched for age, race, and socioeconomic status. They found an increased incidence of behavior problems, particularly in the younger Turner's syndrome patients. The patient group had problems reflecting immaturity and poor attention skills as well as poor peer relationships. Sonis et al. (1983) suggest that the behaviors of these patients possibly reflect the results of delayed central nervous system myelinization.

Other investigators have looked at personality and psychosocial functioning in girls with Turner's syndrome from a different perspective. Perheentupa et al. (1974) and Taipale (1979), in Finland, conducted a study of statural growth and psychological development in 36 Turner's syndrome patients to address the question of optimal timing of hormone treatment. Their psychological assessments revealed adequate self-concepts and peer relationships until the time of puberty. At puberty, girls who were not developing along with their peers became socially withdrawn and immature in their behavior and fantasies. Perheentupa and colleagues suggest that this regression can be avoided if the timing of estrogen replacement is such that Turner's syndrome patients begin pubertal development within the same time frame as their peers. These researchers suggest that the pattern of withdrawn, socially immature behavior is not a characteristic of this genetic syndrome, but is secondary to delayed puberty.

Thus, the existing data suggest that girls and women with Turner's syndrome, as a group, tend to have a particular personality style characterized by immaturity, low arousal and high stress tolerance with short attention span in younger patients. However, there is disagreement about the etiology of this behavior pattern. Some researchers see it as a biologically based result of the genetic anomaly while others view these characteristics as behavioral adaptations to being short statured and sexually immature. Some support for the latter position comes from Nielsen et al.'s (1977) study that found adult women with Turner's syndrome to be similar to short stature, amenorrheic women without a genetic anomaly, in immaturity of social independence and assertiveness. Furthermore, children with constitutional growth delay have been shown to be at higher risk for behavior problems, such as social withdrawal, immaturity and low self-esteem (Gordon et al., 1982; Holmes et al., 1982).

The present paper reports on a study which looks at the social relationships and behavioral characteristics of preadolescent and adolescent girls with Turner's syndrome compared to a control group of short statured girls. The two groups were comparable in terms of age, verbal IQ, height and familial socioeconomic status (SES). The study looks at whether Turner's syndrome patients have fewer friends and poorer social relationships than other short stature girls, and secondly whether there is a higher incidence of behavioral problems in girls with Turner's syndrome. The study has two major advantages: the inclusion of a matched short statured control group and the use of teacher as well as parent and self-report data.

METHOD

Subjects

Subjects were recruited from the patients with Turner's syndrome followed in the Endocrine and Genetics Clinics of a major pediatric hospital. Patients between 9 and 17 years with a verbal IQ of over 79 were included. Twenty-nine patients were contacted and 22 participated in the study. Seven chose not to participate in the study. Of these, one was severely retarded, three did not want to commit the time, and three did not participate because their parents did not want to make an issue of Turner's syndrome. Five of the participants were excluded from the final sample because their verbal IQs were 79 or below.

The final index sample consisted of 17 subjects with karyotypes consistent with a diagnosis of Turner's syndrome. Ten of the patients had 45, X karyotypes; two had 45, X/46, X, r(X); one 45, X/46, XX; one 46, XiX; one 45, X/46, X, i(Xq); one 45, X/46, XXp; and one 46, XX; Xp-. Eight subjects were currently taking replacement hormones. Of these, seven were taking conjugated estrogens (Premarin®) 0.3–0.625 mg on days 1–25 and medroxyprogesterone acetate (Provera®) 5–10 mg on days 15–25. One subject was taking oxandrolone (Anavar®) at the time of assessment and six others had previously had a trial of oxandrolone 3–12.5 mg per day to promote statural growth.

Control subjects were recruited from the population of girls seen in the Endocrine Clinic for an evaluation of short stature. All of the control subjects were below the 5th percentile in height. These patients had received a careful clinical evaluation including genetic studies in 15 cases. Short stature was determined to be familial in 14 cases, secondary to chronic asthma in 1 case, and related to a non-X-linked genetic anomaly in the 16th case. One control child had also received a trial of oxandrolone to stimulate growth but was no longer taking this medication at the time of this study. Twenty-two short stature patients were contacted regarding the study and 17 agreed to participate. One of these was dropped from the final sample because of a verbal IQ below 80. Five chose not to participate, three because of the inconvenience of the study, one because the parents did not want to make an issue of the child's short stature, and the fifth parent agreed but the child refused.

The Turner's syndrome and control subjects were comparable in terms of age, height, verbal IQ, and family SES (see Table 1). The age means were 13.1, s.d. 2.43, for the index group and 12.91, s.d. 2.75, for the controls. The mean height was 52.01 inches for the index group and 52.8 for the control.

Intellectual ability was determined at the time of participation in the study and was measured using the age appropriate Wechsler Intelligence Scale. The mean verbal IQ for the index group was 95.4, s.d. 10.62, and 99.94, s.d. 12.04, for the control group. As would be expected, the Turner's syndrome subjects had significantly lower performance IQs than the control subjects (Turner's syndrome subjects $M = 91.41$, s.d. = 10.92; controls $M = 107.5$, s.d. = 14.01, $t = -3.77$, $p < 0.001$).

Table 1. Sample Characteristics: Turner's Syndrome (TS) and Short Stature (SS) Subjects

	TS (N = 17)		SS (N = 16)		p
	M	S.D.	*M*	S.D.	
Age	13.11	2.43	12.91	2.75	NS
Height (inches)	52.01	4.98	52.80	4.50	NS
Weight (lb)	78.38	22.10	77.30	20.10	NS
Verbal IQ	95.41	10.62	99.94	12.04	NS
SES	40.94	15.79	44.81	14.60	NS

Family SES was determined using the revised Hollingshead Index (1975). The two groups had similar SES profiles with the index group having a mean of 40.94, s.d. 15.79, and the controls having a mean of 44.81, s.d. 14.6. Both means fall into the minor professional/technical social strata according to the Hollingshead system.

Sixteen of the index subjects were Caucasian and one was black. All of the control subjects were Caucasian.

Materials and Procedure

Each subject completed the Friendship Questionnaire (Bierman and McCauley, 1984), the Chumship Checklist (Mannarino, 1978), the Children's Depression Inventory (Kovacs, 1980), and the Piers-Harris Self-Concept Scale (Piers, 1969). The Friendship Questionnaire was designed to include simple, concrete, and specific questions about a child's peer relationships which could be easily and objectively answered by children. Four open-ended questions were included to allow children to describe their friendships in their own words (e.g., number of friends, best friends). Each of these questions was asked twice—once concerning friends at school, and a second time concerning friends at home. Then children were presented with a series of 32 rating items on which they estimated the frequency of specific positive and negative behaviors with peers. They were asked how often specific interactions, such as getting teased by peers, occurred and answered using 5-point Likert scale (0—none of the time, never to 5—all of the time, everyday). Half of the items referred to positive interactions and half to negative; half were interactions typical of school settings and half were interactions likely to occur in home settings; half referred to initiations received from peers while the others referred to behaviors directed toward peers. Scores on these items were summed to form two scores—a positive interaction score and a negative interaction score. The internal psychometric properties of the Friendship Questionnaire were evaluated based upon a total sample of 251 children (Bierman and McCauley, 1984).

The Chumship Checklist asks the child to indicate the number and nature of activities he or she engages in with best friend and then friends in general. The Children's Depression Inventory is a 27-item self-rating scale that assesses symptoms of depression such as sad mood, loss of appetite, and hopelessness. The Piers-Harris is a commonly used self-report, self-concept scale. The scale has 80 items with a total score reflecting overall self-concept and six subfactors; behavior, school status, physical appearance, anxiety, popularity, and happiness. Higher scores indicate a more positive self-concept.

The mother of each child also completed a battery of questionnaires. Mothers completed the Friendship Questionnaire (Bierman and McCauley, 1984), the Child Behavior Checklist (Achenbach, 1978; Achenbach and Edelbrock, 1979), and a Parent-Teacher Questionnaire. The Friendship Questionnaire has been described above. It had not been used with parents before, but we felt it was important to have comparable parent and child reports of peer interactions. The Child Behavior Checklist (CBCL) was developed as a standardized measure of the behavior problems and competencies of children age 4 through 16. The current version has two sections; the first consists of social competency scales concerning school performance and the amount and quality of participation in sports, games, hobbies, chores, organizations, and social relationships. Parents are asked to rate the children's activities in comparison to other same-age children. The second section consists of 113 items covering a variety of behavior problems. The CBCL is filled out by parents who respond by circling 0—indicating that the item is not true of their child, 1—indicating that the item is somewhat or sometimes true, or 2—indicating that the item is often true or very true. The CBCL can be scored for three social competency scales: activities, social, and school, and 10 behavioral problem cluster scales including depressed, aggressive, and somatic complaints. The scales are also divided into two general factors so that Internalizing and Externalizing scores are obtained. The Scale provides information about the prevalence and nature of behavior problems in relation to a normative sample.

Parents also completed the Parent-Teacher Questionnaire, a scale developed for this study to assess areas of behavioral concern that have been identified in the literature for girls with Turner's syndrome. The scale consists of 55 items each rated on a 5-point scale, with a high score reflecting the greatest difference from the same age children. There were 11 subsets consisting of 5 items each covering the following areas: seeks adult help; seeks social approval; need for structure and guidance; maturity; problems with teasing; participation in free play; emotional/social awareness; denial of difficulty; ability to recognize rejection; emotional vulnerability; and popularity. The questionnaire included items such as "This child denies that things bother her," "This child initiates play with other children," etc. Teachers completed this questionnaire also.

Each subject and their parent(s) were seen in an outpatient clinic area of a Child Psychiatry Clinic. All data were collected in a single session. Informed Consent was obtained from all subjects and parents.

RESULTS

Social Relationships

The responses from the Friendship Questionnaires are summarized on Table 2. The results indicated that the Turner's syndrome subjects reported fewer friends ($t = 2.71$, 31 df, $p < 0.01$) and more negative interactions with peers ($t = 2.58$, 31 df, $p < 0.05$) than did the control subjects. The two groups did not differ on number who named a best friend, rating of positive peer interactions, or the number of activities on the Chumship scale. Mothers' responses on the Friendship Questionnaire were significantly different on number of friends ($t = -4.18$, 29 df, $p < 0.001$) as well as number of children with a best friend ($t = -2.57$, 30 df, $p < 0.05$) and positive interaction with peers (-4.6, 27 df, $p < 0.001$). In all cases, the Turner's syndrome sample had scores indicating less positive peer interactions than the short stature controls.

On the three Social Competency scales of the CBCL, mothers of Turner's syndrome subjects indicated poorer adjustment than control mothers: activities ($t = -1.49$, 31 df, NS), social ($t = -3.2$, 31 df, $p < 0.005$), and school performance ($t = -4.29$, 31 df, $p < 0.001$). Table 3 summarizes these findings. Both groups had raw score means which were within the normal range on these scales. However, the index subjects were at the 55th percentile for activities, 16th percentile for social and 7th percentile for school, whereas the short stature girls were at the 68th percentile for social and the 50th percentile for school.

Mothers were also asked to compare the subjects' social relationships with those of their siblings. On these ratings, 12 or 71% of the Turner's

Table 2. Friendship Questionnaire Responses of the Turner's Syndrome (TS) and Short Stature (SS) Subjects and Their Mothers

Friendship Questionnaire	Subjects				Mothers			
	TS		SS		TS		SS	
	M	(s.d.)	M	(s.d.)	M	(s.d.)	M	(s.d.)
Open-ended Questions								
No. of friends	6.4	(3.98)	10.12	(3.88)**	2.9	(2.35)	6.2	(2.1)**
Best friend	0.59	(0.51)	0.87	(0.34)	0.47	(0.51)	0.87	(0.35)*
Behavioral Rating Items								
Positive interactions	5.46	(1.09)	6.37	(1.53)	4.65	(1.62)	6.71	(0.9)*
Negative interactions	3.08	(0.98)	2.41	(0.37)*	2.65	(0.59)	2.47	(0.44)
Chumship								
Best friend	12.3	(2.36)	11.86	(2.21)				
Friends	7.76	(4.01)	9.75	(2.54)				

* $p < 0.05$; ** $p < 0.01$.

Table 3. Social Competency Scales (T Scores) of the Child Behavior Checklist for Turner's Syndrome (TS) and Short Stature (SS) Subjects

Social Competency	TS		SS		p
	M	(S.D.)	M	(S.D.)	
Activities	49.52	(5.44)	52.00	(3.90)	NS
Social	39.39	(10.94)	49.57	(6.37)	0.005
School	35.41	(8.28)	46.81	(6.84)	0.001

syndrome subjects were rated as worse than siblings in contrast to 4 or 25% of the short stature group ($\chi^2 = 7.0$, 2 df, $p < 0.05$).

On the Parent and Teacher Questionnaire, mothers and teachers rated the Turner's sample as having more difficulties than peers (mother— $t = 3.44$, 26 df, $p < 0.01$; teachers—$t = 2.92$, 20 df, $p < 0.01$). Turner's syndrome and control mothers rated their children differently on the following 7 of the 11 clinically derived sets of items: needs guidance and structure ($t = 4.89$, 30 df, $p < 0.001$), maturity ($t = 2.85$, 30 df, $p < 0.01$), seeks social approval ($t = 2.73$, 31 df, $p < 0.01$), participation in unstructured play/activities ($t = 2.97$, 28 df, $p < 0.01$), social emotional perceptiveness ($t = 2.91$, 27 df, $p < 0.01$), emotional vulnerability ($t = 2.22$, 28 df, $p < 0.05$), and popularity ($t = 4.42$, 29 df, $p < 0.001$). Teachers also rated the two groups as significantly different on six of the item sets: needs guidance and structure ($t = 3.16$, 29 df, $p < 0.01$), teased ($t = 2.9$, 29 df, $p < 0.01$), participates in free play (29 df, $p < 0.01$), social emotional perceptiveness ($t = 2.91$, 27 df, $p < 0.01$), emotional vulnerability ($t = 2.22$, 28 df, $p < 0.05$), and popularity ($t = 4.42$, 29 df, $p < 0.001$). Both parents and teachers rated the Turner's syndrome subjects as having more problems in these areas. Parent and teacher reports were positively correlated (Pearson correlation coefficient of 0.62, $p < 0.005$).

Behavior Problems

One the self-report measures, the Turner's syndrome subjects demonstrated significantly lower self-concept on the Piers-Harris Children's Self-Concept Scale. This was reflected in the overall self-image score ($t = -3.7$, df 31, $p < 0.001$), as well as in five of the six factors: intellectual and school status ($t = -2.66$, df 31, $p < 0.01$), physical appearance ($t = -3.92$, df 31, $p < 0.001$), anxiety ($t = -2.03$, df 31, $p < 0.05$), popularity ($t = -4.17$, df 31, $p < 0.001$), and happiness ($t = -3.40$, df 31, $p < 0.01$). The groups did not differ on the behavior factor of the Piers-Harris Scale or on the Children's Depression Inventory. Therefore, although the Turner's syndrome children indicated low self-concept they did not endorse features of clinical depression.

Mothers reported type and frequency of behavior problems in their responses to the CBCL. TheCBCL has norms for children divided by sex and by age groups (6–11 and 12–16 years). This sample spanned both age groups but the majority were in the older age group; therefore, all subjects were analyzed according to the 12–16-year-old norms (Achenbach and Edelbrock, 1983). Turner's syndrome subjects were rated as having more behavior problems on the following scales: Depressed-Withdrawn ($t = 3.31$, df 31, $p < 0.005$), and Immature-Hyperactive ($t = 3.60$, df 31, $p < 0.005$). They also had higher scores on the broader band Externalizing Factor ($t = 2.13$, df 31, $p < 0.05$). See Table 4 for a summary of these CBCL results. All the group means were within the normal range (55–70 T scores), with the Immature-Hyperactive Scale approaching the upper limits of the normal range with a mean T score of 69.06.

An item analysis was performed to identify particular items differentiating the index and control subjects. This was done using the method described by Sonis et al. (1983). Ten items differentiated the two groups and were more frequently reported for the Turner's syndrome subjects. The items were: acts too young, gets teased a lot, secretive, easily jealous, worrying, stubborn, complains of loneliness, can't concentrate, impulsive, not liked by other children.

Table 4. Behavior Problem Scales (T Scores) of the Child Behavior Checklist for Turner's Syndrome (TS) and Short Stature (SS) Subjects

Behavior Problem Scales	TS		SS		p
	M	(s.d.)	M	(s.d.)	
Anxious-Obsessive	65.35	(11.25)	59.94	(5.70)	NS
Somatic Complaints	61.13	(7.39)	66.13	(10.61)	NS
Schizoid	62.71	(8.14)	58.56	(7.34)	NS
Depressed Withdrawn	65.65	(8.65)	56.87	(6.29)	0.005
Immature-Hyperactive	69.06	(10.40)	58.44	(9.19)	0.005
Delinquent	61.76	(7.28)	58.94	(6.35)	NS
Aggressive	60.76	(10.53)	57.25	(3.53)	NS
Cruel	64.76	(9.20)	57.12	(13.27)	NS
Other Problems	5.65	(5.59)	3.12	(2.33)	NS
Internalizing	19.71	(14.38)	11.56	(8.53)	NS
Externalizing	17.24	(15.18)	8.37	(7.68)	0.05

DISCUSSION

The results of the present study consistently depict the Turner's syndrome subjects as doing more poorly in terms of peer relationships and having more behavioral problems than the short stature controls. The Turner's syndrome subjects were described by parents and teachers as having fewer friends, needing more structure to socialize and to complete tasks, and having more difficulty understanding social cues. Concerns were raised about a wide variety of behavioral problems covering all subscales of the CBCL. In general, the results suggest an increased level of overall concern about the behavior of these girls rather than a focused, circumspect problem area. The elevated Immature/Hyperactive scale reflects in great part the poor social relationships and immaturity also reported in the Friendship Questionnaire and the Parent and Teacher Questionnaire. The items most frequently endorsed on the Immature/ Hyperactive scale were: acts too young (14 of 17 index subjects), is teased (14 of 17), prefers younger children (13 of 17). Furthermore, the girls with Turner's syndrome were rated as significantly higher on the Externalizing Scale of the CBCL. This suggests that their parents do not see them as withdrawn and retiring but as having more acting out behaviors. The items most frequently endorsed on the Externalizing dimension were: argues a lot (16 of 17), jealous (12 of 17), impulsive (12 of 17), secretive (12 of 17).

In contrast to previous reports, the present results suggest more compromised social functioning and behavioral distress than that found by Money and Mittenthal (1970) or Nielsen et al. (1977). The present results are generally consistent with those reported by Sonis et al. (1983) with some areas of discrepancy. This sample was rated across raters and a variety of instruments as having serious deficits in social competency, while Sonis et al's. (1983) subjects were not so clearly identified as deficient in these areas. Furthermore, Sonis' subjects are seen as hyperactive where the present sample seems more socially immature with "hyperactivity" specifically being endorsed for only 7 or 41% of the group. Sonis et al. (1983) suggest that hyperactivity is more a problem in younger Turner's syndrome patients and decreases with age and further neurological maturity. In this sample, an item asking about hyperactivity specifically was endorsed for 3 of the 5 (60%) patients in the younger age (11 or below) group as opposed to 4 of 12 older girls (33%). This is consistent with Sonis et al.'s finding; however, data on a greater number of Turner's syndrome subjects would be needed for this finding to be confirmed.

The Parent and Teacher Questionnaire was designed to tap the kinds of problems described for Turner's syndrome patients such as low emotional arousal, immaturity, and unassertiveness. Teachers and mothers see the Turner's syndrome girls as more in need of outside structure to complete tasks and make decisions; as less assertive in terms of participating in spontaneous play and more likely to be involved only in organized group activities; as less aware or sensitive to others' needs, and finally as less popular with peers. Neither mothers or teachers saw the Turner's syndrome subjects as having a greater tendency to deny or ignore difficulties or to be unresponsive to rejection. Thus, the parent and teacher reports and the children's own report of low self-image do not support the hypothesis that these children have unusually high stress tolerance and reduced reaction to negative feedback. They are clearly seen as doing poorly and report feeling badly about themselves. The present sample also does not appear to be correctly characterized by a primary picture of hyperactivity as described by Sonis et al. (1983). Rather the most consistent characteristics are social ineptitude and isolation. This kind of social isolation has been observed in some adult women with Turner's syndrome (McCauley et al., in preparation) as well.

The generalizability of the present results are clearly limited because of sampling issues. Both the Turner's syndrome and short stature samples are small and may be biased. Parents with significant concerns about their children may be more likely to participate in this type of project. The control sample did turn out to include children who appear to be doing well in terms of both intellectual and social skills. Other studies of short stature children have found more behavioral and social concerns (Gordon et al., 1982; Holmes et al., 1982). However, we attempted to minimize the bias by using short stature children who had been of enough concern to their parents to pursue an evaluation into the cause of their slow growth.

The present findings suggest that short stature is not the reason for the social and emotional difficulties of the Turner's syndrome patients. The short stature control sample, although teased about their size, do not show a high prevalence of behavior problems, appear to hold their own with peers and report self-image scores within the normal range.

A number of factors could explain the problems seen in the Turner's syndrome subjects. First is the issue of delayed sexual maturation. Delayed pubertal timing does not appear to completely account for the social deficits found in the present study since only the two oldest subjects had begun hormone treatment later than 13 (one at 15 and the second at 17). The second subject had shown some spontaneous sexual development initially so hormone treatment had been postponed. Of course, hormone replacement only mimics the natural pubertal process but does not completely duplicate the hormone production or fluctuation of the naturally cycling woman. Thus, hormonal differences rather than simply delayed puberty may contribute to the behavioral problems seen.

The second important factor is the other physical anomalies that sometimes accompany Turner's syndrome, such as webbing of the neck and digital and nail defects. These anomalies affect the physical appearance of the Turner's syndrome girls and may lower self-confidence or cause others to react negatively to them. However, many girls with Turner's syndrome have few perceivable physical anomalies other than their short stature. In the present sample, the number of external physical anomalies was not correlated with parent or teacher ratings of social competence but was correlated with the Turner's syndrome subjects ratings on the Piers-Harris Children's Self-Concept Scale. Specifically, a greater number of physical anomalies was significantly correlated with a lower self-image score on the physical appearance ($r = -0.45, p = < 0.05$) and anxiety ($r = -0.52, p = < 0.05$) subscales.

A third critical factor could be differences in brain development and maturation. Research on the cognitive development of Turner's syndrome patients has documented problem solving deficits suggestive of right hemisphere weakness (Alexander and Money, 1965; Alexander et al., 1966; Money, 1963; Silbert et al., 1977), while other research points to more global cross hemisphere deficits (Pennington et al., 1982; Waber, 1979). These defictis have been attributed to delayed brain maturation secondary to the lack of prenatal and pubertal ovarian hormone activity. One study (Buchsbaum et al., 1974) of Turner's syndrome women not taking exogenous hormones found EEG patterns similar to those of prepubescent girls rather than adult women. It is possible that some of the social difficulties these patients have are due to cognitive immaturity which impedes problem solving in both social and intellectual spheres.

In sum, young Turner's syndrome patients present more social and behavioral problems than do other short statured girls with no genetic anomalies. These difficulties do not appear to be behavioral adaptations to short stature nor do they appear to be easily ascribed to delayed puberty. The present sample exhibited significant social difficulties even when hormonal replacement was begun at an age similar to that of the normally developing peer. The results support a need to examine further the impact of delayed neurological development on social and emotional adjustment as well as on cognitive functioning. Moreover, the results highlight the need for clinicians to be sensitive to the social and emotional difficulties these patients and their families may be having. Early identification of behavioral concerns, and therapeutic or educational intervention when appropriate might short circuit the long term negative impact on self-esteem and social involvement.

REFERENCES

Achenbach, T. (1978), The child behavior profile; I. Boys age 6–11. *J. Consult. Psychol.*, 43:478–488.

_____ & Edelbrock, C. (1979), The child behavior profile; II. Boys aged 12–16 and girls aged 6–11 and 12–16. *J. Consult. Clin. Psychol.*, 47:223–233.

_____ (1983), Manual for the Child Behavior Checklist and Revised Child Behavior Profile. Queen City Printers.

Alexander, D., Ehrhardt, A.A. & Money, J. (1966), Defective figure drawing, geometric and human in Turner's syndrome. *J. Nerv. Ment. Dis.*, 42:161–167.

Baekgaard, W., Nyborg, H. & Nielsen, J. (1978), Neuroticism and extroversion in Turner's syndrome. *J. Abnorm. Psychol.*, 87:583–586.

Bierman, K. L. & McCauley, E. (1984), A Standardized child interview to assess social competence and peer relationships. Unpublished paper.

Buchsbaum, M.S., Henkin, R.I, & Christiansen, R.L. (1974), Differences in averaged evoked responses in normal population with observations on patients with gonadal dysgenesis. *Electroencephalog. Clin. Neurophysiol.*, 37:137–144.

Ehrhardt, A.A., Greenberg, N. & Money, J. (1970), Female gender identity and absence of fetal hormones: Turner's syndrome. *Johns Hopkins Med. J.*, 126:234–248.

Garron, D.C. & Vander Stoep, L.R. (1969), Personality and intelligence in Turner's syndrome. *Arch. Gen Psychiat.*, 21:339–346.

Gordon, M. Crouthamel, C., Post, E.M. & Richman, R.A. (1982), Psychosocial aspects of constitutional short stature: social competence, behavior problems, self-esteem, and family functioning. *J. Pediat.*, 101:477–480.

Halmi, K. A. & DeBault, L.E. (1974), Gonosomal aneuploidy in anorexia nervosa. *Amer. J. Hum. Genet.*, 26;195–198.

Hampson, J.L., Hampson, J.C. & Money, J. (1955), The syndrome of gonadal agenesis (ovarian agenesis) and male chromosomal pattern in girls and women: psychologic studies. *Bull. Hopkins Hosp.*, 97:207–226.

Hollingshead, A.B. (1975), Four Factor Index of Social Status. Unpublished Paper.

Holmes, C.S., Hayford, J.T. & Thompson, R.G. (1982), Personality and behavior differences in groups of boys with short stature. *Child. Hlth. Care*, 11:61–64.

Kovacs, M. (1980/81), Rating scales to assess depression in school-aged children. *Acta Paedopsychiat.*, 46:305–315.

Kron, T., Katz, J.L., Gorzynski, G. & Weiner, H. (1977), Anorexia nervosa and gonadal dysgenesis. *Arch. Gen. Psychiat.*, 34:332–335.

Mannarino, A.P. (1978), The interactional process in preadolescent friendships. *Psychiatry*, 41:308–312.

McCauley, E. Ehrhardt, A.A. & Sybert, V. (1984), A reevaluation of the social function of adult women with Turner's syndrome. Paper in preparation.

Money, J. (1963), Cytogenetic and psychosexual incongruities with a note on space form blindness. *Amer. J. Psychiat.*, 119:820–827.

_____ & Alexander, D. (1966), Turner's syndrome: further demonstration of the presence of specific cognitional deficits. *J. Med. Genet.*, 3:47–48.

_____ & Granoff, D. (1965), IQ and the somatic stigma of Turner's syndrome. *Amer. J. Ment. Defic.,* 70:69–77.

_____ & Mittenthal, S. (1970), Lack of personality pathology in Turner's syndrome: relations to cytogenetics, hormones and physique. *Behav. Genet.,* 1:43–56.

Nielsen, J., Nyborg, H. & Dahl, G. (1977), Turner's syndrome: a psychiatric-psychological study of 45 women with Turner's syndrome. *Acta Jutlandica XLV* (whole monograph).

Pennington, B.F., Bender, B., Puck, M., Salbenblatt, J. & Robinson, A. (1982), Learning disabilities in children with sex chromosome anomalies. *Child Develpm.,* 53:1182–1192.

Perheentupa, J., Lenko, H.L., Nevalainen, I., Nittymaki, M., Soderholm, A. & Taipale, V. (1974), Hormone therapy in Turner's syndrome: growth and psychological aspects. Pediatric XIV. *Growth Develpm. Endocrinol.,* 5:121–127.

Piers, E.V. (1969), Manual for the Piers-Harris Children's Self-Concept Scale. Counselor Recordings and Tests, Nashville, Tenn.

Raft, D., Spencer, R.F. & Toomey, T.C. (1976), Ambiguity of gender identity fantasies and aspects of normal and pathology in hypopituitary dwarfism and Turner's syndrome: three cases. *J. Sex Res.,* 12:161–172.

Sabbath, J.C., Morris, T.A., Menzer-Benaron, D. & Sturgis, S.H. (1961), Psychiatric observations in adolescent girls lacking ovarian function. *Psychosom. Med.,* 23:224–231.

Shaffer, J.W. (1962), A specific cognitive deficit observed in gonadal aplasia (Turner's syndrome). *J. Clin. Psychol.* 18:403–406.

Silbert, A., Wolff, D.H. & Lilienthal, J. (1977), Spatial and temporal processing in patients with Turner's syndrome. *Behav. Genet.,* 7:11–21.

Sonis, W.A., Levine-Ross, J., Blue, J., Cutler, G.B., Loriaux, P.L. & Klein, R.P. (1983), Hyperactivity and Turner's Syndrome. Paper presented at American Academy of Child Psychiatry Meetings, San Francisco.

Taipale, V. (1979), Adolescence in Turner's syndrome. Monograph from Children's Hospital, University of Helsinki, Helsinki, Finland.

Waber, D. (1979), Neuropsychological aspects of Turner's syndrome. *Develpm. Med. Child Neurol.,* 21:58–70.

23

An Examination of the Borderline Diagnosis in Children

Deborah A. Greenman, John G. Gunderson,
Melanie Cane, and Peter R. Saltzman

McLean Hospital, Belmont, Massachusetts

A retrospective study of 86 children aged 6–12 years who had been hospitalized for psychiatric reasons revealed that adult criteria for borderline personality disorder could identify a group of children with many of the features attributed in the literature to the borderline child. The relative paucity of significant differences between the children identified as borderline and those identified as nonborderline raises questions about the validity and utility of the term. Further work is necessary to clarify the meaning of a vulnerability to psychotic regression in the disturbed child and the relation of such a vulnerability to the adult borderline personality disorder.

The term "borderline child" is of uncertain meaning and validity, despite its widespread clinical use. While it is the subject of a growing literature (1–4), it is not an accepted child diagnosis in *DSM-III* or the Group for the Advancement of Psychiatry classification. Like the adult borderline concept, the term was developed by clinicians working with patients whose psychopathology seemed to be on the "border" between neurosis and psychosis (5–8); these clinicians' observations were drawn from in-

Reprinted from the *American Journal of Psychiatry*, 1986, Vol. 143, 998–1003. Copyright 1986 by the American Psychiatric Association.
Supported by the Psychosocial Research Fund of McLean Hospital.
The authors thank Jacqueline Olds, M.D., for her contributions to this work.

tensive psychotherapy and psychoanalysis (5–13). Attempts have been made to organize descriptions from the literature into diagnostic criteria (2), but definitions of the syndrome remain a confusing mix of the con cepts and language of developmental psychology, descriptive psychopathology, and psychoanalytic theory. In this paper we report on a study that explored the meaning of the term and its relationship to the adult disorder.

Similarities between the borderline syndrome of childhood and adult borderline personality disorder have been noted in several descriptive studies. Bradley (14) found that Gunderson and Singer's (15) criteria for adult borderline personality disorder could differentiate borderline and nonborderline children. Petti and Law (3) demonstrated that *DSM-III* adult criteria for borderline and schizotypal personality disorder could distinguish the two disorders in 10 latency age children with "borderline psychotic" psychopathology. Pfeffer et al. (16) studied 102 children and found that 54% of those who manifested both suicidal and assaultive behavior (as contrasted with either behavior alone or neither behavior) met *DSM-III* criteria for borderline personality.

Studies of children diagnosed as borderline have begun to report on the presence of nondiagnostic features in these children that have appeared in the adult literature to be associated with borderline psychopathology. Organicity (2, 4, 11, 17), parental neglect and physical abuse (2), and early separations from the mother (14) have been noted for borderline children as they have for adults (18–23). In addition, Petti and Unis (24) observed that depressed "borderline" children, like depressed borderline adults, responded to treatment with antidepressant medication.

The specific aims of this study were to evaluate whether a borderline syndrome similar to that identified in adults can be found in children, to determine whether this syndrome corresponds to the use of the term in the literature on children, and to examine whether children fulfilling adult criteria for borderline personality disorder have other characteristics linked in the literature to the adult syndrome (e.g., organicity, early separations, etc).

METHOD

The subjects were 86 children 6 to 12 years old who had been admitted to McLean Hospital's Hall Mercer Children's Center between 1971 and 1978. Because of the association between borderline disorder and suicidality noted in *DSM-III* and elsewhere (25–27), we included in our study sample 57 children who had either threatened or attempted suicide.

We expected that this subgroup would be a high-risk population in which to find the borderline syndrome. The remaining 29 subjects were non-suicidal children admitted during the same 7-year period. There were no significant differences between the two groups in mean age, ratio of males to females, or socioeconomic status. Overall, the resulting sample was largely white, middle class, and male (72%), with a mean±SD age of 9.9±1.8 years.

The Diagnostic Interview for Borderlines (DIB) (28) has been adapted to allow for retrospective (DIB-R) diagnoses of borderline personality disorder by chart review (29). Minor modifications were made in this study for use with children (available from authors). The DIB-R groups 24 variables in five major areas of psychopathology: social adaptation, impulsivity, affects, psychosis, and interpersonal relations (table 1). Uniformly available sources of information from the charts were used to score the 24 borderline variables. Scores from each of the five areas were scaled and the scaled scores totaled for each subject. The standard cutoff of 7 was used. After establishing adequate interrater reliability (r = .83), two of us (D.A.G. and M.C.) completed independent DIB-R ratings on the 86 records.

In addition to the 24 variables used for diagnosis on the DIB-R, 30 other "independent" variables were rated. Some variables were selected because of a presumed association with the child borderline syndrome, others because of their association with the adult borderline syndrome (table 2). In addition, the diagnosis and degree of improvement on discharge were recorded. *DSM-II* diagnoses were translated to equivalent *DSM-III* diagnoses. Chi-square analyses were used to compare the borderline and nonborderline subjects on both diagnostic and independent variables. A forward stepwise discriminant function analysis was used to identify the diagnostic variables that best differentiated those subjects who met criteria for borderline personality disorder from those who did not.

The concordance between the DIB-R-defined syndrome and the "borderline syndrome" described in the literature on children was examined in three additional ways. Because of the emphasis in the literature on children on "borderline psychotic" thinking and behavior, we asked whether evidence of impaired reality testing on psychological tests (in the absence of a clear-cut psychosis) would predict other features associated with the borderline diagnosis. Second, we examined the group of 27 subjects that we found to be borderline according to the DIB-R to see whether they fulfilled the criteria distilled from the literature by Bemporad et al. (2). Finally, we divided the entire sample into the same four

Table 1. Comparison of Borderline and Nonborderline Hospitalized Children on Variables of the Diagnostic Interview for Borderlines, Revised

Variable[a]	Total (N=86)		Borderline (N=27)		Nonborderline (N=59)		Chi-Square Analysis
	N	%	N	%	N	%	
Social adaptation							
Appropriate presentation	71	82.6	25	92.6	46	79.3	n.s.
Poor school attendance	19	22.1	6	22.2	13	22.0	n.s.
Scholastic underachievement	48	55.8	15	55.6	33	56.9	n.s.
Poor adjustment to group	63	73.3	22	81.5	41	70.7	n.s.
Impulse patterns							
Suicidal thoughts/behaviors	54	64.3	18	69.2	36	62.1	n.s.
Running away behavior	14	16.3	4	15.4	10	16.9	n.s.
Delinquent behavior	44	51.2	20	74.1	24	40.7	$\chi^2=8.27$, df=1, p<.005
Accident proneness	9	10.6	3	11.1	6	10.3	n.s.
Self-destructive behavior	23	26.7	10	37.0	13	22.0	n.s.
Substance abuse	3	3.5	2	8.0	1	1.7	n.s.
Assaultiveness	55	64.0	24	88.9	31	52.5	$\chi^2=10.62$, df=1, p<.005
Affect							
Irritable, hostile, angry	66	77.6	26	96.3	40	69.0	$\chi^2=7.93$, df=1, p<.005
Chronically unhappy, anhedonic	33	38.4	11	42.3	22	37.9	n.s.
Depression	65	75.6	23	85.2	42	71.2	n.s.
Flat affect[b]	1	1.2	1	3.8	0	0.0	n.s.
Psychosis							
Dissociative episodes	5	5.8	2	7.7	3	5.2	n.s.
Episodes of psychotic thinking	9	10.7	7	28.0	2	3.7	$\chi^2=9.99$, df=1, p<.005
Episodes of paranoid thinking	4	4.8	2	7.7	2	3.5	n.s.
Psychotic tendencies on psychological testing	31	36.9	16	59.3	15	27.8	$\chi^2=7.55$, df=1, p<.01
Interpersonal relations							
Demanding/dependent/entitled	68	79.1	26	96.3	42	73.7	$\chi^2=6.08$, df=1, p<.05
Manipulative/devaluing/ argumentative/sadistic	68	79.1	26	100.0	42	71.2	$\chi^2=9.36$, df=1, p<.005
Splitting	30	34.9	15	57.7	15	25.4	$\chi^2=8.23$, df=1, p<.005
Disposed to caretaking	6	7.0	2	7.4	4	6.8	n.s.
Socially isolated, a loner[b]	11	12.8	4	14.8	7	12.3	n.s.

[a]N values vary for some items because variables scored as "?" rather than "yes" or "no" were few in number and were omitted from the chi-square analysis.

[b]Negative scores were given for these traits.

413

Table 2. Comparison of Borderline and Nonborderline Hospitalized Children on Nondiagnostic Variables

Variable[a]	Total (N=86) N	%	Borderline (N=27) N	%	Nonborderline (N=59) N	%	Chi-Square
Abnormal EEG results	26	30.2	6	22.2	20	33.9	n.s.
Abnormal neuropsychological test results	18	20.9	9	33.3	9	15.3	$\chi^2=3.66$, df=1, p<.10
History of learning disability	25	29.4	9	33.3	16	28.1	n.s.
Hyperactivity, abnormal EEG results, learning disorder, or abnormal neuropsychological test results	56	65.1	21	77.8	35	59.3	n.s.
Hyperactivity, abnormal EEG results, or learning disorder	52	60.5	18	66.7	34	57.6	n.s.
History of hyperactivity	33	38.4	15	57.7	18	31.0	$\chi^2=5.35$, df=1, p<.05
Encopresis	4	4.7	1	3.7	3	5.1	n.s.
Enuresis	9	10.5	4	14.8	5	8.5	n.s.
Bizarre behaviors	22	25.9	8	29.6	14	24.6	n.s.
Anorexia	7	8.1	3	11.1	4	6.8	n.s.
Overeating	5	5.8	3	11.1	2	3.4	n.s.
Insomnia	18	20.9	9	33.3	9	15.3	n.s.
Oversleeping	4	4.7	1	3.7	3	5.1	$\chi^2=3.66$, df=1, p<.10
Suicidal behavior[b]							
Threat	25	43.9	11	57.9	14	36.8	n.s.
Attempt	16	28.1	4	21.1	12	31.6	n.s.
Serious attempt	16	28.1	4	21.1	12	31.6	n.s.
Family history of psychiatric illness							
In mother							
Any psychiatric illness	24	27.9	5	18.5	19	32.2	n.s.
Depression	15	17.4	3	11.1	12	20.3	n.s.
Drug/alcohol abuse	5	5.8	0	0.0	5	8.5	n.s.
In father							
Any psychiatric illness	13	15.1	4	14.8	9	15.3	n.s.
Depression	3	3.5	1	3.7	2	3.4	n.s.
Drug/alcohol abuse	9	10.5	4	14.8	5	8.5	n.s.

Parents separated or divorced	38	44.7	13	48.1	25	42.4	n.s.
Verbal fighting between parents	27	31.4	8	29.6	19	32.2	n.s.
Physical fighting between parents	11	12.8	3	11.1	8	13.6	n.s.
Physical abuse of child							
By mother	4	4.7	3	11.1	1	1.7	$\chi^2=3.62$, df=1, p<.10
By father	12	14.0	4	14.8	8	13.6	n.s.
By either parent	13	15.1	5	18.5	8	13.6	n.s.
Child adopted under age 1 month	5	5.8	3	11.1	2	1.7	n.s.
Child adopted over age 1 month	8	9.3	1	3.7	7	11.9	n.s.
Child separated from mother							
0 to 4 years old	13	15.1	3	11.1	10	16.9	n.s.
5 to 10 years old	7	8.1	0	0.0	7	11.9	$\chi^2=3.49$, df=1, p<.10

[a] N values vary for some items because variables scored as "?" rather than "yes" or "no" were few in number and were omitted from the chi-square analysis.
[b] N=57.

415

groups used by Pfeffer et al. (16)—suicidal only, assaultive only, suicidal and assaultive—and then tested whether the coexistence of assaultive and suicidal behaviors would predict the DIB-R borderline diagnosis.

RESULTS

Twenty-seven subjects (31%) were scored as borderline using the DIB-R. The ratio of males to females in the borderline group was the same as for the sample as a whole. The most common *DSM-III* clinical diagnoses given to those designated borderline were conduct disorder (37%) and other personality disorder (15%) (table 3). The percentage of borderline patients in the presumed high-risk group of suicidal patients (33%) was not significantly higher than the percentage of borderline patients in the nonsuicidal group (28%), nor was there any difference in the level or type of suicidal behaviors between the borderline and nonborderline groups. Given these facts as well as the absence of differences in demographic variables between the two groups, we decided to perform all analyses on the sample of 86 children as a whole.

Table 3. Discharge Diagnoses[a] of Borderline and Nonborderline Children Hospitalized for Psychiatric Reasons

	Hospitalized Children					
	Total (N=86)		Borderline (N=27)		Nonborder-line (N=59)	
Diagnosis	N	%	N	%	N	%
Other personality disorder	20	23	4	15	16	27
Conduct disorder	20	23	10	37	10	17
Adjustment disorder	16	19	2	7	14	24
Dysthymic disorder	7	8	0	0	7	12
Borderline personality disorder	5	6	2	7	3	5
Attention deficit disorder with hyper-activity	5	6	2	7	3	5
Overanxious disorder	5	6	3	11	2	3
Other diagnoses[b]	8	9	4	15	4	7

[a]A few patients received more than one diagnosis.
[b]Includes mixed specific developmental disorder, severe mental retardation, major depression, schizophrenia, and intermittent explosive disorder.

Table 1 shows that many of the 24 DIB-R variables were common in both the borderline and nonborderline subjects. There were eight variables that were significantly higher in the borderline group: delinquent behavior, assaultiveness, angry affect, episodes of psychotic thinking, psychotic tendencies on psychological testing, and three variables reflecting disturbed interpersonal behaviors. Three of these variables (psychotic tendencies on psychological testing [r = .73]; demanding, dependent, entitled, or masochistic behavior [r = .67]; and assaultive behavior [r = .41]) also appeared in the discriminant function analysis. The two other variables that added power to the discrimination of the borderline subjects were conventional social presentation (r = .49) and depression (r = .49). With these five variables, 77% of the cases could be separated into borderline and nonborderline groups. This fairly high degree of discriminating power is indicated by the Wilks's lambda value of .60.

A comparison of the borderline and nonborderline subjects on the nondiagnostic variables revealed only one significant difference (table 2). Children in the borderline group were significantly more likely (p < .05) to have been diagnosed as hyperactive at some time before admission. The possible importance of trends (p < .10) in the areas of neuropsychological testing and insomnia was weakened by the failure for other variables in the neurological and depressive areas to be higher in the borderline group.

Contrary to predictions, the borderline children were less likely to have experienced maternal separations or to have mothers who were depressed or who had other psychiatric illnesses, although these differences were not statistically significant.

Characteristics thought to be associated with the adult borderline syndrome (learning disability, abnormal EEG results, family history of psychiatric illness, vegetative signs of depression, bizarre behaviors, parental discord, and adoptions) were high in both borderline and nonborderline groups, without significant differences existing between them.

A comparison of the children who demonstrated psychotic tendencies on psychological testing with those who did not failed to produce two groups with significant differences on any of the diagnostic or independent study variables (with the expectable exception of the other psychotic symptoms of brief paranoid experiences and episodes of psychotic thinking).

Application of Bemporad et al.'s criteria to our group of 27 borderline subjects showed moderate concordance between the two diagnostic methods (table 4). Forty-one percent (11 of 27) of our borderline subjects

Table 4. Concordance of Bemporad et al.'s (2) Child Borderline Criteria in 27 Children Diagnosed According to the Diagnostic Interview for Borderlines, Revised

Bemporad et al.'s Criterion	Children Diagnosed With Diagnostic Interview	
	N	%
1. Fluctuation of functioning	14	51.9
2. Severe anxiety states (evidence of a, b, or c below)	18	66.7
a. Rapid escalation to panic/terror or apparent helplessness in face of mounting anxiety	13	48.2
b. Prominent phobic symptoms	7	25.9
c. Fears of self-annihilation or fantasies/fears of body mutilation or fantasies/fears of impending catastrophe (all three usually found in psychological testing)	10	37.0
3. Disturbed thought content (evidence of symptoms from 3a or 3b)	25	92.6
a. Fluid fantasy reality/boundaries or psychotic thinking shown on psychological tests	22	81.5
b. Underachieves scholastically or displays literal or concrete thinking or has a learning disability or displays poor perceptual/motor skills	18	66.7
4. Disturbed interpersonal relationships (hostile/sadistic and/or demanding/dependent)	26	96.3
5. Poor affective and motoric controls	27	100.0
6. Associated symptoms		
Poor social functioning	23	85.2
Evidence of failure to learn from experience	0	0.0
Lack of personal grooming	4	14.8
Evidence of difficulty adapting to new situations	7	25.9
Evidence of organic impairment	18	66.7
Evidence of one or more associated symptoms	26	96.3

showed evidence of disturbance in all of the five areas outlined by Bemporad et al., and 67% (18 of 27) showed disturbances in at least four of those areas. All or nearly all of our borderline subjects had disturbances in the areas of interpersonal relations, impulse control, and thought processes. Although less common, fluctuation of functioning and pathological anxiety (as defined by Bemporad et al.) were found in about half of our borderline subjects. Of the mixture of heterogenous features that made up Bemporad et al.'s sixth criterion of "associated symptoms," social functioning (85%) and evidence of organic impairment (67%) were common in the borderline subjects. All but one of the borderline subjects (96%) had one or more of the "associated symptoms."

Assaultive and suicidal behavior did occur together at a high frequency in the children diagnosed as borderline by adult (DIB-R) criteria. Sixteen of 27 (59%) of the borderline subjects showed both assaultive and suicidal behaviors, compared to only 30% of the nonborderline subjects (p = .005).

DISCUSSION

This study showed the syndrome of adult borderline personality disorder to be highly prevalent in a selected sample of hospitalized children. Significant differences between borderline and nonborderline groups appeared most often in the areas of psychosis and in both angry actions and hostility-filled interpersonal relations. Unlike adult borderline individuals, our child borderline subjects, diagnosed according to the DIB-R, were significantly more likely to act out against others (assaultiveness) than against themselves (suicidal and self-destructive behaviors). Since the percentages of male and female subjects in the two groups were the same, this result does not reflect sex differences. However, when suicidal behavior (not in itself predictive) and assaultive behavior were both present we found, as did Pfeffer et al., that the likelihood of a borderline diagnosis was significantly increased.

Our finding that psychotic tendencies on psychological testing was the most powerful discriminator of children identified as borderline concurs with the emphasis on the "borderline psychotic" thinking found in the literature on children (2, 5–11). However, the failure of this symptom alone to differentiate two distinct groups suggests that, like suicidal behaviors, this symptom is only weakly predictive of the borderline syndrome. This supports the emphasis on a multiple criteria diagnosis found in both *DSM-III* and the literature on children (2).

Although the prevalence of psychiatric disturbance in the mothers was similar for both borderline and nonborderline groups, the prevalence of physical abuse by the mothers was higher ($p < .10$) in the borderline group. This is in accord with Bemporad et al.'s finding of physical abuse and neglect of the borderline children they studied (2).

In some areas, our failure to find significant differences between the borderline and the nonborderline subjects was at odds with our hypotheses and with previous studies of borderline children. Bradley (14) found a higher prevalence of early maternal separation in borderline children and adolescents than in nonborderline ones. We found the opposite. Her use of less stringently operationalized criteria than the DIB-R could account for this, as could sampling differences. Like Bemporad et al., we observed frequent organic impairment in the borderline children, but because we used a comparison group, we were able to show that this variable's utility in discriminating borderline psychopathology is limited.

This study offered some methodological advances over previous studies. We included stringent and reliable criteria and an unusually standardized set of hospital records from which to make diagnostic ratings. Raters had no prior and confounding knowledge of the subjects and their diagnoses. We also had a relatively homogeneous sample insofar as all subjects were inpatients with a delimited range of age, race, socioeconomic status, and diagnosis. By using a comparison group made up of seriously disturbed but nonpsychotic children, we gave the distinctiveness of the borderline syndrome a particularly tough test. This increases the credibility of the differences we found but also may limit the generalizability of the results.

There are also problems with the study. First, there are limitations to retrospective data. Data from clinical charts sometimes are incomplete and are subject to unknown biases in the recording clinicians. This was a particular problem in applying some criteria that would best be observed in the psychotherapeutic situation, e.g., Bemporad et al.'s fluctuation of functioning and constricted play patterns. Second, we cannot be sure that the variables rated were the most important or would validly tap differences, even if present. For example, the presence of anxiety and fearfulness or phobic behavior prominent in descriptions of the borderline child but not in adults was neither a diagnostic criterion nor an independent variable in our study. The fact that we found that two-thirds of our borderline sample showed evidence of severe anxiety states indicates that this variable merits more study.

Our results take us in two directions. First, they suggest some concordance between the syndrome defined by adult criteria for borderline personality disorder and the syndrome of the borderline child described in the literature. A sizable fraction of this nonpsychotic inpatient sample met adult criteria for borderline personality disorder. The discriminant function analysis further underscored the special importance that the vulnerability to psychotic regression has in children with this syndrome, although this criterion by itself did not seem predictive of a distinct entity. On the other hand, our results do not offer strong evidence that criteria for adult borderline personality disorder define a distinct and meaningful syndrome as tested by a variety of independent variables within this sample of nonpsychotic children. Given that two-thirds of our borderline sample fulfilled most of the Bemporad et al. criteria for the childhood borderline diagnosis, it is likely that the latter criteria define a similarly indistinct group. Hence, we conclude that a more discriminating method for identifying borderline children is still needed for this diagnosis to carry much meaning.

Implicit in the effort to define a group of borderline children who exhibit the same or similar characteristics as the adult borderline subject is the notion that the borderline child has a characteristic way of relating to others and of managing conflicts and anxiety. Important questions are whether patterns of behavior seen in these children are predictive of future performance, whether behaviors and modes of relating endure, and whether the vulnerability to loss of reality testing heals over time, develops into psychosis, or remains stable. We hope to follow these subjects to examine the relationship between the psychopathology seen in childhood and that which will emerge in their young adult years.

REFERENCES

1. Robson KS (ed): The Borderline Child: Approaches to Etiology, Diagnosis, and Treatment. New York, McGraw-Hill, 1983.
2. Bemporad JR, Smith HF, Hanson G, et al: Borderline syndromes in childhood: criteria for diagnosis. Am J. Psychiatry 139:596–602, 1982.
3. Petti TA, Law W: Borderline psychotic behavior in hospitalized children: approaches to assessment and treatment. J Am Acad Child Psychiatry 21:197–202, 1982.
4. Kernberg PF: Update of borderline disorders in children. Psychiatric Hospital 13:137–141, 1982.
5. Weil AP: Certain severe disturbances of ego development in childhood. Psychoanal Study Child 8:271–287, 1953.
6. Geleerd ER: Borderline states in childhood and adolescence. Psychoanal Study Child 13:279–295, 1958.
7. Ekstein R, Wallerstein J: Observations on the psychotherapy of borderline and psychotic children. Psychoanal Study Child 11:303–311, 1956.

8. Ekstein R, Wallerstein J: Observations on the psychology of borderline and psychotic children. Psychoanal Study Child 9:344-369, 1954.

9. Fast I, Chethik M: Some aspects of object relationships in borderline children. Int. J Psychoanal 53:479-485, 1972.

10. Rosenfeld SK, Sprince MP: An attempt to formulate the meaning of the concept "borderline." Psychoanal Study Child 18:603-635, 1963.

11. Pine F: On the concept "borderline" in children. Psychoanal Study Child 29:341-368, 1974.

12. Frijling-Schreuder ECM: Borderline states in children. Psychoanal Study Child 24:307-327, 1970.

13. Chiland C, Lebovici S: Borderline or prepsychotic conditions in childhood—a French point of view, in Borderline Personality Disorders: The Concept, the Syndrome, the Patient. Edited by Hartocollis P. New York, International Universities Press, 1977.

14. Bradley SJ: The relationship of early maternal separation to borderline personality in children and adolescents: a pilot study. Am J. Psychiatry 136:424-426, 1979.

15. Gunderson JG, Singer MT: Defining borderline patients: an overview. Am J Psychiatry 132:1-10, 1975.

16. Pfeffer CR, Plutchik R, Mizruchi MS: Suicidal and assaultive behavior in children: classification, measurement, and interrelations. Am J Psychiatry 140:154-157, 1983.

17. Murray ME: Minimal brain dysfunction and borderline personality adjustment. Am J Psychother 33:391-402, 1979.

18. Andrulonis PA, Glueck BC, Stroebel CF, et al: Organic brain dysfunction and the borderline syndrome. Psychiatr Clin North Am 4:47-66, 1980.

19. Gunderson JG, Kerr J, Englund D: The families of borderlines: a comparative study. Arch Gen Psychiatry 37:27-33, 1980.

20. Walsh F: The family of the borderline patient, in the Borderline Patient. Edited by Grinker R, Werble B. New York, Jason Aronson, 1977.

21. Frank H, Paris J: Recollections of family experience in borderline patients. Arch Gen Psychiatry 38:1031-1034, 1981.

22. Masterson J, Rinsley D: The borderline syndrome; the role of the mother in the genesis and psychic structure of the borderline personality. Int J Psychoanal 56:163-177, 1975.

23. Soloff P, Millward J: Psychiatric disorders in the families of borderline patients. Arch Gen Psychiatry 40:37-44, 1983.

24. Petti TA, Unis A: Imipramine treatment of borderline children: case reports with a controlled study. Am J Psychiatry 138:515-518, 1981.

25. Gunderson JG: Borderline Personality Disorder. Washington, DC, American Psychiatric Press, 1984.

26. Conte H, Plutchik R, Karasu T, et al: A self-report borderline scale: discriminative validity and preliminary norms. J Nerv Ment Dis 168:428-435, 1980.

27. Friedman RC, Aronoff MS, Clarkin JF, et al: History of suicidal behavior in depressed borderline inpatients. Am J Psychiatry 140:1023-1026, 1983.

28. Gunderson JG, Kolb JE, Austin V: The Diagnostic Interview for Borderline Patients. Am J Psychiatry 138:896-903, 1981.

29. Armelius B, Kullgren G, Renberg E: Borderline diagnosis from hospital records: reliability and validity of Gunderson's Diagnostic Interview for Borderlines (DIB). J Nerv Ment Dis 173:32-34, 1985.

24

Long-Term Follow-up of Anorexia Nervosa

Brenda B. Toner
Clarke Institute of Psychiatry, Toronto, Ontario
Paul E. Garfinkel and David M. Garner
Toronto General Hospital, Ontario

This study compared the long-term outcome of restricting and bulimic anorexic women using standardized psychometric instruments in addition to global clinical ratings. Results indicated that, in general, restricting and bulimic anorexic subtypes did not differ in their long-term outcome according to clinical ratings and standardized assessments of anorexic symptoms, psychiatric diagnoses, and psychosocial functioning. The only exception to this pattern was that the bulimic group had a higher incidence of substance use disorders during the last year compared with the restricting group. Findings also indicated that relative to a matched comparison group of women of average weight, a significant percentage of anorexics from both subtypes met DSM-III criteria for an affective or anxiety disorder at some point in their lives as well as at long-term follow-up. Results are discussed in terms of theoretical and methodologic issues involved in the long-term follow-up of anorexia nervosa.

Reprinted with permission of Elsevier Science Publishing Co., Inc., from *Psychosomatic Medicine*, 1986, Vol. 48, No. 7, 520–529. Copyright 1986 by the American Psychosomatic Society, Inc.

This work was funded by a research fellowship from the Ontario Health Foundation to the first author and by grant 866-83/85 from OMHF.

INTRODUCTION

Anorexia nervosa is known to vary widely in its outcome (1). Several recent reviews of follow-up studies (2–5) have reported that the usual method of assessing outcome in anorexia nervosa is by global clinical ratings; assessments of weight and eating parameters are part of these criteria. Other criteria generally include assessments of menstrual function, mental state, sexual adjustment, socioeconomic status, and social adjustment. Few follow-up studies to date have gone beyond global ratings to include a more systematic assessment of attitudes toward eating and body shape as well as other areas of psychologic functioning. Steinhausen and Glanville (4) recommended that outcome research would be improved by the inclusion of objective ratings and standardized scales for anorexic symptoms, psychiatric characteristics, and psychosocial functioning. Inclusion of standardized instruments would reduce the difficulties of cross-study comparisons among investigations employing clinical assessments or other nonstandardized measures of symptoms (3).

The present study involved the follow-up of patients seen between 5 and 14 years earlier with a primary diagnosis of anorexia nervosa. A range of psychologic parameters were investigated using standardized psychometric instruments in addition to global clinical ratings. A minimum follow-up period of 5 years was chosen, since a follow-up period of less than 4 years is considered insufficient for the illness to have taken its full course (6). We were particularly interested in comparing the outcome of anorexics who experienced episodes of bulimia with those who exclusively restricted their caloric intake, since recent studies have documented major differences between these subgroups. For example, bulimic anorexic patients have been found to be more impulsive, extroverted, sexually active and emotionally labile than restricting anorexic patients (7–9). Moreover, several investigators have suggested that bulimia is associated with a less favorable outcome (10–12).

Based on these reports, it was hypothesized that patients with the bulimic subtype of anorexia nervosa would have a less favorable outcome than those with the restricting subtype. Specific hypotheses were not formulated regarding the incidence of various psychiatric disorders among bulimic and restricting anorexics at follow-up and, accordingly, this part of the study was largely exploratory. However, several writers have suggested an association between anorexia nervosa and such psychiatric disorders as affective illness, phobias, and obsessive-compulsive neurosis (e.g., 13–19).

METHODS

Subjects

Of the initial sample of 149 consecutive consultations seen at the Clarke Institute of Psychiatry between 1970 and 1978, 74 were located for follow-up. Of this group, 5 people had died (3 restricters, 2 bulimics), 14 people decided not to participate in the study for a variety of reasons [e.g., no interest, no time, did not want to reopen painful memories, doing better now, and did not want to be reminded of the past, (7 restricters, 7 bulimics)], and 55 former patients agreed to participate in the study. This group consisted of 30 restricting (mean age 28.2 years) and 25 bulimic anorexic women (mean age 28.2 yrs.). A comparison group of 26 women within 90% and 110% of matched population mean weight (20) matched by age, occupational status, and education with no history of anorexia nervosa volunteered for this study. Patients were classified into bulimic and restricting subtypes based upon their symptom picture at the initial consultation. Bulimia was defined as an abnormal increase in one's desire to eat, with episodes of excessive ingestion of large quantities of food that the person viewed as ego-alien and beyond her control (7). Anorexia nervosa was defined according to modified criteria of Feighner et al. (7), as described previously. All participants provided written informed consent and were paid $15.00 to acknowledge their participation.

Measures

Data were derived from three assessment strategies: 1) a structured psychiatric interview; 2) a battery of self-report measures; and 3) a clinical assessment. All participants who were interviewed were weighed. The interview and self-report measures were administered individually by the first author. The clinical assessment was made by clinicians familiar with the present status of the individual. Controls participated in the first two sections of the study.

Structured psychiatric interview

Diagnostic Interview Schedule [DIS]. The DIS, Version III was used for the psychiatric interview (21). The DIS is a structured interview from which psychiatric diagnoses may be systematically obtained in patients and the general population according to three diagnostic systems: DSM-III, Feighner criteria, and Research Diagnostic Criteria. In this study, data are reported according to DSM-III criteria. Validity and reliability for this interview have been well established (e.g., 21).

Self-reports

1. Eating Attitude Test (EAT). The EAT is a 26-item questionnaire designed to assess the broad range of symptoms characteristic of anorexia nervosa (22). Three factors form subscales that are related to dieting, bulimia and food preoccupation, and oral control. The EAT score has been found to be a useful index of improvement, since recovered patients have normal scores (23).

2. Eating Disorder Inventory (EDI). The EDI is a 64-item, self-report questionnaire designed to measure the cognitive and behavioral dimensions characteristic of anorexia nervosa (24). The EDI provides eight subscale scores: Drive for Thinness; Bulimia; Body Dissatisfaction; Ineffectiveness; Perfectionism; Interpersonal Distrust; Interoceptive Awareness; and Maturity Fears. When weight is controlled for, the restricting and bulimic subtypes have been found to be significantly different on Drive for Thinness, Ineffectiveness, and Interoceptive Awareness [higher scores being associated with bulimia].

3. Locus of Control (I-E). The I-E is a 45-item forced-choice questionnaire that yields three factors: the Fatalism factor, which measures the degree to which the person perceives luck or fate as controlling life events; Social Systems control, which measures perceived personal versus sociopolitical control over the environment; and self control, which indicates how much control the individual feels over his or her impulses, desires and emotions (25).

4. Body Dissatisfaction Scale (BDS). The BDS is an adapted version of the Berscheid (26) scale which assesses degree of satisfaction or dissatisfaction for 18 body parts using a 6-point likert scale.

5. Hopkin's Symptoms Checklist (HSCL). The HSCL is comprised of 58 items, which is scored on five underlying symptom dimensions: somatization, obsessive-compulsive, interpersonal sensitivity, anxiety, and depression (27).

6. Janis-Field feelings of ineffectiveness scale (JF) is a 20-item questionnaire designed to assess self-esteem (28).

7. Social Adjustment Self-Report Questionnaire (SAS-SR). The SAS-SR is a 42-item measure designed to assess six major areas of functioning: 1) work as a paid employee, homemaker or student; 2) social and leisure activities; 3) relationship with extended family; 4) marital role as a spouse; 5) parental role; and 6) and membership in the family unit (29). This study reports the overall adjustment score on the SAS-SR which was obtained by summing the scores of all items and dividing by the number of items actually scored [one of two scoring systems recommended by Weissman].

Clinical assessment

Clinical assessment was based on ratings from clinicians familiar with the present status of the individual. Individuals were assigned to one of the following clinical outcome groups: asymptomatic, improved, symptomatic, or deceased. Clinical ratings were based on parameters of eating, weight, menses and social adjustment outlined by Garfinkel et al. (10). For five participants, clinician ratings were unavailable. In these cases, ratings were derived from measures of weight and menses which were obtained at the time of the psychiatric interview.

RESULTS

The hospital charts of 74 patients located (Located group) were compared with hospital charts of the 75 individuals that were not located (Not Located group) in order to determine if the groups initially differed on important variables that might bias the generalizability of the follow-up data. Information obtained from hospital charts were based on data collected from initial patients consultations between 1970 and 1978, which were then coded by a single individual using a standard format (7). Analyses (i.e., *t*-tests, chi-square tests) between Located and Not Located groups indicated that groups did not significantly differ on the following variables: age of onset of anorexia nervosa; duration of illness; age when first seen at the Clarke Institute; frequency of bulimic episodes, vomiting, laxative use, and diuretic use; denial of weight loss; frequency of impulse-related behavior, including stealing, self-mutilation, suicide attempts and other delinquent behaviors; number and quality of friendships; lability of mood; and frequency of alcohol and street drug use. However, *t*-test scores indicated that groups differed on the percentage of the Canadian average weight for their sex, age, and height ($t = 2.7, p < 0.01$), the Located group weighing significantly less at initial assessment than the Not Located group (68.0% vs. 75.2%).

Clinical demographic data on follow-up for restricting anorexic, bulimic anorexic, and comparison groups are presented in Table 1. Age, percent of average weight for age and height, and follow-up duration were analyzed by a one-way analysis of variance (ANOVA). Occupational status and education were subjected to Fisher's exact test.

Table 1. Clinical and Demographic Characteristics of Restricting Anorexic (R), Bulimic Anorexic (B), and Comparison (C) Groups

	R	B	C	P
Age (yr)[a]	28.0 (5.3)	28.2 (4.0)	27.3 (5.3)	NS
Percent of average weight	82.1 (13.7)	84.7 (12.3)	97.8 (12.8)[c]	.001
Follow-up duration (yr)[a]	7.0 (2.2)	7.1 (1.8)	—	NS
Occupational status (%)[b]				
1	4.3	4.8	8.7	NS
2	21.7	28.6	17.4	NS
3	4.3	9.5	4.3	NS
4	26.1	19.0	39.1	NS
5	8.7	9.5	4.3	NS
6	0.0	4.8	4.3	NS
7 (homemaker)	4.3	0.0	0.0	NS
8 (student)	30.4	23.8	21.7	NS
Education (%)				
Postgraduate	8.0	9.5	12.0	NS
University graduate	28.0	33.3	36.0	NS
Partial university	32.0	19.0	40.0	NS
High school	32.0	32.8	12.0	NS
Partial high school	0.0	9.5	0.0	NS
Junior high school	0.0	4.8	0.0	NS

[a]Mean (standard deviation).
[b]Hollingshead occupational scale.
[c]R < C, B < C (Newman-Keuls with p <0.05).

Psychiatric Disorders

The incidence of DSM-III psychiatric disorders among restricting, bulimic, and comparison groups is presented in Table 2. Data for psychiatric diagnoses are presented both in terms of lifetime prevalence and incidence during the last year. Significant overall differences among restricting, bulimic and comparison groups using multiple sample chi-square test are summarized in Table 2. As shown in Table 2, subsequent group comparisons using Fisher's exact test indicated that both bulimic and restricting groups had a significantly higher lifetime prevalence of affective and anxiety disorders and a higher incidence of anxiety disorders during the last year relative to the control group. In contrast, bulimic and restricting groups did not differ in terms of incidence of affective and anxiety disorders. However, as predicted, the bulimic group had a

Table 2. Comparison of Restricting (R), Bulimic Anorexic (B), and Control (C) Groups on DSM-III Disorders: Lifetime Prevalence and Incidence in the Last Year

	Percentage									
	Lifetime Prevalence					Last Year				
Disorder	R	B	C	χ^2	p<	R	B	C	χ^2	p<
Affective Disorders	61.5^e	52.4	11.5	15.0	0.001	38.4^b	28.5	7.7	6.9	0.05
Major depression	46.2^b	28.6	11.5	7.6	0.05	34.6^b	19.0	7.7	5.8	0.05
Bipolar	3.8	9.5	0.0	2.7	NS	3.8	9.5	0.0	2.7	NS
Dysthymia	42.3^e	33.3	0.0	13.7	0.001	—	—	—	—	—
Anxiety Disorders	57.7^e	66.7	7.7	20.4	0.001	42.3^e	52.4	7.7	12.1	0.01
Simple phobia	23.1	23.8	3.8	4.7	NS	19.2	23.8	3.8	4.2	NS
Social phobia	26.9	33.3	3.8	7.2	0.05	23.1	28.6	3.8	5.6	NS
Agoraphobia	11.5^e	42.9	3.8	13.2	0.001	11.5^a	28.5	3.8	6.2	0.05
Panic	19.2^e	33.3	0.0	9.6	0.01	15.3^a	33.3	3.8	10.1	0.01
Obsessive compulsive	38.5^e	28.6	12.0	12.0	0.01	23.0^b	9.6	0.0	7.2	0.05
Substance use disorders	23.1	42.9	15.4	4.7	NS	0.0^c	42.9	7.7	18.4	0.001
Alcohol abuse/dependency	7.7	14.3	0.0	3.8	NS	0.0	10.0	0.0	3.8	NS
Drug abuse/dependency	11.5	9.5	7.7	0.2	NS	0.0	14.3	0.0	7.7	0.05
Tobacco	7.7^d	28.6	11.5	4.3	NS	0.0^d	23.8	7.7	7.8	0.05
Somatization	3.8	4.8	0.0	1.2	NS	3.8	4.8	0.0	1.2	NS
Schizophrenic disorders	0.0	4.8	0.0	—	NS	0.0	4.8	0.0	—	NS
Schizophrenia	0.0	4.8	0.0	—	NS	0.0	4.8	0.0	—	NS
Schizophreniform	0.0	0.0	0.0	—	—	0.0	0.0	0.0	—	—
Antisocial personality	0.0	0.0	0.0	—	—	0.0	0.0	0.0	—	—
Cognitive impairment	0.0	0.0	0.0	—	—	0.0	0.0	0.0	—	—

Multiple Sample Chi Square

[a]R=B>C, Fisher's exact test with p<0.05, [b]B=R>C, [c]B>R, B>C, R=C, [d]C=B>R, [e]B>C, R>C, R=B.

higher incidence of substance use disorders during the last year compared with restricting and comparison groups (42.9% vs. 0.0% and 7.7% respectively). In addition, tobacco use disorder was significantly higher in the bulimic than the restricting group both in terms of lifetime prevalence and incidence of use during the last year.

Self-Report Measures

EDI. A one-way multivariate analysis of variance (MANOVA) indicated overall differences (Wilk's lambda = 0.63, $p < 0.01$) among restricting, bulimic, and comparison groups. This accounted for 37% of the variance in group membership. As indicated in Table 3, subsequent univariate F tests revealed significant group differences on all subscales except Drive for Thinness and Body Dissatisfaction. However, the restricting and bulimic groups did not differ on any of the significant subscales using Scheffe's test ($p < 0.05$). The restricting anorexia nervosa group scored significantly higher than the comparison group on Ineffectiveness, Interoceptive Awareness, and Maturity Fears subscales, while the bulimic group was significantly higher than the comparison group on Bulimia, Perfectionism, and Interpersonal Distrust.

Table 3. Comparison of Restricting Anorexic (R), Bulimic Anorexic (B), and Control (C) Groups on EDI and EAT Subscales

| | Means (Standard Deviations) | | |
	R	B	C
EDI			
Drive for Thinness	5.3(6.7)	5.5(6.2)	2.5(3.6)
Bulimia[a]	1.2(1.9)	2.7(4.3)	0.6(1.5)*
Body Dissatisfaction	8.8(8.6)	7.4(6.4)	7.7(6.1)
Ineffectiveness[b]	7.8(9.1)	5.3(6.7)	1.6(3.0)**
Perfectionism[a]	6.9(4.3)	8.5(4.9)	4.3(3.3)**
Interpersonal distrust[a]	4.0(4.8)	4.2(5.1)	1.2(1.6)*
Interoceptive awareness[b]	5.4(6.9)	3.7(4.2)	2.0(2.9)*
Maturity fears[b]	4.1(4.9)	2.1(2.5)	1.1(1.5)**
EAT			
Dieting	9.6(11.5)	8.3(8.6)	4.9(6.3)
Bulimia[a]	3.0(4.7)	3.2(4.7)	0.5(1.6)*
Oral control[b]	5.0(6.1)	3.7(3.2)	1.0(1.5)**
TOTAL	17.6(20.5)	15.3(14.6)	6.5(7.2)*

*p <0.05, **p <0.01, p <0.001 (one-way analysis of variance).
[a]R = B>C, Scheffe's test with p <0.05.
[b]B = R>C, Scheffe's test with p <0.05.

EAT. A one-way MANOVA again indicated overall differences (Wilk's lambda = 0.82, $p < 0.01$) among restricting, bulimic, and comparison groups. This accounted for 18% of the variance in group membership. As shown in Table 3, subsequent univariate F tests indicated significant group differences on the Bulimia and Oral Control Subscales and the Total EAT score. However, the restricting and bulimic groups did not significantly differ on Bulimia, Oral Control, or Total EAT scores (Scheffe, $p < 0.05$). Compared to the comparison group, the restricting group had significantly higher Oral Control and Total EAT scores and the bulimic group scored significantly higher on the Bulimia subscales.

Janis-Field Scale. A one-way ANOVA indicated a significant difference among restricting, bulimic, and control groups ($F = 3.5$, $p < 0.05$). Although restricting and bulimic groups did not differ from each other, the restricting group had a higher score (indicating less self-esteem) than the comparison group.

Remaining measures. Analyses performed on the remaining self-report measures failed to reveal group differences. Specifically, one-way MANOVAS performed on I-E and HSCL did not indicate overall group differences among restricting, bulimic, and comparison groups. Accordingly, univariate ANOVAs were not conducted for I-E and HSCL subscales. One-way ANOVA also failed to reveal group differences on the BDS and the SAS-SR.

Clinical Assessment

As shown in Table 4, Fisher's exact test failed to reveal significant differences between restricting and bulimic groups on any of the clinical outcome categories.

Table 4. Comparison of Restricting and Bulimic Anorexic Groups on Clinical Outcome

| | Frequency Scores (Percentage) | | |
	Restricting $N = 33$	Bulimic $N = 27$	P^a
Asymptomatic	15 (45)	8 (30)	NS
Improved	8 (24)	8 (30)	NS
Unchanged	7 (21)	9 (33)	NS
Deceased	3 (9)	2 (7)	NS

[a]Group comparisons were subjected to Fisher's exact test.

DISCUSSION

This research compared the long-term outcome of restricting and bulimic anorexic women using standardized psychometric instruments in addition to global clinical ratings. Of interest is the finding that in general, bulimic, and restricting anorexic subtypes did not differ in their long-term outcome according to clinical ratings and standardized assessments of anorexic symptoms, psychiatric diagnoses, and psychosocial functioning. The only exception to this pattern was that the bulimic group had a significantly higher incidence of substance use disorders during the last year compared with the restricting group. The current findings do not support previous suggestions that bulimia is associated with a less favorable outcome (10-12). However, this research differs from previous work in that it represents a long-term follow-up of patients (duration greater than 4 years) using psychometric instruments in addition to clinical assessments. The finding that the bulimic group reported a higher percentage of substance use disorders at follow-up adds support to recent studies which have found that bulimic anorexic patients are more impulsive than their restricting counterparts (7-9).

Although bulimic and restricting subtypes did not generally differ in terms of other psychiatric diagnoses, it is of theoretical and therapeutic interest that both anorexic subtypes had a higher lifetime prevalence of affective and anxiety disorders and a higher incidence of anxiety disorders at follow-up relative to a matched comparison group. In addition, the restricting group had a higher percentage of affective disorders at follow-up relative to the comparison group. The finding that a substantial percentage of anorexic patients met DSM-III criteria for an affective or anxiety disorder at some point in their lives as well as at long-term follow-up lends added support for the suggestion of previous writers for an association between anorexia nervosa and affective/anxiety disorders (13-19). Although most clinicians would currently recognize a core syndrome of primary anorexia nervosa that is distinct from other psychiatric illnesses (1), prospective studies are needed to investigate the relationship between anorexia nervosa and other psychiatric disorders from a longitudinal perspective.

In terms of anorexic symptoms, both anorexic subtypes scored higher on several EDI and EAT subscales relative to the comparison group. It is noteworthy, however, that on some subscales such as Body Dissatisfaction, anorexic and comparison groups did not differ. In fact, group means were remarkably similar (restricting 8.8, bulimic 7.4, comparison 7.7). Although college age norms have been published for the EDI that would suggest that these Body Dissatisfaction means are somewhat elevated (24), there are no available norms for post-college age women that are needed for long-term follow-up studies. This raises a more general methodologic issue in that there is a need for inclusion of matched comparison groups in long-term follow-up studies of anorexia nervosa. To our knowledge, the current study represents the only follow-up investigation of anorexia nervosa that included a comparison group of nonanorexic women. Since the present research included a comparison group, there is a baseline from which to measure anorexic as well as nonanorexic psychologic parameters. Accordingly, in terms of the range of psychologic parameters assessed in this study (i.e., locus of control, body dissatisfaction, psychological symptoms and social adjustment), both anorexic groups do not differ from the comparison group.

Since both psychometric instruments and global clinical ratings indicated that bulimic and restricting subtypes did not differ in their long-term outcome, the question of why the need for psychometric instruments may be raised. As previously mentioned, inclusion of standardized assessments for anorexic symptoms, psychiatric characteristics, and psychosocial functioning would reduce the difficulties of cross-study comparisons (3). Accordingly, although global clinical ratings may be useful, inclusion of standardized psychometric instruments would reduce experimenter bias and increase the comparability of research findings. Further, global clinical ratings provide limited information regarding the presence or absence of eating and weight related symptoms and other areas of psychosocial functioning since information is reduced to a single score or category. A final point concerning psychometric instruments is in their adaptability to comparison groups. Although global clinical ratings (10) have not been used on nonanorexic samples, psychometric instruments such as those administered in the current research have been used in anorexic and nonanorexic samples.

We are aware of the methodologic concerns involved in the failure to follow-up the complete sample of anorexic patients (30). However, we tried to address the problem by comparing the hospital charts of the patients located with the individuals that were not located in order to determine if the groups initially differed on important variables that might bias the generalizability of the follow-up data. In general, results indicated that the groups were similar in terms of both clinical and demographic data.

We are also aware of methodologic concerns regarding whether any of the original restricting anorexic patients eventually became bulimic. Although this study was not designed to address this question directly, the frequency of reported binges can be determined by inspecting critical items on the EDI and the EAT. Accordingly, 14% of the restricting subgroup endorsed item 28 on the EDI, "I have gone on eating binges where I have felt that I could not stop" (⩾often). Moreover, 10% of the restricting subgroup endorsed item 4 on the EAT, "have gone on eating binges where I feel that I may not be able to stop" (⩾ often). These estimates are consistent with Vandereycken and Pierloot's (31) findings that 15% of anorexic dieters reported weekly to daily bulimic episodes at follow-up.

It is also worth noting that in the present study, anorexic patients received their initial bulimic or restricting subgroup classification after an average illness of 3.5 years. In an earlier study, Garfinkel et al. (7) reported that bulimia developed 19.2 + 8.0 (mean + SEM) months after the onset of dieting. Accordingly, in the present study of chronic anorexic patients, bulimic behavior would have largely been established prior to our restricting and bulimic classifications.

In summary, the findings of this study indicate the following: 1) restricting and bulimic subtypes of anorexia nervosa have a similar long-term outcome according to both clinical ratings and standardized assessments of anorexic symptoms, psychiatric diagnoses, and psychosocial functioning; 2) the only exception to this pattern was that the bulimic group had a higher incidence of substance use disorders at follow-up compared with the restricting group; and 3) relative to a matched comparison group of women of average weight, a significant percentage of anorexics from both subtypes met DSM-III criteria for an affective or anxiety disorder at some point in their lives as well as at long-term follow-up.

REFERENCES

1. Garfinkel PE, Garner DM: Anorexia Nervosa: A Multidimensional Perspective. New York, Brunner/Mazel, 1982
2. Hsu LKG: Outcome of anorexia nervosa. Arch Gen Psychiatry 37:1041–1046, 1980
3. Schwartz DM, Thompson MG: do anorectics get well? Current research and future needs. Am J Psychiatry 138:319–323, 1981
4. Steinhausen HC, Glanville K: Retrospective and prospective follow-up studies in anorexia nervosa. Int J Eating Disorders 2:221–235, 1983
5. Swift WJ: The long-term outcome of early onset anorexia nervosa: A critical review. J Am Acad Child Psychiatry 21:38–46, 1982
6. Morgan HG, Russell GFM: Value of family background and clinical features as predictors of long-term outcome in anorexia nervosa: four year follow-up study of 41 patients. Psychol Med 5:355–371, 1975

7. Garfinkel PE, Moldofsky H, Garner DM: The heterogeneity of anorexia nervosa: Bulimia as a distinct subgroup. Arch Gen Psychiatry 37:1036–1040, 1980
8. Casper RC, Eckert ED, Halmi KA, Goldberg SC, Davis JM: Bulimia. Its incidence and clinical importance in patients with anorexia nervosa. Arch Gen Psychiatry 37:1030–1034, 1980
9. Garner DM, Garfinkel PE, O'Shaughnessy M: The validity of the distinction between bulimia with and without anorexia nervosa. Am J Psychiatry 142:581–587
10. Garfinkel PE, Moldofsky H, Garner DM: The outcome of anorexia nervosa: Significance of clinical features, body image and behaviour modification. In Vigersky R (ed), Anorexia Nervosa. New York, Raven, 1977, pp 315–329
11. Selvini Palazzoli MP: Self-Starvation. London, Chaucer, 1974
12. Hsu LKG, Crisp AH, Harding B: Outcome of anorexia nervosa. Lancet 1:61–65, 1979
13. Cantwell DP, Sturzenburger S, Burroughs J, Salkin B, Green JK: Anorexia nervosa: An affective disorder. Arch Gen Psychiatry 34:1087–1093, 1977
14. Crisp AH: Premorbid factors in adult disorders of weight, with particular reference to primary anorexia nervosa (weight phobia). A literature review. J Psychosom Res 14:1–22, 1970
15. Crisp AH, Toms DA: Primary anorexia nervosa or weight phobia in the male: Report on 13 cases. Br Med J 1:334–338, 1972
16. Hasan MK, Tibbetts RW: Primary anorexia nervosa (weight phobia) in males. Postgrad Med J 53:146–151, 1977
17. Schutze G: Anorexia Nervosa. Bern, Huber, 1980
18. Solyom L, Freeman RJ, Thomes CD, Miles JE: The comparative psychopathology of anorexia nervosa: Obsessive-compulsive disorder or phobia. Int J Eating Disorders 3:3–14, 1983
19. Hecht HM, Fichter M, Postpischil F: Obsessive-compulsive neurosis and anorexia nervosa. Int J Eating Disorders 2:69–77, 1983
20. Health and Welfare Canada: Canadian Average Weights for Height, Age and Sex, Nutrition Division of the Department of Health and Welfare, Ottawa, 1954
21. Robins LN, Helzer JE, Croughan J, Ratcliff KS: National Institute of Mental Health Diagnostic Interview Schedule. Arch Gen Psychiatry 38:389, 1981
22. Garner DM, Olmsted MP, Bohr Y, Garfinkel PE: The eating attitude test: Psychometric features and clinical correlates. Psychol Med 12:871–878, 1982
23. Garner DM, Garfinkel PE: The eating attitude test: An index of the symptoms of anorexia nervosa. Psychol Med 9:273–279, 1979
24. Garner DM, Olmsted MP, Polivy J: Development and validation of a multidimensional eating disorder inventory for anorexia nervosa and bulimia. Int J Eating Disorders 2:15–34, 1983
25. Reid DW, Ware EE: Multidimensionality of internal–external control: implications for past and future research. Can J Behav Sci 5:264–271, 1973
26. Berscheid E, Walster E, Hohrnstedt G: The happy American body: A survey report. Psychol Today, November 1973, pp 119–131
27. Derogatis L, Lipman R, Rickels K, Uhlenhath EGH, Covi L: the Hopkins Symptom Checklist (HSCL): A self-report symptoms inventory. Behav Sci 19:1–15, 1974
28. Eagly AH: Involvement as a determinant of response to favourable and unfavourable information. J Pers Soc Psychol 7:1–15, 1967
29. Weissman M, Bothwell S: Assessment of social adjustment by patient self-report. Arch Gen Psychiat 33:1111–1115, 1976

30. Vandereycken W, Pierloot R: Long-term outcome research in anorexia nervosa. Int J Eating Disorders 2:237–242, 1983
31. Vandereycken W, Pierloot R: The significance of subclassification in anorexia nervosa: A comparative study of clinical features in 141 patients. Psychol Med 13: 543–549, 1983

25

Childhood Obsessive Compulsive Disorder

Judith L. Rapoport

National Institute of Mental Health, Washington D.C.

INTRODUCTION

Obsessive compulsive disorder has fascinated clinicians for hundreds of years, but because of the high proportion of cases with childhood onset, the disorder holds particular interest for child psychiatrists. The early clinical descriptions of S. Freud (1955) and Janet (1903) mention children 11 and 5 years of age with classical presentation of the disorder. Systematic studies have affirmed that from half (Pitres & Regis, 1902) to one third (Black, 1978) of adult cases have had their onset by age 15. Moreover, unlike depression and schizophrenia, the disorder appears in virtually identical form in children to that in adults.

Several lines of research, some with psychiatric populations, have served to refocus attention on this disorder. New information derived from epidemiological, pharmacological and clinical descriptive studies, from studies of related disorders and from a large prospective study of children with severe primary obsessive compulsive disorder ongoing at the National Institute of Mental Health, suggest that the disorder is more common than had been thought and reaffirm intriguing neurological links.

Questions equally applicable to adults and child patients are: the continuity with normal development and with personality disorder, the na-

Reprinted with permission from the *Journal of Child Psychology and Psychiatry*, 1986, Vol. 27, No. 3, 289–295. Copyright 1986 by the Association for Child Psychology and Psychiatry, Pergamon Journals Ltd.

ture of the association with other disorders, etiology (with focus on neurobiological components) and long term prognosis—particularly in the light of the newer treatments more widely available.

FREQUENCY OF THE DISORDER OF CHILDREN

The clinical literature describing childhood obsessive compulsive disorder is meagre. The disorder presents itself rarely in clinical populations with a reported incidence of 1% in child psychiatric inpatients (Judd, 1965) and 0.2% of total clinical populations (Hollingsworth, Tanguay, Grossman & Pabst, 1980). However, recent data suggest that the disorder may be more common. While no "pure" cases of obsessive compulsive disorder were described in the survey of over 2000 10- and 11-year olds on the Isle of Wight (Rutter, Tizard & Whitmore, 1970), a total of seven cases were seen with mixed obsessive and anxiety features—an incidence of up to 0.3% depending on how these cases should be classified.

In the United States, epidemiological surveys of the general adult population have suggested prevalence rates of up to 0.3% in the population (Helzer, Robins, McEnvoy, Spitznagel, Stoltzman, Farrer & Brockington, 1985). Only one study to date has specifically examined a large adolescent population for obsessive compulsive disorder (Flament, Rapoport, Whitaker, Berg & Sceery, 1985b). In this study, over 5000 unselected adolescents, the entire high school population of a county in the State of New Jersey, completed a 20 item childhood version of the Leyton Observational Interview as part of a more general survey (Berg, Rapoport & Flament, 1986). Out of the 4451 adolescents who correctly completed the questionnaire, about 2% responded with both high "yes" scores (the number of symptoms reported to be present) and high "interference" scores— a rating of the degree to which these symptoms interfered with their daily activities. The cut-off scores were derived from a clinical population study described below. Follow-up interviews by clinicians experienced with the disorder in childhood revealed 15 "true" cases (those experiencing the symptoms as disturbing and interfering significantly with functioning), about 0.33% of the total population. This is probably a minimal figure because many children with this disorder are secretive, and those most severely disturbed would not have been able to complete the questionnaire (500 children did not do so) or would be too ill to attend school.

THE NIMH STUDY POPULATION

Because of the relative rarity of the disorder, most descriptive information has depended on a case-finding approach. The prospective study at the National Institute of Mental Health is the largest cohort to date of children with this disorder. The sample now consists of 30 cases with an age onset of between 3 and 14 years, having a mean age of 14.5 years on initial referral to the study. The sample is two thirds males, who tended to become ill 2.5 years earlier than females ($P < 0.01$). This appears to be a true difference and not an artifact of initial referral which did not differ by sex.

The patterns of obsessions and compulsions are quite similar to those seen in adults with cleaning rituals most frequently found. Counting and checking rituals are also common, as are repetitive thoughts of violent or sexual events. As with adults, in some cases, differentiation from phobic disorder can be difficult. Other subgroups blend into a Tourette's "spectrum" as discussed below. No case of pure obsessional slowing has been observed.

Because of the relative availability of information about early development from parents, teachers and siblings as well as the child himself, the study provided an opportunity to examine the pre-existing behavioural pattern before the onset of the disorder. As the onset occurred either suddenly or over the period of a few months in most cases, it was relatively easy to distinguish behaviours before the disorder began. Most striking was the absence in early history of obsessive traits for the majority of the group. These children were not particularly noted for their fastidiousness, neatness or superstitious behaviour, nor had they exhibited any exaggeration of normal rituals (meals, bedtime, washing routines) during early childhood. There was however, a predominance of "internalizing" behaviour styles as measured by the Child Behavior Checklist scores (Achenbach & Edelbrock, 1979). The clinical impression, therefore, is clearly that of discontinuity from normal development for these clinically referred subjects.

Examination of the adolescents selected by the epidemiological study of Flament *et al.* (1985b), also suggests a discontinuity from normal personality development even for less severe forms of these behaviours. In this study, 15 children were identified with what were labelled "obsessional features". For example, three of the 15 children would arise some hours earlier than the rest of their family a few days each week in order to wash the walls of their room. This group comprising 0.3% of the total survey population, was "flagged" by the Leyton screening instrument, but received no clinical diagnosis at follow-up interview because their overall functioning was judged to be good and they did not see their behaviours as interfering with their lives in any significant way. However, when asked about the onset of these behaviours, most recalled a rather sudden onset: the subject could often name the month it started, even if this had occurred a year or two before the interview. Thus symptoms did not seem to blend with normal habits.

There was a smaller number of subjects identified on initial screening by the high "yes" and low "interference" scores whom we have called "super normals". These were phenomenally ambitious, energetic youngsters who were carrying out more academic and extracurricular activities and having more responsibilities than most classmates; they led heavily programmed lives, leaving themselves almost no flexibility, sometimes to a remarkable degree. They described a life of teams, jobs, exercise, extra classes, community volunteer work etc. with extraordinarily high performance in all areas. They were concerned about expectations, achievement and worried that they would not meet their heroic list of commitments. Whether "super normals" is at this time, the right term for this group is only a philosophical question. A follow-up study of these subjects as well as those with "obsessional features" is planned.

ASSOCIATION WITH OTHER CONDITIONS

In adults the most commonly associated psychiatric disorder is depression which has occurred either before, concurrently or after the onset of obsessive compulsive disorder in 71% of 149 cases (Welner, Reich & Robins, 1976). This does not seem to be the case in childhood, however, as only three out of 30 subjects met criteria for major affective disorders. In part this difference may be due to the relative infrequency of affective disorders in childhood. In contrast is the striking association with Tourette's Syndrome and anorexia nervosa, which typically have a childhood onset. In a study of children with Tourette's syndrome, obsessional features were found to be prominent (Grad, Peleovitz, Olsen, Mathews & Grad, in press) and family studies have found obsessive disorder to be increased in relatives of Tourette's patients (Nee, Caine, Eldridge & Ebert, 1980; Pauls, Leckman, Towbin, Zahner & Cohen, 1985) even if the proband did not have obsessive symptoms. Clinically, patients with anorexia nervosa often display obsessional symptoms independent of the preoccupation with food. Conversely, women with obsessive compulsive disorder frequently report a past hisory of anorexia nervosa while agrophobics do not have such a history (Kasvikis, Marks, Basoglu & Noshirvani, in press). Four of the 30 children in the NIMH cohort had had motor tics at some time although none of their first degree relatives had a history of tic disorder. Three others had odd "twitches" of the limbs difficult to classify.

It is clear that obsessive disorder can also occur with a variety of other behavioural patterns and this variable pattern of associations may be particulary striking with children. Anna Freud noted that " . . . while in adults symptoms more usually form part of a related personality structure, this is not so for children. In children, symptoms occur just as often in isolation, or are coupled with other symptoms and personality traits of a different nature and unrelated origin" (A. Freud, 1965). This is well-illustrated by the recent report by Bolton & Turner (1984) of two adolescents, both aged 14, with clinically severe obsessive compulsive disorder as well as conduct disorder which appeared to be entirely independent from confrontations over rituals. Similarly, in the NIMH series of 30 cases, six adolescents, four males and two females also met criteria for conduct disorder.

There are a host of neurological links for obsessive compulsive disorder, reviewed elsewhere (Kettle & Marks, in press). Most of these associations have been reported for both adult and adolescent patients but adolescent cases seem particularly well-represented in most series. Aubrey Lewis (1936) for example, noted several cases with childhood onset following encephalitis or febrile seizures. Obsessive phenomena have long been recognised in association with seizures, particularly temporal lobe epilepsy (Bear & Fedio, 1977). Recently, Kettle & Marks (in press) reported two cases with onset of both seizures and obsessive rituals in adolescence; both were aided by behavioural treatment rather than by medical control of seizures. In NIMH series, a variety of "soft" neurological abnormalities have been noted including minor neuromotor disturbances, neuropsychological test deficits similar to those seen in patients with frontal lobe abnormality, and increased ventricular brain ratios on CT scans and abnormal EEG (Rapoport, Elkins, Langer, Sceery, Buchsbaum, Gillin, Murphy, Zahn, Lake, Ludlow & Mendelson, 1981; Behar, Rapoport, Berg, Denckla, Mann, Cox, Fedio, Zahn & Wolfmann, 1984). Unfortunately, these signs did not cluster with a subgroup of patients, but were distributed in various combinations throughout the sample.

TREATMENT

Obsessive compulsive disorder in children, as in adults, generally resists psychodynamic treatment [Zetzel, 1966; Fenichel (quoted in Lewis, 1936); S. Freud, 1958]. While great progress has been made in behavioural treatment with adults (Foa & Goldstein, 1978; Marks, Stern, Mawson, Cobb and McDonald, 1980), relatively few reports have specifically addressed behavioural treatment with obsessive children, although these few indicate that children are able to form useful alliances with behavioural therapists, that family cooperation is even more essential and that failure to enlist this cooperation may be the most difficult aspect of treating children (Weiner, 1967; Bolton, Collins & Steinberg, 1983).

The most promising recent development in the psychopharmacological treatment of obsessive compulsive disorder has been the use of clomipramine hydrochloride (Anafranil). There are now six double-blind studies with adult obsessive compulsive disorder patients, and one study with children and adolescents. Flament, Rapoport, Berg, Sceery, Kilts, Mellstromm & Linnoila (1985c) reported significant improvement in a group of 19 adolescents (mean age 14.5 years) after 5 weeks on clomipramine (mean doses 141 mg/day) compared to their response to a placebo. Few of the children were clinically depressed, and depression at baseline did not predict response to the drug; the effect appeared to be independent of an anti-depressant action. Clinical response did not correlate significantly with plasma concentration of the drug or its metabolites, or with the increase in plasma norepinephrine. However, clinical amelioration when using the drug did correlate significantly with the drug-induced decrease in platelet serotonin (Flament, Rapoport and Murphy, 1985a).

It has become clear from these treatment studies that "symptom substitution" does not occur. That is, once patients are relieved of these symptoms, for the most part they improve their functioning in other areas; new obsessive symptoms do not emerge when the old ones have been improved with either pharmacological or behavioural treatment.

COMMENT AND SPECULATION

Childhood obsessive compulsive disorder is now gaining the attention from child psychiatrists that it deserves. The epidemiological study of Flament *et al.* (1985b) has extended the recent findings with adult populations to adolescents indicating that this is an under-recognized and under-referred disorder. In the light of promising evidence that both behavioural and pharmacological treatments are effective with this age group, greater sensitivity to this diagnosis is important.

The relative specificity of clomipramine's action in blocking neuronal re-uptake of serotonin has led to a "serotonin hypothesis" of obsessive compulsive disorder. This is particularly intriguing in the light of reports of low CSF 5HIAA in suicidally depressed adult individuals, and those with impulsive antisocial behaviours (Asberg, Traskman & Thoren, 1976; Brown, Goodwin, Ballenger, Goyer & Major, 1979) and recent work has extended these relationships to personality measurement in nonclinical populations (Schalling, personal communication). It is tempting to speculate that there is a spectrum of dyscontrol syndromes mediated by serotonergic dysfunction. However, direct evidence for any abnormality of serotonin metabolism in obsessive patients is lacking. Thoren, Asberg, Bertilsson & Traskman (1980) found no difference in CSF 5HIAA between obsessive compulsive patients and matched controls. Insel, Mueller, Alterman, Linnoila & Murphy (1985) found CSF 5HIAA to be slightly higher in patients than in controls. In children platelet serotonin did not differ between 27 unmedicated adolescent patients with obsessive compulsive disorder and matched controls (Flament *et al.,* 1985a).

The relationships between obsessive compulsive disorder, Tourette's Syndrome and conduct disorder are particularly intriguing. Obsessive compulsive disorder might be considered the inverse of Tourette's Syndrome with preoccupation about control of unacceptable gestures or words. Can these be two sides of one neurobiological coin? Animal models are lacking, but studies of basal ganglia lesions in squirrel monkeys suggest that the globus pallidus may mediate some ritual-like behaviours. It is possible that grooming behaviours (in the absence of feeding or defecation) could also be traced to specific brain areas and provide a model for the disorder (McLean, 1978).

As with most aspects of childhood psychopathology, these recent findings bring more questions than answers. Identification of cases is difficult for epidemiological studies as the best instrument to date, the LOI-CV (Berg *et al.,* 1986) has a sensitivity of about 50% (that is, it will only select about 50% of true cases). Epidemiological studies should select populations with symptoms of moderate severity as well as those with "obsessional features" and "supernormals" already discussed. Follow-up of these individuals, including family studies would be of broad interest, for as Aubrey Lewis wrote: "it is difficult to understand some of these problems without also defining the nature of man" (Lewis, 1936).

While the response to clomipramine is intriguing, the clear superiority of this agent over other antidepressants has not yet been conclusively demonstrated. Moreover, other actions of this drug such as its antiparasitic effects also distinguish it from other tricyclic antidepressants (Zilberstein & Dwyer, 1984). Even with the availability of this drug its long-term usefulness is not clear, as preliminary follow-up data suggest wear-off of efficacy with prolonged use in several cases.

Finally, the neurological associations are only suggestive: it is hoped that newer brain-imaging techniques such as positron emission tomography or xenon inhalation may be useful in studying CNS (central nervous system) function in this debilitating disorder.

REFERENCES

Achenbach, T. & Edelbrock, C. (1979). The child behaviour profile—II. Boys aged 12-16 and girls 6-11 and 12-16. *Journal of Consulting Clinical Psychologists,* **47,** 223-233.

Asberg, M., Traskman, L. & Thoren, P. (1976). 5-HIAA in the cerebrospinal fluid—a biochemical suicide predictor? *Archives of General Psychiatry,* **33,** 1193-1197.

Bear, D. & Fedio, P. (1977). Quantitative analysis of interictal behavior in temporal lobe epilepsy. *Archives of Neurology,* **34,** 454-467.

Behar, D., Rapoport, J., Berg, C., Denckla, M., Mann, L., Cox, C., Fedio, P., Zahn, T. & Wolfmann, M. (1984). Computerized tomography and neuropsychological test measures in adolescents with obsessive compulsive disorder. *American Journal of Psychiatry,* **141,** 363-369.

Berg, C., Rapoport, J. & Falment, M. (1986). The Leyton obsessional inventory—child version. *Journal of the American Academy of Child Psychiatry,* **25,** 84-91.

Black A. (1978). The natural history of obsessional neurosis. In H.R. Beech (Ed.), *Obsessional states* (pp. 19-54). London: Methuen.

Bolton, D., & Turner, T. (1984). Obsessive compulsive neurosis with conduct disorder: a report of two cases. *Journal of Child Psychology and Psychiatry,* **25,** 133-139.

Bolton, D., Collins, S. & Steinberg, D. (1983). The treatment of obsessive compulsive disorder in adolescence: a report of 15 cases. *British Journal of Psychiatry,* **142,** 456-464.

Brown, G. L., Goodwin, F., Ballenger, J., Goyer, P. & Major, F. (1979). Aggression in humans correlates with cerebrospinal fluid amine metabolites. *Psychiatry Research,* **1,** 131-139.

Flament, M., Rapoport, J. & Murphy, D. (1985a). Biochemical correlates of response to clomipramine in an adolescent population. Poster presented at Annual Meeting of *American College of Neuropsychopharmacology,* 12 December. Hawaii.

Flament, M., Rapoport, J., Whitaker, A., Berg, C. & Sceery, W. (1985b). Obsessive compulsive disorders in adolescents: an epidemiological study. Presented at the 32nd meeting of the *American Academy of Child Psychiatry,* 27 October, San Antonio, Texas.

Flament, M., Rapoport, J., Berg, C., Screey, W., Kilts, C., Mellstromm, B., & Linnoila, M. (1985c). Clomipramine treatment of childhood obsessive compulsive disorder. *Archives of General Psychiatry,* **42,** 977-983.

Foa, E. & Goldstein, A. (1978). Continuous exposure and complete response prevention of obsessional neuroses. *Behavioural Therapeutics,* **9,** 821-829.

Freud, A. (1965). *Normality and pathology in childhood.* New York: International Universities Press.

Freud, S. (1955). Obsessions and Phobias: "Their psychical mechanism and their aetiology". In J. Strachey (Ed.), *Collected papers I* (standard edn, pp. 128-137). London: Hogarth Press.

Freud, S. (1958). The predisposition to obsessional neurosis. In J. Strachey (Ed.), *The standard edition of the collected works of Sigmund Freud.* London: Hogarth Press.

Grad. L., Pelcovitz, D., Olsen, M., Mathews, M. & Grad, G. The presence of obsessive compulsive symptoms in children with Tourette's disorder. *Journal of the American Academy of Child Psychiatry* (in press).

Helzer, J., Robins, L., McEnvoy, L., Spitznagel, E., Stoltzman, T., Farrer, A. & Brockington, J. (1985). A comparison of clinical and diagnostic interview schedule diagnosis. *Archives of General Psychiatry*, **42**, 657-666.

Hollingsworth, C., Tanguay, P., Grossman, L. & Pabst, P. (1980). Long-term outcome of obsessive compulsive disorder in childhood. *Journal of the American Academy of Child Psychiatry*, **19**, 134-144.

Insel, T., Mueller, E., Alterman, I., Linnoila, M. & Murphy, D. (1985).Obsessive compulsive disorder and serotonin: Is there a connection? *Biological Psychiatry*, **20**, 1174-1188.

Janet, P. (1903). *Les Obsessions et al Psychiasthenie* (Vol. I). Paris: Felix Alcan.

Judd, L. (1965). Obsessive compulsive neurosis in children. *Archives of General Psychiatry*, **12**, 135-144.

Kasvikis, Y., Tsakiris, F., Marks, I., Basoglu, M. & Noshirvani, H. Women with obsessive compulsive disorder frequently report a past history of anorexia nervosa. *International Journal of Eating Disorders* (in press).

Kettle, P. & Marks, I. Neurological factors in an obsessive compulsive disorder. Two case reports and a review of the literature. *British Journal of Psychiatry* (in press).

Lewis, A. (1936). Problems of obsessional illness. *Proceedings of the Royal Society of Medicine*, **29**, 325-336.

Marks, I. (1980). Review of behavioral psychotherapy: I. Obsessive Compulsive Disorders. *American Journal of Psychiatry*, **138**, 584-592.

Marks, I., Stern, R., Mawson, D., Cobb, J. & McDonald, R. (1980). Clomipramine and exposure for obsessive compulsive rituals. *British Journal of Psychiatry*, **136**, 1-25.

McLean, P. (1978) Effects of lesions of the globus pallidus on species typical display behavior in squirrel monkeys. *Brain Research* **149**, 175-196.

Nee, L., Caine, E., Eldridge, R & Ebert, M. (1980). Gilles de la Tourette syndrome: clinical and family study of 50 cases. *Annals of Neurology*, **7**, 41-49.

Pauls, D., Leckman, J., Towbin, K., Zahner, G., & Cohen, D. (1985). Tourette's syndrome and obsessive compulsive disorder; family study evidence for a genetic relationship. Presented at the 32nd annual meeting of the *American Academy of Child Psychiatry*, 27 October, San Antonio, Texas.

Pitres, A. & Regis, E. (1902). *Les obsessions et les impulsions*. Paris: Doin.

Rapoport, J., Elkins, R., Langer, D., Sceery, W., Buchsbaum, M., Gillin, J.C., Murphy, D., Zahn, T., Lake, R., Ludlow, C. & Medelson, W. (1981). Childhood obsessive compulsive disorder, *American Journal of Psychiatry*, **138**, 1545-1553.

Rutter, M., Tizard, J. & Whitmore, K. (1970). *Education Health & Behavior*, London: Longmans.

Thoren, P., Asberg, M., Bertilsson, L. & Traskman, L. (1980). Clomipramine treatment of obsessive compulsive disorder: II. Biochemical aspects. *Archives of General Psychiatry*, **37**, 1289-1295.

Weiner, I. (1967). Behavior therapy in obsessive compulsive neurosis: Treatment of an adolescent boy. Theory resident practice. *Psychotherapy*, **4**, 27-29.

Welner, A., Reich, T. & Robins, E. (1976). Obsessive compulsive neurosis: record follow-up and family studies. *Comprehensive Psychiatry*, **17**, 527-539.

Zetzel, E. (1966). Additional notes upon a case of obsessional neurosis. *International Journal of Psychoanalysis*, **47**, 123-129.

Zilberstein, P. & Dwyer, D. (1984). Antidepressants cause lethal disruption or membrane function in the human protozoan parasite Leishmania. *Science*, **226**, 977-979.

Part VII

OTHER CLINICAL ISSUES

Rachel Gittelman Klein's paper, "Questioning the Clinical Usefulness of Projective Psychological Tests for Children," is timely and pertinent. Examining the major projective tests one by one, she disputes the claims for their accuracy in providing diagnostic reinforcement or in identifying personality characteristics hard to elicit in clinical examination, although the tests may be useful for other purposes. Klein also points out that, despite the great overlap in projective test findings and clinical diagnosis, pharmacological decisions have in fact been made on the sole "evidence" of a projective test report—a practice which she deplores. It is certainly true, as Klein would agree, that projective tests can be clinically useful in certain situations in which the diagnosis is in doubt. But the whole thrust of her argument, which we can reaffirm by our own experiences in clinical practice, is that these projective tests for children are often used so automatically and routinely that the result is an enormous waste of valuable and expensive professional time. As a result, children are frequently denied special tests that they really need and are also deprived of the therapeutic services of expert psychologists whose time is preempted by unnecessary routine projective tests.

We are reprinting three separate articles by Keith D. McDaniel, which appeared in consecutive issues of *Clinical Pediatrics,* entitled "Pharmacologic Treatment of Psychiatric and Neurodevelopmental Disorders in Children and Adolescents (Parts 1, 2, and 3)." Taken together, the McDaniel's articles go systematically from one syndrome to another. In each case we are offered a concise but adequate critical review of the drug treatment issues for each syndrome. In an otherwise splendid guide for clinicians, there is one surprising omission in that no mention is made of tardive dyskinesia, although many other side effects are discussed. (There is a previous excellent review of tardive dyskinesia in children by Gualtieri and Hawk in the 1981 volume of this series).

The effect upon children whose parents have bipolar affective disorder is important for two major reasons. One pertains to the therapist treating the parents whose therapeutic responsibilities should include the attempt to maximize protective factors militating against child pathology. Similarly, the child therapist treating a disturbed child who has a parent with an affective disorder must deal with the specific and special effects such a parental illness can have on the child.

Pellegrini and his group examine these issues and provide specific guidelines and recommendations that can help the child cope with the disruptions and stresses created by the parent's disorder. We are indebted to this study and its findings for practical directions of therapeutic action that will increase the proportion of offspring who, although vulnerable, are able to cope effectively with their stressful home environment.

For decades, the conventional psychiatric wisdom has assumed that accident proneness in children was largely due to intrapsychic factors. The solution, in these terms, was to make psychotherapy available to the child.

The well-known Louisville twin study has been gathering data on home environments, parental features, SES, and child characteristics for many years and also contains information on child injuries. We mourn the recent death of Ronald Wilson whose long-time collaboration with Adam Matheny in the Louisville Twin Study helped maintain its high level. Matheny, in the paper "Injuries Among Toddlers: Contributions from Child, Mother, and Family," has assessed objectively the factors in toddlers aged one to three that increase or decrease the risk of injury. His data derive from maternal self reports and reports on child injuries, direct observations in the home, and child behavior in the laboratory.

Using the statistical method of Regression Analysis, it was possible to find that, when entered first, toddler temperament seemed a significant factor, but as other environmental features were entered and significances adjusted accordingly, the influence of the toddler's characteristics was far outweighed by specific contributions of the environment. Matheny assumes that this is a developmental phenomenon, and its results should not be applied to older children for whom other factors, including within-child characteristics may be of greater importance. In this paper, we are given a clear set of findings that should focus the clinician's attention on those changes in the home environment that can prevent or minimize accidents to toddlers.

Major efforts of mental health professionals regarding child cancer patients have been, until recently, mainly: 1) explaining the symptoms and treatments to children of varying developmental ages; 2) helping children and relatives prepare for an indominantly approaching death;

and 3) helping with the guilt and hindsights of sibs, parents, and others close to the dead child.

Currently, treatment of childhood malignancies has gained in efficacy even though discomforts still prevail, successes remain in the statistical domain, and guilt flourishes for whatever decision has been made if the outcome is unfortunate.

Freund and Siegel, in their paper "Problems in Transition Following Bone Marrow Transplantation: Psychosocial Aspects," based on experiences at Memorial Hospital, report on issues surrounding bone marrow transplants for children with acute leukemia, aplastic anemia, and immune deficiency disease. While positive outcomes are growing in number, mortality is still high. Freund and her associate explore sibs' reactions both to donation and refusal to donate marrow, the patient's and families' reactions to the sick child role while the patient is in danger, as well as during and after recovery. These are matters that will involve clinicians more and more frequently as treatments and survivals mount and the psychological issues become more and more complex.

PART VII: OTHER CLINICAL ISSUES

26

Questioning the Clinical Usefulness of Projective Psychological Tests for Children

Rachel Gittelman Klein

Columbia University, College of Physicians and Surgeons, New York

INTRODUCTION

It is not unusual for psychologists to be asked to assess personality characteristics, such as self-image and esteem, aggressive fantasies and the propensity for their expression, sexual identification, the nature of the child's intrapsychic conflicts, and many more. In order to address these important clinical questions, psychologists often use tests.

Understandably, at times, pediatricians may wish to obtain evaluations other than clinical history to determine the nature of a child's behavioral difficulties and, for this purpose, may refer for psychological testing. The purpose of this paper is to acquaint the reader with the literature on the use of personality and psychodiagnostic testing in children and, thereby, enable pediatricians to reach educated decisions regarding the contribution psychological testing can make in their work with psychiatrically disturbed youngsters.

Psychological testing encompasses various procedures for multiple purposes. The review pertains to projective testing only, and not to psychological testing, in general. Therefore, the value of other psychological assessments such as intelligence and neuropsychological testing should not be inferred from knowledge about the tests discussed here.

Reprinted with permission from *Developmental and Behavioral Pediatrics,* 1986, Vol. 7, No. 6, 378–382. Copyright 1986 by Williams & Wilkins Co.

Rationale of Projective Testing

Most tests used to evaluate children's personality and their conflicts are projective tests. They differ from other tests in that they do not have a correct answer, but allow free rein for response. Their use is rooted in psychoanalytic theory. More specifically, it is predicated on the projective hypothesis, which posits that the interpretation of all experiences is colored by unconscious repressed mental content. Reliance on intrapsychic material is greater when responding to experiences that are ambiguous, rather than well-defined, in content. Consequently, when reacting to test materials that do not have clear content, the child will expose aspects of psychic content not otherwise easily apparent. In this way, a glimpse is offered of the child's unconscious drives or wishes and the nature of the defenses against these drives. The projective tests can be viewed as a controlled form of dream production, or projective play, and the analytic interpretation process of the test responses can proceed in the same vein. A less inferential, more descriptive approach is also used with projective tests in children.

The fact that projective tests are used for evaluating personality, such as the tendency for aggression, feelings about self, sexual conflicts, and more, as well as the presence of a mental disorder, such as a pervasive developmental disorder, schizophrenia, depressive disorders, and so on, rests on the long-held (but unsubstantiated) theory that the same psychological processes account for all aspects of human behavior. Therefore, the same tools can be used to delve into personality traits (which all children have), and psychiatric diagnoses (which, happily, only some have).

There are several levels at which diagnosis can be conducted: one may look for types and levels of personality organization, for specific personality characteristics, and for syndromes or mental disorders. As noted, many believe that there exist dynamic relationships between personality features and psychiatric disorders. Insofar as this model (so far unsubstantiated) of psychopathology is accurate, information regarding personality provides meaningful data for formal diagnostic classification, and for this purpose projective tests might be useful.

PROJECTIVE TESTS

The commonly used projective tests are summarized briefly to familiarize the reader.

Rorschach Test

This is the best-known and least structured personality test; it consists of 10 inkblots, some in colors. The child is told to report what the card looks like to him.

Thematic Apperception Test (TAT)

The TAT consists of 30 cards; all but one blank depict a scene with varying degrees of explicit pictorial content. The examiner selects a number of cards for which the child is asked to make up a complete story.

Children's Apperception Test (CAT)

The CAT is intended to be a child's version of the TAT. It has 10 cards depicting animal scenes that are likely to be more appealing to children than the pictures of the TAT. It shows animals involved in a variety of family type activities intended to reflect parent-child relationships, sibling rivalry. Again, the child is asked to tell a full story for each card.

Blacky Pictures

This test also consists of 10 cards depicting a puppy involved in situations related to the Freudian psychosexual stages of development, especially the oral and anal stages.

Drawings

Among projective drawings are figure drawings, or Draw-a-Person (DAP) test, where the child is asked to draw a person, and the House-Tree-Person, which calls for a drawing of a house and a tree, and drawing of a family as well. Inquiry follows regarding various aspects of the drawing, such as the age and sex of the person, and the child may be asked to talk about the picture. Characteristics such as body image, gender typing, self-esteem, sexual anxiety, capacity for warmth, aggression, and many other personality constructs are inferred from the drawings.

Bender-Gestalt Test

A series of nine geometric designs are copied by the child. Various characteristics of the child's reproductions are used as indices of emotional adjustment.

PERSONALITY TESTING: IS IT VALID?

Personality testing often is requested when there is doubt regarding the significance of the child's symptoms. For example, a child is reported to be aggressive, but the diagnostician wants confirmation of the characterological nature of the aggressive behavior. The assumption underlying projective tests is that, if the child produces aggressive responses, the clinician will be confident that the child's aggression is an important aspect of his personality. If no aggressive themes are present, the significance of the child's overt aggression may be minimized. Conversely, a child who is not aggressive but who produces aggressive themes on the projective testing may be viewed as having great propensity for aggression, or as having a conflict about the expression of hostile feelings. In turn, this trait would be viewed as playing a role in the child's emotional adjustment.

The foregoing assumptions are not rooted in empirical evidence. In fact, there is very little evidence to document the belief that children's personality characteristics are well estimated by projective testing. For example, in a study of the TAT, only one of five ratings of aggression differentiated aggressive and nonaggressive children. In the one discriminant measure, the frequency of response between the two types of children differed by only one response.[1] This magnitude of difference is too small to be applied in a diagnostic fashion. In a study of disturbed children, the Draw-a-Person Test was not found to predict levels of current or future aggression.[2] A large study compared drawings of male delinquents classified as aggressive, withdrawn, and undifferentiated, and nondelinquents, to determine the value of signs that had been previously reported useful to diagnose aggression. Although some signs differentiated the groups, the results are truly puzzling; there were more differences between the types of delinquents than between the delinquents and nondelinquents. Furthermore, the signs occurred only infrequently, therefore providing limited potential for detecting positive cases.[3] Similarly disappointing results were reported with the Bender-Gestalt. The clinical criteria believed to indicate symbolic representation of aggression—heavy drawing over, and progressively larger figures—were unrelated to levels of expressed aggression.[4]

Attempts to identify differences in various aspects of emotional well-being among children whose fathers had died,[5] whose parents had divorced,[6] or who had been placed in foster care[7] also have failed.

The empirical literature dealing with personality assessment in children is surprisingly scant. Therefore, it is not possible to draw definite conclusions concerning the accuracy of personality testing in children. Among the tests, the DAP emerges as an invalid personality test—the indicators of emotional disturbance have not been shown to be reliable.[8]

The TAT has also failed to show satisfactory validity.[9] Too little work has been done with the Rorschach to assess its validity with children. Certainly, given the state of our knowledge, it is unjustified to rely on the test results to rule out the presence of disorders when symptoms are evident, or to assume from the tests that personality deviance is present when it is not evident in the child's behavior.

In addition to describing the current personality pattern, projective tests are sometimes used to reconstruct the child's early developmental psychological history. Statements regarding oral or anal conflicts may be advanced to account for the present clinical picture. This practice is of very dubious merit. Schafer,[10] a leading psychoanalyst, believes that it should be avoided because it provides unreliable historical reconstructions.

Just as questionable is the practice of predicting what is likely to happen to a child on the basis of projective testing. Some report the likelihood of future regression into a psychotic state, or suicide, or sexual maladjustment. There is a total absence of support for the merit of this practice; it is, unfortunately, totally deceptive.

To illustrate concretely the type of unwarranted reconstructions and predictions that are made from projective testing, a few excerpts from actual psychological test reports are quoted:

> The potential for ideas of reference, feelings of depersonalization, are indicated. The groundwork for suicidal ideation has been laid in the desire to retreat back to the maternal womb.
>
> He had achieved a dependent attachment to a mother figure whom he couldn't grasp or understand, but he experienced her as cold and demanding.
>
> A tendency, related perhaps to homosexual strivings, toward severe repression, leading to suicide and imagined rebirth, is evidenced and suicide precautions are indicated.

Statements such as these are extremely seductive; they lead to the belief that heretofore unsuspected events have been revealed. However, these interesting reconstructions and predictions have not fared well when put to the test. Thus, a well-executed longitudinal study of normals tested five times between 8 and 16 years did not find consistency in Rorschach scores over time. The data preclude long-term predictions derived from children's test responses.[11] The study provides documentation for the strong reservations concerning the predictive utility of personality testing in children.

DIAGNOSIS

The practice of classifying patients on the basis of projective tests has a long history. Over the years, many claims have been made regarding the characteristics of schizophrenia, psychopathy, neurosis, and other disorders, on psychological tests. As an example, the presence of "primary-process" responses on projective tests has been used to make a diagnosis of schizophrenia.

The detailed evidence regarding the use of psychological tests for diagnostic purposes leads to the unequivocal conclusion that there is no evidence whatever to support the use of such testing for diagnostic purposes, except in two instances: mental retardation and specific developmental disorders.[12-14]

As an example of what cannot be done, a recent personal observation is reported. The psychological testing of a school-phobic child reportedly indicated psychosis. Because of the test results, the youngster was treated with neuroleptics (in this instance, without success). The ethics of such practice are, at the very best, questionable.

In this anecdote, the use of antipsychotic medication follows logically from the report of schizophrenia. However, the diagnosis is based on the erroneous presumption that psychological tests are diagnostically informative. It is a grave error to make diagnostic or pharmacotherapeutic decisions on the basis of projective testing. This is not to say that the conclusions from the tests should have been ignored completely. They might have raised concern regarding the possible evidence of psychosis and called for a clinical review of the diagnosis. If no evidence for a history of psychosis had been elicited from further interviewing, the test results should have been ignored.

FACTORS COMPLICATING TEST INTERPRETATIONS

Age and IQ have been found to affect test responses. Independent of IQ, reading ability also influences children's Rorschach responses.[15] Clinicians have no means for taking these factors into consideration when they interpret test results, and many studies have failed to control for these factors.

It is important, also, to remember that even when statistically significant results are reported, the overlap in test characteristics among the groups of children studied has been so large that the clinical significance of the findings is nil. The poor showing of the tests is in a context in which the group membership is already established. As explained further on, there is no way to estimate whether the same level of discrimination can be anticipated when the tests are used in clinical situations whose frequency or base rates for the characteristics investigated are very different from those in the samples studied.

Because of the unmet high expectations for personality testing, there has been a devaluing of the merits of making predictions based on their use. The projective tests, although perhaps not very good at predicting, are offered as tools that deepen our understanding. It is obviously true that one can often make predictions without understanding the processes underlying the phonomena observed. However, there is no instance in medicine or psychology where understanding does not facilitate prediction. Therefore, one needs to have serious reservations about procedures that promise understanding but fail to deliver.

An important issue that has been ignored in the use of personality tests in children is the incremental validity of the tests. When a child is referred for testing, much information is already available. The issue then is whether the testing adds further to what is already known. For example, if a diagnosis has been established, does the use of projective testing add to our understanding of the child in a way that will be important in his treatment? Unfortunately, there is a total lack of data from which to derive a rational opinion concerning the incremental validity of projective testing in children. Those who affirm that it exists are expressing a faith, nothing more.

There is a common view that the skill of the psychologist makes up for the inadequacy of the diagnostic tests and that, therefore, in the hands of a talented clinician, projective tests can produce accurate information concerning children's personality and diagnosis. There is no support for this view whatsoever, if one is referring to the interpretation of tests results. As a matter of fact, the evidence points in the opposite direction. When one can make accurate diagnostic interpretations, it is because the deviance is so obvious that most can discern it even in the absence of special training. Subtle inferences by expert clinicians have never been shown to be useful. It is important to keep in mind that I am referring to projective test result interpretations, and not to the observations that can be made from a child's behavior, either during testing or interview. In these situations, it is very likely that talented clinicians make valuable observations and that their judgment is better than that of less capable clinicians.

To conclude, it cannot be emphasized sufficiently that psychiatric diagnosis cannot be made, or even advanced, on the basis of projective test results. This view is echoed even by some with nonambivalent enthusiasm for insights derived from projective tests. For example, a psychoanalyst states, "At present, with current interpretive scoring methods, projective tests should not be used to make important decisions about people."[16]

It is most regrettable that professionals continue to recommend the use of psychological tests to establish a diagnosis, without providing any supporting evidence.[17] Even more deplorable is the allocation of scarce resources to psychodiagnostic testing.

There are some methodological issues that influence the usefulness of psychological tests. The most important, to understand their value in the clinical setting, are the concepts of *sensitivity* and *specificity*. These are touched upon briefly to highlight the pitfalls of noncritical application of personality tests.

Sensitivity and Specificity

Two types of mistakes can occur in the diagnostic process, whether medical or psychological: false-positive and false-negative errors. The terms *sensitivity* and *specificity* are now used to refer to the related concepts of *true positives* and *true negatives*. Sensitivity indicates true positives, that is, diagnosing an illness when it is truly present. Specificity denotes true negatives, i.e., saying that an illness is absent when it is truly absent.

When tests for a type of brain damage are being developed, for example, children with brain damage are compared with those without it. Let us assume, as is often the case, that the groups are roughly equivalent in size; half the children have the disorder and half do not (a base rate of 50% for the disorder). The test is found to select the affected children significantly beyond chance, and is now touted as a good measure for that type of brain damage. (The use of brain damage as an example is purely arbitrary. We could also speak of personality type.) The test now is used with the expectations that it is useful for that particular diagnosis. However, the fact that significant discrimination was found in the experiment with a 50% base rate does not mean that the same degree of accuracy exists in the clinical setting where the base rate for the disorder is different from the ratio in the experiment.[18-21]

In Table 1, the rate of accurate diagnosis is presented for tests with identical sensitivity and specificity; in all instances, the tests are posited to have 60, 70, 80, 90, or 95% accuracy in ruling in (sensitivity) and ruling out (specificity) a disorder. Only the base rate of the disorder has been varied to be either 5 or 50%. The entries in the table represent the percentage of accurate diagnoses in each setting. Note that when only 5% of the clinic patients have a condition, there is extremely poor accuracy, even when both sensitivity and specificity are excellent. For example, if a test has 90% accuracy for establishing the diagnosis when it is present, as well as for dismissing it when it is absent in those diagnosed, only 32% will actually have the disorder. Note that if the tests were not used, and all patients were declared not to have the disorder, a 95% rate of accuracy would be achieved.

Given similarly high sensitivity and specificity (90%) in clinics with a base rate of 50% for the disorder, the percentage correctly diagnosed will improve dramatically. We now reach an 86% accuracy among those diagnosed—a most desirable level, and one far better than if the test had not been used.

In almost all clinical situations, each condition for which a diagnosis is sought has a very low base rate. Therefore, impressively accurate diagnostic statements cannot be derived from tests.

The discussion concerning the poor diagnostic showing of tests when the base rate is low may seem counterintuitive, or even dubious. It is unfortunate that many important issues such as this concerning clinical

Table 1. Percentages of Accurately Identified Cases with Varying Sensitivities and Specificities in Settings with a 5% and 50% Prevalence of Children with a Particular Disorder

Test Specificity (%)	Test Sensitivity (%)									
	60[a]		70[a]		80[a]		90[a]		95[a]	
60	7	50	8	54	10	57	11	60	11	61
70	10	57	11	61	12	64	14	67	14	68
80	14	67	16	70	17	73	19	75	20	76
90	24	80	27	82	30	84	32	86	33	86
95	39	89	42	90	46	91	49	92	50	93

[a]The first and second columns represent accurate diagnostic assignments when the base rate for the diagnosis is 5% and 50%, respectively.

assessment require expert critical review. The well-intentioned clinician does not have the background necessary to judge the diagnostic adequacy of the personality tests available, and, unfortunately, test popularity is not an index of excellence.

CONCLUSIONS

It is important to repeat that the very negative picture presented here pertains only to projective testing. There are other psychological testing procedures, such as tests of cognitive ability, that have great merit. When first introduced, personality tests very understandably carried a tremendous promise, but it remains unfulfilled. However, old convictions die hard. A personal anecdote is a case in point. An eminent physician had referred patients to me regularly for diagnostic evaluation. He called me to ask me to test a young woman to determine whether she had an obsessive compulsive disorder. I agreed to evaluate the patient but informed my colleague that my decision would not rest on her performance on personality tests. He did not refer the patient nor any other subsequently.

Properly trained clinicians can provide very important information about a child's adjustment, his relationships with his family, and his diagnosis. Unfortunately, projective tests do not provide us with sufficient valid information to use them as aids in the diagnostic process of behavior and emotional disorders. The fact that we call them tests is probably most misleading to physicians who have the model of laboratory tests. These are critical to many physical diagnoses, and, in some instances, they may render results of clinical examinations almost superfluous. The same expectation is often held for personality tests. Nothing could be further from reality. They are not tests at all, but procedures from which inferences based on unsubstantiated models of psychological development are made. The whole enterprise would not be troublesome, were it not so expensive, and were it not for the fact that very important decisions are based on them. Perpetuating their use for diagnostic purposes keeps us in the Middle Ages, practicing alchemists trying to turn base metals into precious ones.

REFERENCES

1. Kagan J: The measurement of overt aggression from fantasy. J Abnorm Soc Psychol 52:390–393, 1956
2. Breidenbaugh B, Brozovich R, Matheson L: The hand test and other aggression indicators in emotionally disturbed children. J Pers Assess 38:332–334, 1974

3. Daum JM: Emotional indicators in drawings of aggressive or withdrawn male delinquents. J Pers Assess 47:243–249, 1983
4. Trahan D, Stricklin A: Bender-Gestalt emotional indicators and acting-out behavior in young children. J Pers Assess 43:365–375, 1979
5. Lifshitz M: Social differentiation and organization of the Rorschach in fatherless and two-parented children. J Clin Psychol 31:126–130, 1975
6. Kelly R, Berg B: Measuring children's reactions to divorce. J Clin Psychol 34:215–222, 1978
7. North GE, Keiffer RS: Thematic productions of children in foster homes. Psychol Rep 19:43–46, 1966
8. Hammer M, Kaplan AM: The reliability of children's human figure drawings. J Clin Psychol 22:316–319, 1966
9. Reddy PV: A study of the reliability and validity of the Children's Apperception Test. Br J Educ Psychol 30:182–184, 1960
10. Schafer R: Criteria for judging the adequacy of interpretations, in Jackson DN, Messick S (eds): Problems of Human Assessment. New York, RE Krieger Co, 1978, pp 559–574
11. Exner JE, Thomas EA, Mason B: Children's Rorschachs: Description and prediction. J Pers Assess 49:13–20, 1985
12. Gittelman Klein R: Validity of projective tests for psychodiagnosis in children, in Spitzer RL, Klein DF (eds): Critical Issues in Psychiatric Diagnosis. New York, Raven Press, 1978, pp 141–166
13. Gittelman R: The role of psychological tests for differential diagnosis in child psychiatry: A review. J Am Acad Child Psychiatry 19:413–437, 1980
14. Gittelman R: The use of psychological tests in clinical practice with children, in Shaffer D, Ehrhardt AA, Greenhill LL (eds): The Clinical Guide to Child Psychiatry. New York, The Free Press, 1985, pp 447–474
15. Alheidt P: The effect of reading ability on Rorschach performance. J Pers Assess 44:3–10, 1980
16. Kline P: Psychological Testing. London, Malaby Press, 1976
17. Weiss JL: The clinical use of psychological tests, in Nichol AM (ed): Harvard Guide to Modern Psychiatry. Cambridge, MA, Belknap Press, 1978, pp 41–55
18. Meehl PE: The cognitive activity of the clinician. Am Psychol 15:19–27, 1960
19. Meehl PE: Seer over sign: The first good example. J Exp Res Pers 1:27–32, 1965
20. Meehl PE, Rosen A: Antecedent probability and the efficiency of psychometric signs, patterns, or cutting scores. Psychol Bull 52:194–216, 1955
21. Bernstein DA, Nietzel MT: Introduction to Clinical Psychology. New York, McGraw-Hill, 1980

27

Pharmacologic Treatment of Psychiatric and Neurodevelopmental Disorders in Children and Adolescents (Part 1, Part 2, and Part 3)

Keith D. McDaniel

University of Illinois, Chicago

A review is presented of the diagnosis and drug treatment of the more common psychiatric and developmental disorders in the pediatric population. Where applicable, DSM III (Diagnostic and Statistical Manual of Psychiatric Disorders, III) criteria are utilized to describe the behavioral syndromes. The indications for usage and appropriate dosages of antipsychotics, antidepressants, anxiolytics, stimulants, and lithium are described. Those disorders discussed are attention deficit disorder, conduct disorders, anxiety disorders, sleep disorders, schizophrenia, autism, Tourette's syndrome, mental retardation, depressive illness, manic depressive illness, eating disorders, and enuresis.

Pediatric psychopharmacology offers special challenges. Our selection of psychoactive agents has expanded dramatically. Although the neurosciences have been providing impressive insights into the actions of these

---

Reprinted with permission from *Clinical Pediatrics.* Part 1: 1986, Vol. 25, No. 2, 65–71; Part 2: 1986, Vol. 25, No. 3, 143–146; Part 3: 1986, Vol. 25, No. 4, 198–24. Copyright 1986 by J.B. Lippincott Co.
Editor's Note: This article originally appeared in three consecutive issues of *Clinical Pediatrics,* which are noted above. We are presenting the three installments here as one chapter but have noted where each installment begins. The first installment begins on this page.

agents, pediatric pharmacotherapy has developed more slowly. Because of the lag in psychopharmacologic research in children, the precise indications for drug treatment are not as clearly defined as for adults.

The importance of pediatric psychopharmacology has not passed unnoticed. In *Child Psychiatry: A Plan for the Coming Decade* (1983), the Academy of Child Psychiatry[1] reports that in 1979 the psychopharmacology of childhood received 1.9 percent of Child Mental Health research support. The sparse activity in the field reflects the difficulties of research in this age group related primarily to three factors: (a) the special biology of the developing child, (b) the special psychology of the developing child, and (c) the special place of children in our culture.

Variations in an individual's biology can influence responses to drugs in two ways. There may be differences in the way the biologic system acts on a drug and in the way the drug acts on the biologic system. The first of these sources of variability is referred to as pharmacokinetics. Individuals differ in the way they absorb, metabolize, and eliminate drugs. For example, infants lack enzymes required to metabolize certain drugs. Liver hydroxylation and conjugation of stimulants and benzodiazepines is limited in infants prior to the age of 5 months. However, by 3 years of age, absorption, distribution, protein binding, and metabolism of psychotropic medication is similar to that of an adult.[2] Pharmacodynamics refers to the way the biologic system responds to the drug. This may vary because of changes in a variety of factors. The availability of a drug at a particular location may change. There may be changes in the structure and function of a specific receptor, and there may be changes in the functional organization of systems influenced by the drug. There are clear differences in the way children of different ages respond to a given drug. Not all differences in drug response are due to differences in pharmacodynamics; the developing brain probably does not respond in the same way to a drug as would a fully developed brain. However, the psychotropic effects of most drugs on children are more similar to the effects on adults than they are different.

In the past, large quantities of bodily fluids were needed to carry out some of the assays of drugs and their metabolites so that studies on children were difficult if not impossible. The development of more sensitive and reliable "micro" methods of measurement holds great promise, both for detailed laboratory investigations of pharmacodynamics and for clinical monitoring of drug levels in the individual patient.

The psychology of the developing child also poses two problems in psychopharmacologic research. The first has to do with the reliability of psychiatric diagnosis in children. The second has to do with the evaluation of drug response. Often, it is difficult to obtain useful introspective reports from small children. Additionally, rapid developmental changes make it difficult to describe a stable pattern of psychologic malfunction over time. This has led to a general nosologic vagueness in child psychiatry. Considerable effort is currently being made to remedy the situation, but there is still much work to be done. Here, it is important to remark only that rational psychopharmacology of psychiatric illness is difficult to achieve when the psychiatric illness one proposes to treat is so ill defined that different sorts of disorders are given the same name in different centers.

The same factors that make diagnosis difficult also make evaluation of drug response difficult. Most important is the child's difficulty in verbalizing internal state changes that are necessary data for evaluating and comparing psychoactive drugs.

Finally, the relatively slow progress of pediatric psychopharmacology reflects the special place of the child in our society. Generally, children represent a privileged group in our future-oriented society. Human research committees are strict about permitting research on individuals who cannot give fully informed consent and are particularly stringent when it comes to doing research on normal children. The requirement that research carry potential benefit for the subject almost excludes research on normal subjects and deprives us of some essential information needed to evaluate the responses of pathologic subjects.

The purpose of this review is to provide a description of the more common pediatric psychiatric disorders and the guidelines for appropriate pharmacologic treatment. The orientation of the review is biologic. That is, where appropriate, theories derived from neurochemical, neurophysiologic, and psychobiologic observations are presented, in an effort to lead into the rationale for pharmacologic intervention. There is no intention to undercut the contributions made from psychoanalytic, interpersonal, and psychologic schools of child psychiatry. There is an abundant literature to suggest that psychologic approaches to treatment strategy can be quite effective in subsets of this patient population. Generally, it is accepted that an evaluation of the psychiatrically disturbed child or adolescent should include an assessment of the family, social, educational, and economic environment. This is both important diagnostically and in making treatment recommendations.

Pharmacologic treatment is best carried out concomitantly with non-pharmacologic treatment, which may include individual and family therapy. Because psychopharmacologic treatment of children may require lengthy periods of drug administration, it should only be undertaken when absolutely indicated. It is often helpful to perform an extended evaluation over several weeks or months utilizing some nonpharmalogic methods as trial therapies. This may require referral to a child psychiatrist, child psychologist, family therapist, social worker, and/or educational specialist. If the disorder does not respond to nonpharmacologic treatment or if it is sufficiently severe to be dangerous or disruptive to child and family, the physician should not hesitate to initiate a trial of an appropriate drug, always with careful supervision and monitoring of dosage and effects.

The scope of the treatment approaches presented is limited to pharmacologic. The agents used in the drug management of the disorders discussed are listed in Table 1. For a review of nonpharmacologic forms of treatment the reader is referred elsewhere.[3-15]

BEHAVIORAL SYNDROMES AND THEIR PHARMACOLOGIC TREATMENT (PART 1)

Attention Deficit Disorder

Definition and background. In DSM III,[16] the diagnosis of attention deficit disorder requires that the child show developmentally inappropriate inattention and impulsivity. Inattention is manifested by the failure to finish tasks, easy distractability, apparent poor listening skills, and difficulty concentrating on schoolwork or other tasks requiring sustained attention, including play activities. Impulsivity in these children is characterized by acting before thinking, shifting from one activity to another, difficulty waiting turns, frequently calling out in class and the necessity of close supervision.

The disorder is also subdivided into ADD with hyperactivity and ADD without hyperactivity. To make the diagnosis of ADD with hyperactivity, DSM III requires two of the following signs: (1) runs about or climbs on things excessively, (2) has difficulty sitting still or fidgets excessively, (3) has difficulty staying seated, (4) moves about excessively during sleep, and (5) is always "on the go" or acts as if "driven by a motor." For the diagnosis of ADD, the onset should occur before age 7, the duration should be of at least 6 months, and the symptoms should not be due to schizophrenia or severe mental retardation. In the DSM III manual, affective disorder should also be excluded. That may be a matter of definition. It is rare for a diagnosis of mania to be made before age 7, and when a cyclic affective disorder appears in the former ADD patient, we may wonder if the ADD was not a prodromal or larval form of mania. Even so, follow-up

Table 1. Compendium of Drugs Used in the Pharmacologic Management of Psychiatric and Neurodevelopmental Disorders in Children and Adolescents*

Anticonvulsants
Phenobarbital
Phenytoin (Dilantin)
Antipsychotics
Chlorpromazine (Thorazine)
Fluphenazine (Permitil, Prolixin)
Haloperidol (Haldol)
Thioridazine (Mellaril)
Thiothixene (Navane)
Trifluoperazine (Stelazine)
Anxiolytics and sedatives (including antihistamines)
Chlordiazepoxide (Librium)
Cyproheptadine (Periactin)
Diazapem (Valium)
Diphenhydramine (Benadryl)
Lithium carbonate (Eskalith, Lithane)
Monamine oxidase inhibitors
Phenelzine (Nardil)
Tranylcypromine (Parnate)
Stimulants
Dextroamphetamine (Dexedrine)
Fenfluramine (Pondimin)
Methylphenidate (Ritalin)
Pemoline (Cylert)
Tricyclic antidepressants
Amitriptyline (Elavil, Endep)
Desipramine (Norpramin)
Imipramine (Tofranil, Pramine)
Nortriptyline (Aventyl, Pamelor)

* Only generic names are used in this series of articles; this table adds the more commonly used trade names. All the drugs mentioned have significant side effects. Familiarity with the drug before is important, initiating therapy and careful supervision and monitoring should be continued during usage.

studies have failed to substantiate the conclusions of Menke's[17] report that 25 percent of hyperactive children go on to develop psychoses as adults.

There appears to be a genetic factor in ADD. In the family histories of these children, one finds a higher incidence of alcoholism, psychopathic males, and hysterical females.[18-20] Histories that suggest ADD are common among convicted criminals and prospective studies confirm the impression that ADD children grow up to have a greater normal chance of being arrested for criminal acts.

In pediatrics, attention deficit disorder with hyperactivity is probably the condition most treated with psychoactive drugs. Stimulant drugs, including d-amphetamine, methylphenidate, and magnesium pemoline, can be dramatically effective in reducing the problems these children have in classroom situations.

This disorder and its treatment by stimulants has been known for almost 40 years. Originally, it was noted that these fidgety, impulsive children resembled those with brain damage. Amphetamine was found to improve their behavior and to raise the threshold of these children for electroencephalographic seizures induced by metrazol. This gave further impetus to the notion of some underlying brain damage. Through the years, a vague notion of "minimal brain damage" or "brain dysfunction" has persisted. Some workers, however, have felt that this implication of a mysterious structural abnormality was pejorative and so have offered other alternative explanations.

The notion of maturational lag is one such alternative explanation. Certainly these children are immature for their age. This notion carries with it the hopeful implication that these children will "grow out" of their problems. The gross motor hyperactivity of these children may indeed abate around age 15. Nonetheless, difficulties in attention and problems with general dysphoria persist. This is common enough so that there is now a DSM III recognized adult syndrome referred to as attention deficit disorder, residual type (ADD, RT). These adults also respond well to the short-acting stimulants. Interestingly, while males make up most of the childhood ADD populations, ADD, RT is not uncommon in women. This suggests that many ADD girls go unnoticed, since girls give less trouble to parents and teachers.

Another idea has been that ADD children are underaroused. Fidgeting and irritability can be seen in sleep deprived children, and amphetamine relieves these symptoms in both sleepy children and in ADD children. At one point, it was felt that the improvement in classroom performance brought about by stimulants was paradoxical because the stimulant was not stimulating but rather calming. This presumed paradoxical response was then explained by the further assumption that these children were underaroused. In fact, the effects of stimulants on these children are not paradoxical. Amphetamines will improve performance of normal children in much the same way that it affects those with ADD. Recent electrophysiologic studies have demonstrated differences between normal and ADD children that cannot be attributed to either global underarousal or to immaturity.[21]

Drug Management

In the management of children with ADD and hyperactivity, stimulant drugs are often effective. Stimulants produce impressive short-term results in the classroom and yet are disappointing in the long run. Thus, stimulant-treated children will do more homework and get better grades. Yet at the end of a few years, they will show no more gains on academic achievement tests than an untreated group. Far better results are achieved when drug treatment is supplemented by behavior modification.[22]

In drug treatment, the pediatrician should use the smallest dose that produces satisfactory results. The reports of teachers are essential as the drug is usually administered to cover classroom time and to wear off by bedtime. Thus the parent may see the child only during the period when the drug is wearing off. One may start with 5 mg of methylphenidate in the morning and increase it to doses as high as 20 mg twice a day. If d-amphetamine is used, the dose should be one half that of methylphenidate. The second dose is usually given around noon, if needed, to help the child complete the school day. On an appropriate dose, some children will be calmer, homework will be improved, the amount and quality of classroom work will improve, and among the more active and impulsive ADD children, relationships with peers will improve. Objective testing demonstrates an improvement in short-term memory and in reaction time.

If the dose is increased past this optimum level, classroom behavior may continue to improve, for the child may become even more quiet and compliant. Actual quality of work may not improve, however, and measures of short-term memory and reaction time may deteriorate. Withdrawn children (ADD without hyperactivity) may show better classroom performance, but they may become even more withdrawn and hence less popular with their peers.

An ADD child will have the best hope for the future if provided judicious treatment with stimulants and at the same time be engaged in a program of behavior modification. This should be aimed at teaching social skills and helping the child learn voluntary control of impulsive and intrusive behavior. As can well be imagined, the untreated hyperactive child is not socially popular, and lack of peer acceptance in childhood contributes to inadequate social skills as an adult.

The side effects of stimulant medication are few. The most common is a retardation of growth, even though stimulants generally increase output of human growth hormone. However, a child taken off drug during vacations will usually catch up and maintain expected height and weight. The central nervous system side effects include restlessness, dizziness, tremor, irritability, anorexia, and insomnia. These side effects are dose related and can be controlled with the appropriate adjustments in dosage and schedule of administration. The side effects referable to the autonomic nervous system are hypertension or hypotension, palpitations, flushing, dry mouth, nausea, and abdominal discomfort. With dosages used in clinical practice neither the central or the peripheral side effects are very severe and can be avoided by beginning the treatment regimen at a low dose and gradually tapering up the dose, titrating it to balance therapeutic response and side effects.

The choice of stimulants is to some extent a matter of preference, although methylphenidate is probably the most popular. Methylphenidate is reportedly somewhat more sustained in its effect than d-amphetamine and has fewer cardiovascular side effects. However, the evidence for these differences in cardiovascular side effects is not overwhelming, and these effects are rarely a problem in treating children. A dose of 5 mg d-amphetamine is equivalent to about 10 mg of methylphenidate. Both act around 30 minutes after ingestion, reach peak drug levels at approximately 30 minutes to an hour, and have a duration of action of 4–6 hours.

Magnesium pemoline is longer acting, taking several days to achieve a maximum therapeutic effect. It has the advantage that a dose need be given only once a day, thus sparing the child the embarrassment of having the teacher give him a pill at school. Hepatotoxicity has been reported. Although this is a rare complication, parents should be warned to report epigastric pain or jaundice quickly.

Recently, antidepressants have been shown to be effective in the treatment of ADD,[23] and this treatment approach may be considered if a trial of stimulants proves not to be efficacious. Antidepressants have the advantage of being longer acting and may be given on a once daily basis. Antipsychotics have also been used in treating hyperactivity associated with ADD. In children who do not respond to stimulants, antipsychotic drugs may be tried either alone or in combination with stimulants.[24]

The reason for stimulant effectiveness in these children remains a mystery. Tolerance seems to develop to the euphoriant and anorexic effects of stimulant drugs. By contrast, tolerance does not appear to develop to the therapeutic effects of these drugs in ADD children, nor is there evidence that stopping the drugs results in symptoms of withdrawal. Since these children, untreated, may be at their worst in the classroom and are at their best either alone or in one-to-one situations such as at home, the practice of omitting the drugs on holidays and weekends is recommended, even though this is probably not necessary to prevent the development of tolerance and dependency. In children who demonstrate hyperactive behavior at home as well, medication may be given on weekend days.

CONDUCT DISORDERS

Definition and Background

Conduct disorder is a diagnostic term used to describe antisocial behavior and lack of concern for social norms. Rule breaking is the predominant pattern of behavior. Examples of habitual and antisocial behaviors seen in children with conduct disorder include stealing, lying, truancy, cruelty to animals, physical violence, and destructive behavior such as fire setting. DSM III classification has divided this diagnosis into (a) undersocialized, aggressive, (2) undersocialized, nonaggressive, (3) socialized, aggressive, and (4) socialized, nonaggressive. The undersocialized classification is used if the child demonstrates failure to establish a normal degree of affection, empathy, or bond with others, thereby resulting in poor peer relationships, lack of appropriate guilt, and inability to show concern for the welfare of friends or companions. For a child to be classified as having an aggressive component to the conduct disorder, he would have to demonstrate physical violence against persons or property or thefts involving confrontation with the victim such as purse-snatching, mugging, etc.

Some investigators believe that conduct disorders, especially as they appear in early adolescence, represent the evolution of attention deficit disorder.[25] Because both diagnostic categories are composed of a heterogenous and somewhat overlapping set of symptoms, it is difficult to validate this hypothesis.[25-27] Additionally, the diagnoses are not mutually exclusive, and it is possible for a child to have a clear cluster of behavioral abnormalities that would meet the criteria for both of the disorders. The specific descriptive behavioral symptoms of each patient are important, because the treatment of the conduct disorders depends not so much on the general diagnosis as on the specific symptoms that may respond to pharmacologic intervention.

Drug Management

There is no established pharmacologic regimen for the management of the conduct disorders as a general diagnostic entity. However, the two behavioral symptoms that may respond to medication are hyperactivity and aggression. These will be considered separately, as the treatment approach is different.

The literature on the pharmacotherapy of conduct disorders is scant and confusing. Effective pharmacotherapy has been reported when signs of attention deficit disorder accompany the diagnosis of conduct disorder. When features of impulsivity, short attention span, and hyperkinesis are present in a child with a clear conduct disorder, there is reason to believe that the use of stimulants will be effective in aiding the management. Maletsky[28] treated 23 outpatient boys with conduct disorders with dextroamphetamine (up to 40 mg/day) for a 3-month period and found significant improvement not only in hyperkinetic symptoms but antisocial behaviors as well. However, some drug-treated children continued to be violent. Although there is a paucity of studies performed that control for hyperkinesis, it appears from clinical observation that the use of stimulants in children with conduct disorders is warranted only if the following symptoms accompany the sociopathy: impulsivity, lack of forethought, restlessness, and difficulty sustaining attention. There has been no success with the use of stimulants in treating antisocial children without these associated symptoms.

The presence of aggressive behavior in conduct disorders guides the clinician toward a different pharmacologic approach. Anticonvulsants, antipsychotics, and lithium have all been used. Earlier studies examined the effectiveness of phenytoin and phenobarbital in aggressive behavior and found no benefit. There is no evidence that these agents control aggressive behavior in children not suffering from a clinical seizure disorder. In fact, phenobarbital may aggravate the hyperactivity in some cases.

Antipsychotic drugs are effective in reducing aggressiveness. Chlorpromazine or thioridazine in dosages of 50–200 mg/day given in divided doses decrease the frequency of aggressive behavior; however, these agents are associated with sedation. In a recent study Campbell *et al.*[29] found that haloperidol in dosages of 4–16 mg/day reduced scores on a variety of scales including angry affect, bullying, fighting, negativism, and temper tantrums. Generally the incidence of sedation is lower with haloperidol than chlorpromazine and thioridazine, which points to haloperidol as preferable.

Clinical researchers have examined the role of lithium in the control of aggressive behavior in children.[29,30] These investigators studied a heterogeneous diagnostic population, ranging in ages from 4 to 14 years, all having aggression as a common symptom. Lithium, at plasma levels of 0.5–1.24, was shown to decrease symptoms of rage and aggression in the majority of the patients studied. The incidence of sedation with lithium was found to be similar to haloperidol and slightly less than chlorpromazine.

In summary, for conduct disorders without features of attention deficit disorder or aggressiveness, pharmacotherapy is not indicated. If a child with a conduct disorder demonstrates symptoms of a concomitant attention deficit disorder, a trial of one of the stimulants is warranted. The dosage range and introduction of medication is the same as with that of attention deficit disorders. For this group of children, a trial of antipsychotic medication may be indicated if there is no response to the stimulant trial. In children with conduct disorders and associated aggression, both antipsychotic medication and lithium have been shown to decrease aggression. Current clinical standards would probably dictate the use of antipsychotic medication rather than lithium. Antipsychotics have been used more extensively than lithium in children with aggression, and the clinical effectiveness has been well demonstrated. Recent studies demonstrate that lithium has potential for future use in controlling aggressive behavior in children; however, more studies will be needed to substantiate this claim and confirm the safety for the use in children. At the time of this writing, the package insert for lithium does not recommend its use in children under the age of 12 years.

ANXIETY DISORDERS

Definition and Background

The origins and manifestations of anxiety are complex. Anxiety can best be understood as a derivative of fear. Fear is an adaptive reaction to a situation of immediate danger in which an organism prepares to engage in either "fight or flight" behaviors. Anxiety is a subjective and physiologic state associated with either anticipatory fear or situational fear in which there is not sufficient danger to warrant such a reaction. It has long been thought that anxiety is a learned or conditioned phenomenon, brought about by a series of experiences linked to aversive environmental contingencies. Recent investigation of benzodiazepine receptors, endogenous benzodiazepine ligands, and anxiogenic agents have shed light on the biology of anxiety. Evidence is mounting that anxiety disorders, panic attacks, and possibly phobias may represent a specific neurobiologic state.[31-33] Despite the high incidence of separation anxiety disorder, there is a paucity of controlled studies, especially using a homogeneous patient population. There is lack of diagnostic rigor in many therapeutic studies. There have been numerous studies investigating the role of antianxiety agents (benzodiazepine and antihistamines) in patients labeled "neurotic" or "overly anxious." Conclusions are difficult to make because these groups have included children with attention deficit disorders and conduct disorders.

In children, *separation anxiety* is a normal developmental response. However, when it becomes so severe or occurs in middle childhood and beyond, thereby rendering the child dysfunctional in one or multiple areas, it falls into the realm of psychopathology. Separation anxiety disorder is diagnosed when the child has excessive anxiety concerning separation from those to whom the child is attached. The child may display unrealistic worries, persistent avoidance of being alone, repeated separation nightmares, reluctance to go to sleep without being next to an attachment figure, and/or refusal to go to school. School refusal is a common manifestation of separation anxiety. Unlike many childhood disorders such as attention deficit disorders, conduct disorders, pervasive developmental disorder, and others, separation anxiety disorder is usually self-limited with a high rate of spontaneous remission. If the disorder persists and is not ameliorated by psychosocial intervention, pharmacotherapy should be considered.

Drug Management

A review of the literature reveals three different pharmacologic approaches to separation anxiety disorders. Success has been reported with thioridazine, benzodiazepines, and imipramine. White[34] recommends thioridazine for school refusal. Thioridazine 10 mg prior to going to school in the morning and 10 mg at night has been reported to be successful. Chlordiazepoxide and diazepam have reportedly been used successfully in case reports of school refusal as well. No systematized controlled studies have been conducted using a homogeneous patient population however.

The use of imipramine in separation anxiety disorder, in particular school refusal, deserves some discussion. Imipramine is the only drug that has been subjected to a placebo comparison in a large homogeneous sample of children with school refusal.[35] The children selected had all been absent from school for 2 weeks, and psychosocial intervention had failed to improve symptomatology. A maximum dose of 200 mg/day of imipramine was used with a mean dose of 159 mg/day. A total of 81 percent of the drug-treated children returned to school, whereas only 47 percent of the placebo treated children returned to school. All of the children on imipramine, but only 21 percent of children on placebo reported feeling better. Klein reports that children with school phobia respond to 75–200 mg/day of imipramine. If no detectable sign of clinical response is seen at 125 mg/day, children do not gain any additional benefit from increasing the dose to 200 mg/day. Children who do respond to imipramine should be continued on the drug for an additional 8 weeks after remission. Children with marked separation anxiety but not school refusal, generally show responses at lower doses of imipramine (25–50 mg/day). Imipramine therapy should be initiated at a low dose, in divided dosages or at bedtime, and the dose increased by 10–50 mg/week depending upon the age of the child. For children ages 6–8 years, 10 mg at bedtime is the starting dose. For children older than 8 years, 25 mg at bedtime is the initiating dose.

SLEEP DISORDERS

Definition and Background

The usual disorders of sleep that may require pharmacologic intervention are insomnia and pavor nocturnus, or night terrors. Night terrors are differentiated from nightmares in the following ways. Nightmares are frightening dreams from which the child wakes, can engage in physical activity, and is easily aroused. Because nightmares occur during REM sleep, the child after waking has memory for the dream content. After night terrors, a child does not wake, although there may be considerable activity such as sitting up in bed, crying, and screaming inarticulately. The child is asleep throughout the entire episode, and is amnesic for all the events, which include perspiration, tachypnea, tachycardia, and apparent hallucinations. Following the attack the child generally falls asleep. Night terrors are a non-REM phenomenon and generally occur as a result of arousal from stage-4 sleep. This accounts for the dissociative behavior, physiologic arousal, and lack of memory for the episode.

Drug Management

The decision to treat these disorders depends on the duration, frequency, and severity of the symptoms. If insomnia is not amenable to nonpharmacologic interventions and continues, producing conflict between the child and his parents, a short course for medication is indicated. Drug treatment should probably be considered if night terrors occur with a frequency of once a week or more. The disorders of sleep may be treated with one of a variety of drugs. An antihistamine such as diphenhydramine is the agent of first choice for insomnia. For a child under the age of 6 years, the dose range of diphenhydramine is 12.5 mg at bedtime, with 6.5 mg increment increases every 2–3 days if needed. Children between the ages of 6 and 12 years should be given 25 mg at bedtime and may require up to 50–75 mg. Children over the age of 12 years require 50-mg doses at bedtime with 25–50 mg increments until the desired result is achieved. For night terrors, both diazepam and imipramine have been shown to be effective. Diazepam is considered the drug of first choice, only because it is associated with fewer side effects. The dosage range for diazepam in the 5–12-year range is 2–20 mg, and in the over 12 years group, it is 4–30 mg at bedtime. The initial dose should be 1 mg at bedtime for the younger group with 2–5 mg increments. For the older age group, twice this starting dose is recommended, with 5–10 mg increases as necessary. Imipramine should be started at 10 mg at bedtime in children between the ages of 6 and 8 years with 10 mg increments each week. These dosages can be doubled in treating children over the age of 8 years.

SCHIZOPHRENIA*

Definition and Background

If the validity and reliability of the diagnosis of schizophrenia in adults has long been a source of debate among psychiatrists, the confusion and disagreement surrounding the concept of childhood schizophrenia is even greater. Indeed, there are no diagnostic criteria in DSM III for childhood schizophrenia. The diagnostic criteria for schizophrenia designate no age limit, which suggests that in order to make the diagnosis of child or adolescent schizophrenia, those signs and symptoms referable to the adult diagnosis must be present.

A major diagnostic distinction to be made when presented with a psychotic child is between childhood autism and schizophrenia. The diagnosis of schizophrenia hinges upon the presence of ideas, verbalizations, and behaviors that fall outside the range of normality, such as delusions of religious, grandiose, somatic, or persecutory nature, auditory hallu-

---

*The second installment (Part 2) begins here.

cinations, and illogical speech. The speech in schizophrenia is marked by incoherence, loosening of association, or marked poverty of content. Schizophrenics often display odd behavior such as hoarding, collecting garbage, and marked impairment in personal hygiene. Magical thinking is not uncommon in schizophrenia, with superstitiousness, clairvoyance, and ideas of reference being common forms of bizarre ideation. It is not hard to understand why the diagnosis of schizophrenia is difficult to make in children. Many of the symptoms of schizophrenia involve abnormal speech and bizarre ideas. In children, whose language development may be delayed or whose syntactic structure may be underdeveloped, the speech may show characteristics of incoherence. Children can rarely report ideas abstractly because their verbal abilities and level of cognitive development are not sufficiently advanced. Therefore, a child has difficulty communicating his inner experiences that may involve delusions, reality distortions, and hallucinations. Often these psychotic processes can only be inferred in children from reports from parents and close observation over a long period of time. It is evident that adolescent schizophrenia more closely approximates DSM III criteria than does childhood schizophrenia.

Drug Management

There are no well-controlled studies that show that drug treatment is more effective in schizophrenia than other types of treatment as far as long-term outcome is concerned. Medication, however, can be a valuable addition, and at times an essential treatment modality, in the total management of the schizophrenic child. Sedatives, anxiolytics, stimulants, and antipsychotics have all been tried in this patient population, and there is agreement that only the antipsychotic drugs are beneficial. Antipsychotics are most effective in diminishing psychomotor excitement that may be secondary to psychotic thinking. Other symptoms that respond well to antipsychotic medication are hallucinations, insomnia, severe anxiety, agitation, impulsivity, irritability, and disorganized behavior. The behaviors that generally are little affected by medication are social withdrawal, isolation, and blunted affect.

Chlorpromazine was the first neuroleptic to be used in psychotic children. Both chlorpromazine and thioridazine have proved to be of great value in managing the bizarre behavior of acutely psychotic children. A major problem with these low potency agents is the degree of sedation they produce, which makes concurrent educational therapy difficult. Even at low dosages, children often exhibit sleepiness and psychomotor retardation. Because of this, the high potency neuroleptics are often used in psychotic children of school age. The agents most commonly used are trifluoperazine, fluphenazine, thiothixene, and haloperidol. Haloperidol is generally used for adolescents rather than younger children.

Treatment with an antipsychotic agent should be started at a low dose and administered in a divided dose schedule. A usual starting dose for children under the age of 12 is 25–50 mg of chlorpromazine or thioridazine twice daily, or 1–2 mg of any of the high potency agents twice daily. The drug should be increased in small increments every 3–4 days and changes in objective target symptoms defined and noted. The full range of therapeutic dosages should be explored prior to setting a fixed dose. Although the neuroleptic drugs demonstrate equal overall efficacy in controlling psychotic symptomatology, different individuals show different responses. For this reason, if one agent appears not to have any therapeutic benefit for a child, another neuroleptic selected from a different class should be tried. Each drug should be given a full 4–8 week trial at adequate doses before it is considered ineffectual. It should, of course, be kept in mind that there are individual patients whose symptoms are refractory to drug treatment.

Duration of medication should be individualized. Four to six weeks may suffice for the treatment of an acute psychosis. More frequently, patients require longer periods of time on maintenance medication. Each 3–4 months, after gradually lowering the dose, the drug should be discontinued for 2–3 weeks and the patient's clinical status reassessed. Should symptoms recur, medication may be reinstated. The multidisciplinary approach necessary for the management of all childhood disorders is particularly important here, as observations from multiple informants, including school teacher, aides, nurses, relatives and parents, are helpful to the physician in making rational decisions concerning pharmacotherapy.

AUTISM

Definition and Background

The term "pervasive developmental disorders" is now used to refer to conditions previously classified as autism, childhood schizophrenia, atypical children, and so on. In the current statistical manual (DSM III), a distinction is still drawn between infantile autism and childhood schizophrenia; however, even experienced clinicians have difficulty making the distinction. The diagnosis of infantile autism requires an onset before 30 months of age, a lack of responsiveness to other people, and gross deficits of language development. When speech does develop, it tends to be peculiar, with echolalia and unusual word usage. There are bizarre responses to the environment, attachment to inanimate objects, and resistance to change. One differentiation between infantile autism and childhood schizophrenia is the absence in autism of delusions, hallucinations, loosening of associations, and incoherence, but this is obviously difficult to evaluate when there are gross deficits in language development.

To date, there is no unifying theory that can account for the array of neurobehavioral abnormalities detected in autistic children. As has been proposed with some other major psychiatric disorders, infantile autism may represent a behavioral syndrome that has as its origin a heterogeneous set of neurobiologic abnormalities. Biological hypotheses are based on genetic, biochemical, EEG, and neuropsychologic data.

Infantile autism is more common in boys than girls and about 50 times more common in siblings of autistic children than in the general population. Autistic children have a higher incidence of reverse asymmetry of the two cerebral hemispheres. Hier *et al.*[36] found the parietal–occipital region of the right hemisphere was wider than the left in 57 percent of the autistic patients, a deviation of the usual 5 percent asymmetry in a normal population. Cognitive testing of autistic children demonstrates generally low I.Q. scores (mean 70), and impairment in tasks that require left hemisphere mediated approaches.[37]

Deykin and MacMahon[38] found a higher incidence of seizures and EEG abnormalities in autistic children than in normal controls. These investigators suggest that one fifth of autistic children will manifest a seizure disorder by the time they reach adolescence.

There are similarities between symptoms of autism and those of damage to the temporal lobes. Hetzler and Griffin[39] state, "The main autistic symptoms are most consistent with a neurologic model involving bilateral dysfunction of the temporal lobes. Individual differences in the extent of bilateral involvement and/or coexistent neuropathologies could contribute to the heterogeneity of the autistic population." Pneumoencephalography performed on a group of autistic children demonstrated anatomic abnormalities consisting primarily of dilatation of the left temporal horn.[40]

Drug Management

So far the psychopharmacologic management of these children has not been successful. Painstaking educational efforts that make use of operant conditioning principles can improve social skills and increase language facility. Some of these children can develop to the point where they live relatively normal lives, although they generally remain odd and aloof. The majority, however, require continuing care.

Antipsychotic medication tends to be of little value. When sedation is required, the benzodiazepines seem more useful. In some of these children, there appears to be a disorder of serotonin metabolism. At least in some cases, blood serotonin and urine 5-HIAA are increased.[41] At one time, there was a flurry of interest in treating these children with fenfluramine, an amphetamine-like compound that is more serotonergic than D-amphetamine or methylphenidate. There have also been repeated reports that high doses of pyridoxin (Vitamin B_6) are beneficial to a subset of autistic children. Although no cures have been reported, improvement has been noted in communication and in relationship with humans.[42] Unfortunately, very high doses of B_6 can produce neuronal damage. Further investigation of B_6 and autism has been hampered by the extreme claims made by the megavitamin enthusiasts and the methodologic and statistical flaws in existing studies. Thus, there is little in the literature to offer much hope for pharmacological approaches to autism at this time.

GILLES DE LA TOURETTE'S SYNDROME

Definition and Background

The DSM III diagnosis of Tourette's disorder is based on the presence of recurrent involuntary, repetitive, rapid, purposeless motor movements affecting multiple muscle groups. Multiple vocal tics are another feature of the syndrome. The age of onset of this disorder is between 2 and 15 years, and for the diagnosis to be made, the tics must be present for more than 1 year, according to DSM III. Ordinarily, there is a variation in the intensity of the symptoms over weeks or months.

The age of onset of the disorder is usually between the ages of 4 and 9 years, with a peak at age 5. Typically, the first signs of the disorder resemble the common transient tics of young children. These include face and head tics such as grimacing, raising eyebrows, blinking, wrinkling nose, as well as other body movements such as jerking hands, shrugging shoulders, etc. Within several years, vocal noises develop, such as throat clearing, coughs or grunts, and later barking sounds. Finally, usually during puberty, coprolalia and sudden outbursts of obscenities occur. Interestingly, conscious suppression of coprolalia markedly aggravates tics and other noises. The clinical course of the disorder is punctuated with remissions and exacerbations of varying duration.

Drug Management

Haloperidol provides the greatest degree of improvement in terms of amelioration of the frequency and severity of the tics and vocalizations. Other antipsychotic medications provide similar results but without the same degree of success. Most children respond to daily doses of haloperidol in the range of 2–6 mg. Treatment should be initiated with 0.5 mg and increased daily by 0.5 mg until the desired clinical effect is obtained. The drug should be administered twice daily. Doses greater than 10–15 mg/day are not generally needed, although there have been reports of patients requiring up to 50–80 mg/day. It is not known whether haloperidol influences the natural course of the illness. Psychostimulant drugs, such as methylphenidate, may aggravate the clinical picture and, obviously, should not be used.

It should be noted that prior to making the diagnosis of Tourette's disorder and initiating treatment, a complete work-up is required to rule out other illness such as Wilson's disease, Sydenham's and Huntington's chorea, cerebrovascular accidents, multiple sclerosis, amphetamine intoxication, or other organic mental disorders.

MENTAL RETARDATION

Mental retardation is a diagnostic term referring to children with I.Q.s less than 70. The severity of mental retardation is determined by the I.Q. Mild, moderate, severe, and profound are classified according to I.Q.s less than 70, 50, 30, and 20, respectively. Children with mental retardation often have behavioral problems, not infrequently severe. They may display hyperactivity, aggression, destructiveness, and self-damage (hitting, head banging, biting). Behavioral problems of the child with mild mental retardation may develop because he cannot achieve or do the same things as others his age. Children with any degree of retardation, but most frequently those who are severely or profoundly retarded, may resemble those with childhood schizophrenia and appear psychotic. The most common signs are motor dysfunction, impulsivity, distractibility, restlessness, hyperactivity, aggressiveness, and rage outbursts.

Drug Management

Psychopharmacologic agents do not improve I.Q. or cognitive func
tion in this population. The only indication for medication, then, is to
modify the disturbing and disruptive behaviors mentioned above.
Although any of the antipsychotic medications may be given, thioridazine seems to be the most frequently prescribed. Thioridazine in
divided doses of 20–100 mg/day is generally effective for managing
behavioral problems. The dosage should be initially low (10 mg twice
daily) and gradually increased according to clinical response. If another
antipsychotic medication is selected, the appropriate dose can be determined according to known dosage equivalents. Often the choice of antipsychotic medication is made according to the degree of sedation desired
and the particular side effects to be avoided.

There are case reports of effective treatment of hyperactivity associated
with mental retardation with methylphenidate. Clinical observation has
led to the conclusion that antipsychotic medication is more likely to control hyperactivity in this population of patients. If a trial of antipsychotic
medication proves not to be effective in controlling hyperactivity and distractability, methylphenidate may be considered the second drug of
choice with prescription guidelines similar to those in treating attention
deficit disorder.

Several investigators have found lithium carbonate to be beneficial in
the management of behavioral disorders that may accompany mental
retardation. Self-mutilation can be a common associated symptom and
has been found to be responsive to lithium in up to 50 percent of
cases.[43,44] Aggressiveness, hyperactivity, and destructive behavior in mentally retarded patients may decrease with lithium treatment. A therapeutic trial of lithium should be considered if other pharmacologic
measures have failed.

DEPRESSION*

Definition and Background

The depressions in childhood are similar to the depressions in adult
life in more ways than they are different.[45] However, only in the last
decade or so has the importance of childhood depression received wide-

---

*The third and final installment (Part 3) begins here.

spread acceptance. Investigations into the pharmacologic management of childhood depression are even more recent.

In making the diagnosis of childhood depression, it is important to consider the duration and severity of symptoms. A depressive disorder must be differentiated from a feeling state such as disappointment or transient periods of unhappiness that occur during childhood. Philips[46] has drawn attention to the different forms depression may take according to the child's developmental level. In infancy, an anaclitic depression [47] with failure to thrive may predominate. In the preschool age, there may be passive aggressive behaviors, severe separation anxiety, and somatizations. In early school age, associated symptoms of depression may be school refusal, aggression, depressed affect, and somatizations. In late school age and adolescence, typically adult symptoms emerge, such as self-deprecatory feelings, depressed affect, psychomotor retardation, social isolation, and vegetative signs of insomnia and appetite loss.

The prevalence of childhood depression has been difficult to ascertain. As in adults, depressions often remit spontaneously. In a child, when a disturbance remits after a year, it is easy to assume that the child is "passing through a stage" and has outgrown the difficulty. Theoretic biases have made it difficult to acknowledge childhood depressions. Some psychoanalytic theorists have argued that, since depression results from a harsh superego, depression can not be a problem until the superego is fully developed. The public in general likes to think of childhood as a time of happy innocence, and hence children are viewed as relatively immune to depression. The younger the child, the more difficult it may be to obtain introspective reports of sadness, despair, anxiety, and feelings of worthlessness. Instead, there may be complaints of somatic symptoms, such as headache, upset stomach, etc. There may be withdrawal, loss of customary interest, and school phobias.

The biologic manifestations of depression seen in the adult are also found in childhood depression.[48] There is frequently a dysregulation of the hypothalamic-pituitary-adrenal system that results in escape from dexamethasone suppression of cortisol secretion. Growth hormone responses to insulin may be blunted. It must be emphasized, however, that neuroendocrine abnormalities do not indicate that the primary etiology of the depression is biologic (*e.g.,* due to some genetic factor or to some chemical insult). Psychosocial factors can themselves cause profound neuroendocrine changes, but the resulting disease can nonetheless respond to pharmacologic intervention when psychosocial causes cannot be adequately remedied. Psychosocial dwarfism is a case in point. Either the removal of the child from the depriving environment or treatment with growth hormone can cause a resumption of growth. The decision of whether or not to treat childhood depression with an antidepressant cannot be made on theoretic grounds. Unfortunately, empirical guidelines are only now being developed.[49]

Drug Management

The DST (dexamethasone suppression test) has been shown to be a possible biologic marker for depression.[50] It now appears the test is not as specific as was originally thought, but it still provides evidence for altered neuroendocrine function in this patient population.[51] Although the dexamethasone suppression test (DST) can be negative in some depressives, and yields false positives (for example when there was been weight loss from any cause), it can provide diagnostic and management aid if antidepressant medication is being considered.[52] The test is considered valid after 6 years of age. A baseline cortisol is drawn at 4 pm, then 1.0 mg dexamethasone is given orally at 11 pm. The following day 4 pm and 11 pm cortisol levels are drawn. The most important value is the 4 pm cortisol on the day after dexamethasone, but 11 am and 11 pm values add information. A cortisol level above 5 mc/L indicates escape from suppression and suggests a depression.

Although there are genetic factors in depression, neuroendocrine changes both result from and contribute to the disease. Pharmacologic treatment can produce dramatic improvement although we lack an adequate understanding of the mechanisms involved. Serotonergic and catecholaminergic systems are probably involved, but it is not clear whether there are abnormalities in neurotransmitter metabolism, in receptor sensitivity, or in both.

If the pharmacologic treatment of depression in childhood is to be undertaken, tricyclic antidepressants are the drugs of choice. Control of dose by measuring blood levels is more important in the child than in the adult, since children may not report side effects.

In initiating antidepressant treatment, the drug of choice should be started slowly to evaluate side effects. Generally, antidepressants with less anticholinergic action are tolerated best. Blood levels are particularly important with imipramine and nortriptyline. The relationship between blood levels of imipramine (and its metabolite desipramine) and therapeutic response is a sigmoidal, curvilinear one. Responses of children with levels above 200 ng/ml are superior to those with low levels. Nortriptyline however, has a therapeutic window between 50 and 150 nanograms/ml. That is, blood levels below 50 ng/ml or above 150 ng/ml are associated with a poor response rate. Blood levels between 50 and 150 ng/ ml are positively correlated with a good therapeutic response.[45] The drug should be tapered off slowly when the depression remits, as rapid cessation of tricyclics, particularly one with anticholinergic side effects, can produce unpleasant withdrawal symptoms. The DST test can be used to provide additional evidence that a remission has indeed occurred.

MANIC DEPRESSIVE DISORDER

Definition and Background

Like schizophrenia, the DSM III diagnostic criteria for manic depressive illness (bipolar affective disorder) do not include an age limit. A child who demonstrates the cluster of behaviors so outlined in DSM III could conceivably be diagnosed as manic depressive. The diagnosis requires cyclic episodes of manic behavior and depressed behavior and affect, separated by relatively normal periods of symptom free euthymia. Manifestations of bipolar affective states may present differently in children than in adults. There is considerable controversy surrounding the diagnosis of manic depressive illness in children. As evidence mounts for a fundamental neurobiologic dysregulation of affective disorders and the known importance of genetic factors, there is a resurgence of interest in the concept of childhood manic-depressive illness. The problem of diagnosis is like that of childhood schizophrenia. Children, by virtue of their limited behavioral repertoire and verbal and cognitive abilities, may display different behaviors than an adult with a similar disorder.

There are numerous reports of presumed manic depressive illness in childhood and adolescence. Weinberg *et al.*[53] cited five patients between the ages of 5 and 12 years who had episolic disorders characterized by marked irritability and agitation, hyperactivity, pressure of speech, insomnia, distractibility, and mood instability. These symptoms persisted for longer than 1 month and abated either spontaneously or with the aid of medication, often returning in a cyclical pattern. Euphoria was a common finding and was sometimes manifested as denial of any problem or illness. Carlson *et al.*[54] studied retrospectively the phenomenology and course of illness in six young adolescents with bipolar manic depressive illness. All six met adult criteria for manic depressive illness. However, chart reviews revealed a diagnosis of childhood schizophrenia at previous hospitalizations. Carlson concluded that symptoms present in the early course of their illness were indicative of an affective illness. These included symptoms of both depression and mania. Common depressive symptoms were dysphoric mood, psychomotor retardation, self-deprecatory thoughts, feelings of guilt, and social withdrawal. Episodes of mania in these patients were characterized by euphoria, expansiveness, hyperverbosity, hyperactivity, hypersexuality, and at times irritability and aggressiveness. DeLong[30] described 12 children with severe chronic behavior disorders who he suggested suffered from manic depressive illness. Behavioral features common to his groups consisted of hostility, aggressiveness, and distractibility. Nine of the patients had cyclic mood swings with periods of withdrawal and periods of manic excitement. Family histories of these patients were strongly positive for manic depressive illness, depression, and alcoholism. All of DeLong's patients responded to treatment with lithium carbonate.

Drug Management

As noted, lithium carbonate has not been effective in children with attention deficit disorder with hyperactivity. Similarly, lithium treatment is only minimally effective in children with conduct disorders with hyperactivity and aggressiveness. Many investigators, however, including DeLong as noted above, have shown that lithium provides significant benefits to children with symptoms consistent with manic depressive illness.

Some common observations by multiple investigators have led to preliminary conclusions regarding the nature of manic depressive illness in children and the role of lithium therapy in these patients. First, childhood psychiatric disorders can be carefully classified and examined using genetic, behavioral, pharmacologic response, and pathophysiologic criteria. Manic depressive illness in childhood is characterized by similar behavioral abnormalities as in adult manic depressives. Manic symptomalogy includes euphoria, grandiosity, hyperverbalization, hyperactivity, affective instability, and often irritability and aggressiveness. There may be agitation and insomnia. Characteristic depressive symptomalogy consists of dysphoric mood, psychomotor retardation, social withdrawal, and at times vegetative signs including insomnia and decreased appetite. Cyclical variation in symptomatology is common. A strong family history of manic depressive illness or depression makes the diagnosis more likely. Finally, response to lithium carbonate, in part, can aid the diagnosis. When the above symptoms are noted with a positive family history, there is strong evidence that lithium treatment will be effective.

Lithium treatment, like other psychopharmacologic agents, is initiated with low doses and gradually increased. Final lithium dosage is determined by plasma lithium levels and clinical response. Plasma lithium levels should be between 0.6 and 1.2 MEq/liter. Plasma lithium reaches steady state 5-7 days after initiating a new dose, and blood samples may be obtained accordingly. Because the usage of lithium in the pediatric population has been limited, there are no firm guidelines for duration of treatment or prophylaxis. Little is known about side effects associated with long-term treatment. Some children have been maintained on lithium for up to 3 years with good results and no adverse side effects. As the diagnosis of childhood manic depressive illness gains acceptance, the indications for lithium treatment can be better delineated, and the guidelines for lithium maintenance will be better defined.

Eating Disorders

The eating disorders discussed in this section are anorexia nervosa and bulimia. Although these are separate diagnostic entities, it is clear that there are features of each disorder that may overlap in a given patient, leading to the term bulimia nervosa. For the purposes of treatment strategies, the disorders will be considered separately.

Definition and Background—Anorexia Nervosa

Anorexia nervosa is a disorder predominantly of females in which there is an intense fear of becoming obese with a disturbance of body image, *e.g.,* claiming to "feel fat," although actually emaciated. The patient must have lost 25 percent of her original body weight or of her projected normal body weight to meet the diagnostic criteria for anorexia nervosa. The age of onset of anorexia nervosa is usually 10-30 years, with a mean age of 19 years. This disorder may appear during early adolescence but not be characterized by the full spectrum of symptomatology. The etiology of anorexia nervosa is unknown; however, most investigators have focused on psychologic theories and hence treatment traditionally has not been pharmacologic in nature, both psychologic (individual and family) and behavioral (behavior modification techniques).

There is an abundance of literature on the physical and metabolic abnormalities that accompany anorexia nervosa; however, most of these findings are judged to be a result of the weight loss.[55] The neuroendocrine abnormalities in anorexia nervosa are particularly interesting, and many investigators have proposed that anorexia nervosa should be considered a primary hypothalamic disorder. Abnormalities have been described in almost every endocrine system that has been carefully studied. Patients with anorexia nervosa show disorders in luteinizing hormone releasing hormone (LHRH), nonsuppression following dexamethasone suppression test (DST), elevation of plasma levels of triiodothyronine (T3), elevation of plasma growth hormone (GH), and disorders of urine concentrating ability associated with abnormal cerebral spinal fluid antidiuretic hormone (ADH) levels. Amenorrhea is common in anorexia nervosa and the menstrual cycle frequently does not return to normal following weight gain. The hypothalamus is known to play a critical role in the regulation of eating, activity, temperature, fluid balance, and in the control of the release of pituitary hormones. Although the specific etiology and pathophysiology is unclear, it appears as if in anorexia nervosa there is a simultaneous disruption of multiple hypothalamically regulated functions.[56]

Drug Management

Recently, investigators have suggested that anorexia nervosa can best be thought of as an affective disorder with a particular behavioral expression. Results of genetic and family studies, symptom and mood rating scales, and neurochemical abnormalities support this construct. The pharmacologic treatment of anorexia nervosa is based in part on this evidence. Numerous clinicians have reported successful treatment of anorexia nervosa using both amitriptyline and imipramine. In one controlled study of 36 patients, amitriptyline was found superior to placebo in producing weight gain.[57] A double-blind controlled study demonstrated lithium to have beneficial effects in patients with anorexia nervosa on a variety of measures.[58] Halmi[57] found cyproheptadine to be slightly more effective than amitriptyline and significantly better than placebo in producing weight gain in anorectic patients. Others have reported mixed results with cyproheptadine in anorectics.

Definition and Background—Bulimia

Bulimia is an eating disorder characterized by recurrent episodes of binge eating usually of high calorie foods, following by self-induced vomiting or purging. Patients frequently attempt to lose weight by diets, vomiting, use of cathartics and/or diuretics, or enemas. The disorder is associated with depressed mood and self-deprecating thoughts following binge eating, with an awareness that the eating pattern is abnormal. As in anorexia nervosa, bulimia is limited almost exclusively to females and generally the age of onset is during late adolescence. The etiology of this disorder is unknown, and psychologic treatment modalities have a low rate of success. Like anorexia nervosa, acute treatment may lead to amelioration of symptoms; however, the disorder is usually chronic with frequent exacerbations.

Psychobiologic research on bulimia has led to two theoretic positions concerning the core pathology. The first proposes a cerebral electrophysiologic disturbance; the second includes bulimia with the affective disorders. EEG abnormalities have been found in a subset of patients with eating disorders, predominantly those suffering from bulimia. Rau *et al.*[59, 60] found bulimic patients to have 14- and 6-per second positive spikes in temporal and occipital lobes. Many have argued that this pattern reflects thalamic and hypothalamic dysfunction. Grebb *et al.*[61] studied five patients with eating disorders using a computer analyzed EEG and found abnormalities in % alpha, % beta, % asymmetry and % coherence between homologous leads (reflecting degree of wave shape symmetry and synchrony). These findings were more prevalent in patients with the most abnormal DSTs.

Drug Management

The EEG data in bulimia have prompted clinicians to try anticonvulsants in some patients. Phenytoin has been shown to be effective in controlling binging in a subpopulation of such patients; however, the efficacy of the anticonvulsant is not well correlated with the type or degree of EEG abnormalities.[62, 63]

The association between bulimia and atypical depression has been made by a number of investigators. Symptoms of depression and anxiety are more predominant in bulimic patients than anorectics. Tricyclic antidepressants have limited success in a percentage of bulimics. Recently, focus has turned to the use of monoamine oxidase inhibitors in the treatment of bulimia. Walsh[64] and others have reported improvement in mood and eating behavior in patients treated with both phenelzine and tranylcypromine.

In summary, the pharmacologic treatment of eating disorders is in its infancy. It is clear that not all patients respond to drug treatment; however, there are reports of therapeutic effects in a certain percentage of patients with eating disorders. Future research is needed to identify those psychologic and biologic variables in patient subpopulations that will provide predictive value in selecting a particular drug to aid in treatment. Currently, in anorexia nervosa, cyproheptadine and the tricyclic antidepressants have been shown to have beneficial effects in some patients. Further work is required to assess the differential efficacy of antidepressants acting preferentially on noradrenergic versus serotonergic re-uptake systems. Certain bulimic patients respond to phenytoin treatment. Correlations between EEG abnormalities and anticonvulsant treatment response will aid in rational selection of drug therapy. Increasing evidence suggests that MAO inhibitors may come to have an important role in the treatment of bulimia.

Enuresis

Functional enuresis is classified in DSM III as "other disorders with physical manifestations" and refers to the involuntary voiding of urine by day or night. This disorder is diagnosed only when organic genitourinary abnormalities have been ruled out and when the child is 5 years of age or older.

A good deal of research has been conducted on the pharmacotherapy of enuresis, and the following conclusions have been reached. First, a number of compounds have been found not to be effective; these include dextroamphetamine, anticholinergic drugs, and MAO inhibitors. The only effective class of drugs for treating enuresis are the tricyclic antidepressants.

In 1960, imipramine was found to be effective for enuresis in low dosages (25 mg at bedtime).[35] In that report, the symptoms reappeared on discontinuation of the drug. Subsequent studies have demonstrated that imipramine is significantly superior to placebo, producing 85 percent improvement rates. In up to 50 percent of these responders, total elimination of bedwetting is obtained; in the remainder, bedwetting is reduced. The dosage range studied for imipramine has been 20–100 mg given at bedtime. Most children respond to low dosages, 25–50 mg, and high dosages are only required in the small percentage of children who become refractory to lowered doses during the treatment period. Other tricyclics studied have been found to be equally effective. These include imipramine, amitriptyline, desipramine, and nortriptyline. Because the greatest amount of data has been collected for imipramine, clinicians routinely use this drug.

It was initially thought that imipramine affects bedwetting by altering sleep stages, but this view has been refuted. Enuretic episodes are not related to any one sleep stage, and drug-induced inhibition of rapid eye movement has been shown not to mediate the therapeutic effect. The mechanism of tricyclic action on enuresis is not clearly understood.

Treatment should be initiated with 25 mg given at bedtime. Beneficial results may be seen immediately but generally take between 5 and 7 days.

If no response occurs within this time, the dose should be increased by 25 mg increments. Obviously, a record of frequency of bedwetting is needed prior to initiation of drug treatment in order to assess the effectiveness of the medication accurately. After a response has occurred, it is recommended that medication be continued for no more than 6 months prior to tapering off the medication.

It should be noted that there are effective treatments for enuresis other than pharmacotherapy, and these approaches should be considered in the management of this symptom. Behavioral techniques using conditioning known as "the bell and the pad" have yielded the best results of the nonpharmacologic methods. Additionally, enuresis often spontaneously disappears without any intervention. Therefore, the severity and duration of the symptom as well as the specifics of the clinical presentation should guide the clinician in developing the most logical treatment plan.

REFERENCES

1. American Academy of Child Psychiatry. Child Psychiatry: A Plan for the Coming Decades. Washington DC: Academy of Child Psychiatry, 1983
2. Coffey B, Shader RI, Greenblatt DJ. Pharmacokinetics of benzodiazepines and psychostimulants in children. J. Clin Psychopharmacol 1983;3:217
3. Atkeson BM, Forehand R. Home-based reinforcement programs designed to modify classroom behavior: a review and methodological evaluation. Psychol Bull 1979;86:1298
4. Barker P. Basic Family Therapy. London: Grandu, 1981
5. Bornstein MR, Bellack AS, Hersen M. Social skills training for unassertive children: a multiple baseline analysis. J Appl Behav Anal 1977;19:983
6. Bruch H. Management of anorexia nervosa. Resident and Staff Physician 1976;19:61
7. Burns WJ, Lavigne JV, eds. Progress in Pediatric Psychology. New York: Grune and Stratton, Inc., 1984
8. Cytryn L, McKnew DH. Treatment issues in childhood depression. Psychiatric Annals 1985;15:401
9. Eysenck HJ. Learning theory and behavior therapy. In: Eysenck HJ, ed. Behavior Therapy and the Neuroses. Oxford: Pergamon Press, 1960
10. Garfinkel PE, Garner DM. Anorexia Nervosa. A Multidimensional Perspective. New York: Brunner/Mazel, Inc., 1982
11. Graziano AM, DeGiovanni IS, Garcia KA. Behavioral treatment of children's fears: a review. Psychol Bull 1979;86:804
12. Guze SB, Earls FJ, Barrett JE, eds. Childhood Psychopathology and Development. New York: Raven Press, 1983
13. McCord J. A thirty-year follow-up of treatment effects. Am Psychol 1978;33:284
14. Rutter M, ed. Infantile Autism: Concepts, Characteristics, and Treatment. New York: Churchill Livingstone, 1971

15. Sholevar GP, Benson RM, Blinder BJ, eds. Emotional Disorders in Children and Adolescents, Medical and Psychological Approaches to Treatment. New York: Spectrum Publications, Inc., 1980

16. American Psychiatric Association. Diagnostic and Statistical Manual of Mental Disorders. 3rd ed. Washington, DC, 1980

17. Menkes MM, Rowe JS, Menkes JH. A 25-year follow up study on the hyperactive child with minimal brain dysfunction. Pediatrics 1967;39:273

18. Cantwell D. Genetic studies of hyperactive children: psychiatric illness in biologic and adopting parents. In: Fieve R, Rosenthal D, Brills H, eds. Genetic Research in Psychiatry. Baltimore: Johns Hopkins University Press, 1975

19. Cantwell D. Psychiatric illness in the families of hyperactive children. Arch Gen Psychiatry 1972;70:414

20. Morrison J, Stewart M. A family study of the hyperactive child syndrome. Biol Psychiatry 1971;3:189

21. Callaway E, Halliday R, Naylor H. Hyperactive children's event-related potentials fail to support underarousal and maturational lag theories. Arch Gen Psychiatry 1983;40:1243

22. Pelham WE, Bender ME. Peer relationships in hyperactive children: description and treatment. In: Advances in Learning and Behavioral Disabilities. Vol. 1, 365, JAI Press, 1982

23. Garfinkel BD, Wender PH, Sloman L, et al. Tricyclic antidepressant and methylphenidate treatment of attention deficit disorder in children. J Am Acad Child Psychiatry 1983;22:343

24. Gittelman-Klein R, Klein DF, Katz S, et al. Comparative effects of methylphenidate and thioridazine in hyperactive children. I: Clinical Results. Arch Gen Psychiatry 1976;33:1217

25. Schuckit MA, Petrich J, Chiles J. Hyperactivity: diagnostic confusion. J Nerv Ment Dis 1978;166:79

26. El-Guebaly N, Offord DR. The offspring of alcoholics: a critical review. Am J Psychiatry 1977; 134:357

27. Rutter M, Hersov L, eds. Child Psychiatry: Modern Approaches. Philadelphia: J.B. Lippincott, 1977

28. Maletsky BM. D-amphetamine and delinquency: hyperkinesis persisting? Dis Nerv Syst 1974;35:543

29. Campbell M, Cohen IL, Small AM. Drugs in aggressive behavior J Am Acad Child Psychiatry 1982;21:107

30. DeLong GR. Lithium carbonate treatment of select behavior disorders in children suggesting manic-depressive illness. J Pedatr 1978;93:689

31. Braestrup C, Petersen EN, Nielsen M. Biochemical and behavioral studies of anxiety: convulsive benzodiazepine receptor ligands. Psychopharmacol Bull 1982; 18:8

32. Ninun PT, et al. Benzodiazepine receptor-mediated experimental "anxiety" in primates. Science 1982;218:1332

33. Uhde TW, Boulenger JP, Siever LJ. Animal models of anxiety: implications for research in humans. Psychopharmacol Bull 1982;18:47

34. White JH. Pediatric Psychopharmacology: A Practical Guide to Clinical Application. Baltimore: Williams & Wilkins Co., 1977

35. Klein DF, Gittelman R, Quitkin F, et al. Diagnosis and Drug Treatment of Psychiatric Disorders. 2nd ed. Baltimore: Williams and Wilkins, 1980

36.	Hier DB, LeMay M, Rosenberger PB. Autism and unfavorable left-right asymmetries of the brain. J Autism Dev Disorder 1979;9:153
37.	Hoffman W, Prior M. Neuropsychological dimensions of autism in children: a test of the hemispheric dysfunction hypothesis. J Clin Neuropsychol 1982;4:27
38.	Deykin EY, MacMahon B. The incidence of seizures among children with autistic symptoms. Am J Psychiatry 1979;136:1310
39.	Hetzler BE, Griffin J. Infantile autism and the temporal lobe of the brain. J Autism Dev Disord 1981;11:317
40.	DeLong GR. A neuropsychologic interpretation of infantile autism. In: Rutter M, Schopler E, eds. Autism: A Reappraisal of Concepts and Treatment. New York: Plenum Press, 1978
41.	Hanley HG, Stahl SM, Freedman DX. Hyperserotonenemia and amine metabolites in autistic and retarded children. Arch Gen Psychiatry 1977;34:521
42.	Martineau J, Garreau B, Barthelmy C, et al. Effects of vitamin B6 on averaged evoked potentials in infantile autism. Biol Psychiatry 1981;16:627
43.	Cooper AF, Fowlie HC. Control of gross self-mutilation with lithium carbonate. Br J Psychiatry 1973;122:37
44.	Micev U, Lynch DM. Effect of lithium on disturbed severely mentally retarded patients. Br J Psychiatry 1974;125:110
45.	Work HH. Depression in childhood and adolescence. In: Grinspoon L, ed. The American Psychiatric Association Annual Review. Washington, DC: American Psychiatric Press, 1982
46.	Philips I. Childhood depression: interpersonal interactions and depressive phenomena. Am J Psychiatry 1979;136:511
47.	Spitz R. Anaclitic depression. In: Psychoanalytic Study of the Child. Vol. 2. New York: International University Press: 1947
48.	Lowe TL, Cohen DJ. Biological research on depression in childhood. In: Cantwell DP, Carlson GA, eds. Affective Disorders in Childhood and Adolescence: An Update. Jamaica, NY: Spectrum Publications, 1983
49.	Kashani JH, Husain A, Shekim WO. Current perspectives on childhood depression: an overview. Am J Psychiatry 1981;138:143
50.	Carroll BJ, Feinberg M, Greden JF. A specific laboratory test for the diagnosis of melancholia. Arch Gen Psychiatry 1981;38:15
51.	Targum SD. The application of serial neuroendocrine challenge studies in the management of depressive disorder. Biol Psychiatry 1983;18:3
52.	Poznanski EO, Carroll BJ, Banegas MC, et al. The dexamethasone suppression test in prepubital depressed children. Am J Psychiatry 1982;139:321-4
53.	Weinberg WA, Brumback RA. Mania in childhood. J Dis Child 1976;130:380
54.	Carlson GA, Strober M. Manic depressive illness in early adolescence. J Am Acad Child Psychiatry 1978;17:138
55.	Borson S, Katon W. Chronic anorexia nervosa: medical mimic. West J Med 1981;135:257
56.	Walsh BT. The endocrinology of anorexia nervosa. In: Sachar EJ, ed. The Psychiatric Clinics of North America: Advances in Psychoneuroendocrinology. Philadelphia: W.B. Saunders Co., 1980
57.	Halmi KA, Eckert E, Falk JR. Cyproheptadine for anorexia nervosa. Lancet 1357, 1982
58.	Gross HA, Ebert MH, Faden VB, et al. A double-blind controlled trial of lithium carbonate in primary anorexia nervosa. J Clin Psychopharmacol 1981;1:376

59. Rau HJ, Green RS. Compulsive eating: a neurophysiologic approach to certain eating disorders. Compr Psychiatry 1975;16:223
60. Rau JH, et al. Electroencephalographic correlates of compulsive eating. Clin Electroencephalography 1979;10:180
61. Grebb JA, Struve FA, Green RS. Electrophysiologic abnormalities in patients with eating disorders. Compr Psychiatry 1984;25:216
62. Moore SL, Rakes SM. Binge eating—therapeutic response to diphenylhydantoin: case report. J Clin Psychiatry 1974;131:428
63. Wermuth BM, Davis KL, Hollister LE, et al. Phenytoin treatment of the binge-eating syndrome. Am J Psychiatry 1977;134;1244
64. Walsh BT, Stewart JW, Wright L, et al. Treatment of bulimia with monoamine oxidase inhibitors. Am J Psychiatry 1982;139:12

28

Personal and Social Resources in Children of Patients with Bipolar Affective Disorder and Children of Normal Control Subjects

David Pellegrini, Shelley Kosisky, Debra Nackman, Leon Cytryn, Donald H. McKnew, Elliot Gershon, Joel Hamovit, and Karen Cammuso

Catholic University of America, Washington, D.C., and National Institute of Mental Health, Bethesda, Maryland

The authors examined the personal resources (social problem-solving ability, internal locus of control, self-esteem, and self-perceived competence) and social resources (social network structure and support) in 23 children of patients with bipolar affective disorder (probands) and 33 children of normal control parents. Positive resource profiles were related to psychiatric well-being in the offspring. Nondisordered probands, in particular, demonstrated a strikingly positive profile of personal resources as well as a wide range of peer, sibling, and other kin supporters. Disordered probands had a strikingly negative set of personal resources and a relatively greater reliance on nonkin adult supporters. The absence of a supportive best friend was associated with affective disorder across offspring groups.

In a number of studies, striking rates of depression and other forms of emotional and behavioral disturbance have been observed among the

---

Reprinted with permission from the *American Journal of Psychiatry*, 1986, Vol. 143, No. 7, 856–861. Copyright 1986 by the American Psychiatric Association.

children of affectively ill parents. The regularity of these observations has led to a consensus that such children are at increased risk for psychiatric disorders which may represent the antecedents of adult affective illness (1). However, few of these findings have been derived from studies that used an offspring control group, standardized assessment interviews, and explicit diagnostic criteria. Moreover, most studies of risk for affective disorder to date have examined parental groups with mixed illnesses, typically combining the offspring of patients with unipolar and bipolar affective disorder (2) or severe and minor depression (3) for data-analytic purposes. Considerable evidence suggests the etiological heterogeneity of such types of affective disorder (4), and the adaptive challenges to their offspring undoubtedly differ in important, although largely unexplored, ways as well. Finally, only minimal attention has been directed so far toward the psychosocial characteristics of those children who maintain psychiatric well-being in the context of risk for affective disorder. Such characteristics represent potential protective factors whose identification would contribute to the development of effective programs of prevention and remediation.

In the present study we address the nature of these psychosocial characteristics in the offspring of patients with bipolar I affective disorder compared with the offspring of normal control subjects. Our efforts represent a further investigation of a relatively small sample previously described (5). Here we test the hypothesis that psychiatric well-being in children is related to a specific array of psychosocial characteristics which constitute a core set of personal resources (social problem-solving ability, internal locus of control, general self-esteem, and self-perceived competence) and social resources (extensiveness of social contacts and self-perceived availability of social support). A substantial body of literature links deficits in each of the personal resources examined to a wide variety of adjustment difficulties in childhood (6–8). Moreover, each presumably constitutes a central component of cognitive-affective functioning that should be specifically implicated in a child's psychological vulnerability to or development of affective disorder. Although largely unexplored in childhood, social networks that are perceived to be constricted or disharmonious and unsupportive have also been closely linked to the development of adult depression (9).

METHOD

Subjects

Subjects included 23 probands (11 boys, 12 girls) from 16 families in which one parent met diagnostic criteria for bipolar I affective disorder and 33 control subjects (16 boys, 17 girls) from 19 families in which both parents had lifetimes free of psychiatric disorder. All subjects were recruited from a slightly larger pool of participants in an ongoing investigation of the familial transmission of affective disorder (5) (three proband families with six offspring and three control families with four offspring had declined further participation). All subjects provided informed consent after the nature of the study had been explained.

Probands and control subjects were further divided according to whether they had experienced some psychiatric disorder at any time, thereby yielding four groups for investigation. Sixteen (70%) of the 23 probands and 15 (45%) of the 33 control subjects met *DSM-III* criteria for one or more lifetime psychiatric disorders. Of the 16 disordered probands, 11 (69%) had manifested some form of affective disturbance (major depression, atypical/minor depression, dysthymia, cyclothymia, or mania), in comparison with nine (60%) of the 15 disordered control subjects. (See Gershon et al. [5] for an analysis of diagnostic findings in the full set of offspring.)

All subjects were between 7 and 18 years of age, with a mean of 12 years, 8 months. Of the 56 children, 38 (68%) were from families in social class 2 or 3 as defined by the Hollingshead-Redlich scale. An additional 17 (30%) were from social class 1. Only one child was from social class 4. All subjects were white, with the exception of one disordered black male proband. Six (38%) of the 16 probands' families but none of the 19 control subjects' families had divorced parents.

Diagnostic Procedures

Parental psychiatric status was ascertained with a systematic lifetime diagnostic interview, the Schedule for Affective Disorders and Schizophrenia (SADS-L) (10), modified to screen for anorexia and bulimia. In addition, each parent supplied systematically obtained family history information on the other parent. All parental diagnoses were made blindly according to modified Research Diagnostic Criteria (RDC) (11, 12) by using procedures described elsewhere (4, 11, 13).

To ascertain the psychiatric status of offspring, each child and a parent were interviewed separately with an analogous instrument, the KIDDIE-SADS-E (14), modified to assess functional impairment and incapacitation (5). Both sources of information were considered to derive a blind, consensual diagnosis for each child in accord with *DSM-III* criteria (5).

Psychosocial Assessment

Each child was individually administered a battery of measures by an interviewer who was blind to parentage and psychiatric status.

Intellectual ability. The vocabulary subtest of the WISC-R (for 7–16-year-olds) or the WAIS-R (for 17–18-year-olds) was used to estimate intellectual ability, a potentially important although relatively immutable covariate of psychiatric functioning in offspring.

Social problem-solving ability. A modified version of the Means-Ends Problem-Solving Test (7) was used to measure "alternative solutions thinking," a central component of the problem-solving process. Children were asked to generate multiple alternative solutions to four hypothetical social dilemmas concerning peer conflict over a toy, provocation of the mother's anger, loneliness in a new neighborhood, and peer teasing. Responses were scored for 1) the sum of relevant, unique solutions generated per dilemma, 2) the sum of irrelevant responses, and 3) the variety of solutions used (defined in terms of 13 mutually exclusive content categories). Scores for the number of irrelevant solutions generated were inverted so that higher scores were reflective of more competent performance, in keeping with other variables, all of which were scored in a positive direction. Interrater reliabilities of .89 to .96 were obtained for five randomly selected response protocols.

Locus of control. The 26-item Nowicki-Duke Control Scale (15) (for 5–8-year-olds) or the 40 item Nowicki-Strickland Control Scale (16) (for 9–18-year-olds) was administered to assess locus of control. Each item was designed to reflect either an internal or an external locus of control. The two self-report scales were equated by converting total scores to the proportion of internally oriented items endorsed.

Self-esteem and self-perceived competence. Harter's 28-item Perceived Competence Scale for Children (17) was administered to assess children's general feelings of self-worth as well as their perceptions regarding their skill in academic, social, and physical performance domains (four subscales of seven items each). For each item, children were asked to judge, on an underlying 4-point scale, the degree to which an evaluative statement reflected their own feelings about themselves or their abilities. Subscale scores index the overall positivity of a child's self-perceptions in a given domain.

Social network structure and support. A structured clinical interview was devised and administered to assess the composition and diversity of a child's social network and the child's perception of the availability of social support. First, systematic inquiries were made regarding peers, immediate family members (i.e., parents and siblings), extended kin (i.e., aunts, uncles, cousins, grandparents), and nonkin adults (e.g., teachers bosses, doctors, ministers, neighbors, friends of parents). With regard to peers, children were asked if they had a "best friend" (i.e., a person they liked more than anyone else and who also seemed to feel the same way about them). To be included as a network member, a designated individual had to be living in the same household as the child or be someone whom the child liked to see and to whom the child felt close. Except for parents, stepparents, and siblings, face-to-face contact within the previous 12 months was also required.

After we had determined the core composition of a child's perceived social network, a series of four commonplace situations was presented. These concerned 1) mother being ill, 2) father being ill, 3) getting into trouble with a neighbor, and 4) difficulty getting along with a friend. Children were asked about which network members, if any, they could confide in if they were facing such a situation (i.e., emotional supporters) and which they could count on for advice or practical assistance (i.e., instrumental supporters). Finally, children were asked about which network members, if any, shared worries or sought help from them. Network members who could be counted on as helpful providers of emotional or instrumental support in any one of the four problem contexts were designated as supporters. Those who also reportedly received support were designated as reciprocal supporters.

Five scores reflecting the structural diversity of a child's social network were derived: the number of peers, kin residing in the home, nonresiding kin, nonkin adults, and special peer groups (i.e., clubs or organizations) to which the child belonged. A corresponding set of five additional scores reflected the child's perception of the availability of social support: the number of supporters who were peers, residing kin, nonresiding kin, nonkin adults, and reciprocal supporters.

RESULTS

Preliminary Analyses

A series of two-way ANOVAs failed to reveal significant main or interaction effects for risk status (proband versus control) or psychiatric status (no lifetime *DSM-III* disorder versus any such disorder) with respect to either age or vocabulary performance (the sample mean±SD for vocabulary was 12.5 ± 3.12, indicative of above average intellectual ability). A significant main effect for risk status was apparent, however, with regard to social class: F = 6.33, df = 1, 49, p < .02. The mean±SD social class of control subjects (1.79 ± .74) was significantly higher than that of probands (2.39 ± .84). Finally, a three-way log-linear analysis of risk status, psychiatric status, and sex suggested that the proportion of boys to girls was not significantly different across the four groups.

Analyses of Personal and Social Resources

Group differences in the quality of resources were examined principally by means of profile analysis of covariance (18). This multivariate statistical approach (akin to analysis of covariance with repeated measures) allows one to consider the overall patterning of group characteristics while controlling for experiment-wise error. As a preliminary step, all raw scores were standardized within the sample as a whole (i.e., Z scores were computed, yielding a sample mean of zero and a standard deviation of one for each variable). This procedure facilitates within-subject comparisons across variables or resource dimensions. Three separate profile analyses were undertaken. In each case, two grouping factors and their interaction were considered: risk status (proband versus control) and lifetime psychiatric status (disordered versus nondisordered), with socioeconomic status treated as a covariate to control for preexisting group differences.

The first profile analysis considered the eight scores reflecting social problem-solving ability, internality, self-esteem, and self-perceived competence. This analysis revealed a significant Risk Status × Psychiatric Status interaction (F = 7.23, df = 1,51, p < .01), suggesting that the four groups differed significantly with respect to the overall quality of their personal resources (figure 1).

The post hoc comparisons (Tukey's procedure) required to clarify this interaction effect indicated that nondisordered probands exhibited a significantly more positive profile of personal resources (mean±SD composite Z = 4.27 ± 3.97) than did nondisordered control subjects (composite Z = −.18 ± 3.59), disordered control subjects (composite Z = .08 ± 4.45), or disordered probands (composite Z = −1.72 ± 2.59) (p < .01 for all pairwise comparisons). Disordered probands also showed a less positive profile than did either control group (p < .01). The two control groups did not significantly differ from each other in this regard.

The second analysis considered the profile of five social resource variables related to network structure. This analysis revealed a significant Variable × Risk Status interaction (F = 6.32, df = 4,208, p < .001), sug-

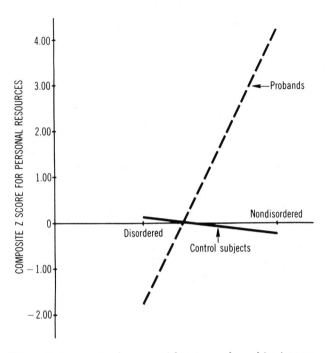

Figure 1. Interaction between risk status and psychiatric status for composited personal resources of 22 children of patients with bipolar affective disorder (probands) and 33 children of normal parents (control subjects).

gesting that all probands combined (i.e., disordered and nondisordered) differed significantly from all control subjects combined in the overall composition of their social networks (figure 2). No main or interaction effects were evident with regard to offspring's psychiatric status. That is, the network structure of disordered subjects was comparable to that of nondisordered subjects within both the proband and control subsamples and across the sample as a whole.

Post hoc comparisons undertaken to clarify the Variable × Risk Status interaction indicated that control subjects reported significantly more peers (p < .01) and residing kin (p < .01) in their networks as well as more group affiliations (p < .01) than did probands. On the other hand, probands reported being close to and having contact with significantly more nonresiding kin (p < .01). No such differences were evident with respect to nonkin adult network members.

The final analysis considered the profile of five social resource

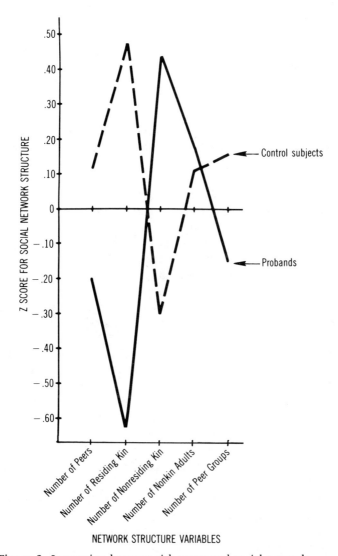

Figure 2. Interaction between risk status and social network structure profiles of 22 children of patients with bipolar affective disorder (probands) and 33 children of normal parents (control subjects).

variables related to social support. This analysis revealed a significant main effect with regard to psychiatric status (F = 5.82, df = 1,51, p < .02). Overall, nondisordered subjects (regardless of risk status) reported significantly more available supporters (mean±SD composite Z = .85 ± 2.33) than did disordered subjects (composite Z = .78 ± 2.36). However, a Variable × Psychiatric Status interaction effect also approached significance (F = 2.05, df = 4, 208, p < .10). This finding reflected a tendency for nondisordered subjects in general and nondisordered probands in particular to report having fewer nonkin adult supporters than did disordered subjects.

No main or interaction effects on network support were evident with regard to offspring's risk status. That is, the amount of support available to probands and control subjects was comparable within both the disordered and nondisordered subsamples and across the sample as a whole. However, a significant Variable × Risk Status interaction (F = 3.23, df = 4, 208, p < .02) indicated that probands (regardless of psychiatric status) differed significantly from control subjects in the sources of their perceived support (figure 3). Post hoc comparisons indicated that control subjects reported a significantly greater number of residing kin supporters (p < .01), nonkin adult supporter (p < .01), and reciprocal supporters (p < .05) than did probands. Probands, on the other hand, reported significantly more nonresiding kin supporters (p < .01). No differences were evident with respect to the number of available peer supporters.

Affective Disorder and the Availability of a Supportive Best Friend

A number of previous studies have implicated the absence of an intimate relationship as a risk factor specific to adult depression (9). Thus, although statistical analyses were otherwise restricted to treating offspring with different psychiatric disorders together because of small samples, we considered the association between having a best friend as a supporter and having experienced an episode of affective disorder. No association between having a best friend supporter and general psychiatric disorder was evident (χ^2 = 2.13, df = 1, N = 56, n.s.). However, when nondisordered and affectively disordered children were compared, an association was observed: χ^2 = 4.72, df = 1, N = 45, p < .03. Of the 11 youngsters who reported that they did not have a best friend, eight (73%) were affectively disordered and only three (27%) were normal (i.e., the relative odds for an affective disorder were 2.67 to 1 for this group). In comparison, 12 (35%) of the 34 youngsters who did claim such a friend

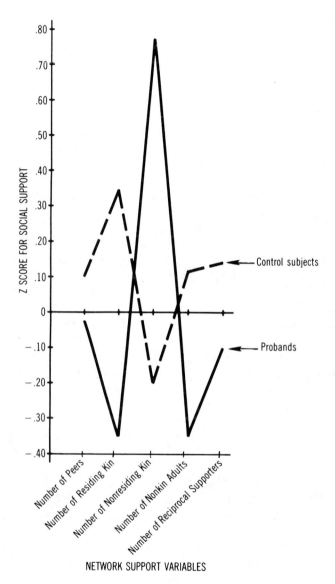

Figure 3. Interaction between risk status and social support profiles of 22 children of patients with bipolar affective disorder (probands) and 33 children of normal parents (control subjects).

were affectively disordered, and 22 (65%) were normal (i.e., the relative odds here were .55 to 1). Thus, the risk (odds ratio) for having an affective disorder relative to no disorder was 4.9 times as great for youngsters with no best friend than for those who did have a best friend.

DISCUSSION

A number of conclusions and observations seem warranted on the basis of the present findings. First, the expectation that psychiatric well-being would be related to a more positive profile of personal and social resources was generally confirmed. A low level of perceived social support was clearly associated with lifetime psychiatric disorder in the children of both bipolar patients and normal parents. This is in keeping with a growing body of literature regarding social support and adult psychiatric disturbance. Particularly striking was evidence suggesting that the absence of a supportive relationship with a best friend may be a particular risk factor associated with affective disorder in childhood, as the absence of an intimate and confiding marital relationship seems to be in adulthood (9).

Rutter (19) has suggested that, in the context of parental mental illness, supportive relationships with nondisordered family members as well as with nonkin adults might be protective in childhood. The present data provide more support for the former idea than for the latter. Perceived availability of a wide range of peer, sibling, and other kin supporters was associated with well-being in both probands and control subjects. In contrast, reliance on a multiplicity of nonkin adult supporters was associated with psychiatric disorder. This link between support from nonkin adults and psychiatric disorder apeared to be especially characteristic of probands.

It is not clear from the present data, of course, whether nondisordered children were better able to establish supportive, intimate relationships with kin and peers alike and that such significant others were, in turn, most effective in mediating life stress and genetic vulnerability, or whether such children were simply more fortunate in having receptive and responsive supporters close at hand. The superior personal resources of the nondisordered probands suggest that, at least, they may have been more adept at extracting the maximum benefit from their social milieu. Again, however, a fortuitously supportive environment must certainly have fostered such skills.

The picture with regard to the relationship between psychiatric well-being and personal resources was more complex. Nondisordered probands demonstrated a strikingly superior profile of personal resources, while disordered probands demonstrated a strikingly inferior one. However, the profile of personal resources considered in the present study failed to differentiate disordered and nondisordered control children. These findings are reminiscent of the "invulnerability" or "resiliency" phenomenon that a number of investigators speculate is characteristic of a considerable proportion of children exposed to stressful life circumstances (20).

Striking and more uniform differences were also evident between the offspring of bipolar and normal parents with regard to how these children perceived their own social networks. These differences were apparent in overall network structure as well as in the nature and sources of social support and appeared to operate independently of offspring's psychiatric functioning. It is likely that parental mental illness exerts a direct effect on the structure of a child's social relationships. Such direct effects may account, in part, for observed proband-control differences in both kin and peer relationships. For example, whereas control parents in the present sample did not display the high divorce rate evident in the general population (none was divorced), 38% of the probands had divorced parents. Parental illness is likely to provoke marital separations as well as to elicit substitute caretaking efforts from extended kin, especially from grandparents, aunts and uncles, and older siblings who may have previously moved out of the house in an effort to escape the discord and disruptions that frequently characterize life with a parent who has bipolar disorder (21). Such findings, taken together, probably account for the higher concentration of nonresiding kin and the lower concentration of residing kin in the perceived networks of both disordered and nondisordered probands. Finally, adults with bipolar affective disorder are generally known to have difficulties maintaining intimate relationships outside the family (21). Thus, the diminished involvement of probands with their peers may partially reflect the modeling of parental interpersonal difficulties and/or attitudes toward interpersonal involvement and support exchange.

Obviously, retrospective risk research of this kind does not allow one to sort out causes from consequences. The possibly confounding influence of clinical status further compounds the problem of causal interpretation in retrospective research. For example, psychiatric difficulties clearly may contribute to perceptions of unsupportiveness in one's family environment and to the felt need to seek a sympathetic ear from a friend's parent, a neighbor, or some other such adult. Nevertheless, the present findings provide some worthwhile clues regarding the impact of parental bipolar disorder on the social networks of offsprings, as well as clues regarding the relationship of personal and social resources to psychiatric disturbance in children. The disruption of social networks in childhood and the fostering of inadequate problem-solving skills and a diminished sense of personal control, competence, and self-worth may represent primary mechanisms through which parental psychiatric disorder leads to increased rates of psychiatric disorder in offspring. The psychosocial attributes considered in the present study clearly warrant further investigation to clarify the extent to which they simply mirror or actually mediate vulnerability to psychiatric disorder in children at risk.

REFERENCES

1. Beardslee WR, Bemporad J, Keller MB, et al: Children of parents with major affective disorder: a review. Am J Psychiatry 140:825–832, 1983
2. Cytryn L, McKnew DH Jr, Bartko JJ, et al: Offspring of patients with affective disorders, II. J Am Acad Child Psychiatry 21:389–391, 1982
3. Orvaschel H, Weissman MM, Padian N, et al: Assessing psychopathology in children of psychiatrically disturbed parents: a pilot study. J Am Acad Child Psychiatry 20:112–122, 1981
4. Gershon ES, Hamovit J, Guroff JJ, et al: A family study of schizoaffective, bipolar I, bipolar II, unipolar, and normal control probands. Arch Gen Psychiatry 39:1157–1167, 1982
5. Gershon ES, McKnew D, Cytryn L, et al: Diagnoses in school-age children of bipolar affective disorder patients and normal controls. J Affective Disord 8:283–291, 1985
6. Lefcourt HM (ed): Research with the Locus of Control Construct. New York, Academic Press, 1981
7. Spivack C, Platt J, Shure MB: The Problem-Solving Approach to Adjustment. San Francisco, Jossey-Bass, 1976
8. Wilcox A, Fritz B: Actual-ideal discrepancies and adjustment. J Counseling Psychol 18:166-169, 1971
9. Hirschfeld RMA, Cross CK: Epidemiology of affective disorders: psychosocial risk factors. Arch Gen Psychiatry 39:35–46, 1982
10. Spitzer RL, Endicott J: Schedule for Affective Disorders and Schizophrenia—Lifetime Version. New York, New York State Psychiatric Institute, Biometrics Research, 1975
11. Mazure C, Gershon ES: Blindness and reliability in lifetime psychiatric diagnosis. Arch Gen Psychiatry 36:521–525, 1979
12. Spitzer RL, Endicott J, Robins E: Research Diagnostic Criteria (RDC) for a Selected Group of Functional Disorders, 2nd ed. New York, New York State Psychiatric Institute, Biometrics Research, 1975
13. Gershon ES, Guroff JJ: Information from relatives: diagnosis of affective disorders. Arch Gen Psychiatry 41:173–180, 1984
14. Orvaschel H, Weissman M: Adaptation of the Schedule for Affective Disorders and Schizophrenia for School Age Children, Epidemiologic Version, KIDDIE-SADS-E with DSM-III (Addenda). New Haven, Yale Depression Center, June 1982

15. Nowicki S, Duke MP: A preschool and primary internal-external control scale. Developmental Psychol 10:874–880, 1974
16. Nowicki S, Strickland BR: A locus of control scales for children. J Consult Clin Psychol 40:148–154, 1973
17. Harter S: The Perceived Competence Scale for Children. Child Dev 53:87–97, 1982
18. Kirk RE: Experimental Design: Procedures for the Behavioral Sciences. Belmont, Mass, Brooks/Cole, 1968
19. Rutter M: Protective factors in children's responses to stress and disadvantage, in Primary Prevention of Psychopathology, vol 3. Edited by Kent MW, Rolf JE. Hanover, NH, Hanover University Press of New England, 1979
20. Rutter M, Garmezy N: Developmental psychopathology, in Handbook of Child Psychiatry, vol 4. Edited by Mussen P. New York, John Wiley & Sons, 1983
21. Davenport YB, Adland ML, Gold PW, et al: Manic-depressive illness: psychodynamic features of multigenerational families. Am J Orthopsychiatry 49:24–35, 1979

29

Problems in Transition Following Bone Marrow Transplantation: Psychosocial Aspects

Barbara L. Freund and Karolynn Siegel
Memorial Sloan-Kettering Cancer Center, New York

The number of patients achieving long-term survival following bone marrow transplantation is increasing. Psychosocial issues that may arise for the pediatric patient and for the family following discharge from the hospital are described. Implications for other situations in which there is a lengthy hospitalization for an organ transplant or life-threatening condition are highlighted.

Bone marrow transplantation has become an accepted form of therapy for acute leukemia, aplastic anemia, and immune deficiency diseases.[8] While the number of patients achieving long-term survival after transplant is increasing, the risk of mortality is still relatively high and transplantation is often complicated by significant morbidity. Transplantation patients require prolonged hospitalization with intensive supportive systems which include protected isolation in a laminar air flow environment, administration of oral nonabsorbable antibiotics, total body radiation, intravenous administration of chemotherapy and blood products, nutritional support due to therapy-induced mucasitis and anorexia, and skilled nursing care around the clock.

Reprinted with permission from the *American Journal of Orthopsychiatry*, 1986, Vol. 56, No. 2, 244–252. Copyright 1986 by the American Orthopsychiatric Association, Inc.

While there has been some recent discussion in the literature concerning the psychosocial stresses experienced by patients and their families during the period of transplantation and isolation, [3-5, 7, 9-11] the difficulties they face during the first weeks following discharge from the hospital have received less attention. It is this period of readjustment that is the focus of this paper.

While this paper focuses on the global issues of readjustment that may occur in any family with a child undergoing the transplant procedure, there are special concerns associated with each of the different diseases treated by bone marrow transplantation. We will begin by addressing some of the specific concerns associated with three diagnostic groups—leukemia, aplastic anemia, and severe combined immunologic deficiency. A number of the generic psychosocial concerns faced by the patient and the family in the transition from the hospital to the home environment will then be examined. Interventions that we have found helpful in alleviating some of these problems will be outlined. Although the issues will be discussed in the context of bone marrow transplantation, they have potential relevance to other situations that require extended hospitalization for an organ transplant or life-threatening condition.

Our observations are based on clinical work over a three-year period with 83 pediatric patients who underwent the transplant and were discharged to their homes. Of these, 56 were diagnosed with leukemia, 13 with aplastic anemia, and 14 with severe combined immunologic deficiency (SCID).

DISEASE-SPECIFIC ISSUES

For children with leukemia, the bone marrow transplant represents the culmination of earlier courses of treatment. These patients and their families have usually had time to begin to accept the illness, integrate it into their lives, and assign some meaning to it. Many of the stresses and changes associated with the transplant procedure—such as living with uncertainty, a disproportionate focus on the sick child, a disruption of usual family routines—have already been confronted by these families. At the same time, however, many such families arrive at the transplant stage with a sense of desperation, feeling that this is truly their last hope. Having experienced so many vicissitudes of the disease in the past, most families manifest an "acquired vigilance" that makes it difficult for them to trust their perception that recovery is proceeding well. Having lived with the disease for so long, these families have an especially difficult time suspending their preoccupation with the illness.

Aplastic anemia cases present a different set of circumstances. In most instances these patients have learned of their diagnosis only weeks before the transplant procedure is begun. The patients and their families have had little opportunity to assimilate the shocking news of the diagnosis or to redefine their situation before they must direct their full energies to getting through the various stages of the complex procedure. For many, the work of trying to integrate the illness into their lives must be put in abeyance until after the first critical phases of the procedure and the isolation are passed. This can significantly complicate the task of readjusting to the home environment. On the one hand, there is the need to work through the complex feelings of shock, anger, and despair associated with the realization that a potentially fatal illness has threatened the patient and the unity of the family. At the same time, they must cope with the expected physical and psychological consequences of the bone marrow transplantation.

Since SCID is a genetically transmitted disease, parents of children in this third patient group often experience a prominent sense of guilt. Until recently SCID patients may have required up to a few years of hospitalization following the transplant. As a result of recent advances in this procedure the average length of hospitalization has been dramatically reduced. Currently, most will be discharged within several months.

These patients are usually infants and in some instances the parents have already lost another child to the disease. While these families can be better prepared for the stresses of the treatment, they may also experience more anxiety in the period of transition because of their earlier loss. In addition, because this genetic condition may be diagnosed in the first few weeks of the infant's life, the parents may have had little time caring for the child at home. A child who had been home for a period of months before the diagnosis of SCID and the transplant may have manifested symptoms of irritability, eating difficulties, and frequent vomiting. Fears that even more of these problems, and the distress they created, might recur can make the parents apprehensive about the post-discharge period. In either case, ambivalence about leaving the hospital may be particularly pronounced in these cases.

REINTEGRATION OF PATIENT AND FAMILY

Ambivalence

Patients and their families often experience ambivalence when it is time to leave the protective atmosphere of the marrow transplant unit.[5, 6, 10] The nature of the experience can often evoke intense dependency needs in both the patient and the parents. Furthermore, the isolation room is often invested with magical qualities and there is apprehension on the part of both the parents and the child about whether a sufficiently safe environment can be maintained in the home.[5, 6] The parents, especially mothers, may welcome the opportunity to resume their role as the child's principal caretaker. Yet they may be reluctant to take on full responsibility once again for the child's well-being, and to relinquish the intensive support and assistance they received from the hospital staff. Parents may also fear and regret the loss, once they return home, of the support they received from staff and relatives of other transplant patients on the unit. As part of an attempt to deal with their anxiety about the child's safety at home, parents often observe precautions that exceed those required in the post-discharge period.

The child too may feel anxious about the parents' capacity to keep the child "well" at home, and as a result may be ambivalent about leaving the protective care of the hospital staff. Some patients—especially the younger ones—form very strong emotional attachments to members of the staff.[1] Such an outcome is understandable given the extended nature of the relationship, the life-threatening aspect of the illness, and the close and limited social contacts of the patient during hospitalization. Thus, the patient may resent and worry about the possibility that this special relationship with the staff will be superceded by the next patient.[1] The patient's dual task at this stage is to decathect not only from the staff, but from the insular environment of the transplant unit as well.

It is common for patients and staff members to exchange photographs or small gifts at the time of discharge. On a symbolic level these serve as a kind of "transitional object" that mitigates separation anxiety for the patient and family. This exchange is also emotionally comforting for staff members who are susceptible to similar feelings. Having cared for a child through the many weeks of the hospitalization required by the transplant procedure, staff can have difficulty relinquishing this primary caretaking role. Separation anxiety and a reluctance to give up the care of the child are frequent manifestations experienced by staff during the period the family is preparing to take the child home.

Expectations

Notwithstanding the ambivalence of leaving the safe haven of the hospital, once home some patients and families are also likely to experience unrealistic expectations for a transition period without its inherent difficulties. While in the hospital, most patients and their families are single-mindedly focused on completing the isolation and hospitalization phase of the process. A prevalent fantasy is that if they can effectively endure hospitalization with minimal medical and emotional complications, a successful course of recovery is virtually guaranteed. Although maintaining an emphasis on mastering each day of the hospitalization period can be effective on one level, it may be maladaptive in the long run if it leads to inadequate psychological and practical preparation for problems that may occur later. Without such preparation, patients and their families are particularly vulnerable to a profound sense of disappointment and despair should subsequent setbacks occur.

In addition, while the patients may feel well and want to think of themselves as recovered, they are confronted with the physical and emotional differences between themselves and their siblings and peers.[10] A full resumption of previously enjoyed peer group activities and a return to school must be postponed. Disappointed expectations coupled with the realization of persistent illness-related differences can result in a period of significant depression. It can also perpetuate a sense of ambiguity about the patients' medical status.

The potential for severe disappointment is present from another source as well. Some patients and family members equate discharge with cure. This is often not the case. Serious, life-threatening medical complications, such as graft-versus-host disease (GVHD), life-threatening infections, particularly pneumonia, and recurrence of the original disease remain salient dangers for some patients. Even in the absence of such complications patients cannot resume a "normal" life for at least five to six months following transplantation due to heightened susceptibility to infection. During this period, they must still remain in a relatively clean environment, and avoid close interaction with large groups of nonfamily members in school, restaurants, theaters, etc.

On a more personal level, the meaning that patients assign to their illness and to the transplant may also influence their expectations of how the family will treat them upon their return home. Many patients and their families view bone marrow transplantation as a complex and extraordinarily advanced procedure. It has been noted that this construction can lead to feelings of entitlement associated with being the survivor of this demanding experience.[1] Patients may imagine that only a small, select group of eligible individuals are offered this treatment. This contributes to their tendency to view themselves as among the "chosen." Upon returning home, therefore, these patients may expect family and friends to affirm their new sense of themselves as different and special.

Having spent months, sometime years, integrating and adapting to their disease, some patients have been observed to experience significant difficulty abandoning the sick role. The family, on the other hand, may feel frustrated and angry with the patient who refuses to give up the dependencies inherent in the patient role and who expects to be treated as he or she was treated throughout the critical times of the illness and hospitalization.

Sibling Transition Issues

Frequently it is a sibling who serves as the donor for the transplant. At the time of tissue typing, competition among siblings for the role of donor may occur. Those who do not serve as donors may feel further excluded from events that have been the focus of the family's energies since the illness was diagnosed. They may feel ashamed and inadequate for having been unable to play a more important role in the process.

The relationship between the patient and the donor-sibling may change significantly in the post-transplant period. Families often comment on the special sense of closeness and uniqueness that characterizes the patient-donor relationship. Comments and jokes about how the patient has taken on qualities and characteristics of the donor reflect a perception of the process as magical and potent. Although patients often feel deeply indebted to their donors, some donors may feel that they have not received adequate recognition for their "heroic" contribution.[10] If medical complications develop, however, donors may continually worry about the part played by their marrow. In the event of the death of a patient, the donor may experience a profound sense of guilt at having let down the sibling and the family.[8]

In most cases, at least one parent has had to leave the family to go with the patient to a distant medical center for the transplant. Siblings often experience a sense of abandonment during their parents' absence. This can lead to anger as well as feelings of bitterness and jealousy over what they regard as the exclusive parental attention received by the patient. Coexisting with sibling feelings of jealousy, anger, and resentment may be guilt about these feelings and about being the well one. The aggressive impulses a sibling may experience toward the patient as a normal developmental expression of sibling rivalry may be imagined to be responsible for the patient's illness.

In an attempt to assuage these strong sibling reactions parents sometimes make unrealistic promises that once the family is reunited illness-related stresses will no longer occur. These sibling expectations are inevitably disappointed. Patients typically continue to receive a disproportionate share of the parents' energies and attention after their return.

Such things as the necessary concerns for cleanliness and the fear of exposure to infection contribute to a continuing focus on the patient. Furthermore, parental demands requiring that siblings restrict their activities to certain areas of the house or apartment and forego the home visits of some friends further exacerbate the siblings' feelings of disappointment and loss.

CONSEQUENCES FOR THE MARITAL RELATIONSHIP

Usually one parent travels with the patient to the distant medical center for the transplant while the other remains home to continue working to assume child care responsibilities. Thus, the period of hospitalization for the transplantation usually necessitates prolonged separation of the spouses. This extended separation brings about changes in the division of responsibilities within the family, forcing both partners to give up roles that had been exclusively theirs and to assume new ones. Although both may recognize the practical necessity of these shifts, they continue to be emotionally invested in their relinquished roles. Parents may feel anger at having to defer to their spouse decision-making that was once either shared or held autonomously.

This period of separation may also bring about considerable changes in each spouse's self-image. Prior to coming to the transplant center, the mother may have maintained a traditional, dependent relationship with the father. Having weathered the many stresses and responsibilities related to caring for her child throughout the hospitalization, she may have developed a new sense of herself as a competent individual capable of making independent decisions. In the same way, the father's view of himself as an effective emotional caretaker may have grown significantly during this period. Once the family is reunited, he may insist on retaining a central role in this area. If either partner is unable to encompass the changes in the relationship required by the other's new sense of self, marital tension is likely to ensue.

Extended periods of separation can also contribute to "dis-synchrony" of coping between the parents.[2] Dis-synchrony refers to an incongruence in specific cognitive appraisals or affective states. That is, when the parents are differentially involved in the day-to-day events concerning the illness and its treatment, considerable differences between them may emerge in their understanding of what is happening, the meaning they assign to events, and the timing of their emotional responses. This dis-synchrony can create enormous tension and distress between family members.[2]

Additionally, the experience of having gone through this extraordinary procedure together tends to forge a strong and intimate bond between the child and the parent who stayed with the child during the period of isolation. Given the insular nature of the hospitalization experience and the lack of normal daily interaction with other family members, each depends exclusively on the other for the satisfaction of their needs for emotional and physical closeness. This bond often endures once the family is reunited and can cause the other parent to feel both jealous and excluded. Confronted with these feelings, that parent struggles to regain a sense of primacy in meeting the spouse's needs and to restore the emotional intimacy shared before the illness. Often a long period of time may be necessary for the parents to establish a new equilibrium in their marriage.

INTERVENTIONS

Various aspects of psychosocial adjustment for patients and their families associated with the transition from hospital to home following bone marrow transplantation have been described. Based on our clinical work, we have identified a number of interventions that can facilitate this period of transition following hospitalization. While in our own setting the interventions discussed below are usually initiated by the social worker on the transplant team, any mental health professional working with this population may find it useful to consider their application.

Assisting Patient and Family to Approach Discharge Realistically

The mental health professional, in consultation with the medical nursing team, should try to ensure that the patient and family enter the discharge period with realistic expectations. Without deflating hope or a positive attitude toward the patient's recovery, the patient and family must nevertheless be given a full understanding of possible eventualities. All patients ad their families are vulnerable to a profound sense of disappointment later if they expect a return to normalcy faster than is likely.

The mental health professional and a nurse should meet with the patient and the parents near the end of hospitalization specifically to assess if they are adequately prepared for the events that may ensue in the post-discharge period. If siblings are available to participate in this session, they should be included. Both the patient and family members should be encouraged to articulate their expectations so that appropriate modifications may be suggested. If siblings are not available to participate in these sessions the parents and the patient should be asked to speculate about their likely expectations.

Providing a Framework for Resumption of Prior Activities

Given the uncertain and variable course of the recovery it is difficult to provide parents with firm guidelines concerning the post-discharge period. As a result families often leave the hospital uncertain about such issues as when the child should return to school or resume participation in peer group activities. Some families are overly cautious and unnecessarily delay resumption of the patients' former pursuits; others— possibly as part of their need to view the patient as cured—encourage the patient prematurely to take up these activities. While definitive answers may not be possible, the provision of at least a tentative timetable would provide patients and families with a framework that enables them to begin to plan for the future.

Sensitizing Parents to Feelings of the Well Siblings

We have outlined above some of the conflictual feelings that well siblings may experience toward the patient and their parents. Sensitizing parents to the possible presence of these feelings and the ways they might be expressed behaviorally will better prepare the parents to deal with these feelings when they materialize. Our clinical experience indicates that parents tend to be aware of the potential concerns of the donor sibling but are less aware of the feelings their other children may harbor. With the almost exclusive family focus on the patient, parents should be made aware, prior to the hospital discharge, of possible reactions on the part of siblings who have not made a tangible contribution to the transplant process. They, too, long for recognition and acceptance during the potentially awkward period of family reintegration.

Assisting Parents in Accepting Changes in Their Relationship

In most cases, both parents come to the medical center on the day of discharge to take the child home. At this time, or on an earlier occasion close to discharge, the mental health worker should try to meet with both parents, should help them explore how the intense experiences they have gone through may have altered the way they feel about themselves and their relationship, and should encourage them to express any anxieties or concerns they have about how their relationship may have been altered. Individuals who have been confronted by the extraordinary demands and adaptions of this experience are inevitably going to be changed by it. It should be pointed out that while change in a long-standing relationship can be frightening it can also be an opportunity for growth and development.

Parents should also be encouraged to make an effort to be together by themselves for some time each week in the period following discharge. They need time to reestablish a sense of contact and unity as spouses, as well as parents. Finally, they should be offered some reassurance that, although their relationship will have changed somewhat, in time a new equilibrium will be reached. The strengths and resources they have demonstrated in the past should be identified so that they can draw on these in the period of transition. Above all the importance of maintaining good communication during this difficult period should be stressed.

Community Outreach

Often, when a child returns home, follow-up may be largely assumed by a community hospital, where the staff will generally have had little or no prior experience with transplant cases. The mental health worker who was involved with the family during the transplant should contact the appropriate staff member at the facility and explain the nature of the difficulties patient and family are likely to experience in the period of transition. The worker at the local hospital should also be apprised of any specific psychosocial problems the family experienced and relevant information about how they coped with the stress of the procedure.

If a community mental health worker who had contact with the family before the transplant or will be involved with them afterward can be identified, it may be helpful if that person can meet periodically during the period of hospitalization with the well siblings and the parent who has remained at home to care for them. This will prevent these family members from feeling excluded from the main events and help them to confront and resolve any ambivalent feelings toward the patient and other parent before they return home.

Finally, the transplant team social worker should contact the patient's teacher or school counselor before the child returns to class. They should be informed about the kinds of concerns the child may have about returning to school and peer group acceptance. The teacher may also be concerned about how to treat the former patient and how to deal with issues that may be raised by classmates. Taking time to discuss these concerns and provide some guidelines and concrete suggestions may better enable the teacher to assist the child in readjusting to school.

Clergy in the patient's community can also be an important source of support to some families during the period of transition. Typically, the member of the clergy at the cancer center who has been most involved with the family will initiate this communication.

Family Follow-up

The close ties with the staff that develop during the period of the transplantation and isolation have already been described. It is important for the patient and the family not to feel abandoned by the hospital team after discharge. The mental health professional on the transplant team should assume responsibility for following up on cases to see if the family is experiencing any serious psychosocial problems as well as to maintain contact for the family with the hospital. In the period immediately following discharge, when the parents may be apprehensive about their ability to care for the child on their own, the sense that the hospital staff is still available for support is very important.

Providing an Outlet for Staff Reactions

As mentioned, the feelings of the transplant team constitute an important component of the transition process and should not be overlooked. The staff must be assisted to acknowledge feelings of loss and to resolve them so as not to complicate the process of transition for the patient and family. At our center, ongoing staff support groups have proven to be a relaxed and effective means of expressing the staff's thoughts and wishes about their role with patients following discharge.

Follow-up contact with the family is important for the staff. Staff members are vulnerable to a sense of abandonment or rejection if the relationship with the family ends abruptly at the time of discharge. They were intensely involved in the care of the critically ill patient for many weeks and it is important for them to learn that the child is home, well cared for, and recovering satisfactorily. Nursing staff is encouraged to make contact with patients and families when they come to the hospital for their outpatient clinic visits. Similarly, during their clinic appointments, patients and families are encouraged to visit the floor where they received their treatment.

CONCLUSION

It is hard to explain what it is like when you have been closed in one room for so long. I was excited and nervous thinking about going back to the real world of people, germs, touching and feeling. I couldn't seem to absorb it all. I was looking at everything not knowing if I should touch anything. Then I began to wonder how is my new environment going to affect me?

This was written by a bone marrow transplant patient as she was preparing for discharge following an eight-week hospitalization. Her feelings reflect those of many of our patients as they anticipate leaving the hospital and beginning the readjustment phase of their illness. Until now attention has been predominantly focused on the hospitalization phase of the procedure. We have found most patients and their families are receptive to talking about their day-to-day anxieties and concerns associated with the illness and their hospital stay. There is a marked difference in their willingness to address their thoughts and worries as they approach discharge and prepare to return home. The task of helping patients and their families to prepare psychologically for discharge and their adjustment to home is a difficult one. This is an area of psychosocial practice in bone marrow transplantation that requires ongoing analysis and development.

REFERENCES

1. Brown, H. and Kelly, M. 1976. Stages of bone marrow transplantation. Psychosomat. Med. 38(6):439–446.
2. Christ, G. 1982. Dis-synchrony of coping among children with cancer, their families and the treating staff. *In* Psychosocial Family Interventions in Chronic Pediatric Illness, A. Christ and K. Flomenshaft, eds., Plenum, New York.
3. Holland, J. et al. 1977. Psychological response of patients with acute leukemia to germ-free environments. Cancer 40(2):871–879.
4. Kellerman, J., Rigler, D. and Siegel, S. 1977. The psychological effects of isolation in protected environments. Amer. J. Psychiat. 134(5):563–565.
5. Kellerman, J. et al. 1976. Psychological evaluation and management of pediatric oncology patients in protected environments. Med. Pediat. Oncol. 2(3):353–360.
6. Kellerman, J., Siegel, S. and Rigler, D. 1980. Special treatment modalities: laminar airflow rooms. *In* Psychological Aspects of Childhood Cancer, J. Kellerman, ed., Charles C Thomas, Springfield, Ill.
7. Kutsanellou-Meyer, M. and Christ, G. 1978. Factors affecting coping of adolescents and infants on a reverse isolation unit. Soc. Wk. Hlth Care 4(2):125–137.

8. O'Reilly, R. 1983. Allogeneic bone marrow transplantation: current status and future directions. Blood 62(5):941–961.

9. Patenaude, A. and Rappeport, J. 1982. Surviving bone marrow transplantation: the patient in the other bed. Ann. Intern. Med. 97(6):915–918.

10. Patenaude, A., Szymanski, L. and Rappeport, J. 1979. Psychological costs of bone marrow transplantation in children. Amer. J. Orthopsychiat. 49(3):409–422.

11. Pfefferbaum, B., Lindamood, M. and Wiley, F. 1977. Pediatric bone marrow transplantation: psychological aspects. Amer. J. Psychiat. 134(11):1299–1301.

30

Injuries Among Toddlers: Contributions from Child, Mother, and Family

Adam P. Matheny, Jr.

University of Louisville School of Medicine, Kentucky

Mothers' reports of injuries among 116 toddlers followed longitudinally from 1 to 3 years were used to designate one group (n = 32) as having higher injury liability and one group (n = 84) as having lower injury liability. The self-reported temperament of the mothers, directly appraised aspects of the toddlers' homes, and directly observed characteristics of the toddlers were correlated with injury liability. Higher injury liability was signified by features from all three sources. The mothers tended to be less educated and depicted themselves as more emotionally overwhelmed and less energetic; the homes tended to be less optimal for child development, of lower socioeconomic status, and marked by higher levels of noise and disorder; and the toddlers, who were likely to be male, were observed to be less tractable and manageable. Regression analyses indicated that a combination of characteristics of the mother and home provided a moderately strong multiple R with toddler's injury liability, and the toddler's characteristics made no additional significant contributions. The results are in-

Reprinted with permission from the *Journal of Pediatric Psychology*, 1986, Vol. 11, No. 2, 163–176. Copyright 1986 by Plenum Publishing Corporation.

This study was supported in part by the U.S. Public Health Service research grants OCD 90-C-922, HD 03217, and HD 14352, and by a research grant from the John D. and Catherine T. Mac Arthur Foundation (R. S. Wilson, Principal Investigator). A research grant from the Graduate School, University of Louisville fostered the completion of data and analyses. The assistance of R. Arbegust, P. Gefert, M. Hinkle, J. Lechleiter, B. Moss, S. Nuss, D. Sanders, and A. Thoben is gratefully acknowledged.

*terpreted as indicating that the injury liability of toddlers can be better es-
tablished by considering foremost those social and environmental conditions extrinsic to the child. However, that same emphasis may not apply
to older children and adolescents. It is suggested that pediatric psychologists take a developmental perspective when evaluating factors pertaining to children's injuries.*

In comparison with all other problems of childhood, injuries make the
largest contribution to mortality and morbidity rates from the end of the
first year on. That epidemiological fact has reawakened interest in
research on the behavioral aspects of childhood injuries. Earlier research, dating back to around 1950, consisted largely of exploratory
studies limited by sample size, inadequate assessment tools, and a
reliance on somewhat rudimentary analyses. The limitations and methodological problems (Haddon, Suchman, & Klein, 1964) of those studies
fostered the impression that behavioral research on childhood injuries
was a narrow preoccupation of little consequence. Yet, there has been a
gradual accumulation of more sophisticated studies attempting to
demonstrate that systematic variations in children's injuries can be
related to systematic variations in the behaviors of the individuals involved (Matheny & Fisher, 1984).

Manheimer and Mellinger (1967) examined the personality characteristics of about 700 boys and girls distributed into three levels of injury
according to the frequency of medically attended injuries reported during 4-year intervals. The investigators conceptualized two behavioral
domains as underlying accident liability: behaviors that govern exposure
to hazards, and behaviors that impair coping with hazards. They found a
significant relation between injury liability and mothers' or teachers'
ratings of activity, extroversion, exploring/independent, daring, rough-
housing, and athletic prowess—characteristics presumed to increase exposure to hazards. For boys, and to lesser extent, for girls, there was also a
clear set of relations between liability and discipline problems, aggression, competitiveness, showing off, tenacity, frustration tolerance, impulsivity, carelessness, unreliability, and inattentiveness—characteristics
that might impair coping with hazards.

Later investigations (Langley, McGee, Silva, & Williams, 1983; Langley,
Silva, & Williams, 1980; Matheny, Brown, & Wilson, 1971) examined the
history of injuries of children in longitudinal samples and found largely
similar sets of behaviors related to injury liability. Children reported as
being more active, emotionally reactive or temperamental, inattentive,
disobedient, or management problems tended to have more injuries

than children rated as having contrasting characteristics. Thus, the combined results from these investigations indicated that when behavioral assessments focused on the child, there was a somewhat refined set of children's behaviors associated with liability for injuries.

For the most part, the previous studies have concentrated on older children. It is less certain whether injuries of the infant and toddler are associated with their behavioral characteristics. Moreover, because of the importance of parental behavior and the home environment for the safety of the young child, it is not clear which of the various components—child, parents, or home—contributes the most to the links, if there are any, with childhood injuries.

The present study was undertaken to explore these considerations. Longitudinal assessments of children, mothers, and home environments provided a body of data describing behavioral characteristics of children and their mothers and extensive observations of the children's home environments. From the longitudinal sample the assessments pertaining to all children reaching age 3 years were taken to examine two questions: Are there any characteristics of the toddler, mother, or home that are associated with injury liability from the child's first to the child's third year of life? Among the same characteristics, which ones contribute the most to a prediction of childhood injuries for the same 2-year period?

METHOD

Subjects

The children in this study were selected from pairs of twins participating in an ongoing longitudinal study of temperament. The twins were recruited from families representing the entire socioeconomic range found in the Louisville metropolitan area. Occupations of the heads of household were converted to Duncan's scores for socioeconomic status (Reiss, 1961). According to this classification of socioeconomic status (SES), there were almost 30% of the families in the lowest two deciles of the 100-point range of scores; the remaining families were distributed in somewhat equal proportions among the other deciles.

At the time of study 51 male and 65 female children from 47 same-sex and 11 opposite-sex twin pairs were selected. The selection of the 116 children from the total sample was made on the following basis: (a) Visits had been made to the children's homes during the children's infancy; (b) the mothers had completed a self-report of their own adult temperament as measured by the Thurstone Temperament Schedule; and (c) direct observations of the children's temperament were available when the children were toddlers.

Measures

Injury criterion. The reports of the children's injuries were obtained from interviews with parents who were asked about the nature, severity, and circumstances surrounding all injuries, and whether or not medical attention had been sought. The interviews were conducted during each visit to the laboratory and the history of injuries for the interval from the last visit was brought up to date. For this study, the interviews at 18, 24, 30, and 36 months were used for the injury histories from 12 to 36 months.

According to the history of injuries for the 2-year period, each toddler was assigned to one of two groups representing injury liability. A toddler reported to have had two or more injuries, with at least one of the injuries receiving medical attention, was placed in the "higher liability" group. A toddler with one injury not receiving medical attention or no injury at all was placed in the "lower liability" group.* Injuries related to moving vehicles were considered only if the toddler was a pedestrian.

The application of this scheme resulted in 32 toddlers (19 male, 13 female) being assigned to the higher liability group, and 84 toddlers (32 male, 52 female) being assigned to the lower liability group. There were proportionately more males than females in the higher liability group, and the sex difference was significant, $\chi^2 = 4.25, df = 1, p < .05$. Because of sample size, the analyses were not applied to male and female toddlers as separate groups; however, the sex of the child was entered in the analyses as an independent variable.

Maternal characteristics. During the first year of participation in the study, mothers completed the Thurstone Temperament Schedule (Thurstone, 1953), a self-administered inventory composed of 140 items in a "Yes," "?," "No" format. The items are scored to represent seven aspects

---

*The term *medical attention*, applied to the "higher liability" group, refers to a child's injury having been brought to the attention of any member(s) of the health care delivery systems in the metropolitan area, even if the child was not seen or treated directly by a physician. Because there are scores of emergency centers, walk-in clinics, private physicians, health maintenance groups, and other forms of access to medical treatment, direct verification of parental reports, however desirable, was beyond the scope of the study. In view of the sustained contact with the participants in the research program, there is no reason to believe that a systematic bias affects parental reports of the severity of the injury or the treatment sought.

of adult temperament: Active (the tendency to participate and be actively engaged with the world); Vigorous (liking physical activities and energetic occupations); Impulsive (the tendency to make quick decisions or change from one activity to another); Dominant (taking initiative, responsibility, or leadership); Stable (steady in mood and not easily overwhelmed by crisis); Sociable (liking and adapting to other people); and Reflective (liking quiet work and reflective thinking).

In addition, the number of years of schooling completed by the mother was included as an indirect indicant of her realized intellectual attainments.

Characteristics of home environment. When the children were between 6 and 9 months old, a social worker made home visits scheduled to take place at a time when they would be awake for at least part of the visit. Throughout the visit, usually lasting from 1 to 2 hr, the social worker completed an extensive protocol based on direct observations and an interview. The protocol contained items representing two sets of measures: (a) items from an inventory, Appraisals of Opportunities for Developmental Experiences (ABODE; Matheny, Thoben, & Wilson, 1982), specifically compiled for assessing twins' homes; and (b) items constituting Home Observation for Measurement of the Environment (HOME; Caldwell, 1978).

The key items from ABODE were drawn from several sources (Matheny, Wilson, Dolan, & Krantz, 1981; Wachs, Uzgiris, & Hunt, 1971; White & Watts, 1973; Wilson, Brown, & Matheny, 1971; Yarrow, Rubenstein, & Pedersen, 1975), and the items were condensed by principal components factor analysis with varimax rotation. The analyses yielded three factors with eigenvalues > 1.00. The factors and the factor loadings for each item are shown in Table 1.

The first factor pertained to the general physical and social features of the home environment for fostering both intellectual and social development of the child. The factor was labeled Adequacy of the Home Environment. The second factor consisted of a high loading from a single item referring to the number of books in the household, but there were additional moderate loadings from items referring to the child's personal space. Consequently, the second factor was labeled Books/personal space. The third factor, identified by items pertaining to noise, confusion and clutter in the household, was labeled Noise/confusion. Standardized factor scores (mean = 0, SD = 1.00) from these three factors became the first set of measures of the home environment.*

---

*The factor analysis was determined for a large sample (n = 121) of families including the families in the present study. There were no significant differences between the three fac-

Table 1. Factor Loadings for Measures of Home and Neighborhood[a]

	Factors		
Measures	I	II	III
Global rating: Physical environment for adequacy in fostering social development	.88		
Adequacy of indoor play space	.84		
Global rating: Physical environment for adequacy in fostering intellectual development	.83	.41	
Global rating: Total environment for adequacy in fostering intellectual development	.78	.38	
Provision of indoor play materials	.76	.39	
Global rating: Total environment for adequacy in fostering social development	.76		− .32
Parental interest in and control of nutrition	.65		
Provision of children's equipment	.62		.41
Appliance score	.58	.45	
Number of books		.84	
Stimulus shelter: Child's own space	.38	.58	
Ratio: rooms/people	.43	.53	
Decorations in child's room	.33	.51	
Quality of the interior of the home	.35	.51	− .40
Noise and confusion in the home			.78
Cleanliness and lack of clutter in the home	.43		− .66
Total variance %	36.6	16.8	10.8

[a]Factor loadings < .30 omitted.

The second set of measures of the home environment was represented by scores for the six scales comprising Caldwell's HOME (1978). The scales are identified as the following: (a) emotional and verbal responsivity of the mother; (b) avoidance of restriction and punishment; (c) organization of the physical and temporal environment; (d) provision of appropriate play materials; (e) maternal involvement with the child; and (f) opportunities for variety in daily stimulation.

Toddler temperament. A key feature of the longitudinal temperament study was the direct assessment of temperament in a laboratory setting. Visits to the laboratory were scheduled at 6-month intervals from 1 to 3 years of age. In the laboratory setting, the toddlers were confronted with a succession of age-related activities and challenges presented systemati-

---

tor scores from the sample in this study and the large sample. For 21 families, interobserver reliabilities were computed on scores generated by the social worker and a graduate student acting as an independent observer. The mean interobserver reliability for the rating scales comprising ABODE was .89. Agreement on categorical items was in the range from 90 to 95%. For the six HOME scales, the mean interobserver reliability was .86.

cally in a standardized manner. The laboratory sessions were videotaped, and raters worked from the tapes to rate a toddler's predominant behaviors observed during 2-min periods for a total of 15 periods. The behaviors rated, on 9-point bipolar scales, were the following: emotional tone, activity, attentiveness, social orientation, and amount of vocalizations. The ratings were combined for all of the 15 periods to yield a single composite score for each behavior. To that set of composite scores were added two additional composite scores: variability of activity (a reflection of the change in activity over the course of fifteen 2-min periods); and resistance to restraint (an indication of the toddler's upset and struggle with procedures involving physical measurements). A complete description of the laboratory procedures, rating scales, and creation of the composite scores has been provided elsewhere (Matheny & Wilson, 1981; Wilson & Matheny, 1983a).

Previous factor analyses of the laboratory ratings have shown that five of the seven composite scores provided recurrent markers of the toddler's temperament (Matheny, Wilson, & Nuss, 1984). The scores— emotional tone, attentiveness, social orientation, activity variability, and resistance to restraint—contributed to a factor that was moderately stable over 6-month intervals and moderately correlated with parental reports of the toddler's temperament. The factor was labeled Lab-Tractability because higher factor scores depicted a toddler relatively more positive in emotional tone, approachful, attentive, accepting of procedures involving physical measurements, and less variable in activity from one observation period to the next.

For the present study, Lab-Tractability factor scores were available for laboratory observations at 12, 18, 24, and 30 months. In view of the fact that the injury criterion was based on a summary of injuries for the entire interval from 12 to 36 months, we decided to create a summary measure of the toddler's temperament for the same 2-year interval. That was accomplished simply by adding the four factor scores (extracted from visits at 12, 18, 24, and 30 months) and using the mean of the four scores as the best single description of the toddler's temperament observed directly in the laboratory.*

---

*Interrater reliabilities for the laboratory observations were determined by two raters independently rating the observations made on every third child. For this sample, the mean interrater reliability for the five scales comprising the Lab-Tractability factor was .84.

RESULTS

Table 2 provides the direct correlations between each set—mother, home environment, or toddler—of characteristics and injury liability. The significant correlations for characteristics within each set are described in the following sections. It must be recalled, however, that the characteristics were not necessarily independent measures, either within a set or between sets. Therefore, as a multiple regression analysis will demonstrate, the characteristics associated independently with injury liability are fewer in number than those listed in Table 2.

Characteristics of mother. It is apparent that several attributes of the mother, as obtained from the mother's self-assessment by the Thurstone, were related to injury liability. Mothers who reported themselves to be more emotionally stable (Stable), or more actively engaged with the world (Active), or more energetic (Vigor) were mothers whose toddlers were reported to have lower injury liabilities. In addition, mothers with higher levels of education had toddlers with lower injury liability. Although each of the significant associations was modest, the correlations indicated that maternal characteristics assessed before the child's first birthday were linked with the toddler's liability for injuries reported between 1 and 3 years.

Home environment. Here again, the correlations were modest, with the strongest correlation (.33) being found for a link between a factor representing noise, confusion, and clutter, and injury liability. In general, toddlers with lower liability for injury tended to live in home environments marked by less noise, confusion, and clutter, where there was more maternal involvement with the toddler, or where the physical and social environment was more adequate for the child development.

The contribution of SES was anticipated because of its link with mother's education as well as a number of specific features of the home (Wilson & Matheny, 1983b). However, SES becomes relatively unimportant once characteristics of the mother and home are accounted for.

Toddler. The single measure of the toddler's observed temperament was significantly correlated with injury liability; the more tractable toddlers, as denoted by the Lab-Tractability factor scores, sustained fewer injuries. If we consider the behaviors composing the factor, the correlation indicated that toddlers who were positive in mood, attentive, approachful, and generally manageable in the laboratory setting were less likely to sustain more frequent and serious injuries from ages 1 to 3 years.

The sex difference for injury liability is shown by the marginal but

Table 2. Children's Injury Liability: Correlations with Characteristics of Mother, Home, and Child[a]

Mother		Home environment		Child	
Thurstone Temperament Schedule		ABODE factors		Tractability	$-.27^c$
Activity	$-.22^b$	I. Adequacy home environment	$-.22^b$	Sex	$.19^b$
Vigor	$-.20^b$	II. Books/personal space	$-.04$		
Impulsive	$-.13$	III. Noise/confusion	$.33^c$		
Dominant	$-.09$				
Stable	$-.26^c$	HOME			
Social	$-.13$	Emotional-verbal responsivity	$-.11$		
Reflective	$-.17$	Avoidance of restriction	$-.12$		
		Organization of environment	$-.15$		
Education	$-.28^c$	Provision of play materials	$-.10$		
		Maternal involvement	$-.20^b$		
		Opportunities for variety	$-.12$		
		Socioeconomic status	$-.26^c$		

[a]Injury liability is a classification for which 1 = lower liability and 2 = higher liability for injuries. Sex is classified with female = 1, male = 2.

[b]$p \leq .05$.

[c]$p \leq .01$.

significant correlation of .19. As noted before, the male toddlers were more likely to belong to the higher liability group.

Multiple Regression Analysis

In view of the fact that almost all of the significant correlations in Table 2 were low order, the next step was to determine what combination of variables would maximize the prediction of injury liability. Many of the variables were intercorrelated, however. Therefore, a multiple regression program (BMD P2R) was used to identify the variables making independent and significant contributions to the prediction. The variables were entered in hierarchical order with the presumption that first, the seven maternal characteristics, and second, the nine features of the home environment would be more influential than the toddler's own behavior. At the third level of entry were the temperamental factors that represented the toddler's behavior and sex. The background variables, maternal education and family SES, were entered at the final level.

The regression program examines the variables according to the order specified and extracts each variable that contributes significantly to the multiple regression. As each variable is entered, the remaining variables are adjusted to take into account the predictive variance shared with the variable entered. The program continues to recycle in this manner until all of the variables with significant contributions to the predictive equation have been considered.

The results of the regression analysis are presented in Table 3. It is evident that the multiple R is a substantial improvement over the prediction afforded by the variables considered singly. Moreover, some of the 20 discrete variables did not contribute to the multiple R once other variables had been entered. For example, the toddler's own behavior had a higher correlation with the toddler's injury liability than many of the characteristics of the mother and home. However, after those significant contributions had been entered, the toddler's tractability made no additional independent contribution to the multiple R.

One of the chief reasons for arranging the multiple regression analysis in the order specified was that characteristics extrinsic to the toddler were presumed to be largely influential for creating safe or unsafe conditions. However, one cannot ignore the results that show features of the toddler to be correlated with injury liability. With that fact in mind, the regression analysis was run again, with the toddler's characteristics entered first, followed by maternal, and background measures in that order. The supplementary analysis indicated that the toddler's tractability was entered

Table 3. Multiple Correlations of Mother, Home, and Child Variables with Child Injury Liability from 1 to 3 Years

Step no.	Assigned level of entry	Variables and source	Original R	Partial R	Multiple R
1.	1.	Mother: stable (Thurstone)	-.26		.26
2.	1.	Mother: activity (Thurstone)	-.22	-.20	.32
3.	2.	Home: noise-confusion factor (ABODE)	.33	.41	.50
4.	1.	Mother: vigor (Thurstone)	-.20	-.19	.53
5.	4.	Mother: education	-.28	-.24	.57

in the multiple *R*, but once the maternal and home measures were entered, toddler's tractability was removed as a significant contributor. Therefore, the supplementary analysis confirmed the original result: After the contributions of the mother and the home environment were accounted for, the toddler's characteristics provided no significant addition to the prediction of injury liability.

DISCUSSION

The results of this study indicated that a higher liability for injuries among toddlers is signified by features from three sources: mothers, home environments, and the toddlers themselves. For the injury-liable toddlers, the mothers tended to have a lower level of education and depicted themselves as more emotionally overwhelmed and less energetic; the home and family environments tended to be generally less optimal for child development, of lower SES, and marked by higher levels of noise and disorder; and finally the toddlers themselves, who were more likely to be male, were observed to be less tractable and manageable. Taken one at a time, each feature provided only a modest association with the injury criterion; however, certain combinations of features, namely, those from the mother and home, provided a moderately strong relation with the toddler's history of injuries from 1 to 3 years. From a developmental perspective, the results indicate that the antecedents of the injuries of the young child might be understood best by focusing on the characteristics of the supervising adult and the more immediate environment. By and large, the toddler's behavior contributes to the injury equation but appears to be less important. One might have anticipated these results, given the influence of parents and home environments on a toddler's behavior. Yet, there are no multivariate studies available that could buttress such a sensible view with empirical findings.

The fact that the toddler's behavior did not make a significantly large contribution to the multiple regression analysis does not mean that the toddler's characteristics are unimportant, however. As noted elsewhere (Langley et al., 1983), there appear to be linear relations between childhood injuries by age 3 years and parental reports of the child's activity level. Moreover, through application of the method of co-twin control, the toddler's reported temperament has been associated with injury liability once parental and environmental variables were equated within pairs of twins (Matheny, 1985). Twins who were toddlers with a higher liability for injuries were reported by their mothers to be less adaptable, more negative in mood, and more withdrawn than their co-twins. Therefore, these and other sparse reports (Matheny & Fisher, 1984) suggest that characteristics of the toddler may contribute to injury liability, and as a consequence, they should not be neglected either for the design of intervention programs or for research. However, after examining the injuries of most toddlers, it is clear that parental attributes and features of the home are the factors related to injury liability that largely surpass those more intrinsic to the child.

In view of the developmental features of childhood injuries (Matheny, in press), the present results should be interpreted narrowly only insofar as they apply to the toddler. Older children have expanding access to an increasingly wider range of environments. We might anticipate that the correlates of injury liability will change with developmental progress, and the contributions of parents and home environments might become less salient. There is evidence that the behaviors of the older child are more associated with injury histories (Langley et al., 1983; Manheimer & Mellinger, 1967; Matheny, 1980), and it has been firmly established that the differential injury liability for male and female children becomes more pronounced with age (Matheny, in press). Therefore, one should be cautious in generalizing the present results to other periods of childhood and especially to adolescence.

McFarland (1963) has reminded us that injuries involve multiple causes, with mutual interactions, and the understanding of the injury equation requires the identification of a variety of variables and their interactions. That reminder, as applied to childhood injuries, is worth repeating, providing that a developmental view is maintained. Pediatric psychologists are in a position uniquely suited to hold that view, largely because they are mindful of the fact that developmental progress is represented by change—in the child and in the conditions successively impinging on the child.

A commonplace observation is that many behavioral and environmental conditions are not equally hazardous to all children regardless of age. The age-dependent changes in the types of injuries reported attests to that fact (Matheny & Fisher, 1984). Consequently, ideal strategies for injury prevention should evolve from a series of empirically verified risk registries that are developmentally specific. In the context of the present study, the risk registry would include attributes of the mother and home that relate directly to the increased potential for injury. Surveillance, anticipatory guidance, or perhaps more routinized contact with the family—all within the purview of pediatric psychologists—can be brought to bear upon the families at risk for this developmental epoch. Therefore, the strategies for prevention are applied when they are developmentally appropriate. We further presume that a risk registry for another epoch would comprise different attributes to be considered for developing different strategies. For example, we might find that attributes of the home environment are not as related to the injuries of teen-agers, but attributes of the neighborhood or community are.

At the moment, the sources of systematic variations in childhood injuries still remain undefined because so many aspects of childhood are neither uniform nor stable over long reaches of time. Yet, placing childhood injuries within a developmental context offers the chance of avoiding a concentration on traits (accident proneness) alone or a concentration on environments alone. Perhaps in that way we can settle the disputatious concerns (Barry, 1975; Klein, 1980; Matheny & Fisher, 1984) about the utility of examining the characteristics of individuals for designing effective injury-prevention strategies.

REFERENCES

Barry, P.Z. (1975). Individual versus community orientation in the prevention of injuries. *Preventive Medicine, 4,* 47–56.

Caldwell, B.M. (1978). *Home observation for the measurement of the environment.* Little Rock: University of Arkansas.

Haddon, W., Suchman, E.A., & Klein, D. (1964). *Accident research methods and approaches.* New York: Harper & Row.

Klein, D. (1980). Societal influences on childhood accidents. *Accident Analysis and Prevention, 12,* 275–281.

Langley, J., McGee, R., Silva, P., & Williams, S. (1983). Child behavior and accidents. *Journal of Pediatric Psychology, 8,* 181–189.

Langley, J., Silva, P.A., & Williams, S. (1980). A study of the relationship of ninety background, developmental, behavioural and medical factors to childhood accidents. A report from the Dunedin Multidisciplinary Child Development Study. *Australian Paediatric Journal, 16,* 244–247.

Manheimer, D.E., & Mellinger, G.D. (1967). Personality characteristics of the child accident repeater. *Child Development, 38,* 491–513.

Matheny, A.P., Jr. (1980). Visual-perceptual exploration and accident liability in children. *Journal of Pediatric Psychology, 5,* 343–351.

Matheny, A.P., Jr. (1985, April). *Toddler temperament and accident liability within twinships.* Paper presented at the biennial meeting of the Society for Research in Child Development, Toronto.

Matheny, A.P., Jr. (in press). Accidents and injuries. In D. Routh (Ed.), *Handbook of pediatric psychology.* New York: Guilford Press.

Matheny, A.P., Jr., Brown, A., & Wilson, R.S. (1971). Behavioral antecedents of accidental injuries in early childhood: A study of twins. *Journal of Pediatrics, 79,* 122–124.

Matheny, A.P., Jr., & Fisher, J.E. (1984). Behavioral perspectives on children's accidents. In M. Wolraich & D. Routh (Eds.), *Advances in behavioral pediatrics* (vol. 5, pp. 221–263). Greenwich, CT: JAI Press.

Matheny, A.P., Jr., Thoben, A.S., & Wilson, R.S. (1982). Appraisals of basic opportunities for developmental experiences (ABODE): Manual for home assessments of twin children. *JSAS Catalog of Selected Documents in Psychology, 12,* 31 (Ms. No. 2472).

Matheny, A.P., & Wilson, R.S. (1981). Developmental tasks and rating scales for the laboratory assessment of infant temperament. *JSAS Catalog of Selected Documents in Psychology, 11,* 81–82 (Ms. No. 2367).

Matheny, A.P., Jr., Wilson, R.S., Dolan, A.B., & Krantz, J.Z. (1981). Behavioral contrasts in twinships: Stability and patterns of differences in childhood. *Child Development, 52,* 579–588.

Matheny, A.P., Jr., Wilson, R.S., & Nuss, S.M. (1984). Toddler temperament: Stability across settings and over ages. *Child Development, 55,* 1200–1211.

McFarland, R.A. (1963). A critique of accident research. *Annals of New York Academy of Sciences, 107,* 686–695.

Reiss, A.J., Jr. (1961). *Occupations and social status.* New York: Free Press of Glencoe.

Thurstone, L.L. (1953). *Examiner manual for the Thurstone Temperament Schedule,* (2nd ed.). Chicago: Science Research Associates.

Wachs, T.D., Uzgiris, I., & Hunt, J. McV. (1971). Cognitive development in infants of difference age levels and from different environmental background. *Merrill-Palmer Quarterly, 17,* 283–317.

White, B., & Watts, JU. (1973). *Experience and environment: Major influences on the development of the young child* (Vol. 1). Englewood Cliffs, NJ: Prentice Hall.

Wilson, R.S., Brown, A.M., & Matheny, A.P., Jr. (1971). Emergence and persistence of behavioral differences in twins. *Child Development, 42,* 1381–1389.

Wilson, R.S., & Matheny, A.P., Jr. (1983a). Assessment of temperament in infant twins. *Developmental Psychology, 19,* 172–183.

Wilson, R.S., & Matheny, A.P., Jr. (1983b). Mental development: Family environment and genetic influences. *Intelligence, 7,* 195–215.

Yarrow, L.J., Rubenstein, J., & Pedersen, F. (1975). *Infant and environment.* New York: Wiley.

Part VIII

CHILD ABUSE

It becomes increasingly clear with the passing years that widespread child abuse constitutes a shameful blot on our society and makes a mockery of the oft-repeated cliché that we are a "child-centered country." We also assume that our concern for our children contrasts with the brutality and neglect suffered by children in the "Dark Ages" of early medieval Europe. Kroll and Bachrach challenge this assumption in an ingenious and scholarly study of the available historical data regarding the treatment of sick children in the Middle Ages. They conclude that parents in pre-Crusade Europe made serious efforts to secure the health and well-being even of sick and handicapped children. They leave us with the sobering possibility that "Western" civilization may indeed have regressed rather than progressed since the "Dark Ages."

It is only in recent years that mental health professionals have begun to accept the horrendous fact that child sexual abuse is widespread and requires both empirical study of its impact on the child victim and the formulation of programs of prevention and treatment. The attention given to this serious question is so recent that it is only now possible to review the relevant literature systematically. This task has been undertaken by Browne and Finkelhor who present an excellent, thorough, and critical analysis of the studies thus far reported. They find that research on child sexual abuse is still in its infancy and that most of the available studies have substantial sample, design, and measurement problems. But there can be no doubt, even from these flawed reports, that child sexual abuse can have serious psychological consequences. Browne and Finkelhor offer a number of pertinent suggestions for improving methodological and conceptual approaches so that research in this important psychosocial problem can be effective.

PART VIII: CHILD ABUSE

31

Child Care and Child Abuse in Early Medieval Europe

Jerome Kroll and Bernard Bachrach

University of Minnesota Hospitals, Minneapolis

The concern about widespread abuse of children in modern Western society has led historians and health care professionals to examine the past for evidence of similar abusive practices. The expectation has been that the past, especially the Middle Ages, will reveal even worse attitudes and practices toward children. Our research, based upon analysis of care given to sick children in early medieval Europe, suggests that considerable attention, effort, and expense were devoted to seeking help for sick and crippled children. At the same time, there is no body of evidence to sustain the notion of widespread child abuse during these Dark Ages of Western civilization.

The landmark article by Kempe et al. (1962), which forced into our consciousness the modern epidemic of child abuse and neglect, moved pediatricians, child psychiatrists, and child welfare workers to consult the history books in order to discover how children in earlier and more primitive societies were treated. The virtual absence of serious historical studies on children in general and the problem of child abuse in particular prior to the 19th century has now been remedied.

Indeed, during the past two decades, the general thrust of both the scholarly and popular treatment of childhood in the Middle Ages, with a

Reprinted with permission from the *Journal of the American Academy of Child Psychiatry*, 1986, Vol. 25, No. 4, 562–568. Copyright 1986 by the American Academy of Child and Adolescent Psychiatry.

few exceptions that have not been given great attention, has been to emphasize abuse, neglect, abandonment, and infanticide (Bakan, 1971; Heins, 1984; Robin, 1981; Smith, 1975; Solomon, 1973). Two grand designs have served to inform this enterprise: Aries' (1962) thesis that the notion of childhood as a developmental phase distinct from adulthood was not conceptualized until after the Middle Ages, and DeMause's theories, published in book form in 1974 and echoed frequently in later articles in the *History of Childhood Quarterly* which he founded in 1973, that Western society has undergone distinct modes in its concepts of childhood and its actual child rearing practices, beginning with infanticide (ancient Greeks and Romans), *progressing* upward toward abandonment (medieval) and intrusiveness (17th century), and finally evolving to our more enlightened helping mode (mid-20th century).

The prominence of Aries' *L'Enfant et la vie familiale sous l'ancien regime* inspired medievalists to examine his thesis, "in medieval society the idea of childhood did not exist," in detail. After two decades of scholarly research (DeMaitre, 1977; Forsythe, 1976; Kroll, 1977; McLaughlin, 1974), Aries' grand thesis has been undermined, but it has spun off tangents that offer even greater distortions of the Middle Ages than did the original idea. The scholarly rebuttal, based upon research data largely in Latin and often published in relatively obscure journals that are not generally read by physicians or even historians of medicine, has not succeeded in capturing the popular imagination as had Aries' more spectacular, although unsound claims. Starting with Aries' conclusions that children received no special recognition or care *qua* children, and adding to it the common though largely unjustified perception of the Middle Ages as a long period of unrelieved obscurantism and brutality, readers are propelled toward the conclusion that infants and children, being the most helpless members of medieval society, must have been, to a greater extent than in our progressive society, victimized in a most brutal fashion. This case is secured for the naive reader with a few adroitly selected anecdotes.

DeMause (1974) enlarged Aries' grand thesis into an even grander design, corresponding to a Whiggish notion that the history of mankind is one of inexorable progress. This is linked to his psychohistorical thesis that infants and children of all eras have suffered from the unconscious hostility of parents directed toward their offspring. DeMause asserts that these children, in turn, grow up to have unconscious hostility, based upon their own experience with their aggressive parents, toward their children, and so this cycle is perpetuated through the generations of mankind. According to DeMause, the story of civilization is the progress which societies achieve in controlling, subjugating, and finally "sublimating" this almost instinctual hostility between generations.

Despite the fundamental difficulty in developing compelling evidence to sustain these characterizations, DeMause has found substantial sympathy from workers in the field of child abuse who, in turn, find their educational and legislative tasks greatly strengthened by "discoveries" that all societies have resisted attempts to protect children from parental viciousness. These "discoveries" have fit in so perfectly with present attempts to reform heinous social practices toward children that there has been little incentive to examine the historical evidence upon which the generalizations are based.

Historical evidence does not support either sweeping claims for brutality and indifference to children in early medieval Europe or more simplistic notions which stigmatize the childrearing practices of entire civilizations. Indeed, it has been seen that the "same" society may treat children differently as economic conditions fluctuate (deVries, 1984). As sociobiological theory would predict, for example, infanticide may have increased in the Middle Ages during famine years and decreased during the post-plague years of 1350–1400 when there was a great shortage of farm laborers (Dickeman, 1975). In this vein, an account of the terrible famine in the Loire valley from 1031–1034 describes both the norm of tenderness and concern of parents in raising children and the devastating effect of extended starvation upon this relationship. This famine reduced people to eating such things as mice, dogs, green twigs and tree roots, and sent large crowds of starving men, women, and children wandering over the countryside in a mad search for food. As Andre of Fleury (*Les miracles de Saint Benoit,* 1853), an 11th century contemporary, observes, some parents were said to have killed and eaten their children:

> At the height of such calamity . . . the sweet delicate children who nursed at the breast . . . in the midst of their meals were slaughtered by the impious hands of their parents, whose disordered minds with menacing eyes and threatening faces did not fear to stuff themselves with this superlative feast.

Andre makes it clear that parents who did such things, even under these dire circumstances, had become deranged by their physical condition and mental stress. The text leaves no doubt which is the norm and which the aberration, nor is its obvious sarcasm sparing in its condemnation of the parents' actions.

Furthermore, when one looks toward the phenomenal growth in population of medieval Europe (Genicot, 1964; Krause, 1957; Russell, 1958; 1965; Titow, 1961) despite a *natural* infant mortality rate of at least 30–40% (Hollingsworth, 1969; Kelly and Snedden, 1960; WHO, 1973), it seems highly unlikely on the face of it that the surviving children, who carried the promise of the future, were the specific targets for society's aggressions, frustrations, and neurotic conflicts. Rather, it may be suggested that such *assumptions* of widespread brutality toward children may well reflect the well-ingrained prejudice concerning virtually anything Medieval. Indeed DeMause's grand design, as medievalists have shown, is but a recent manifestation of this orientation which tends to support the needs of many health care professionals and lobbyists who have looked to "historians with a conscience" to provide a usable past.

A HYPOTHESIS REEXAMINED

The general thesis for which confirmatory, supportive, or contradictory evidence must be sought is as follows:

> In the Middle Ages, children were treated poorly. They were generally given none of the special care, consideration, and attention which modern society considers essential for normal child development. Furthermore, children were the object of widespread neglect, abuse, abandonment, and murder (via infanticide and lethal neglect).

What is the evidence to support this general thesis which informs the historical comments found in medical textbooks and journals? Many serious scholars, while accepting the broad outline of the abuse and infanticide thesis, acknowledge that the picture has been built upon fragmentary evidence because of the consensus that children are poorly documented in the medieval sources. Herlihy (1978) stated that for the pre-Crusade era we must rely principally on law codes, penitentials, and theological commentaries which are presumed to represent norms of some sort. More recently Arnold (1980) has argued that there is insufficient evidence to prove widespread infanticide, much less other forms of child abuse. Ende (1983) concurs with Arnold but nevertheless appears to feel that the early Middle Ages should not be exempted from the universal conclusion that infanticide and child abuse were widespread phenomena throughout all periods of history.

Despite this general assumption that there is a scarcity of evidence about medieval childhood, there remains, in fact, a relative abundance of largely untapped material in various genres of narrative sources which even permit a rough type of quantitative evaluation. In light of a sample of these generally neglected source materials, it will be suggested here that the prevailing view of treatment of medieval children, and more particularly, of those who were at grave risk due to illness, conforms more closely to our contemporary view of how such children should be treated than to the stereotype suggested by Aries, DeMause, and subsequent writers.

We have chosen to look at sick children as a "worst case" example; that is, if child abuse were endemic in medieval Europe, one would expect this phenomenon to be seen most glaringly in the treatment of sick children: those suffering from birth defects, the crippled, the blind, and the damaged, all of whom could be expected to contribute less to the productivity and security of a family. Since access to medical care was difficult and the general effectiveness of medical care was not likely to inspire confidence in those responsible for the welfare of children, the vulnerability of sick children and the statistical likelihood that they would perish—a likelihood that the medieval parent would not be able to quantify but surely understood on the basis of life's experiences—might be thought to militate strongly against parental efforts to secure treatment for their sick children. We suggest that if significant efforts were made in a quantitative sense to seek relief for sick children, then the focus in understanding the care of children should be placed toward the positive rather than upon largely undocumented allegations of rampant child abuse, abandonment, and infanticide. We further suggest that an index of how medieval parents felt toward their children can be developed in relation to the efforts they made and the costs they incurred to protect the weakest and most vulnerable among them.

METHOD

There are three major methodological problems to consider in investigating the question: how were sick children treated in medieval Europe? The first is to designate, and to some extent, delimit, the temporal and geographical boundaries of the subject matter. The second is the selection of sources, since there is no single collection of early medieval material focused primarily upon infants and children. The third is to obtain a sufficiently large sample of cases in order to eliminate or attenuate the potential bias that may be present in any single source and to avoid the technique of "proof by anecdote," which so obviously lacks methodological soundness.

We have chosen to restrict our sources to pre-Crusade (pre-1100) England and the Frankish kingdoms, encompassing the so-called Dark Ages of the 1000-year medieval period. We have restricted our inquiry to narrative sources (saints' lives and chronicles). These sources contain much incidental material about childhood and child-rearing practices. Our finding that between 15 and 20% of miracle cures concern children brought for medical care indicates that this cannot have been a practice that was out of the ordinary. The purpose of hagiography was to tell a believable story for the glory of the saint, and if care for sick children were unusual, the credibility of the tale would be undermined.

Although the population of sick children who are described in the biographies of saints is obviously not a random sample of sick children in pre-Crusade Europe, there is little reason to believe that we cannot obtain a reasonably accurate picture of some aspects of childhood illnesses and care in the early Middle Ages from such sources. Although many of the illnesses are mentioned primarily to record a very complicated social pattern of religious and secular values (which we will discuss later), the actual descriptions of the symptoms and signs of the children's illnesses are often naturalistic and accurate. Thus, our hagiographic and chronicle sources are adequate to develop a reasonably good idea of the range of illnesses described in children, the behaviors of those caring for sick children, the types of treatments or interventions, and the outcomes of the illnesses.

In a sense, the incidental nature of most of the references to childhood illnesses seems to provide some confidence that the medieval authors have not intentionally or systematically distorted the technical details of the presentation, progress, or outcome of the illnesses, even if the choice of what was presented may on occasion be politically or religiously motivated. Thus the anonymous author of the 8th century *Liber Historia Francorum* (1973) may have a religious point to make in mentioning that one of Clovis' newborn sons succumbed to an illness shortly after baptism, but we can accept the fact of the neonatal death independently of doctrinal disputes.

Finally, although general categories of illnesses (e.g., paralysis, traumatic injuries, dysentery, plague, madness) can be recognized by their descriptions, these medieval authors overwhelmingly appear medically naive insofar as there is no reason to believe that they are committed to a particular medical doctrine, such as the humoral theory, which might bias their descriptions of illnesses in a systematic way. On the other hand, neither is there evidence that they are committed to doctrines of sin and punishment as the causal factors of mental or physical diseases (Kroll and Bachrach, 1984).

We reviewed 22 saints' lives, 5 secular biographies, and 5 chronicles. These were not preselected to support our viewpoint, but are part of a larger survey of medical and psychiatric conditions in early medieval Europe. We extracted for examination *all* references to sick children and tabulated these along a number of parameters. The broad categories are *demographic, medical,* and *parental behavior* (the latter an index of effort expended in seeking treatment for the sick child).

Determination of gender and broad social class are relatively straightforward. Ages of children are rarely given. We used the conventions of language as set forth in the 7th century by Isidore of Seville (1964), whose work provided the basic guide on this topic throughout the Middle Ages: *infans,* birth to age 7; *puer et puella*, ages 7–14; *adolescens,* ages 14–28. The medical data are classified much as described in the sources. We have not tried to superimpose modern diagnoses upon the data, except for purposes of broad categorizations. For example, a description is provided in Bede's *History of the English Church and People* (1974) of a young nun, daughter of the abbess, who had recently been bled in the arm. Within a few days the arm was painful and swollen, and the young girl was very ill and likely to die. She is cured by the ministrations of St. John of Beverly. We classified this illness as an infection, although the text does not literally refer to it as such (Book V, p. 3).

The area which required the greatest subjective judgment was estimating what we termed "index of effort." By this construct we hope to give some measure of the effort expended by caregivers in attempting to obtain treatment for the child. We examined such indices as whether a physician was sought, the number of shrines visited, the costs of traveling to the shrines, and obligations the parents might incur in asking a holy man or woman to intervene on behalf of their child.

RESULTS

Sixty-four episodes of illnesses in children are mentioned in the source material. Eight of the saints' lives, five secular biographies, and one chronicle make no reference to children's illnesses and are not further discussed in this article. There are a total of 371 references to all illnesses (adult and childhood) in the sources. Thus 17% (64/371) of the reported illnesses occur in children. Table 1 presents the number of cases described in each source.

Table 2 presents the data on age, gender, and social class. There were 44 boys and 19 girls. The gender of the one case of infanticide is not given in the text. There is some indication of age for 75% of the boys and slightly

Table 1. Episodes of Childhood Illnesses in Pre-Crusade
Sources[a]

Source	Illnesses in Children	All Illnesses Mentioned	Percentage Illnesses in Children
Arnulf	1	9	11
Berarius	2	5	40
Bertuinus	1	3	33
Jonas: Columbanus	2	9	22
Adamnan: Columba	1	20	5
Anon: Cuthbert	7	15	47
Bede: Cuthbert	2	21	10
Walafrid: Gall	6	27	22
Rudolf: Leoba	1	4	25
Romaricus	2	3	67
Walaricus	2	11	18
Eddius: Wilfrid	1	10	10
Aldegunda	1	4	25
Corbinianus	1	6	17
Bede: Historia	10	38	26
Flodoard: Annals	2	27	7
Gregory: Historia	18	92	20
Liber Hist Francorum	4	13	31
Totals	64	317[b]	20

[a] References available upon request.

[b] In addition, there were 14 sources which described 54 cases of illnesses in adults, but none in children. If we add these 54 cases to the 317 cases listed above, we arrive at $N = 371$. Of this total, 64 cases (17%) are of childhood illnesses.

less than 50% of the girls. All the illnesses in babies under age 2 are in reference to boys. Although approximately 50% of the children are from the nobility or clergy (often both), the other 50% are descriptions of illnesses in the children of townspeople and peasants.

Table 3 presents the data on diagnoses, gender, and mortality. Thirteen children were mad or possessed, 9 were crippled or paralyzed, 9 had fever or infections, 6 had dysentery, and 4 had plague. Dysentery was fatal in all cases, plague in 3 of 4 cases, and fever or infection in 22% of cases. Most other conditions were not fatal. Overall, 16 (25%) of the 64 sick children died, 14 of the fatalities occurring in boys.

Table 4 presents an index of effort made on behalf of the sick child. The categories are not mutually exclusive; a child may be represented under several categories. There was no information for many cases, whereas in

Table 2. Gender, Age, and Social Class of Sample (N = 64)

Sample	Male	Female	Total
Age			
Under 2	9	0	10[a]
2–14	17	6	23
Over 14	8	1	9
Unknown age	10	12	22
Total	44 (70%)	19 (30%)	63
Social Class			
Nobility	18	3	21
Clerical	5	5	10
Other (town, peasant)	15	4	20[a]
Unknown	6	7	13
Total	44	19	64

[a] The gender of the single case of infanticide is not given in the text. The infant was born to a "begger-girl."

others the child may have taken sick and died before help could be sought. In slightly over half the cases (53%), the parents either brought the sick child to a holy man or shrine or the holy man was requested to travel to the child. The distance traveled varied from a short walk across town to an arduous journey, or in a sense, a pilgrimage, of several hundred kilometers. This will be discussed more fully in the next section.

DISCUSSION

The purpose of this paper is to examine the question of how were sick children treated in the Middle Ages. Phrased as an inquiry of the dominant theory, it would be: What is the evidence that children were abused, neglected, and murdered on a large scale in the Middle Ages, and what is the evidence to the contrary?

We have strongly emphasized that any useful answers to these questions must depend upon the validity of the methodology employed. The usual method, which seems to rely upon the selection of a few horrible examples of child abuse, taken out of context and interpreted as the norm, is of dubious validity. It is also our position that no positive conclusions should be drawn from sources that provide no information. Some scholars would perhaps suggest that silence is significant (Kellum, 1974). At this point in our research, we are not persuaded. Thus the goals of this paper are *both* to demonstrate that source material for a study of early medieval childhood is available for at least quantitative analysis, and to suggest some specific answers to the questions posed above.

Table 3. Diagnoses and Gender

Diagnosis	Male	Female	Total	No. of Deaths	Percent Mortality
Plague	4	0	4	3	75
Dysentery	6	0	6	6	100
Fever, infection	8	1	9	2	22
Dying, unspecified	10	5	15	4	27
Injury	2	0	2	—	—
Blindness	0	3	3	—	—
Mutism	2	0	2	—	—
Crippled, paralyzed	6	3	9	—	—
Mad/Possessed	6	7	13	—	—
Infanticide	0	0	1[a]	1	100
Totals	44	9	64	16	25

[a] Gender not given in text.

Table 4. Index of Effort to Obtain Help for Sick Child
(N = 64)[a]

Action Taken	Male	Female	Total
Parents bring child to saint, shrine, or church	18	10	28
Nobility requests assistance of saint	4	3	7
Saint or bishop travel to sick child	3	3	6
Saint stays up all night praying	1	—	1
Already in monastery, special care given	1	4	5
Total	27	20	47

[a] Categories are not mutually exclusive. An episode of illness may appear under more than one category.

Much of the data are fairly clear: more male than female children are described; male children have a higher mortality rate than female; although the children of the nobility are represented disproportionately to their presumed percentage of the population, there is considerable attention paid to illnesses in the children of townspeople and peasants; dysentery and plague have a high mortality in children. Although each of these observations could serve as a starting point for a detailed discussion of some specific aspect of medieval child care, we will confine our remarks to the concept of an index of effort as a way of measuring parental concern for their children.

There are many ways of measuring the efforts which parents undertake to obtain care for their sick children. This method of judging parental concern has the advantage that it is based upon parental behavior, not verbal expressions of concern. It is true that parental solicitude may have been motivated by other than love for the child, concerns such as dynastic survival, formation of political alliances through marriage, and shortage of labor. The divining of parental motivation, however, is problematic in all cultures and is beyond the scope of this paper. Therefore we are proposing that an index of effort based upon manifest behavior can serve as a heuristic tool for an examination of early medieval child care.

The first thing to note is that there are direct and indirect costs to be tallied in an index of effort. Direct costs are theoretically measurable, if sufficient information is available. Direct costs could be calculated in money, goods, land, and labor or loss of labor. A gift of money (gold or silver) may be promised or given in return for a cure, or resources may be expended directly in bringing a child to a shrine. Similarly, a donation of goods (candle wax, linen, hides, grain, cattle, iron or other metals) or land may be made in return for a cure. A more difficult computation would involve the costs of transporting a sick child to a distant shrine. Thus even a journey to a shrine 50 or 60 kilometers away (a long trip to strange territory, by medieval standards) involves a minimum of a week's travel for the round trip calculated on a rate of ox cart travel at best of less than 20 kilometers per day (Leighton, 1970); to this must be added the cost of fodder for the oxen and food for the humans, the cost of labor in removing oxen from the field, the loss of the human labor of those who accompany the cart carrying the child, all multiplied by the number of additional days spent at the shrine or church. There were also risks of robbery and death while on the journey, as well as the risks of leaving the home a little less protected and secure. In addition, anxiety about travel was always present.

Indirect costs are obviously more difficult to calculate, but infinitely more interesting, since they primarily involve important shifts in a person's personal, social, and political relationships. For example, a local magnate, especially one who has been hostile to local ecclesiastics and missionaries, would incur obligations involving matters of status and prestige by obtaining help for his children from a saint. In Walafrid's 9th century *Life of St. Gall* (1927), Duke Gunzo sided with his subjects when they resumed their pagan worship and complained to him that St. Gall had destroyed their idols and interfered with their hunting. Gunzo ordered Gall to depart from his territory and did not punish the villagers when they murdered two of the missionary's monks. Then, however, Duke Gunzo's only daughter, Fridiburga, became ill and "was possessed by an evil spirit which tormented her in many ways, so that she remained almost wholly without food and would often roll on the ground, foaming at the mouth and in such a dire frenzy that four men could scarcely hold her with all their efforts" (Chapter 15). Two bishops arrive to find the girl in a violent frenzy and her parents, kinfolk and the entire household weeping over her and weighed down with grief. The bishops begin their prayers, but Fridiburga breaks free from the hands holding her, snatches a sword, and tries to kill the bishops.

Duke Gunzo then sent his men to fetch St. Gall for help. The holy man, still offended at the shabby treatment he had previously received from the Duke, refused to come. Finally after much negotiation, Gall agreed to help and set out on the journey. On the way, he receives a message from the Duke, urging him to come more quickly, for the girl has now been 3 days without food. When Gall arrived, he found the sick girl "lying in her mother's lap, with closed eyes, gaping mouth and limbs relaxed, like one already dead" (Chapter 18). The holy man exorcised the demon and brought the girl back to health.

As a result of this process, Duke Gunzo was publicly obligated to St. Gall. Personal obligations incurred in such a manner could not be ignored, but were essential components of the formal social structure of early medieval Europe, a matter of honor. Duke Gunzo had to accept Gall and his monks in his territory. He had to protect Gall and his monks. He had to reverse his previous policies toward Gall and the monastic settlement. He had to risk alienating his own pagan subjects. All of these concessions by the Duke are to be considered the price he paid for the cure of his daughter. This is certainly tangible evidence of Gunzo's concern for his child, and a girl child at that, who are often characterized by scholars as having very limited value in medieval society (Bullough and Campbell, 1980; Coleman, 1976; Herlihy, 1975). We would of course undermine our own methodological arguments were we to claim that this anecdote could provide the basis for a sweeping generalization about the great value of little girls, or even little noble girls in early medieval Europe. However, we offer this episode merely as an illustration of behavior that is supported by the quantitative evidence we have developed.

Another form of a combined direct and indirect cost is the promise by the parents of a sick child to give the child to the church if the saint will heal the child. That this promise is not a subterfuge by which parents unload a sickly child onto the monastery is clearly seen in those cases in which the parents break their promise once the child is healed. The parents manifestly have other plans for their offspring and quickly ignore the rash offer they made under the duress of trying to save their child's life. From our evidence, it is clear that families of the "middle class" and petty nobility are seen to object more frequently than one might expect to their children entering church or monastic service. We are informed about cases of broken promises because the child is reported to relapse, or some other calamity, such as the death of the father who broke his oath, results (Bernard of Clairvaux, 1978).

CONCLUSIONS

In the working out of the complex relationships between secular and religious interests in the early Middle Ages, assuring the health and well-being of children was one of the important services that the church had to offer. There is often evidence that secular remedies were tried first, and when these were unsuccessful, as we know they were in the face of infantile diarrhea, plague, abscesses, wound infections, neurologic diseases, and other childhood ailments, then the intervention of God was sought, most often in the person of a local holy man or woman or a local shrine with putatively potent relics. Brown (1981) commented on the "medical pluralism" of late antique-early medieval society and the tight bond of personal obligation that one incurred in shifting from a relatively impersonal medical system to seek healing from a holy person or shrine. A rough estimate of parental valuation and concern for a child can be obtained by examining the persistence with which parents sought help for the sick child and the costs which they bore in this endeavor.

Some observations can now be made about the history of child abuse and infanticide in pre-Crusade Europe. First, we are not suggesting that child abuse and infanticide did not occur in the Middle Ages. We are stating unequivocally, however, that the evidence for child abuse and infanticide being widespread phenomena, by any reasonable understanding of such phraseology, is utterly lacking. We further suggest that the evidence is lacking for such heinous behavior *not* because there is no evidence about the care and concern for children. We have demonstrated that there is rich source material about children. The argument that the absence of evidence for child abuse and infanticide reflects a conspiracy of silence which only proves child abuse was widespread may be sufficient for conspiracy buffs, but cannot be entertained by serious historians. Generalizations about the universality of violence against children unfortunately assume as fact the very premise that requires demonstration, namely, that *all* societies have, on a large scale, gravely abused their children.

We have provided evidence which is more than anecdotal in nature that parents in pre-Crusade Europe regularly expended substantial efforts and resources to secure the health and well-being even of sick and damaged children. These putatively less valuable members of society, one might conclude, should have been the primary targets for abuse and destruction if early medieval society truly was inclined toward such ends. Whether parents of the early Middle Ages were more concerned about their children than were parents of ancient Greece and Rome, the later Middle Ages, or early modern industrial society remains to be examined. If the abuse of children in the United States is as widespread as some would argue (*National Study,* 1981), then we must consider entertaining the possibility that Western civilization may indeed have regressed rather than progressed since the Dark Ages.

REFERENCES

Anonymous (1973), *Liber Historiae Francorum.* (Ed. and trans. B. Bachrach.) Lawrence, Kan.: Coronado Press.

Aries, P. (1962), *Centuries of Childhood.* New York: Random House.

Arnold, K. (1980), *Kind und Gesellschaft in Mittelalter und Renaissance.* Paderborn: Schoenengh.

Bakan, D. (1971), *Slaughter of the Innocents.* San Francisco: Jossey-Bass.

Bede (c.672-735 A.D.), *A History of the English Church and People.* Harmondsworth: Penguin Books, 1974.

Bernard of Clairvaux (1978), *The Life and Death of Saint Malachy the Irishman.* Kalamazoo, Mich.: Cistercian Publications, Chapter 23.

Brown, P. (1981), *The Cult of the Saints.* Chicago: University of Chicago Press, pp. 112-120.

Bullough, V. & Campbell, C. (1980), Female longevity and diet in the Middle Ages. *Speculum,* 50:317-325.

Coleman, E. (1976), Infanticide in the early Middle Ages. In: *Women in Medieval Society,* ed. S. M. Stuard. Philadelphia: University of Pennsylvania Press, pp. 47-70.

Demaitre, L. (1977), The idea of childhood and child care in medical writings of the Middle Ages. *J. Psychohist.,* 4:461-490.

DeMause, L. (1974), The evolution of childhood. In: *The History of Childhood,* ed. L. DeMause. New York: Harper & Row.

DeVries, M.W. (1984), Temperament and infant mortality among the Masai of East Africa. *Amer. J. Psychiat.,* 141:1189-1194.

Dickeman, M. (1975), Infanticide and demographic consequences. *Ann. Rev. Ecol. Systemat.,* 6:107-137.

Ende, A. (1983), Children in history: a personal review of the past decade's published research. *J. Psychohist.,* 11:65-88.

Forsythe, I. H. (1976), Children in early medieval art: ninth through twelfth centuries. *J. Psychohist.,* 4:31-70.

Genicot, L. (1964), On the evidence of growth of population in the west. In: *Change in Medieval Society,* ed. S. Thrupp. New York: Appleton, pp. 14-39.

Heins, M. (1984), The "battered child" revisited. *J. Amer. Med. Assn.,* 251:3295-3300.

Herlihy, D. (1975), Life expectations for women in medieval society. In: *The Role of Women in the Middle Ages,* ed. R.T. Morewedge, Albany NY.: State Univerisity of New York Press.

————— (1978), Medieval children. In: *Essays on Medieval Civilization,* ed. B.K. Lackner & K.R. Philip. Austin, Tex.: University of Texas Press.

Hollingsworth, T.H. (1969), *Historical Demography.* London: The Sources of History.

Isidorus of Seville (d. 636 A.D.), *The Medical Writings* (transl. W.D. Sharpe). *Trans. Amer. Philos. Soc.* (New Series), 54:1-75, 1964.

Kelley, F. & Snedden, W. (1960), Prevalence and geographic distribution of goitre. In: *Endemic Goitre.* Geneva: WHO.

Kellum, B. (1974), Infanticide in England in the later Middle Ages. *Hist. Childhood Q.,* 1:367-388.

Kempe, C.H., Silverman, F. N., Steele, B.F., et al. (1962), The battered-child syndrome. *J. Amer. Med. Assn.,* 181:17-24.

Krause, J. (1957), The medieval household: large or small? *Econ. Hist. Rev.* (Series 2), 9:420–432.

Kroll, J. (1977), The concept of childhood in the Middle Ages. *J. Hist. Behav. Sci.,* 13:384–393.

———— & Bachrach, B. (1984), Sin and mental illness in early medieval Europe. *Psychol. Med.,* 14:507–514.

Leighton, A.C. (1970), *Transport and Communications in Early Medieval Europe, A.D. 500–1000.* New York: Barnes & Nobel.

Les miracles de Saint Benoit (1853), ed. E. deCertain. Paris: Jules Renouard.

McLaughlin, M.M. (1974), Survivors and surrogates: child and parents from the ninth to the thirteenth centuries. In: *The History of Childhood,* ed. L. DeMause. New York: Harper & Row.

National Study of the Incidence and Severity of Child Abuse and Neglect (1981), DHHS Publication Number 81-30325. Washington, D.C.: Department of Health and Human Services.

Robin, M. (1981), Sheltering arms: the roots of child protection. In: *Child Abuse,* ed. E.H. Newberger. Boston: Little Brown, pp. 1–21.

Russell, J.C. (1958), *Late Ancient and Medieval Population.* Philadelphia: American Philosophical Society.

———— (1965), Recent advances in medieval demography. *Speculum,* 40:84–101.

Smith, S.M. (1975), *The Battered Child Syndrome.* London: Butterworths.

Solomon, T. (1973), History and demography of child abuse. *Pediatrics,* 51:773–776.

Titow, J.Z. (1961), Some evidence of the thirteenth century population increase. *Econ. Hist. Rev.* (Series 2), 14:218–224.

Walafrid Strabo (807–849 A.D.), *Life of St. Gall.* London: Society for Promoting Christian Knowledge, 1927.

WHO (1973), *Statistics Report,* Volume 26. Geneva: World Health Organization.

32

Impact of Child Sexual Abuse: A Review of the Research

Angela Browne and David Finkelhor
University of New Hampshire, Durham

This article reviews studies that have tried to confirm empirically the effects of child sexual abuse cited in the clinical literature. In regard to initial effects, empirical studies have indicated reactions—in at least some portion of the victim population—of fear, anxiety, depression, anger and hostility, aggression, and sexually inappropriate behavior, anxiety, feelings of isolation and stigma, poor self-esteem, difficulty in trusting others, a tendency toward revictimization, substance abuse, and sexual maladjustment. The kinds of abuse that appear to be most damaging, according to the empirical studies, are experiences involving father figures, genital contact, and force. The controversy over the impact of child sexual abuse is discussed, and recommendations for future research efforts are suggested.

Although clinical literature suggests that sexual abuse during childhood plays a role in the development of other problems ranging from

Reprinted with permission from *Psychological Bulletin,* 1986, Vol. 99, No. 1, 66–77. Copyright 1986 by the American Psychological Association, Inc.

This research was supported by National Institute of Mental Health Grant (MH15161), National Center for Child Abuse and Neglect Grant 90CA 0936/01, and the Eden Hall Farm Foundation.

The authors would like to thank the following people for their assistance and comments during the preparation of this article: Christopher Bagley, Larry Baron, John Briere, Jean Ellison, William Friedrich, Mary Ellen Fromuth, Linda Gott, Judith Herman, Karin Meiselman, Diana Russell, and the members of the Family Violence Research Seminar. This article is one of a series on child sexual abuse and family violence published by the Family Violence Research Program at the University of New Hampshire.

anorexia nervosa to prostitution, empirical evidence about its actual effects is sparse. In this article we review the expanding empirical literature on the effects of child sexual abuse, discuss its initial and long-term effects, review studies on the impact of different kinds of abuse, and conclude with a critique of the current literature and some suggestions for future research.

Child sexual abuse consists of two overlapping but distinguishable types of interaction: (a) forced or coerced sexual behavior imposed on a child, and (b) sexual activity between a child and a much older person, whether or not obvious coercion is involved (a common definition of "much older" is 5 or more years). As might be expected, not all studies relevant to our purposes share these parameters. Some have focused on experiences with older partners only, excluding coerced sexual experiences with peers. Others have looked only at sexual abuse that was perpetrated by family members. Such differences in samples make comparisons among these studies difficult. However, we include all the studies that looked at some portion of the range of experiences that are bounded by these two criteria. (See Table 1 for a breakdown of sample composition of the studies reviewed.)

Two areas of the literature are not included in our review. A small number of studies on the effects of incest (e.g., Farrell, 1982; Nelson, 1981), as well as one review of the effects of child sexual experiences (Constantine, 1980), combine data on consensual, peer experiences with data that involve either coercion or age disparity. Because we were unable to isolate sexual abuse in these studies, we had to exclude them. Secondly, we decided to limit our review to female victims. Few clinical, and even fewer empirical, studies have been done on male victims (for exceptions, see Finkelhor, 1979; Rogers & Terry, 1984; Sandfort, 1981; Woods & Dean, 1984), and it seems premature to draw conclusions at this point.* Under "empirical" studies, we include any research that attempted to quantify the extent to which a sequelae to sexual abuse appeared in a specific population. Some of these studies used objective measures, whereas others were based primarily on the judgments of clinicians.

---

*The whole literature on sexual abuse poses problems for differentiating according to gender of victims. As Table 1 shows, many studies contain a small number of men included in a larger sample of women. Unfortunately, many of these studies do not specifically mention which effects apply to men, so it is possible that some of the sequelae described apply only to the men. However, we believe that most of the sequelae described relate primarily to women.

Table 1. Studies of Effects of Sexual Abuse

Study	Source of sample	N	Gender	Age of respondents	Focus of study	Comparison group
Anderson, Bach, & Griffith, 1981	Sexual assault center	227	F = 155 M = 72	Ad	I, E	No
Bagley & Ramsay, 1985	Random sample	679	F = 401 M = 278	A	I, E	Yes
Benward & Densen-Gerber, 1975	Drug treatment center	118	F = 118	Ad, A	I	No
Briere, 1984	Community health center	153	F = 153	A	I, E	Yes
Briere & Runtz, 1985	College students	278	F = 278	Ad, A	I, E	Yes
Courtois, 1979	Ads and mental health agencies	31	F = 31	A	I	No
DeFrancis, 1969	Court cases	250	F = 217 M = 33	C, Ad	I, E	No
DeYoung, 1982	College students, therapy patients, and others	80	F = 72 M = 8	C, Ad, A	I	No
Fields, 1981	Prostitutes recruited after arrest	85	F = 85	A	I	Yes
Finkelhor, 1979	College students	796	F = 530 M = 266	Ad, A	I, E	Yes
Friedrich, Urquiza, & Beilke, (in press)	Sexual assault center, group therapy	64	F = 49 M = 15	C	I, E	No
Fromuth, 1983	College students	482	F = 482	Ad, A	I, E	Yes
Harrison, Lumry, & Claypatch, 1984	Dual disorder treatment program	62	F = 62	A	I, E	Yes
Herman, 1981	Clients in therapy	60	F = 60	Ad, A	I	Yes

(continued)

Table 1. *(Continued)*

Study	Source of sample	N	Gender	Age of respondents	Focus of study	Comparison group
James & Meyerding, 1977	Prostitutes selected from arrest records					
Study 1		92	F = 92	Ad, A	I, E	No
Study 2		136	F = 136	A	I, E	No
Landis, 1956	College students	950	F = 726 M = 224	A	I, E	Yes
Langmade, 1983	Mental health centers, private clinics	68	F = 68	A	I	Yes
Meiselman, 1978	Clinical records, psychiatric clinic	108	F = 97 M = 11	C, Ad, A	I	Yes
Peters, J., 1976	Rape crisis center	100	—	C	I	No
Peters, S., 1984	Follow-up, community random sample	119	F = 119	A	I, E	Yes
Russell, in press	Random sample	930	F = 930	A	I, E	Yes
Sedney & Brooks, 1984	College students	301	F = 301	Ad, A	I, E	Yes
Seidner & Calhoun, 1984	College students	152	F = 118 M = 34	A	I, E	Yes
Silbert & Pines, 1981	Prostitutes recruited by ads	200	F = 200	Ad, A	I, E	No
Tsai, Feldman-Summers, & Edgar, 1979	Ads	90	F = 90	A	I, E	Yes
Tufts study, 1984	Clinical referrals	156	F = 122 M = 34	C, Ad	I, E	No

Note. F = female and M = male. C = child, Ad = adolescent, and A = adult. I = intrafamilial and E = extrafamilial.

INITIAL EFFECTS

By initial effects, we mean those reactions occurring within 2 years of the termination of abuse. These early reactions are often called *short-term* effects in the literature. We prefer the term *initial* effects, however, because "short-term" implies that the reactions do not persist—an assumption that has yet to be substantiated.

Emotional Reactions and Self-Perceptions

Although several empirical studies have given support to clinical observations of generally negative emotional effects resulting from childhood sexual abuse, only two used standardized measures and compared subjects' scores to general population norms. In an early study of the effects of sexual abuse on children, DeFrancis (1969) reported that 66% of the victims were emotionally disturbed by the molestation: 52% mildly to moderately disturbed, and 14% seriously disturbed. Only 24% were judged to be emotionally stable after the abuse. However, because this sample was drawn from court cases known to Prevention of Cruelty to Children services or to the police, and because the subjects came primarily from low income and multiple-problem families who were on public assistance, these findings may have little generalizability.

In investigating a different type of special population, Anderson, Bach, and Griffith (1981) reviewed clinical charts of 155 female adolescent sexual assault victims who had been treated at the Harborview Medical Center in Washington and reported psychosocial complications in 63% of them. Reports of "internalized psychosocial sequelae" (e.g., sleep and eating disturbances, fears and phobias, depression, guilt, shame, and anger) were noted in 67% of female victims when the abuse was intrafamilial and 49% when the offender was not a family member. "Externalized sequelae" (including school problems and running away) were noted in 66% of intrafamilial victims and 21% of extrafamilial victims. However, no standardized outcome measures were used, so the judgments of these effects may be subjective.

In what is probably the best study to date, researchers affiliated with the Division of Child Psychiatry at the Tufts New England Medical Center gathered data on families involved in a treatment program restricted to those children who had been victimized or revealed their victimization in the prior 6 months. Standardized self-report measures—the Louisville Behavior Checklist (LBC), the Piers-Harris Self-Concept Scale, the Purdue Self-Concept Scale, and the Gottschalk Glesser Content Analysis

Scales (GGCA)—with published norms and test validation data were used, so that characteristics of sexually abused children could be contrasted with norms for general and psychiatric populations. Subjects ranged in age from infancy to 18 years and were divided into preschool, latency, and adolescence age groups. Data were gathered on four areas: overt behavior, somaticized reactions, internalized emotional states, and self-esteem.

In evaluating the initial psychological effects of child sexual abuse, Tufts (1984) researchers found differences in the amount of pathology reported for different age groups. Seventeen percent of 4- to 6-year-olds in the study met the criteria for "clinically significant pathology," demonstrating more overall disturbance than a normal population but less than the norms for other children their age who were in psychiatric care. The highest incidence of psychopathology was found in the 7- to 13-year-old age group, with 40% scoring in the seriously disturbed range. Interestingly, few of the adolescent victims exhibited severe psychopathology, except on a measure of neuroticism.

Friedrich, Urquiza, and Beilke (in press) also used a standardized measure in their study of 61 sexually abused girls. Subjects were referred by a local sexual assault center for evaluation or by the outpatient department of a local hospital. Children in this sample had been abused within a 24-month period prior to the study. Using the Child Behavior Check List (CBCL; see Achenbach & Edelbrock, 1983, for a description of this measure), Friedrich et al. reported that 46% of their subjects had significantly elevated scores on its Internalizing scale (including fearful, inhibited, depressed, and overcontrolled behaviors) and 39% had elevated scores on its Externalizing scale (aggressive, antisocial, and undercontrolled behaviors). This was compared with only 2% of the normative sample who would be expected to score in this range. Younger children (up to age 5) demonstrated a tendency to score high on the Internalizing scale, whereas older children (ages 6–12) were more likely to have elevated scores on the Externalizing scale.

Breaking down emotional impact into specific reactions, we find that the most common initial effect noted in empirical studies, similar to reports in the clinical literature, is that of fear. However, exact proportions vary from a high of 83% reported by DeFrancis (1969) to 40% reported by Anderson et al. (1981). Because of its use of standardized measures, we would give the most credence to the Tufts (1984) study, which found that 45% of the 7- to 13-year-olds manifested severe fears as measured by the LBCs, compared with 13% of the 4- to 6-year-olds. On the adolescent version of the LBC, 36% of the 14- to 18-year-olds had elevated scores on "ambivalent hostility," or the fear of being harmed.

Another initial effect in children is reactions of anger and hostility. Tufts (1984) researchers found that 45% to 50% of the 7- to 13-year-olds showed hostility levels that were substantially elevated on measures of aggression and antisocial behavior (LBC), as did 35% on the measure of hostility directed outward (GGCA). Thirteen percent to 17% of 4- to 6-year-olds scored above the norms on aggression and antisocial behavior (LBC), whereas 25% of 4- to 6-year-olds and 23% of the adolescents had elevated scores on hostility directed outward (GGCA). In his study of court cases, DeFrancis (1969) noted that 55% of the children showed behavioral disturbances such as active defiance, disruptive behavior within the family, and quarreling or fighting with siblings or classmates. DeFrancis' sample might have been thought to overselect for hostile reactions; however, these findings are not very different from findings of the Tufts study for school-age children.

Guilt and shame are other frequently observed reactions to child sexual abuse, but few studies give clear percentages. DeFrancis (1969) observed that 64% of his sample expressed guilt, although this was more about the problems created by disclosure than about the molestation itself. Anderson et al. (1981) reported guilt reactions in 25% of the victims. Similarly, depression is frequently reported in the clinical literature, but here too, specific figures are rarely given. Anderson et al. (1981) found that 25% of female sexual assault victims were depressed after the abuse.

Sexual abuse is also cited as having an effect on self-esteem, but this effect has not yet been established by empirical studies. Fifty-eight percent of the victims in the DeFrancis (1969) study expressed feelings of inferiority or lack of worth as a result of having been victimized. However in a surprising finding, Tufts (1984) researchers, using the Purdue Self-Concept Scale, found no evidence that sexually abused children in any of the age groups had consistently lower self-esteem than a normal population of children.

Physical Consequences and Somatic Complaints

Physical symptoms indicative of anxiety and distress are noted in the empirical literature as well as in clinical reports. In their chart review of female adolescent victims, Anderson et al. (1981) found that 17% had experienced sleep disturbances and 5%–7% showed changes in eating habits after the victimization. J. Peters (1976), in a study of child victims of intrafamilial sexual abuse, reported that 31% had difficulty sleeping and 20% experienced eating disturbances. However, without a comparison group, it is hard to know if this is seriously pathological for any group of children, or for clinical populations in particular. Adolescent pregnancy is another physical consequence sometimes mentioned in empirical literature. DeFrancis (1969) reported that 11% of the child victims in his study became pregnant as a result of the sexual offense; however, this figure seems far too high for a contemporary sample. Meiselman (1978), in analyzing records from a Los Angeles psychiatric clinic, found only 1 out of 47 incest cases in which a victim was impregnated by her father.

Effects of Sexuality

Reactions of inappropriate sexual behavior in child victims have been confirmed by two studies using standardized measures (Friedrich et al., in press; Tufts, 1984). In the Tufts (1984) study, 27% of 4- to 6-year-old children scored significantly above clinical and general population norms on a sexual behavior scale that included having had sexual relations (possibly a confounding variable in these findings), open masturbation, excessive sexual curiosity, and frequent exposure of the genitals. Thirty-six percent of the 7- to 13-year-olds also demonstrated high levels of disturbance on the sexual behavior measure when contrasted to norms for either general or clinical school-age populations. Similarly, Friedrich et al. (in press), using the CBCL to evaluate 3- to 12-year-olds, found that 70% of the boys and 44% of the girls scored at least one standard deviation above a normal population of that age group on the scale measuring sexual problems. Interestingly, sexual problems were most common among the younger girls and the older boys.

Effects on Social Functioning

Other aftereffects of child sexual abuse mentioned in the literature include difficulties at school, truancy, running away from home, and early marriages by adolescent victims. Herman (1981) interviewed 40 patients in therapy who had been victims of father-daughter incest, and compared their reports with those from a group of 20 therapy clients with seductive, but not incestuous, fathers. Of the incest victims, 33% attempted to run away as adolescents, compared with 5% of the comparison group. Similarly, Meiselman (1978) found that 50% of the incest victims in her sample had left home before the age of 18, compared with 20% of women in a comparison group of nonvictimized female patients. Younger children often went to a relative, whereas older daughters ran away or eloped, sometimes making early marriages in order to escape the abuse. Two studies, neither with comparison groups, mentioned school problems and truancy. Ten percent of the child victims in J. Peters's (1976) study quit school, although all of his subjects were under the age of 12 at the time. Anderson et al. found that 20% of the girls in their sample experienced problems at school, including truancy or dropping out.

A connection between sexual abuse, running away, and delinquency is also suggested by several studies of children in special treatment or delinquency programs. Reich and Gutierres (1979) reported that 55% of the children in Maricopa County, Arizona who were charged with running away, truancy, or listed as missing persons were incest victims. In addition, in a study of female juvenile offenders in Wisconsin (1982), researchers found that 32% had been sexually abused by a relative or other person close to them.

Summary of Initial Effects of Child Sexual Abuse

The empirical literature on child sexual abuse, then, does suggest the presence—in some portion of the victim population—of many of the initial effects reported in the clinical literature, especially reactions of fear, anxiety, depression, anger and hostility, and inappropriate sexual behavior. However, because many of the studies lacked standardized outcome measures and adequate comparison groups, it is not clear that these findings reflect the experience of all child victims of sexual abuse or are even representative of those children currently being seen in clinical settings. At this point, the empirical literature on the initial effects of child sexual abuse would have to be considered sketchy.

LONG-TERM EFFECTS

Emotional Reactions and Self-Perceptions

In the clinical literature, depression is the symptom most commonly reported among adults molested as children, and empirical findings seem to confirm this. Two excellent community studies are indicative of this. Bagley and Ramsay (1985), in a community mental health study in Calgary utilizing a random sample of 387 women, found that subjects with a history of child sexual abuse scored more depressed on the Centre for Environmental Studies Depression Scale (CES-D) than did nonabused women (17% vs. 9% with clinical symptoms of depression in the last week), as well as on the Middlesex Hospital Questionnaire's measure of depression (15% vs. 7%). S. Peters (1984), in a community study in Los Angeles also based on a random sample, interviewed 119 women and found that sexual abuse in which there was physical contact was associated with a higher incidence of depression and a greater number of depressive episodes over time, and that women who had been sexually abused were more likely to have been hospitalized for depression than nonvictims. In a multiple regression that included both sexual abuse and family background factors (e.g., a poor relationship with the mother), the variable of child sexual abuse made an independent contribution to depression.

The link between child sexual abuse and depression has been confirmed in other nonclinical samples as well. Sedney and Brooks (1984), in a study of 301 college women, found a greater likelihood for subjects with childhood sexual experiences to report symptoms of depression (65% vs. 43% of the control group) and to have been hospitalized for it (18% of those depressed in the childhood experience group vs. 4% of women in the control group). These positive findings are surprising, in that the researchers used an overly inclusive definition of sexual experiences that may not have screened out some consensual experiences with peers. Their results are consistent, however, with those from a carefully controlled survey of 278 undergraduate women by Briere and Runtz (1985) using 72 items of the Hopkins Symptom Checklist, which indicated that sexual abuse victims reported that they experienced more depressive symptoms during the 12 months prior to the study than did nonabused subjects.

Studies based on clinical samples (Herman, 1981; Meiselman, 1978) have not shown such clear differences in depression between victims and nonvictims. For example, although Herman (1981) noted major depressive symptoms in 60% of the incest victims in her study, 55% of the comparison group also reported depression. Meiselman (1978) reported depressive symptoms in 35% of the incest victims whose psychiatric records she reviewed, compared with 23% of the comparison group; again, this difference was not significant.

Both clinical and nonclinical samples have shown victims of child sexual abuse to be more self-destructive, however. In an extensive study of 153 "walk-ins" to a community health counseling center, Briere (1984) reported that 51% of the sexual abuse victims, versus 34% of nonabused clients, had a history of suicide attempts. Thirty-one percent of victims, compared with 19% of nonabused clients, exhibited a desire to hurt themselves. A high incidence of suicide attempts among victims of child sexual abuse has been found by other clinical researchers as well (e.g., Harrison, Lumry, & Claypatch, 1984; Herman, 1981). Bagley and Ramsay (1985), in their community study, noted an association between childhood sexual abuse and suicide ideation or deliberate attempts at self-harm. And Sedney and Brooks (1984) found that 39% of their college student sample with child sexual experiences reported having thoughts of hurting themselves, compared with 16% of the control group. Sixteen percent of these respondents had made at least one suicide attempt (vs. 6% of their peers).

Another reaction observed in adults who were sexually victimized as children is symptoms of anxiety or tension. Briere (1984) reported that 54% of the sexual abuse victims in his clinical sample experienced anxiety attacks (compared with 28% of the nonvictims), 54% reported nightmares (vs. 23%), and 72% had difficulty sleeping (compared with 55% of the nonvictims). In their college sample, Sedney and Brooks (1984) found 59% with symptoms indicating nervousness and anxiety (compared with 41% of the controls); 41% indicated extreme tension (vs. 29% of the controls), and 51% had trouble sleeping (compared with 29% of the controls). These findings are supported by results from community samples, with Bagley and Ramsay (1985) noting that 19% of their subjects who had experienced child sexual abuse reported symptoms indicating somatic anxiety on the Middlesex Hospital Questionnaire, compared with 9% of the nonabused subjects.

The idea that sexual abuse victims continue to feel isolated and stigmatized as adults also has some support in the empirical literature, although these findings come only from the clinical populations. Sixty-four percent of the victimized women in Briere's (1984) study reported feelings of isolation, compared with 49% of the controls. With incest victims, the figures are even higher: Herman (1981) reported that all of the women who had experienced father-daughter incest in her clinical sample had a sense of being branded, marked, or stigmatized by the victimization. Even in a community sample of incest victims, Courtois (1979) found that 73% reported they still suffered from moderate to severe feelings of isolation and alienation.

Although a negative self-concept was not confirmed as an initial effect, evidence for it as long-term effect is much stronger. Bagley and Ramsay (1985) found that 19% of the child sexual abuse victims in their random sample scored in the "very poor" category on the Coopersmith self-esteem inventory (vs. 5% of the control group), whereas only 9% of the victims demonstrated "very good" levels of self-esteem (compared with 20%

of the controls). Women with very poor self-esteem were nearly four times as likely to report a history of child sexual abuse as were the other subjects. As might be expected, self-esteem problems among clinical samples of incest victims tended to be much greater: Eighty-seven percent of Courtois's (1979) community sample reported that their sense of self had been moderately to severely affected by the experience of sexual abuse from a family member. Similarly, Herman (1981) found that 60% of the incest victims in her clinical sample were reported to have a "predominantly negative self-image," as compared with 10% of the comparison group with seductive but not incestuous fathers.

Impact on Interpersonal Relating

Women who have been sexually victimized as children report problems in relating both to women and men, continuing problems with their parents, and difficulty in parenting and responding to their own children. In DeYoung's (1982) sample, 79% of the incest victims had predominantly hostile feelings toward their mothers, whereas 52% were hostile toward the abuser. Meiselman (1978) found that 60% of the incest victims in her psychotherapy sample disliked their mothers and 40% continued to experience strong negative feelings toward their fathers. Herman (1981) also noted that the rage of incest victims in her sample was often directed toward the mother and observed that they seemed to regard all women, including themselves, with contempt.

In addition, victims reported difficulty trusting others that included reactions of fear, hostility, and a sense of betrayal. Briere (1984) noted fear of men in 48% of his clinical subjects (vs. 15% of the nonvictims), and fear of women in 12% (vs. 4% of those who had not been sexually victimized). Incest victims seem especially likely to experience difficulty in close relationships: Sixty-four percent of the victims in Meiselman's (1978) clinical study, compared with 40% of the control group, complained of conflict with or fear of their husbands or sex partners, and 39% of the sample had never married. These results are supported by findings from Courtois's (1979) sample, in which 79% of the incest victims experienced moderate or severe problems in relating to men, and 40% had never married.

There is at least one empirical study that lends support to the idea that childhood sexual abuse also affects later parenting. Goodwin, McCarthy, and Divasto (1981) found that 24% of mothers in the child abusing families they studied reported incest experiences in their childhoods, compared with 3% of a nonabusive control group. They suggested that difficulty in parenting results when closeness and affection is endowed with a sexual meaning, and observed that these mothers maintained an emotional and physical distance from their children, thus potentially setting the stage for abuse.

Another effect on which the empirical literature agrees is the apparent vulnerability of women who have been sexually abused as children to be revictimized later in life. Russell (in press), in her probability sample of 930 women, found that between 33% and 68% of the sexual abuse victims (depending on the seriousness of the abuse they suffered) were raped later on, compared with 17% of women who were not childhood victims. Fromuth (1983), in surveying 482 female college students, found evidence that women who had been sexually abused before the age of 13 were especially likely to later become victims of nonconsensual sexual experiences. Further evidence of a tendency toward revictimization comes from a study conducted at the University of New Mexico School of Medicine on 341 sexual assault admittances (Miller et al., 1978). In comparing women who had been raped on more than one occasion with those who were reporting a first-time rape, researchers found that 18% of the repeat victims had incest histories, compared with only 4% of first-time victims.

In addition to rape, victims of child sexual abuse also seem more likely to be abused later by husbands or other adult partners. Russell (in press) found that between 38% and 48% of the child sexual abuse victims in her community sample had physically violent husbands, compared with 17% of women who were not victims; in addition, between 40% and 62% of the abused women had later been sexually assaulted by their husbands, compared with 21% of nonvictims. Similarly, Briere (1984) noted that 49% of his clinical sexual abuse sample reported being battered in adult relationships, compared with 18% of the nonvictim group.

Effects on Sexuality

One of the areas receiving the most attention in the empirical literature on long-term effects concerns the impact of early sexual abuse on later sexual functioning. Almost all clinically based studies show later sexual problems among child sexual abuse victims, particularly among the victims of incest. However, there have not yet been community-based studies on the sexual functioning of adults molested as children, as there have been of other mental health areas such as depression.

Of the clinical studies, Meiselman (1978) found the highest percentage of incest victims reporting problems with sexual adjustment. Eighty-seven percent of her sample were classified as having had a serious problem with sexual adjustment at some time since the molestation, compared with 20% of the comparison group (women who had been in therapy at the same clinic, but had not been sexually victimized as children). Results from Herman's (1981) study are somewhat less extreme: Fifty-five percent of the incest victims reported later sexual problems, although they were not significantly different from women with seductive fathers on this measure. Langmade (1983) compared a group of women in therapy who had been incest victims with a matched control group of nonvictimized women and found that the incest victims were more sexually anxious, experienced more sexual guilt, and reported greater dissatisfaction with their sexual relationships than the controls. In his study of walk-in sample to a community health clinic, Briere (1984) found that 45% of women who had been sexually abused as children reported difficulties with sexual adjustment as adults, compared with 15% of the control group. Briere also noted a decreased sex drive in 42% of the victims studied, versus 29% of the nonvictims.

Two nonclinical studies show effects on sexual functioning as well. Courtois noted that 80% of the former incest victims in her sample reported an inability to relax and enjoy sexual activity, avoidance of or abstention from sex, or, conversely, a compulsive desire for sex. Finkelhor (1979), studying college students, developed a measure of sexual self-esteem and found that child sexual abuse victims reported significantly lower levels of sexual self-esteem than their nonabused classmates. However, Fromuth (1983), in a similar study also with a college student sample, found no correlation between sexual abuse and sexual self-esteem, desire for intercourse, or students' self-ratings of their sexual adjustment. Virtually all (96%) of Fromuth's respondents were unmarried and their average age was 19, so it is possible that some of the long-term sexual adjustment problems reported by women in the clinical and community samples were not yet in evidence in this younger population. Still, this does not explain the discrepancy from the Finkelhor findings.

In another study, Tsai, Feldman-Summers, and Edgar (1979) compared three groups of women on sexual adjustment measures: sexual abuse victims seeking therapy, sexual abuse victims who considered themselves well-adjusted and had not sought therapy, and a nonvictimized matched control group. Results indicated that the "well-adjusted" victims were not significantly different from the control group on measures of overall and sexual adjustment, but the victims seeking therapy did show a difference. They experienced orgasm less often, reported themselves to be less sexually responsive, obtained less satisfaction from their sexual relationships, were less satisified with the quality of their close relationships with men, and reported a greater number of sexual partners. It is hard to know how to interpret findings from a group of victims solicited on the basis of feeling "well-adjusted." This seems far different from a comparison group of victims who were not in therapy, and thus these results are questionable.

A long-term effect of child sexual abuse that has also received a great deal of attention in the literature is an increased level of sexual behavior among victims, usually called promiscuity (e.g., Courtois, 1979; De-Young, 1982; Herman, 1981; Meiselman, 1978). Herman noted that 35% of the incest victims in her sample reported promiscuity and observed that some victims seemed to have a "repertoire of sexually stylized behavior" that they used as a way of getting affection and attention (p. 40). DeYoung (1982) reported that 28% of the victims in her sample had engaged in activities that could be considered promiscuous; Meiselman (1978) found 25%. However, in her study of 482 female college students, Fromuth (1983) found no differences in this variable and observed that having experienced child sexual abuse only predicted whether subjects would describe themselves as promiscuous, not their actual number of partners. This potentially very important finding suggests that the "promiscuity" of sexual abuse victims may be more a function of their negative self-attributions, already well documented in the empirical literature, than their actual sexual behavior; thus researchers should be careful to combine objective behavioral measures with this type of self-report.

Another question that has received comment but little empirical confirmation concerns the possibility that sexual abuse may be associated with later homosexuality in victims. Although one study of lesbians found molestation in their backgrounds (Gundlach, 1977), Bell and Weinberg (1981), in a large-scale, sophisticated study of the origin of sexual preference, found no such association. Studies from the sexual abuse literature have also found little connection (Finkelhor, 1984; Fromuth, 1983; Meiselman, 1978).

Effects on Social Functioning

Several studies of special populations suggest a connection between child sexual abuse and later prostitution. James and Meyerding (1977) interviewed 136 prostitutes and found that 55% had been sexually abused as children by someone 10 or more years older, prior to their first intercourse. Among adolescents in the sample, 65% had been forced into sexual activity before they were 16 years old. Similarly, Silbert and Pines (1981) found that 60% of the prostitutes they interviewed had been sexually abused before the age of 16 by an average of two people for an average of 20 months. (The mean age of these children at the time of their first victimization was 10.) They concluded that, "The evidence linking juvenile sexual abuse to prostitution is overwhelming" (p. 410). However, Fields (1981) noted that, although 45% of the prostitutes in her sample had been sexually abused as children, this did not differentiate them from a comparison group of nonprostitutes matched on age, race, and education, of which 37% had been abused. Although there was no difference in prevalence between the two groups, Fields did find that the prostitutes were sexually abused at a younger age—14.5 versus 16.5— and were more apt to have been physically forced.

An association between child sexual abuse and later substance abuse has also received empirical support. S. Peters (1984), in a carefully controlled community study, found that 17% of the victimized women had symptoms of alcohol abuse (vs. 4% of nonvictimized women), and 27% abused at least one type of drug (compared with 12% of nonvictimized women). Herman (1981) noted that 35% of the women in her clinical sample with incestuous fathers abused drugs and alcohol (vs. 5% of the women with seductive fathers). Similarly, Briere (1984), in his walk-in sample from a community health center, found that 27% of the childhood sexual abuse victims had a history of alcoholism (compared with 11% of nonvictims), and 21% had a history of drug addiction (vs. 2% of the nonvictims). College student samples appear more homogeneous: Sedney and Brooks (1984) found a surprisingly low reported incidence of substance abuse, and no significant differences between groups.

Summary of Long-Term Effects

Empirical studies with adults confirm many of the long-term effects of sexual abuse mentioned in the clinical literature. Adult women victimized as children are more likely to manifest depression, self-destructive behavior, anxiety, feelings of isolation and stigma, poor self-esteem, a tendency toward revictimization, and substance abuse. Difficulty in trusting others and sexual maladjustment in such areas as sexual dysphoria, sexual dysfunction, impaired sexual self-esteem, and avoidance of or abstention from sexual activity have also been reported by empirical researchers, although agreement between studies is less consistent for the variables on sexual functioning.

IMPACT OF SEXUAL ABUSE

In light of the studies just reviewed, it is appropriate to evaluate the persistent controversy over the impact of sexual abuse on victims. It has been the continuing view of some that sexual abuse is not traumatic or that its traumatic impact has been greatly overstated (Constantine, 1977; Henderson, 1983; Ramey, 1979). Proponents of this view contend that the evidence for trauma is meager and based on inadequate samples and unwarranted inferences. Because of the general lack of research in this field, clinicians have only recently been able to substantiate their impressions that sexual abuse is traumatic with evidence from strong scientific studies. However, as evidence now accumulates, it conveys a clear suggestion that sexual abuse is a serious mental health problem, consistently associated with very disturbing subsequent problems in some important portion of its victims.

Findings of long-term impact are especially persuasive. Eight nonclinical studies of adults (Bagley & Ramsay, 1985; Briere & Runtz, 1985; Finkelhor, 1979; Fromuth, 1983; S. Peters, 1984; Russell, in press; Sedney & Brooks, 1984; Seidner & Calhoun, 1984), including three random sample community surveys, found that child sexual abuse victims in the "normal" population had identifiable degrees of impairment when compared with nonvictims. Although impairments in these nonclinical victims are not necessarily severe, all the studies that have looked for long-term impairment have found it, with the exception of one (Tsai et al., 1979).

These findings are particularly noteworthy in that the studies were identifying differences associated with an event that occurred from 5 to 25 years previously. Moreover, all these studies used fairly broad definitions of sexual abuse that included single episodes, experiences in which no actual physical contact occurred, and experiences with individuals who were not related to or emotionally close to the subjects. In all four studies that used multivariate analyses (Bagley & Ramsay, 1985; Finkelhor, 1984; Fromuth, 1983; S. Peters, 1984), differences in the victimized group remained after a variety of background and other factors had been controlled. The implication of these studies is that a history of childhood sexual abuse is associated with greater risk for mental health and adjustment problems in adulthood.

Unfortunately, although the studies indicate higher risk, they are not so informative about the actual extent of impairment. In terms of simple self-assessments, 53% of intrafamilial sexual abuse victims in Russell's (in press) community survey reported that the experience resulted in "some" or "great" long-term effects on their lives. Assessments with standardized clinical measures show a more modest incidence of impairment: In Bagley & Ramsay's (1985) community survey, 17% of sexual abuse victims were clinically depressed as measured by the CES-D, and 18% were seriously psychoneurotic. Thus, most sexual abuse victims in the community, when evaluated in surveys, show up as slightly impaired or normal. It is possible, however, that some of the impairment associated with childhood molestation is not tapped by these survey evaluations.

Summarizing, then, from studies of clinical and nonclinical populations, the findings concerning the trauma of child sexual abuse appear to be as follows: In the immediate aftermath of sexual abuse, from one-fifth to two-fifths of abused children seen by clinicians manifest pathological disturbance (Tufts, 1984). When studied as adults, victims as a group demonstrate impairment when compared with their nonvictimized counterparts, but under one-fifth evidence serious psychopathology. These findings give reassurance to victims that extreme long-term effects are not inevitable. Nonetheless, they also suggest that the risk of initial and long-term mental health impairment for victims of child sexual abuse should be taken very seriously.

EFFECTS BY TYPE OF ABUSE

Although the foregoing sections have been concerned with the various effects of abuse, there are also important research questions concerning the effects of various kinds of abuse. These have usually appeared in the form of speculation about what types of abuse have the most serious impact on victims. Groth (1978), for example, on the basis of his clinical experience, contended that the greatest trauma occurs in sexual abuse that (a) continues for a longer period of time, (b) occurs with a more closely related person, (c) involves penetration, and (d) is accompanied by aggression. To that list, MacFarlane (1978) added experiences in which (e) the child participates to some degree, (f) the parents have an unsupportive reaction to disclosure of the abuse, and (g) the child is older and thus cognizant of the cultural taboos that have been violated. Such speculations offer fruitful directions for research. Unfortunately, however, only a few studies on the effects of sexual abuse have had enough cases and been sophisticated enough methodologically to look at these questions empirically. Furthermore, the studies addressing these issues have reached little consensus in their findings.

Duration and Frequency of Abuse

Although many clinicians take for granted that the longer an experience goes on, the more traumatic it is, this conclusion is not clearly supported by the available studies. Of nine studies, only four found duration associated with greater trauma. (We are treating duration and frequency synonymously here because they tend to be so highly correlated.) Three found no relation, and two even found some evidence that longer duration is associated with less trauma.

Russell's (in press) study reported the clearest association: In her survey of adult women, 73% of sexual abuse that lasted for more than 5 years was self-rated as extremely or considerably traumatic by the victims, compared with 62% of abuse lasting 1 week to 5 years and 46% of abuse occurring only once. Tsai et al. (1979) found duration and frequency associated with greater negative effects, when measured with the Minnesota Multiphasic Personality Inventory and a problems checklist, at least in their group of adult sexual abuse victims who sought counseling. Bagley and Ramsay (1985) found that the general mental health status of adult victims—measured by a composite of indicators concerning depression, psychoneurosis, suicidal ideation, psychiatric consultation, and self-concept—was worse for longer lasting experiences. Finally, Friedrich, Urguiza, and Beilke (in press), studying children, found that both duration and frequency predicted disturbances measured by the CBCL, even in multivariate analysis.

However, other studies have not found such relations. Finkelhor (1979), in a retrospective survey of college students, used a self-rating of how negative the experience was in retrospect and found no association with duration. Langmade (1983) reported that adult women seeking treatment who had had long or short duration experiences did not differ on measures of sexual anxiety, sexual guilt, or sexual dissatisfaction. In addition, the Tufts (1984) study, looking at child victims with more comprehensive measures than Friedrich et al. (in press), could find no association between duration of abuse and measures of distress, using the Louisville Behavior Checklist and the Purdue Self-Concept Scale, as well as other measures.

Finally, some studies indicated a completely reversed relation. Courtois (1979), surprisingly, found that adult victims with the longest lasting experiences reported the least trauma. In addition, in their college student sample, Seidner and Calhoun (1984) reported that a high frequency of abuse was associated with higher self-acceptance (but lower social maturity) scores on the California Psychological Inventory.

In summary, then, the available studies reach quite contradictory conclusions about the relation between duration and trauma. However, duration is closely related to other aspects of the abuse experience—e.g., age at onset, a family relationship between victim and offender, and the nature of the sexual activity. Some of the contradictions may be cleared up when we have better studies with well-defined multivariate analyses that can accurately assess the independent effect of duration.

Relationship to the Offender

Popular and clinical wisdom holds that sexual abuse by a close relative is more traumatic than abuse by someone outside the family. Empirical findings suggest that this may be the case, at least for some types of family abuse. Three studies have found more trauma resulting from abuse by relatives than by nonrelatives: Landis (1956), in an early study asking students about how they had recovered; Anderson et al. (1981), in a chart review of adolescents in a hospital treatment setting; and Friedrich et al. (in press), in their evaluation of young victims. However, other researchers (Finkelhor, 1979; Russell, in press; Seidner & Calhoun, 1984; Tufts, 1984) found no difference in the impact of abuse by family members versus abuse by others.

It must be kept in mind that how closely related a victim is to the offender does not necessarily reflect how much betrayal is involved in the abuse. Abuse by a trusted neighbor may be more devastating than abuse by a distant uncle or grandfather. Also, whereas abuse by a trusted person involves betrayal, abuse by a stranger or more distant person may involve more fear, and thus be rated more negatively. These factors may help explain why the relative-nonrelative distinction is not necessarily a consistent predictor of trauma.

What has been more consistently reported is greater trauma from experiences involving fathers or father figures compared with all other types of perpetrators, when these have been separated out. Russell (in press) and Finkelhor (1979) both found that abuse by a father or stepfather was significantly more traumatic for victims than other abuse occurring either inside or outside the family. The Tufts (1984) study also reported that children abused by stepfathers showed more distress, but for some reason it did not find the same elevated level of distress among victims abused by natural fathers. Bagley and Ramsay (1985) found a small but nonsignificantly greater amount of impairment in women molested by fathers and stepfathers.

Type of Sexual Act

Results of empirical studies generally suggest, with a couple of important exceptions, that the type of sexual activity is related to the degree of trauma in victims. Russell's findings on long-term effects in adult women are the most clear-cut: Fifty-nine percent of those reporting completed or attempted intercourse, fellatio, cunnilingus, analingus, or anal intercourse said they were extremely traumatized, compared with only 36% of those who experienced manual touching of unclothed breasts or genitals and 22% of those who reported unwanted kissing or touching of clothed parts of the body. The community study by Bagley and Ramsay (1985) confirms this, in a multivariate analysis that found penetration to be the single most powerful variable explaining severity of mental health impairment, using a composite of standardized instruments.

Moreover, four other studies confirm the relation between type of sexual contact and subsequent effects by demonstrating that the least serious forms of sexual contact are associated with less trauma (Landis, 1956; S. Peters, 1984; Seidner & Calhoun, 1984; Tufts, 1984). However, some of these studies did not find the clear differentiation that Russell and Bagley and Ramsay did between intercourse and genital touching. The Tufts (1984) study, for example, using measures of children's anxiety, found children who had been fondled without penetration to be more anxious than those who actually suffered penetration. Moreover, there are three additional studies (Anderson et al., 1981; Finkelhor, 1979; Fromuth, 1983) that do not show any consistent relation between type of sexual activity and effect. Thus, a number of studies concur that molestation involving more intimate contact is more traumatic than less intimate contact. However, there is some disagreement about whether intercourse and penetration are demonstrably more serious than simple manual contact.

Force and Aggression

Five studies, three of which had difficulty finding expected associations between trauma and many other variables, did find an association between trauma and the presence of force. With Finkelhor's (1979) student samples, use of force by an abuser explained more of a victim's negative reactions than any other variable, and this finding held up in multivariate analysis. Fromuth (1983), in a replication of the Finkelhor study, found similar results. In Russell's (in press) study 71% of the victims of force rated themselves as extremely or considerably traumatized, compared with 47% of the other victims.

The Tufts (1984) study found force to be one of the few variables associated with children's initial reactions: Children subjected to coercive experiences showed greater hostility and were more fearful of aggressive behavior in others. Tufts researchers reported that physical injury (i.e., the consequence of force) was the aspect of sexual abuse that was most consistently related to the degree of behavioral disturbances manifested in the child, as indicated by the LBC and other measures. Similarly, Friedrich et al. (in press) found the use of physical force to be strongly correlated with both internalizing and externalizing symptoms on the CBCL.

Three other studies present dissenting findings, however. Anderson et al. (1981), in studying initial effects, concluded that, "the degree of force or coercion used did not appear to be related to presence or absence of psychosocial sequelae" in the adolescents they evaluated (p. 7). Seidner and Calhoun (1984), in an ambiguous finding, noted that force was associated with lower social maturity but higher self-acceptance. In addition, Bagley and Ramsay (1985) found that force was associated with greater impairment, but this association diminished to just below the significance level in multivariate analysis. Despite these findings, we are inclined to give credence to the studies showing force to be a major traumagenic influence especially given the strong relation found by Finkelhor, Friedrich et al., Fromuth, Russell, and the Tufts study. Although some have argued that victims of forced abuse should suffer less long-term trauma because they could more easily attribute blame for abuse to the abuser (MacFarlane, 1978), empirical studies do not seem to provide support for this supposition.

Age at Onset

There has been a continuing controversy in the literature about how a child's age might affect his or her reactions to a sexually abusive experience. Some have contended that younger children are more vulnerable to trauma because of their impressionability. Others have felt that their naiveté may protect them from some negative effects, especially if they are ignorant of the social stigma surrounding the kind of victimization they have suffered. Unfortunately, findings from the available studies do not resolve this dispute.

Two studies of long-term effects do suggest that younger children are somewhat more vulnerable to trauma. Meiselman (1978), in her chart review of adults in treatment, found that 37% of those who experienced incest prior to puberty were seriously disturbed, compared with only

17% of those who were victimized after puberty. Similarly, Courtois (1979), in her community sample, assessed the impact of child sexual abuse on long-term relationships with men and the women's sense of self, and also found more effects from prepubertal experiences.

However, four other studies found no significant relation between age at onset and impact. Finkelhor (1979), in a multivariate analysis, found a small but nonsignificant tendency for younger age to be associated with trauma. Russell (in press) also found a small but nonsignificant trend for experiences before age 9 to be associated with more long-term trauma. Langmade (1983) could find no difference in sexual anxiety, sexual guilt, or sexual dissatisfaction in adults related to the age at which they were abused. Bagley and Ramsay (1985) found an association between younger age and trauma, but that association dropped out in multivariate analysis, especially when controlling for acts involving penetration.

The Tufts (1984) study gave particular attention to children's reactions to abuse at different ages. Tufts researchers concluded that age at onset bore no systematic relation to the degree of disturbance. They did note that latency-age children were the most disturbed, but this finding appeared more related to the age at which the children were evaluated than the age at which they were first abused. They concluded that the age at which abuse begins may be less important than the stages of development through which the abuse persists.

In summary, studies tend to show little clear relation between age of onset and trauma, especially when they control for other factors. If there is a trend, it is for abuse at younger ages to be more traumatic. Both of the initial hypotheses about age of onset may have some validity, however: Some younger children may be protected by naiveté, whereas others are more seriously traumatized by impressionability. However, age interacts with other factors like relationship to offender, and until more sophisticated analytical studies are done, we cannot say whether these current findings of a weak relation mean that age has little independent effect or is simply still masked in complexity.

Sex of Offender

Perhaps because there are so few female offenders (Finkelhor & Russell, 1984), very few studies have looked at impact according to the sex of the offender. Two studies that did (Finkelhor, 1984; Russell, in press) both found that adults rated experiences with male perpetrators as being much more traumatic than those with female perpetrators. A third study (Seidner & Calhoun, 1984) found male perpetrators linked with lower self-acceptance, but higher social maturity, in college-age victims.

Adolescent and Adult Perpetrators

There are also very few studies that have looked at the question of whether age of the perpetrator makes any difference in the impact of sexual abuse on victims. However, two studies using college student samples (Finkelhor, 1979; Fromuth, 1983) found that victims felt significantly more traumatized when abused by older perpetrators. In Finkelhor's multivariate analysis (which controlled for other factors such as force, sex of perpetrator, type of sex act, and age of the offender), age of the offender was the second most important factor predicting trauma. Fromuth (1983) replicated these findings. Russell (in press), with a community sample, reported consistent, but qualifying, results: In her survey, lower levels of trauma were reported for abuse with perpetrators who were younger than 26 or older than 50. The conclusion that experiences with adolescent perpetrators are less traumatic seems supported by all three studies.

Telling or Not Telling

There is a general clinical assumption that children who feel compelled to keep the abuse a secret in the aftermath suffer greater psychic distress as a result. However, studies have not confirmed this theory. Bagley and Ramsay (1985) did find a simple zero-order relation between not telling and a composite measure of impairment based on depression, suicidal ideas, psychiatric consultation, and self-esteem. However, the association became nonsignificant when controlled for other factors. Finkelhor (1979), in a multivariate analysis, also found that telling or not telling was essentially unrelated to a self-rated sense of trauma. Further, the Tufts (1984) researchers, evaluating child subjects, reported that the children who had taken a long time to disclose the abuse had the least anxiety and the least hostility. Undoubtedly, the decision to disclose is related to many factors about the experience, which prevents a clear assessment of its effects alone. For example, although silence may cause suffering for a child, social reactions to disclosure may be less intense if the event is long past. Moreover, the conditions for disclosure may be substantially different for the current generation than they were for past generations. Thus, any good empirical evaluation of the effects of disclosure versus secrecy needs to take into account the possibility of many interrelationships.

Parental Reaction

Only two studies have looked at children's trauma as a function of parental reaction, even though this is often hypothesized to be related to trauma. The Tufts (1984) study found that when mothers reacted to disclosure with anger and punishment, children manifested more behavioral disturbances. However, the same study did not find that positive responses by mothers were systematically related to better adjustment. Negative responses seemed to aggravate, but positive responses did not ameliorate, the trauma. Anderson et al. (1981) found similar results: They noted 2½ times the number of symptoms in the children who had encountered negative reactions from their parents. Thus, although only based on two studies of initial effects, the available evidence indicates that negative parental reactions aggravate trauma in sexually abused children.

Institutional Response

There is a great deal of interest in how institutional response may affect children's reactions to abuse, but little research has been done. Tufts (1984) researchers found that children removed from their homes following sexual abuse exhibited more overall behavior problems, particularly aggression, than children who remained with their families. However, the children who were removed in the Tufts study were also children who had experienced negative reactions from their mothers, so this result may be confounded with other factors related to the home environment.

Summary of Contributing Factors

From this review of empirical studies, it would appear that there is no contributing factor that all studies agree on as being consistently associated with a worse prognosis. However, there are trends in the findings. The preponderance of studies indicate that abuse by fathers or stepfathers has a more negative impact than abuse by other perpetrators. Experiences involving genital contact seem to be more serious. Presence of force seems to result in more trauma for the victim. In addition, when the perpetrators are men rather than women, and adults rather than teenagers, the effects of sexual abuse appear to be more disturbing. These findings should be considered tentative, however, being based on only two studies apiece. When families are unsupportive of the victims, and/or victims are removed from their homes, the prognosis has also been shown to be worse; again, these findings are based on only two studies.

Concerning the age of onset, the more sophisticated studies found no significant relation, especially when controlling for other factors; however, the relation between age and trauma is especially complex and has not yet been carefully studied. In regard to the impact of revealing the abuse, as opposed to the child keeping it a secret, current studies also suggest no simple relation. Of all these areas, there is the least consensus on the effect of duration of abuse on impact.

DISCUSSION

Conclusions from the foregoing review must be tempered by the fact that they are based on a body of research that is still in its infancy. Most of the available studies have sample, design, and measurement problems that could invalidate their findings. The study of the sexual abuse of children would greatly benefit from some basic methodological improvements.

Samples. Many of the available studies are based on samples of either adult women seeking treatment or children whose molestation has been reported. These subjects may be very self-selected. Especially if sexual abuse is so stigmatizing that only the most seriously affected victims seek help, such samples could distort our sense of the pathology most victims experience as a result of this abuse. New studies should take pains to expand the size and diversity of their samples, and particularly to study victims who have not sought treatment or been reported. Advertising in the media for "well-adjusted" victims, as Tsai et al. (1979) did, however, does not seem an adequate solution, as this injects a different selection bias into the study.

We favor sampling for sexual abuse victims within the general population, using whole communities—as in Russell's (in press), S. Peters's (1984) and Bagley and Ramsay's (1985) designs—or other natural collectivities (high school students, college students, persons belonging to a health plan, etc.). Obtaining such samples may be easier with adult than with child victims. If identified child victims must be used, care should be taken to sample from all such identified children, not just the ones that get referred for clinical assessment and treatment and who may therefore represent the most traumatized group.

Control groups. Some of the empirical studies cited here did not have comparison groups of any sort. Such a control is obviously important, even if it is only a group of other persons in treatment who were not sexually victimized (e.g., Briere, 1984; Meiselman, 1978). In some respects, however, this control procedure may actually underestimate the types and severities of pathology associated with sexual abuse, because problems that sexual abuse victims share with other clinical populations will not show up as distinctive effects. An as yet untried, but we believe fruitful, approach is to match victims from clinical sources with other persons who grew up with them: that is, schoolmates, relatives, or even unvictimized siblings.

Measurement. Most of the studies we reviewed used fairly subjective measures of the outcome variables in question (e.g., guilt feelings, fears, etc.). We are encouraged by the appearance of studies such as the Tufts study and Bagley and Ramsay's survey, which used batteries of objective measures. However, empirical investigations need to go even further. To test for the specific and diverse sequelae that have been associated with child sexual abuse, it would appear that special sexual abuse outcome instruments now need to be developed. Instruments designed specifically to measure the aftereffects noted by clinicians might be more successful at showing the true extent of pathology related to the experience of sexual abuse in childhood.

Sexual abuse in deviant subpopulations. Some of the studies purporting to show effects of child sexual abuse are actually reports of prevalence among specialized populations, such as prostitutes (James & Meyerding, 1977; Silbert & Pines, 1981), sex offenders (Groth & Burgess, 1979), or psychiatric patients (Carmen, Rieker, & Mills, 1984). To conclude from high rates of abuse in deviant populations that sexual abuse causes the deviance can be a misleading inference. Care needs to be taken to demonstrate that the discovered rate of sexual abuse in the deviant group is actually greater than in a relevant comparison group. In at least one study of sex offenders, for example, although abuse was frequent in their backgrounds, even higher rates of prior abuse were found for prisoners who had not committed sex crimes (Gebhard, Gagnon, Pomeroy, & Christenson, 1965). It is important to recognize that such data do not indicate that sexual abuse caused the deviance, only that many such offenders have abuse in their backgrounds.

Developmentally specific effects. In studying the initial and long-term effects of sexual abuse, researchers must also keep in mind that some effects of the molestation may be delayed. Although no sexual difficulties may be manifest in a group of college student victims (as in Fromuth, 1983), such effects may be yet to appear and may manifest themselves in studies of older groups. Similarly, developmentally specific effects may be seen among children that do not persist into adulthood, or that may assume a different form as an individual matures. The Tufts (1984) study clearly demonstrated the usefulness of looking at effects by defined age groupings.

Disentangling sources of trauma. One of the most imposing challenges for researchers is to explore the sources of trauma in sexual abuse. Some of the apparent effects of sexual abuse may be due to premorbid conditions, such as family conflict or emotional neglect, that actually contributed to a vulnerability to abuse and exacerbated later trauma. Other effects may be due less to the experience itself than to later social reactions to disclosure. Such questions need to be approached using careful multivariate analyses in large and diverse samples, or in small studies that match cases of sexual abuse that are similar except for one or two factors. Unfortunately, these questions are difficult to address in retrospective long-term impact studies, as it may be difficult or impossible to get accurate information about some of the key variables (e.g., how much family pathology predated the abuse).

Preoccupation with long-term effects. Finally, there is an unfortunate tendency in interpreting the effects of sexual abuse (as well as in studies of other childhood trauma) to overemphasize long-term impact as the ultimate criterion. Effects seem to be considered less "serious" if their impact is transient and disappears in the course of development. However, this tendency to assess everything in terms of its long-term effect betrays an "adulto-centric" bias. Adult traumas such as rape are not assessed ultimately in terms of whether they will have an impact on old age: They are acknowledged to be painful and alarming events, whether their impact lasts 1 year or 10. Similarly, childhood traumas should not be dismissed because no "long-term effects" can be demonstrated. Child sexual abuse needs to be recognized as a serious problem of childhood, if only for the immediate pain, confusion, and upset that can ensue.

REFERENCES

Achenbach, T.M, & Edelbrock, C. (1983). *Manual for the child behavior checklist.* Burlington: University of Vermont.

Anderson, S.C., Bach, C.M., & Griffith, S. (1981, April). *Psychosocial sequelae in intrafamilial victims of sexual assault and abuse.* Paper presented at the Third International Conference on Child Abuse and Neglect, Amsterdam, The Netherlands.

Bagley, C., & Ramsay, R. (1985, February). *Disrupted childhood and vulnerability to sexual assault: Long-term sequels with implications for counseling.* Paper presented at the Conference on Counseling the Sexual Abuse Survivor, Winnipeg, Canada.

Bell, A., & Weinberg, M. (1981). *Sexual preference: Its development among men and women.* Bloomington: Indiana University Press.

Benward, J., & Densen-Gerber, J. (1975, February) *Incest as a causative factor in anti-social behavior: An exploratory study.* Paper presented at the meeting of the American Academy of Forensic Science, Chicago, IL.

Briere, J. (1984, April). *The effects of childhood sexual abuse on later psychological functioning: Defining a "post sexual abuse syndrome."* Paper presented at the Third National Conference on Sexual Victimization of Children, Washington, DC.

Briere, J., & Runtz, M. (1985, August). *Symptomatology associated with prior sexual abuse in a non-clinical sample.* Paper presented at the annual meeting of the American Psychological Association, Los Angeles, CA.

Carmen, E., Rieker, P.P., & Mills, T. (1984). Victims of violence and psychiatric illness. *American Journal of Psychiatry, 141,* 378–383.

Constantine, L. (1977). *The sexual rights of children: Implications of a radical perspective.* Paper presented at the International Conference on Love and Attraction, Swansea, Wales.

Constantine, L. (1980). Effects of early sexual experience: A review and synthesis of research. In L. Constantine & F.M. Martinson (Eds.), *Children and sex* (pp. 217–244). Boston: Little, Brown.

Courtois, C. (1979). The incest experience and its aftermath. *Victimology: An International Journal. 4,* 337–347.

DeFrancis, V. (1969). *Protecting the child victim of sex crimes committed by adults.* Denver, CO: American Humane Association.

DeYoung, M. (1982). *The sexual victimization of children.* Jefferson, NC: McFarland.

Farrell, W. (1982). *Myths of incest: Implications for the helping professional.* Paper presented at the International Symposium on Family Sexuality, Minneapolis, MN.

Fields, P.J. (1981, November), Parent-child relationships, childhood sexual abuse, and adult interpersonal behavior in female prostitutes. *Dissertation Abstracts International, 42,* 2053B.

Finkelhor, D. (1979). *Sexually victimized children.* New York: Free Press.

Finkelhor, D. (1984). *Child Sexual abuse: New theory and research.* New York: Free Press.

Finkelhor, D., & Russell, D. (1984). Women as perpetrators of sexual abuse: Review of the evidence. In D. Finkelhor (Ed.), *Child sexual abuse: New theory and research* (pp. 171–187). New York: Free Press.

Friedrich, W.N. Urquiza, A.J., & Beilke, R. (in press). Behavioral problems in sexually abused young children. *Journal of Pediatric Psychology.*

Fromuth, M.E. (1983, August). *The long term psychological impact of chldhood sexual abuse.* Unpublished doctoral dissertation, Auburn University, Auburn, AL.

Gebhard, P., Gagnon, J., Pomeroy, W., & Christenson, C. (1965). *Sex offenders: An analysis of types.* New York: Harper & Row.

Goodwin J., McCarthy, T., & Divasto, P. (1981). Prior incest in mothers of abused children. *Child Abuse and Neglect, 5,* 87–96.

Groth, N.A., (1978). Guidelines for assessment and management of the offender. In A. Burgess, N. Groth, S. Holmstrom, & S. Sgroi (Eds), *Sexual assault of children and adolescents* (pp. 25–42). Lexington, MA: Lexington Books.

Groth, N.A., & Burgess, A.W. (1979). Sexual trauma in the life histories of rapists and child molesters. *Victimology: An international Journal 4,* 10–16.

Gundlach, R. (1977). Sexual molestation and rape reported by homosexual and heterosexual women. *Journal of Homosexuality, 2,* 367–384.

Harrison, P.A., Lumry, A.E., & Claypatch, C. (1984, August). *Female sexual abuse victims: Perspectives on family dysfunction, substance use and psychiatric disorders.* Paper presented at the Second National Conference for Family Violence Researchers, Durham, NH.

Henderson, J. (1983). Is incest harmful? *Canadian Journal of Psychiatry, 28,* 34–39.

Herman, J.L. (1981). *Father-daughter incest.* Cambridge, MA: Harvard University Press.

James, J., & Meyerding, J. (1977). Early sexual experiences and prostitution. *American Journal of Psychiatry, 134,* 1381–1385.

Landis, J. (1956). Experiences of 500 children with adult sexual deviation. *Psychiatric Quarterly Supplement, 30,* 91–109.

Langmade, C.J. (1983). The impact of pre- and postpubertal onset of incest experiences in adult women as measured by sex anxiety, sex guilt, sexual satisfaction and sexual behavior. *Dissertation Abstracts International, 44,* 917B. (University Microfilms No. 3592)

MacFarlane, K. (1978). Sexual abuse of children. In J.R. Chapman & M. Gates (Eds.), *The victimization of women* (pp. 81–109). Beverly Hills, CA: Sage.

Meiselman, K. (1978). *Incest.* San Francisco: Jossey-Bass.

Miller, J., Moeller, D., Kaufman, A., Divasto, P., Fitzsimmons, P., Pather, D., & Christy, J. (1978). Recidivism among sexual assault victims. *American Journal of Psychiatry, 135,* 1103–1104.

Nelson, J. (1981). The impact of incest: Factors in self-evaluation. In L. Zakus & F. Mahlon (Eds.), *Children and sex* (pp. 163–174). Boston: Little, Brown.

Peters, J.J. (1976). Children who are victims of sexual assault and the psychology of offenders. *American Journal of Psychotherapy, 30,* 398–421.

Peters, S.D. (1984). *The relationship between childhood sexual victimization and adult depression among Afro-American and white women.* Unpublished doctoral dissertation, University of California, Los Angeles, CA.

Ramey, J. (1979). Dealing with the last taboo. *Sex Information and Education Council of the United States, 7,* 1–2, 6–7.

Reich, J.W., & Gutierres, S.E. (1979). Escape/aggression incidence in sexually abused juvenile delinquents. *Criminal Justice and Behavior, 6,* 239–243.

Rogers, C.M., & Terry, T. (1984). Clinical intervention with boy victims of sexual abuse. In I. Stewart and J. Greer (Eds.), *Victims of Sexual Aggression* (pp. 1–104). New York: Van Nostrand, Reinhold.

Russell, D.E.H. (in press). *The secret trauma: Incest in the lives of girls and women.* New York: Basic Books.

Sandfort, T. (1981). *The sexual aspect of paedophile relations.* Amsterdam: Pan/Spartacus.

Sedney, M.A., & Brooks, B. (1984). Factors associated with a history of childhood sexual experience in a nonclinical female population. *Journal of the American Academy of Child Psychiatry, 23,* 215–218.

Seidner, A., & Calhoun, K.S. (1984, August). *Childhood sexual abuse: Factors related to differential adult adjustment.* Paper presented at the Second National Conference for Family Violence Researchers, Durham, NH.

Silbert, M.H., & Pines, A.M. (1981). Sexual child abuse as an antecedent to prostitution. *Child Abuse and Neglect, 5,* 407–411.

Tsai, M., Feldman-Summers, S., & Edgar, M. (1979). Childhood molestation: Variables related to differential impact of psychosexual functioning in adult women. *Journal of Abnormal Psychology, 88,* 407–417.

Tufts' New England Medical Center Division of Child Psychiatry (1984). *Sexually exploited children: Service and research project.* Final report for the Office of Juvenile Justice and Delinquency Prevention. Washington, DC: U.S. Department of Justice.

Wisconsin Female Juvenile Offender Study (1982). *Sex abuse among juvenile offenders and runaways. Summary report.* Madison, WI: Author.

Woods, S.C., & Dean, K.S. (1984). *Final report: Sexual abuse of males research project* (Contract No. 90 CA/812). Washington, DC: National Center on Child Abuse and Neglect.

TWENTY-YEAR AUTHOR INDEX

Best, D.L., 1976: 123
Beytagh, L.A.M., 1970: 195
Bianchi, E.C., 1980: 583
Bicknell, J., 1984: 346
Biller, H.B., 1971: 120
Billingsley, A., 1971: 323
Birch, H., 1976: 34
Birch, H.G., 1968: 212, 335; 1969: 265, 611; 1971: 166; 1972: 96, 165; 1973: 156, 321; 1975: 255
Birns, B., 1969: 24; 1972: 139; 1977: 261
Black, F.W., 1982: 344
Blank, M., 1969: 217; 1971: 286
Bloch, E.L., 1972: 275
Bloom, W., 1972: 457
Bohman, M., 1973: 489; 1980: 148; 1981: 217
Bolling, J.L., 1975: 232
Borelli, J., 1984: 133
Bornstein, M.H., 1977: 44
Borowitz, G.H., 1971: 335
Bortner, M., 1968: 212; 1971: 166
Boswell, J.J., 1973: 285
Boudreault, M., 1985: 374; 1986: 397; 1987: 291
Boutin, P., 1986: 397; 1987: 241
Bowlby, J., 1983: 29
Brackbill, Y., 1972: 3; 1973: 18; 1977: 3
Braun, J., 1973: 358
Brazelton, T.B., 1977: 665
Breitenbucher, M., 1981: 666
Breslau, N., 1982: 397
Bretherton, I., 1979: 78
Breton, J.-J., 1978: 319; 1979: 540
Bridger, W.H., 1969: 217; 1972: 139
Briggs, J.L., 1973: 139
Bronfenbrenner, U., 1971: 210; 1975: 12
Brooke, E., 1970: 351
Brown, G., 1982; 525
Brown, J.V., 1981: 17
Brown Dolan, A., 1982: 229
Browne, A., 1986: 632; 1987: 555
Brozovsky, M., 1976: 710
Brunner, J.S., 1972: 47; 1974: 53
Brunnquell, D., 1983: 430
Bruun, R., 1975: 468
Bryant, B., 1977: 677
Bryson, C.Q., 1973: 503, 576
Bucknam, F.G., 1971: 581
Bullard, D.M., 1968: 540
Bunney, W.E., 1981: 581
Burgess, D., 1985: 235
Burkes, L., 1979: 476
Burstein, B., 1981: 144
Burton, N., 1979: 450

Butterfield, E.C., 1969: 137; 1971: 526
Butterfield, P., 1987: 26

Cadoret, R.J., 1976: 232, 258; 1981: 447
Cadwell, J., 1983: 337, 345
Cain, A.C., 1970: 417
Cain, C., 1981: 447
Caldwell, B.M, 1968: 149; 1971: 3; 1973: 232
Cameron, J.R., 1978: 233; 1979: 271
Cammuso, K., 1987: 494
Campbell, M., 1973: 589
Campbell, S.B., 1979: 392
Campos, J.J., 1980: 95; 1981: 49; 1987: 26
Cane, M., 1987: 410
Cantwell, D.P., 1972: 554; 1975: 311; 1980: 418; 1983: 205
Caparulo, B.K., 1977: 204, 545; 1982: 550
Capéraà, P., 1985: 374; 1986: 397
Capobianco, F., 1971: 526
Carey, W.B., 1973: 639; 1975: 79, 87; 1979: 263; 1980: 265; 1981: 589; 1984: 230
Carlsmith, J.M., 1982: 620
Carlson, G., 1980: 418
Case, Q., 1973: 619
Chadwick, O., 1982: 525
Chadwick, O.F.D., 1976: 358
Chamberlin, R.W., 1975: 63
Chambers, S., 1976: 34
Chang, Pi-Nian, 1982: 182
Char, W.F., 1975: 483; 1984: 145, 155; 1986: 314
Charlesworth, W.R., 1969: 1
Charnov, E.L., 1985: 53
Chavez, C.J., 1977: 108
Chess, S., 1968: 335; 1969: 125, 185; 1970: 540; 1971: 353; 1972: 539; 1973: 172, 405; 1975: 150; 1976: 341; 1977: 489; 1978: 223, 486; 1979: 168; 467; 1980: 3; 1981: 295; 1982: 448; 1983: 48; 1984: 281; 1985: 140
Chick, J., 1980: 386; 1981: 555
Chihara, T., 1981: 494
Chiles, J., 1979: 377
Chivian, E., 1986: 289
Chmura Kraemer, H., 1982: 421
Churchill, D.W., 1970: 436; 1973: 576
Cicci, R., 1972: 407
Clark, K.B., 1970: 279
Clarke, A.D.B., 1973: 459; 1979: 105; 1982: 94; 1985: 27
Clarke, A.M., 1982: 94; 1983: 230; 1985: 27
Clarke, C., 1985: 280
Clements, M., 1972: 554
Clemmens, R.L., 1972: 407

Minde, K.K., 1972: 415; 1979: 677; 1981:
    58; 1982: 463; 1987: 40
Minde, R., 1982: 463
Minuchin, S. 1976: 319
Mishler, E.G., 1972: 568
Mitchell, A.C., 1971: 513
Mittelman, M., 1984: 281; 1985: 304
Mo, A., 1986: 549
Money, J., 1973: 435; 1977: 215, 240; 1980:
    203
Moore, M., 1979: 46
Morgan, G.A., 1983: 217
Morrison, B., 1979: 612
Moss, A., 1972: 139
Moss, H.A., 1968: 73
Mosteller, S., 1975: 498
Muenchow, S., 1980: 574; 1984: 466; 1985:
    603
Muir, D., 1980: 85
Murdock, C.W., 1974: 590
Murphy, A., 1973: 479
Murphy, M.A., 1986: 140
Mussen, P., 1970: 195
Myers, R.A., 1975: 79

Nackman, D., 1987: 494
Nadas, A.S., 1974: 370
Nadelson, C.C., 1980: 305
Nagy Jacklin, C., 1986: 587
Nair, P., 1972: 407
Needleman, H.L., 1974: 359
Nelson, K., 1982: 249
Nelson, K.E., 1978: 165
Nelson, R., 1982: 344
Nelson, S.H., 1975: 199
Nemeth, E., 1972: 415
Nestler, V., 1983: 492
Nettles, M., 1986: 24
Neubauer, P.B., 1971: 84; 1977: 121
Nevis, S., 1968: 22
Newberger, E.H., 1974: 569; 1978: 547
Newman, C.J., 1977: 149
Newman, L.E., 1977: 230
Newman, S., 1976: 448
Nichols, P.L., 1985: 560
Nichtern, S., 1974: 545
Niskanen, P., 1979: 331
Nolan, T., 1986: 386
Novotny, E.S., 1971: 543
Nuss, S.M., 1985: 332
Nyhan, W.L., 1977: 175

O'Connor, N., 1968: 516
O'Malley, J.E., 1980: 543; 1981: 263
Oberklaid, F., 1980: 234; 1986: 386

Offer, D., 1982: 593
Ogbu, J.U., 1982: 113
Ollendick, T.H., 1985: 570
Onesti, S., 1970: 551
Orasanu, J., 1980: 157
Orgun, I.N., 1971: 581
Ornitz, E.M., 1969: 411; 1977: 501; 1985:
    452; 1986: 505
Osborn, M., 1980: 583
Osofsky, H.J., 1971: 556
Osofsky, J.D., 1971: 556
Ostrea, E.M., 1977: 108
Ostrov, E., 1982: 593
Otnow Lewis, D., 1980: 591; 1981: 508;
    1985: 586
Owens, R., 1981: 306

Palisin, H., 1981: 36
Palmer, F.B., 1977: 455
Pandoni, C., 1978: 209
Pannabecker, B.J., 1983: 144
Parmelee, A.H., 1987: 63
Parry, M.H., 1970: 14
Parton, D.A., 1977: 51
Paternite, C.E., 1977: 327, 342
Paul, R., 1985: 413
Paulauskas, S.L., 1985: 520
Payne, D.T., 1968: 166
Pearsall, D., 1974: 521
Pedersen, F.A., 1973: 3
Pellegrini, D., 1987: 494
Penman, R., 1983: 156
Perez-Reyes, M.G., 1974: 480
Perlstein, A., 1976: 710
Perry, C., 1969: 196
Person, E.S., 1986: 197
Persson-Blennow, I., 1980: 217; 1982: 317
Pescovitz, O.H., 1987: 140
Peters-Martin, P., 1985: 315
Peterson, R.E., 1980: 192
Petrich, J., 1979: 377
Petti, T.A., 1979: 476
Pettit, M.G., 1970: 261
Petty, L.K., 1985: 452
Pfeifer, C.M., 1972: 457
Philips, I., 1968: 311; 1976: 373
Pichel, J.I., 1975: 189
Piggott, L.R., 1974: 349; 1980: 519
Pinard, G., 1978: 319
Pincus, J.H., 1975: 281; 1980: 591
Pivchik, E.C., 1968: 540
Pivchik, G., 1968: 540
Pless, I.B., 1972: 589; 1980: 554
Plomin, R., 1978: 216; 1981: 133; 1985:
    253; 1986: 24

Wolins, M., 1970: 218
Wollersheim, J.P., 1968: 356
Woodrow, K.M., 1975: 459
Woodson, R., 1983: 119
Wright, S.W., 197: 279

Yando, R., 1973: 729
Yarrow, L.J., 1973: 3; 1980: 31; 1983: 217
Yarrow, M.R., 1974: 95
Young, J.G., 1977: 204; 1978: 102; 1982: 550
Young, R.D., 1977: 409
Yule, W., 1977: 359

Zastowny, T.R., 1985: 475
Zelson, C., 1972: 25
Ziegler, M.G., 1978: 209
Zigler, E., 1968: 281; 1969: 137, 352; 1971: 185, 526; 1972: 325; 1973: 729; 1974: 154, 199; 1978: 417, 613; 1979: 407, 559; 1980: 574; 1982: 502; 1984: 466; 1985: 603; 1986: 669
Zimmerman, E.G., 1985: 452
Zimmerman, I.L., 1984: 166
Zingale Ilfeld, H., 1983: 545
Zrull, J.P., 1971: 455

TWENTY-YEAR ARTICLE INDEX

Adolescence

Volume 2: 1969

The Psychiatric Significance of Adolescent Turmoil *(J. F. Masterson)*
Neurologic Organization in Psychiatrically Disturbed Adolescents *(M. E. Hertzig and H. G. Birch)*
Chinese-American Child-Rearing Practices and Juvenile Delinquency *(R. T. Sollenberger)*

Volume 4: 1971

Ego Disorganization and Recidivism in Delinquent Boys *(J. Satten, E. S. Novotny, S. L. Ginsparg, and S. Averill)*
Adolescents as Mothers: Results of a Program for Low-Income Pregnant Teenagers with Some Emphasis upon Infants' Development *(H. J. Osofsky and J. D. Osofsky)*
Psychiatric Problems in Adolescents with Cerebral Palsy *(R. D. Freeman)*

Volume 7: 1974

Sex Counseling on Campus: Short-Term Treatment Techniques *(R. Bauer and J. Stein)*
Follow-Up after Therapeutic Abortion in Early Adolescence *(M. G. Perez-Reyes and R. Falk)*
The Indian Adolescent: Psychosocial Tasks of the Plains Indian of Western Oklahoma *(J. R. Allen)*
The Adolescent Patient's Decision to Die *(J. E. Schowalter, J. B. Fernholt, and N. M. Mann)*

Volume 8: 1975

A Long-Term Follow-Up Study of Sixty Adolescent Psychiatric Outpatients *(J. I. Pichel)*
A National Study of the Knowledge, Attitudes and Patterns of Use of Drugs by Disadvantaged Adolescents *(S. H. Nelson, D. P. Kraft, and J. Fielding)*

Volume 9: 1976

The Ego and the Integration of Violence in Homicidal Youth *(C. H. King)*
Hospitalized Suicidal Adolescents *(H. I. Schneer, A. Perlstein, and M. Brozovsky)*

Volume 10: 1977

Psychopathology in Adolescence *(I. B. Weiner and A. C. Del Gaudio)*
Evolution of Behavior Disorders into Adolescence *(A. Thomas and S. Chess)*
School-Related Problems of Mexican-American Adolescents *(B. Bryant and A. Meadow)*

Volume 12: 1979

Current Contradictions in Adolescent Theory *(J. C. Coleman)*
Adolescent Rebellion in the Kibbutz *(M. Kaffman)*
Coping Styles of 34 Adolescents with Cerebral Palsy *(K. K. Minde)*

Volume 13: 1980

Phenomenology Associated with Depressed Moods in Adolescents *(S. C. Inamdar, G. Siomopoulos, M. Osborn, and E. C. Bianchi)*
Violent Juvenile Delinquents: Psychiatric, Neurological, Psychological, and Abuse Factors *(D. O. Lewis, S. S. Shanok, J. H. Pincus, and G. H. Glaser)*

Volume 14: 1981

The Psychological Impact of Menarche: Integrative Versus Disruptive Changes *(J. Rierdan and E. Koff)*
Self-Concept, Self-Esteem, and Body Attitudes Among Japanese Male and Female Adolescents *(R. M. Lerner, S. Iwawaki, T. Chihara, and G. T. Sorell)*
Race Bias in the Diagnosis and Disposition of Violent Adolescents *(D. O. Lewis, S. S. Shanok, R. J. Cohen, M. Kligfeld, and G. Frisone)*
Critical Review of Research on Psychotherapy Outcome with Adolescents: 1967-1977 *(M. G. Tramontana)*

Volume 15: 1982

The Mental Health Professional's Concept of the Normal Adolescent *(D. Offer, E. Ostrov, and K. I. Howard)*
Natural History of Male Psychological Health, X: Work as a Predictor of Positive Mental Health *(G. E. Vaillant and C. O. Vaillant)*
Sexual Development, Age, and Dating: A Comparison of Biological and Social Influences Upon One Set of Behaviors *(S. M. Dornbusch, J. M. Carlsmith, R. T. Gross, J. A. Martin, D. Jennings, A. Rosenberg, and P. Duke)*
Antisocial Adolescents: Our Treatments Do Not Work—Where Do We Go From Here? *(S. J. Shamsie)*

Volume 17: 1984

Reexamining the Concept of Adolescence: Differences Between Adolescent Boys and Girls in the Context of Their Families *(J. F. McDermott, Jr., A. B. Robillard, W. F. Char, J. Hsu, W. S. Tseng, and G. C. Ashton)*

Brain Damage and Cerebral Dysfunction

Child Abuse

Child Abuse and Neglect: The Rights of Parents and the Needs of Their Children *(A. P. Derdeyn)*
A Case for Permanent Foster Placement of Dependent, Neglected and Abused Children *(A. P. Derdeyn)*

Volume 14: 1981

Child Maltreatment: An Ecological Integration *(J. Belsky)*
Prospective Study of the Significance of Life Stress in the Etiology of Child Abuse *(B. Egeland, M. Breitenbucher, and D. Rosenberg)*

Volume 15: 1982

Failure of "Bond Formation" as a Cause of Abuse, Neglect, and Maltreatment *(B. Egeland and B. Vaughn)*

Volume 20: 1987

Child Care and Child Abuse in Early Medieval Europe *(J. Kroll and B. Bachrach)*
Impact of Child Sexual Abuse: A Review of the Research *(A. Browne and D. Finkelhor)*

Clinical Psychiatry

Volume 1: 1968

The Contribution of Obstetric Complications to the Etiology of Behavior Disorders in Childhood *(S. Wolff)*
Behavior Problems Revisited: Findings of an Anterospective Study *(S. Chess, A. Thomas, and H. Birch)*
Masked Depression in Children and Adolescents *(K. Glaser)*
Emotional Reactions of Handicapped Children *(R. D. Freeman)*
The Home Visit in Child Psychiatry *(R. D. Freeman)*

Volume 2: 1969

The Two Camps in Child Psychiatry: A Report from a Psychiatrist-Father of an Autistic and Retarded Child *(J. E. Kysar)*
Passivity *(I. M. Josselyn)*
Male Childhood Transsexualism *(R. J. Stoller)*
A Study of Anorexia Nervosa in Young Girls *(W. Warren)*
Phobias of Childhood: Etiology and Treatment *(M. Berecz)*

Volume 3: 1970

The Children Haven't Read Those Books: Reflections on Differential Diagnosis *(L. Kanner)*
A Tri-Axial Classification of Mental Disorders in Childhood *(M. Rutter, et al.)*
A Clincial Evaluation of Children with Psychotic Parents *(E. J. Anthony)*
Suicidal Behavior as a Child Psychiatric Emergency *(A. Mattsson, L. S. Seese, and J. W. Hawkins)*
On Borrowed Time: Observations on Children with Implanted Cardiac Pacemakers and Their Families *(R. Galdston and W. J. Gamble)*

Volume 4: 1971

Volume 5: 1972

Volume 6: 1973

Volume 7: 1974

Volume 8: 1975

Volume 9: 1976

Volume 10: 1977

Volume 11: 1978

Volume 12: 1979

Volume 13: 1980

Volume 14: 1981

A Prospective, Longitudinal Study of Children Registered for Adoption: A 15-Year Follow-up *(M. Bohman and S. Sigvardsson)*

Parental Death in Childhood and Risk of Adult Depressive Disorders: A Review *(C. Tennant, P. Bebbington, and J. Hurry)*

Schizoid Personality in Childhood: A Controlled Follow-up Study *(S. Wolff and J. Chick)*

Diagnosis of Depression in Children: A Reassessment *(L. Cytryn, D. H. McKnew, Jr., and W. E. Bunney, Jr.)*

Minimal Brain Dysfunction and Hyperkinesis *(W. B. Carey and S. C. McDevitt)*

Hyperkinesis Comes of Age: What Do We Know and Where Should We Go? *(J. Loney)*

Tardive Dyskinesia and Other Drug-Induced Movement Disorders Among Handicapped Children and Youth *(C. T. Gualtieri and B. Hawk)*

Volume 15: 1982

Behavioral Contrasts in Twinships: Stability and Patterns of Differences in Childhood *(A. P. Matheny, Jr., R. S. Wilson, A. Brown Dolan, and J. Z. Krantz)*

Coping Strategies in Psychiatric Clinical Research *(H. C. Kraemer)*

Ecological Variables and Examiner Biases in Assessing Handicapped Preschool Children *(T. Field)*

Elective Mute Children: Psychological Development and Background Factors *(I. Kolvin and T. Fundudis)*

Neurological "Soft" Signs in Low-birthweight Children *(M. E. Hertzig)*

A Prospective Study of Children with Head Injuries: III. Psychiatric Sequelae *(G. Brown, O. Chadwick, D. Shaffer, M. Rutter, and M. Traub)*

Computed Tomographic Brain Scanning in Children with Developmental Neuropsychiatric Disorders *(B. K. Caparulo, D. J. Cohen, S. L. Rothman, J. G. Young, J. D. Katz, S. E. Shaywitz, and B. A. Shaywitz)*

Biological Validation of the Hyperkinetic Syndrome *(J. L. Rapoport and H. B. Ferguson)*

Volume 16: 1983

Biological Research in Child Psychiatry: The Interplay of Theory and Investigation *(J. L. Rapoport and D. R. Ismond)*

Chronic Malnutrition and Child Behavior: Effects of Early Caloric Supplementation on Social and Emotional Functioning at School Age *(D. E. Barrett, M. R. Yarrow, and R. E. Klein)*

Issues in the Psychological Care of Pediatric Oncology Patients *(D. Brunnquell and M. D. Hall)*

Psychiatric Consultation to the Child with Acute Physical Trauma *(K. Ravenscroft)*

Somnambulism in Childhood—Prevalence, Course and Behavioral Correlations *(G. Klackenberg)*

Volume 17: 1984

How People Make Their Own Environments: A Theory of Genotype → Environment Effects *(S. Scarr and K. McCartney)*

Environmental Effects on Intelligence: The Forgotten Realm of Discontinuous Nonshared Within-Family Factors *(R. B. McCall)*

The Psychopathology of Handicap *(J. Bicknell)*

Developmental Issues

Volume 1: 1968

Child Development: A Basic Science for Pediatrics *(I. B. Richmond)*

Volume 3: 1970

Industrialization, Child-Rearing Practices, and Children's Personality *(P. Mussen and L. A. M. Beytagh)*
Group Care: Friend or Foe? *(M. Wolins)*

Volume 4: 1971

Behavior-Genetic Analysis and Its Biosocial Consequences *(J. Hirsch)*
Issues in Assessing Development *(D. Flapan and P. B. Neubauer)*
Psychological Development—Predictions from Infancy *(M. Rutter)*
Father Absence and the Personality Development of the Male Child *(H. B. Biller)*
Growth in Social Competence in Institutionalized Mentally Retarded Children *(A. C. Mitchell and V. Smeriglio)*
Institutionalization and the Effectiveness of Social Reinforcement: a Five- and Eight-Year Follow-Up Study *(E. Zigler, E. C. Butterfield, and F. Capobianco)*

Volume 5: 1972

Cultural Differences and Inferences about Psychological Processes *(M. Cole and J. S. Bruner)*
Normal Psychosexual Development *(M. Rutter)*
Functional Effects of Fetal Malnutrition *(H. G. Birch)*
Child Work and Social Class *(M. Engel, G. Marsden, and S. W. Pollock)*

Volume 6: 1973

Learning and the Concept of Critical Periods in Infancy *(K. Connolly)*
On the First Three Subphases of the Separation-Individuation Process *(M. S. Mahler)*
The Issues of Autonomy and Aggression in the Three-Year-Old: The Uktu Eskimo Case *(J. L. Briggs)*
Intellectual Levels of School Children Severely Malnourished During the First Two Years of Life *(M. E. Hertzig, H. G. Birch, S. A. Richardson, and J. Tizard)*
Development in Middle Childhood *(A. Thomas and S. Chess)*
Coping and Growth in Adolescence *(S. H. King)*
Relationships Between Child and Adult Psychiatric Disorders *(M. L. Rutter)*
Psychiatric Patients Seen as Children and Adults: Childhood Predictors of Adult Illness *(G. W. Mellsop)*
Environmental Effects on Language Development: A Study of Young Children in Long-Stay Residential Nurseries *(B. Tizard, O. Cooperman, A. Joseph, and J. Tizard)*
Outerdirectedness and Imitative Behavior in Institutionalized and Noninstitutionalized Younger and Older Children *(E. Zigler and R. Yando)*

Volume 11: 1978

Volume 12: 1979

Volume 13: 1980

Volume 15: 1982

Volume 20: 1987

Child Psychology: The Future *(H. R. Schaffer)*
Environmental Context of Child Development *(A. J. Samcroff)*
Childhood Parental Death and Adult Psychopathology *(P. V. Ragan and T. H. McGlashan)*
Biobehavioral Aspects of Precocious Puberty *(W. A. Sonis, F. Comite, O. H. Pescovitz, K. Hench, C. W. Rahn, G. B. Cutler, Jr., D. L. Loriaux, and R. P. Klein)*
Minor Neurological Indicators and Developmental Function in Preschool Children *(G. B. Landman, M. D. Levine, T. Fenton, and B. Solomon)*
Stability (and Instability) of Type A Behavior from Childhood to Young Adulthood *(L. Steinberg)*

Drug Abuse

Volume 7: 1974

A Survey of Adolescent Drug Use Patterns *(V. A. Gelineau, M. Johnson, and D. Pearsall)*
Youth Who Use Drugs: Psychodynamic Diagnosis and Treatment Planning *(S. Proskauer and R. S. Rolland)*
The Children of Drug Users *(S. Nichtern)*

Volume 9: 1976

A Hierarchy of Drug Use in Adolescence: Behavioral and Attitudinal Correlates of Substantial Drug Use *(B. A. Hamburg, H. C. Kraemer, and W. Jahnke)*
Sequence and Stages in Patterns of Adolescent Drug Use *(D. Kandel and R. Faust)*
Parental Failure and Consequences for Children. The Drug-Abusing Mother Whose Children Are in Foster Care *(D. Fanshel)*

Volume 12: 1979

Antecedents of Adolescent Initiation into Stages of Drug Use: A Developmental Analysis *(D. B. Kandel, R. C. Kessler, and R. Z. Margulies)*

Volume 13: 1980

Illicit Drug Use Among Urban Adolescents: A Decade in Retrospect *(K. Hein, M. I. Cohen, and I. F. Litt)*

Volume 16: 1983

Differential Motor and State Functioning in Newborns of Women on Methadone *(J. Marcus, S. L. Hans, and R. Jeruchimowicz Jeremy)*
Children of Methadone-maintained Mothers: Follow-up to 18 Months of Age *(T. S. Rosen and H. L. Johnson)*
Development and Psychopathology of Children With the Fetal Alcohol Syndrome *(H. C. Steinhausen, V. Nestler, and H. L. Spohr)*

Hyperactive Child

Volume 19: 1986

Neuropharmacology of Methylphenidate and a Neural Substrate for Childhood Hyperactivity *(C. T. Gualtieri and R. E. Hicks)*

Infancy Studies

Volume 1: 1968

The Role of Biological Rhythms in Early Psychological Development *(P. H. Wolff)*
Pattern Preferences and Perceptual-Cognitive Development in Early Infancy *(R. L. Fantz and S. Nevis)*
Nonnutritive Sucking and Response Threshholds in Young Infants *(P. H. Wolff and M. A. Simmons)*
Comparative Development of Negro and White Infants *(C. E. Walters)*

Volume 2: 1969

Cognition in Infancy: Where Do We Stand in the Mid-Sixties? *(W. R. Charlesworth)*
Social Class and Cognitive Development in Infancy *(M. Golden and B. Birns)*
Consistent Individual Differences in the Nutritive Sucking Behavior of the Human Newborn *(R. E. Kron, J. Ipsen, and K. E. Goddard)*
Social and Emotional Behavior in Infancy *(H. N. Ricciuti)*

Volume 3: 1970

Maintaining the Positive Behavior of Infants by Increased Stimulation *(H. L. Rheingold and H. R. Samuels)*
Perceptual-Motor Behavior in Infancy as a function of Age and Stimulus Familiarity *(H. R. Schaffer and M. H. Parry)*
Perceptual-Cognitive Development in Infancy: A Generalized Expectancy Model as a Function of the Mother-Infant Interaction *(M. Lewis and S. Goldberg)*
A Case of Congenital Sensory Neuropathy Diagnosed in Infancy *(J. L. Rapoport)*
On the Meaning of Behavior: Illustrations from the Infant *(J. Kagan)*

Volume 4: 1971

The Effects of Psychosocial Deprivation on Human Development in Infancy *(B. M. Caldwell)*
The Infant Separates Himself from His Mother *(H. L. Rheingold and C. O. Eckerman)*
Attachment, Exploration, and Separation: Illustrated by the Behavior of One-Year-Olds in a Strange Situation *(M. D. S. Ainsworth and S. M. Bell)*

Volume 5: 1972

Cumulative Effects of Continuous Stimulation on Arousal Level in Infants *(Y. Brackbill)*
Parental, Birth, and Infancy Factors in Infant Twin Development *(M. G. Allen, W. Pollin, and A. Hoffer)*
Neonatal Narcotic Addiction: 10-Year Observation *(C. Zelson, E. Rubio, and E. Wasserman)*

Volume 6: 1973

Dimensions of Early Stimulation and Their Differential Effects on Infant Development *(I. J. Yarrow, J. L. Rubinstein, F. A. Pedersen, and J. J. Jankowski)*
Stereotype Temporal Conditioning in Infants *(Y. Brackbill and H. E. Fitzgerald)*
The Relative Efficacy of Contact and Vestibular-Proprioceptive Stimulation in Soothing Neonates *(A. F. Korner and E. B. Thoman)*
Evaluation of Infant Intelligence: Infant Intelligence Scores—True or False? *(M. Lewis and H. McGurk)*
Transitions in Infant Sensorimotor Development and the Prediction of Childhood IQ *(R. B. McCall, P. S. Hogarty, and N. Hurlburt)*
Infants Around the World: Cross-Cultural Studies of Psychomotor Development from Birth to Two Years *(E. E. Werner)*

Volume 10: 1977

Classical Conditioning in Infancy: Development and Constraints *(H. E. Fitzgerald and Y. Brackbill)*
The Categories of Hue in Infancy *(M. H. Bornstein, W. Kessen, and S. Weiskopf)*
Learning to Imitate in Infancy *(D. A. Parton)*
The Fathers (Not the Mothers): Their Importance and Influence with Infants and Young Children *(F. Earls)*
Behavioral Concomitants of Prenatal Addiction to Narcotics *((M. E. Strauss, R. H. Starr, Jr., E. M. Ostrea, C. J. Chavez, and J. Stryker)*

Volume 12: 1979

Neonatal Assessment Procedures: A Historical Review *(K. L. St. Clair)*
State and Rhythmic Processes *(T. F. Anders)*
Infant Antecedents of Cognitive Functioning: A Longitudinal Study *(J. Kagan, D. R. Lapidus, and M. Moore)*
Making Friends With One-Year Olds: An Experimental Study of Infant-Stranger Interaction *(I. Bretherton)*

Volume 13: 1980

Newborn Infants Orient to Sounds *(D. Muir and J. Field)*
Facial Patterning and Infant Emotional Expression: Happiness, Surprise and Fear *(S. W. Hiatt, J. J. Campos, and R. N. Emde)*
Night-Waking in Infants During the First Year of Life *(T. F. Anders)*

Volume 14: 1981

The Significance of Speech to Newborns *(H. L. Rheingold and J. L. Adams)*
Early Interaction: Consequences for Social and Mental Development at Three Years *(R. Bakeman and J. V. Brown)*
The Neonatal Perception Inventory: Failure to Replicate *(H. Palisin)*
Two Methods of Studying Stranger Reactivity in Infants: A Review *(T. M. Horner)*
Infant Wariness Toward Strangers Reconsidered: Infants' and Mothers' Reactions to Unfamiliar Persons *(K. Kaltenbach, M. Weinraub, and W. Fullard)*
Multiple Functions of Proximity Seeking in Infancy *(D. F. Hay)*

Volume 15: 1982

Volume 16: 1983

Volume 17: 1984

Volume 18: 1985

Volume 19: 1986

Volume 20: 1987

Language—Cognition—Learning

Volume 5: 1972

Volume 6: 1973

Volume 7: 1974

Volume 8: 1975

Volume 9: 1976

Dyslexia in Children and Young Adults: Three Independent Neuropsychological Syndromes *(S. Mattis, J. H. French, and I. Rapid)*
Admission and Follow-up Status of Reading Disabled Children Referred to a Medical Clinic *(R. Gottesman, I. Belmont, and R. Kaminer)*

Volume 10: 1977

Twins with Academic Learning Problems: Antecedent Characteristics *(A. P. Matheny, Jr., A. B. Dolan, and R. S. Wilson)*
Utilization of a Psychiatric-Social Work Team in an Alaskan Native Secondary Boarding School *(E. B. Harvey, L. Gazay, and B. Samuels)*

Volume 11: 1978

Aspects of Language Acquisition and Use From Age 2 to Age 20 *(K. E. Nelson)*
Language, Cognitive Development and Personality *(M. Lewis)*

Volume 12: 1979

On the Acquisition of Nonverbal Communication: A Review *(C. Mayo and M. La France)*
Stability of Change in Reading Achievement Over Time: Developmental and Educational Implications *(I. Belmont and L. Belmont)*
Kaspar Hauser's Recovery and Autopsy: A Perspective on Neurological and Sociological Requirements for Language Development *(N. Simon)*
Improving Cognitive Ability in Chronically Deprived Children *(H. McKay, L. Sinisterra, A. McKay, H. Gomez, and P. Lloreda)*

Volume 14: 1981

Genetics and Intelligence: Recent Data *(R. Plomin and J. C. DeFries)*
Sex Differences in Cognitive Functioning: Evidence, Determinants, Implications *(B. Burstein, L. Bank, and L. F. Jarvik)*
School Influences on Children's Behavior and Development: The 1979 Kenneth Blackfan Lecture, Children's Hospital Medical Center, Boston *(M. Rutter)*
Self-Perception and Academic Achievement: Variations in a Desegregated Setting *(B. R. Hare)*

Volume 15: 1982

Individual Differences in Language Development: Implications for Development and Language *(K. Nelson)*
Testing for Children: Assessment and the Many Determinants of Intellectual Competence *(S. Scarr)*
The Changed Social Context of Testing *(E. W. Gordon and M. D. Terrell)*
Language, Social, and Cognitive Impairments in Autism and Severe Mental Retardation *(L. Wing)*

Volume 16: 1983

Developmental, Social and Behavioral Characteristics of Speech and Language Disordered Children *(L. Baker and D. P. Cantwell)*
Infants' Persistence at Tasks: Relationships to Cognitive Functioning and Early Experience *(L. J. Yarrow, G. A. Morgan, K. D. Jennings, R. J. Harmon, and J. L. Gaiter)*
Psychology and Education *(A. M. Clarke)*

Volume 18: 1985

Outcomes of Severe Disorders of Language Acquisition *(R. Paul and D. J. Cohen)*
The Search for Subtypes of Specific Learning Disability *(J. D. McKinney)*

Volume 19: 1986

Cognitive Performance and Academic Achievement of Japanese, Chinese, and American Children *(H. W. Stevenson, J. W. Stigler, S. Lee, G. W. Lucker, S. Kitamura, and C. Hsu)*

Volume 20: 1987

Inside Intelligence *(R. J. Sternberg)*
Future of the LD Field: Research and Practice *(B. K. Keogh)*
Mathematics Achievement of Chinese, Japanese, and American Children *(H. W. Stevenson, S. Lee, and J. W. Stigler)*

Mental Retardation

Volume 1: 1968

Familial Mental Retardation: A Continuing Dilemma *(E. Zigler)*
Social Class and Mental Illness: The Diagnosis of Organicity and Mental Retardation *(J. F. McDermott, Jr., S. I. Harrison, A. Schrager, P. Wilson, E. Killins, J. Lindy, and R. W. Waggoner, Jr.)*
Psychopathology and Mental Retardation *(I. Philips)*

Volume 2: 1969

Expectancy of Success and the Probability Learning of Middle-Class, Lower-Class, and Retarded Children *(G. Gruen and E. Zigler)*
Medical Counseling of Parents of the Retarded *(G. Solomons and F. J. Menolascino)*

Volume 3: 1970

Emotional Disturbances in Mentally Retarded Children *(F. J. Menolascino)*
Parents of the Mentally Retarded Child: Emotionally Overwhelmed or Informationally Deprived? *(A. P. Matheny and J. Vernick)*

Volume 4: 1971

Behavior Deviations in Mentally Retarded Children *(S. Chess and M. Hassibi)*
Mutability of Intelligence and Epidemiology of Mild Mental Retardation *(Z. Stein and M. Susser)*
Intelligence Quotients and Intelligence Loss in Patients with Phenylketonuria and Some Variant States *(J. L. Berman and R. Ford)*

Volume 5: 1972

Luria's Verbal Deficiency Theory of Mental Retardation and Performance on Sameness, Symmetry, and Opposition Tasks: A Critique *(E. Zigler and D. Balla)*
Reinforcement Therapy for Behavior Problems in Severly Retarded Children *(B. L. Baker and M. H. Ward)*
Does Malnutrition Cause Permanent Mental Retardation in Human Beings? *(R. E. Frisch)*

Volume 6: 1973

Repeat Evaluations of Retarded Children *(A. Murphy and L. Pounds)*

Volume 7: 1974

Natural History of Mental Retardation: Some Aspects of Epidemiology *(G. Tarjan, S. W. Wright, R. K. Eyman, and C. V. Keeran)*
Intellectual Consequences of Perinatal Anoxia *(A. W. Gottfried)*
Self Concept and the Retarded: Research and Issues *(E. A. Lawrence and J. F. Winschel)*
Primitive, Atypical, and Abnormal-Psychotic Behavior in Institutionalized Mentally Retarded Children *(F. J. Menolascino)*
Civil Rights of the Mentally Retarded—Some Critical Issues *(C. W. Murdock)*

Volume 9: 1976

Psychopathology and Mental Retardation: A Study of 100 Mentally Retarded Children: I. Psychopathology *(I. Philips and N. Williams)*

Volume 11: 1978

Genetic Disorders and Mental Retardation *(B. F. Crandall)*
Impact of Institutional Experience on the Behavior and Development of Retarded Persons *(E. Zigler and D. A. Balla)*

Volume 12: 1979

National Crisis in Mental Retardation Research *(E. Zigler)*

Parent-Child Interaction

Volume 1: 1968

Sex, Age, and State as Determinants of Mother-Infant Reaction *(H. A. Moss)*
The Role of Eye-to-Eye Contact in Maternal-Infant Attachment *(K. S. Robson)*
On Human Symbiosis and the Vicissitudes of Individuation *(M. S. Mahler)*

Volume 6: 1973

Maternal Deprivation Reconsidered *(M. Rutter)*
Removing Infant Rhesus from Mother for 13 Days Compared with Removing Mother from Infant *(R. A. Hinde and L. Davies)*
What Does Research Teach Us About Day Care: For Children Under Three *(B. M. Caldwell)*
Characteristics of the Emotional Pathology of the Kibbutz Child *(M. Kaffman)*

Volume 7: 1974

Research on Child Rearing as a Basis for Practice *(M. R. Yarrow)*
The Effects of Maternal Employment on Children *(B. Wallston)*

Volume 8: 1975

Authoritarian and Accommodative Child-Bearing Styles: Their Relationships with the Behavior Patterns of Two-Year-Old Children and with Other Variables *(R. W. Chamberlin)*
Temperament in Adopted and Foster Babies *(W. B. Carey, W. L. Lipton, and A. Myers)*
Night Waking and Temperament in Infancy *(W. B. Carey)*

Volume 9: 1976

Parent-Child Relationships and Psychopathological Disorder in the Child *(D. Rosenthal, P. H. Wender, S. Kety, F. Schulsinger, J. Welner, and R. O. Rieder)*
Mother-Child Interaction Observed at Home *(A. Schlieper)*

Volume 11: 1978

Social Competence in Infancy: A Model of Parent-Infant Interaction *(S. Golberg)*
Family Structure and the Mental Health of Children *(S. G. Kellam, M. E. Ensminger, and R. J. Turner)*
The Kibbutz as a Social Experiment and as a Child-Rearing Laboratory *(B. Beit-Hallahmi and A. I. Rabin)*
Infant Day Care and Attachment Behaviors Toward Mothers and Teachers *(D. C. Farran and C. T. Ramey)*
The Mother-Child Relationship and the Development of Autonomy and Self-Assertion in Young (14-30 Months) Asthmatic Children *(Y. Gauthier, C. Fortin, P. Drapeau, J. J. Breton, J. Gosselin, L. Quintal, J. Weisnagel, L. Tetreault, and G. Pinard)*

Volume 12: 1979

Children of Divorce *(S. Jenkins)*
Father Absence and Children's Cognitive Development *(M. Shinn)*
Prenatal Loss of Father and Psychiatric Disorders *(M. O. Huttunen and P. Niskanen)*
Sexual Identity of 37 Children Raised by Homosexual or Transsexual Parents *(R. Green)*
Adoption: Legal Resolution or Legal Fraud? *(R. G. Andrews)*

Volume 13: 1980

Divorce, A Child's Perspective *(E. M. Hetherington)*
Fathers, Children and Joint Custody *(J. B. Greif)*
Fantasy and Reality in Patients' Reports of Incest *(A. A. Rosenfeld, C. C. Nadelson, and M. Krieger)*

Volume 14: 1981

Mother-Infant "Bonding": Failure to Generalize *(M. J. Svejda, J. J. Campos, and R. N. Emde)*
Some Determinants of Mother-Infant Interaction in the Premature Nusery *(K. K. Minde, P. Marton, D. Manning, and B. Hines)*
Are Women More Responsive Than Men to the Young? A Review of Developmental and Situational Variables *(P. W. Berman)*
The Arrival of a Sibling: Changes in Patterns of Interaction Between Mother and First-born Child *(J. Dunn and C. Kendrick)*
Effects of Divorce on the Visiting Father-Child Relationship *(J. S. Wallerstein and J. B. Kelly)*
Effects of Nonmaternal Care on Children: Research Evidence and Popular Views *(C. Etaugh)*

Volume 17: 1984

Cultural Variations in Family Attitudes and Their Implications for Therapy *(J. F. McDermott, Jr., W. F. Char, A. B. Robillard, J. Hsu, W. S. Tseng, and G. C. Ashton)*
Parental Work Patterns in Alternative Families: Influence on Child Development *(I. L. Zimmerman and M. Bernstein)*
Attachment Behavior of Deaf Children with Deaf Parents *(K. P. Meadow, M. T. Greenberg, and C. Erting)*

Volume 18: 1985

Institutional Rearing, Parenting Difficulties, and Marital Support *(D. Quinton, M. Rutter, and C. Liddle)*
Joint Custody: A Critical Analysis and Appraisal *(A. P. Derdeyn and E. Scott)*
Working Mothers and Their Children *(A. E. Siegel)*
The Mother Working Outside the Home *(American Academy of Pediatrics Committee on Psychosocial Aspects of Child and Family Health)*
Mothers Who Work Outside of the Home and Their Children: A Survey of Health Professionals' Attitudes *(H. P. Martin, D. Burgess, and L. S. Crnic)*

Physical Illness

Volume 1: 1968

Volume 3: 1970

Volume 5: 1972

Volume 6: 1973

Volume 7: 1974

Volume 11: 1978

Volume 13: 1980

Volume 14: 1981

Visible Physical Impairment and Psychological Adjustment Among Pediatric Cancer Survivors *(J. E. O'Malley, D. Foster, G. Koocher, and L. Slavin)*
Psychosocial Factors in Juvenile Diabetes: A Review *(S. B. Johnson)*
Do Deaf Children Have a Typical Personality? *(S. Chess and P. Fernandez)*
Personality Adjustment of Children and Adolescents with Hypopituitarism *(D. Drotar, R. Owens, and J. Gotthold)*

Volume 20: 1987

Problems in Transition Following Bone Marrow Transplantation: Psychosocial Aspects *(B. L. Freund and K. Siegel)*
Injuries Among Toddlers: Contributions from Child, Mother, and Family *(A. P. Matheny, Jr.)*

Psychosis and Autism

Volume 1: 1968

Social Class and Mental Illness: The Question of Childhood Psychosis *(J. F. McDermott, Jr., S. I. Harrison, J. Schrager, P. Wilson, E. Killins, J. Lindy, and R. W. Waggoner, Jr.)*
Early Characteristics of Monozygotic Twins Discordant for Schizophrenia *(J. R. Stabenau and W. Pollin)*
Perceptual and Motor Discrimination in Psychotic and Normal Children *(B. Hermelin and N. O'Connor)*
Psychosis of Childhood: A Five Year Follow-up of Experiences in a Mental Retardation Clinic *(F. J. Menolascino and L. Eaton)*

Volume 2: 1969

Concepts of Autism: A Review of Research *(M. Rutter)*
Perceptual Inconstancy in Early Infantile Autism *(E. M. Ornitz and E. R. Ritvo)*
Avoiding Institutionalization of Psychotic Children *(R. M. Silberstein, W. Mandell, J. D. Dalack, and A. Cooper)*

Volume 3: 1970

A Longitudinal Study of Schizophrenic Children with Autism *(L. Bender)*
Special "Isolated" Abilities in Severely Psychotic Young Children *(A. C. Cain)*
Psychotic Children and Behavior Modification *(D. W. Churchill)*
A Five-to-Fifteen-Year Follow-Up Study of Infantile Psychosis—III. Psychological Aspects *(L. Lockyer and M. Rutter)*
Thought Disorders in Parents of Psychotic Children *(L. Schopler and J. Loftin)*

Volume 4: 1971

Imitation and Echoing in Young Schizophrenic Children *(T. Shapiro, A. Roberts, and B. Fish)*
Epidemiology of Infantile Autism *(D. A. Treffert)*

Volume 5: 1972

Volume 6: 1973

Volume 7: 1974

Volume 8: 1975

Volume 9: 1976

Volume 10: 1977

Volume 11: 1978

Follow-Up Report on Autism in Congenital Rubella *(S. Chess)*
Genetic Theories and the Validation of Psychiatric Diagnoses: Implications for the Study of Children of Schizophrenics *(D. R. Hanson, I. I. Gottesman, and P. E. Meehl)*

Volume 13: 1980

Do Autistic Children Come From Upper-Middle-Class Parents? *(E. Schopler, C. E. Andrews, and K. Strupp)*
Pre-, Peri-, and Neonatal Factors and Infantile Autism *(J.-A. Finegan and B. Quarrington)*
The Incidence of Seizures Among Children with Autistic Symptoms *(E. Y. Deykin and B. MacMahon)*
Overview of Selected Basic Research in Autism *(L. R. Piggott)*

Volume 17: 1984

Cognitive Deficits in the Pathogenesis of Autism *(M. Rutter)*

Volume 18: 1985

Developing Concepts of Childhood Autism: The Influence of Experimental Cognitive Research *(M. Prior)*
Autistic Children Who Become Schizophrenic *(L. K. Petty, E. M. Ornitz, J. D. Michelman, and E. G. Zimmerman)*

Volume 19: 1986

Neurophysiology of Infantile Autism *(E. M. Ornitz)*
Autistic Children as Adults: Psychiatric, Social, and Behavioral Outcomes *(J. M. Rumsey, J. L. Rapoport, and W. R. Sceery)*
Concordance for the Syndrome of Autism in 40 Pairs of Afflicted Twins *(E. R. Ritvo, B. J. Freeman, A. Mason-Brothers, A. Mo, and A. M. Ritvo)*

Social Issues

Volume 1: 1968

Learning Patterns in the Disadvantaged *(S. S. Stodolsky and G. Lesser)*
Violence in Ghetto Children *(R. Coles)*

Volume 2: 1969

Racism, the Family, and Society: A Crisis inValues *(L. Eisenberg)*
Health and the Education of Socially Disadvantaged Children *(H. G. Birch)*
Family and Social Pathology in the Ghetto *(H. Rodman)*
Compensatory Education? *(D. A. Wilkerson)*
Northern Children Under Desegregation *(R. Coles)*
Fatherless Homes: A Review of Research *(E. Herzog and C. E. Sudia)*

Volume 3: 1970

Early Malnutrition and Central Nervous System Function *(N. S. Scrimshaw)*

Volume 4: 1971

Volume 6: 1973

Volume 7: 1974

Volume 8: 1975

Volume 9: 1976

Differential Self-Concept in American Indian Children as a Function of Language and Examiner *(H. P. Lefley)*
New Perspectives on Old Issues in Education for the Minority Poor *(E. W. Gordon)*
Arrests and Delinquency in Two Generations: A Study of Black Urban Families and Their Children *(N. Robins, P. A. West, and B. L. Herjanic)*
Child Custody Consultation *(A. P. Derdeyn)*

Volume 10: 1977

The Emergence and Socialization of Sex Differences in the Earliest Years *(B. Birns)*
Sex Differences: A Study in the Eye of the Beholder *(J. Condry and S. Condry)*
Child Advocacy: A Perspective *(J. E. Knitzer)*
Ethnicity, Geographic Locale, Age, Sex and Urban-Rural Residence in Variables in the Prevalence of Mild Retardation *(D. J. Reschly and F. J. Jipson)*
Status Changes of Children in Foster Care: Final Results of the Columbia Longitudinal Study *(D. Fanshel)*
The Murdered Child and His Killers *(D. Kaplun and R. Reich)*
Child Custody Contests in Historical Perspective *(A. P. Derdeyn)*
A Consideration of Legal Issues in Child Custody Contests *(A. P. Derdeyn)*
The Changing Legal Status of Foster parents *(S. N. Katz)*

Volume 16: 1983

Growing Up With the Threat of Nuclear War: Some Indirect Effects on Personality Development *(S. K. Escalona)*
Effects of the Nuclear War Threat on Children and Teenagers: Implications for Professionals *(M. Schwebel)*
Prevention of Children's Psychosocial Disorders: Myth and Substance *(M. Rutter)*
Adolescent Development and Public Policy *(N. Hobbs and S. Robinson)*
Prevention of Emotional Problems Among Native-American Children: Overview of Developmental Issues *(I. N. Berlin)*
The "Competence" of Children: No Longer All or None *(W. Gaylin)*
Children's Rights in the Family and Society: Dilemmas and Realities *(J. Knitzer)*
Does Joint Custody Work? A First Look at Outcome Data of Relitigation *(F. W. Ilfeld, Jr., H. Z. Ilfeld, and J. R. Alexander)*

Volume 17: 1984

Psychologists Look at Television: Cognitive, Developmental, Personality and Social Policy Implications *(J. L. Singer and D. G. Singer)*

Volume 18: 1985

How to Influence Social Policy Affecting Children and Families *(E. Zigler and S. Muenchow)*
Black Children's Race Awareness, Racial Attitudes, and Self-Concept: A Reinterpretation *(M. B. Spencer)*
Holocaust Survivors and Their Children: Comments on Psychiatric Consequences and Psychiatric Terminology *(R. Krell)*
Response Patterns in Children and Adolescents Exploited Through Sex Rings and Pornography *(A. W. Burgess, C. R. Hartman, M. P. McCausland, and P. Powers)*

Volume 19: 1986

Special Stress and Coping

Volume 15: 1982

Volume 17: 1984

Volume 19: 1986

Volume 20: 1987

Temperament Studies

Volume 11: 1978

Volume 12: 1979

Volume 13: 1980

Volume 14: 1981

Volume 15: 1982

Volume 16: 1983

Volume 17: 1984

Volume 18: 1985

Volume 19: 1986

Treatment and Delivery of Services

Volume 5: 1972

Principles of Drug Therapy in Child Psychiatry with Special Reference to Stimulant Drugs *(L. Eisenberg)*

The Behavioral Treatment of School Phobia: Current Techniques *(M. Hersen)*

Brief Psychotherapy with Children: Process of Therapy *(A. J. Rosenthal and S. V. Levine)*

Intervention in Infancy: A Program for Blind Infants *(S. Fraiberg)*

Parents as Cotherapists in the Treatment of Psychotic Children *(E. Schopler and R. J. Reichler)*

Advocacy and the Children's Crisis *(J. Knitzer)*

Community Child Psychiatry: Evolution and Direction *(W. Hetznecker and M. A. Forman)*

Volume 6: 1973

Lithium and Chlorpromazine: A Controlled Crossover Study of Hyperactive Severely Disturbed Young Children *(M. Campbell, B. Fish, J. Korein, T. Shapiro, P. Collins, and C. Koh)*

Effects of Prolonged Phenothiazine Intake on Psychotic and Other Hospitalized Children *(J. B. McAndrew, Q. Case, and D. A. Treffert)*

Volume 7: 1974

Amphetamines in the Treatment of Hyperkinetic Children *(L. Grinspoon and S. B. Singer)*

Volume 8: 1975

Presynaptic Catecholamine Antagonists as Treatment for Tourette Syndrome: Effects of Alpha Methyl Para Tyrosine and Tetrabenazine *(R. D. Sweet, R. Bruun, E. Shapiro, and A. K. Shapiro)*

The Undeclared War Between Child and Family Therapy *(J. F. McDermott, Jr., and W. F. Char)*

Family Therapy with Multiproblem, Multichildren Families in a Court Clinic Setting *(P. A. Rosenthal, S. Mosteller, J. L. Wells, and R. S. Rolland)*

Volume 9: 1976

The Treatment of Adopted Versus Neglected Delinquent Children in the Court: A Problem of Reciprocal Attachment? *(D. O. Lewis, D. Balla, M. Lewis, and R. Gore)*

Sisterhood-Brotherhood Is Powerful: Sibling Sub-Systems and Family Therapy *(S. Bank and M. D. Kahn)*

Professional Abuse of Children: Responsibility for the Delivery of Services *(H. J. W. Polier)*

Utilization of Mental Health Services for Children Relative to Social Class. A Pilot Study *(H. K. von Brauchitsch)*

Volume 11: 1978

External and Internal Roadblocks to Effective Child Advocacy *(J. W. Polier)*

Human Diversity, Program Evaluation and Pupil Assessment *(E. W. Gordon)*

Federal Day Care Standards: Rationale and Recommendations *(D. J. Cohen and E. Zigler)*

The Health Status of Foster Children *(M. R. Swire and F. Kavaler)*

Volume 12: 1979

IQ, Social Competence, and Evaluation of Early Childhood Intervention Programs *(E. Zigler and P. K. Trickett)*
The Effects of Day Care: A Critical Review *(J. Belsky and L. D. Steinberg)*
Ethnicity and Service Delivery *(S. Jenkins and B. Morrison)*

Volume 15: 1982

Selectivity of Treatment Modalities *(S. Chess)*
A Plea to End the Use of the Patterning Treatment for Retarded Children *(E. Zigler)*
Comments on Some Ethical, Legal, and Clinical Issues Affecting Consent in Treatment, Organ Transplants, and Research in Children *(M. Lewis)*
Language Patterns of Opponents to a Child Protection Program *(P. L. Adams and G. J. Roddey)*

Volume 17: 1984

The Role of Psychological Research in the Formation of Policies Affecting Children *(E. E. Maccoby, A. J. Kahn, and B. A. Everett)*
Infant Day Care and Infant-Care Leaves: A Policy Vacuum *(E. Zigler and S. Muenchow)*
Child Custody and Divorce: A Lawyer's View *(H. H. Foster)*

Volume 19: 1986

Assessing Head Start at 20: An Invited Commentary *(E. Zigler)*
On the Efficacy of Early Intervention Programs *(S. Provence)*
The Clinician as Advocate—Interventions in Court Settings: Opportunities, Responsibilities, and Hazards *(M. F. Shore)*